Psychopathy:
Theory, Research
and Implications for Society

NATO ASI Series

Advanced Science Institutes Series

A Series presenting the results of activities sponsored by the NATO Science Committee, which aims at the dissemination of advanced scientific and technological knowledge, with a view to strengthening links between scientific communities.

The Series is published by an international board of publishers in conjunction with the NATO Scientific Affairs Division

A Life Sciences	Plenum Publishing Corporation
B Physics	London and New York
C Mathematical and Physical Sciences	Kluwer Academic Publishers
D Behavioural and Social Sciences	Dordrecht, Boston and London
E Applied Sciences	
F Computer and Systems Sciences	Springer-Verlag
G Ecological Sciences	Berlin, Heidelberg, New York, London,
H Cell Biology	Paris and Tokyo
I Global Environmental Change	

PARTNERSHIP SUB-SERIES

1. Disarmament Technologies	Kluwer Academic Publishers
2. Environment	Springer-Verlag / Kluwer Academic Publishers
3. High Technology	Kluwer Academic Publishers
4. Science and Technology Policy	Kluwer Academic Publishers
5. Computer Networking	Kluwer Academic Publishers

The Partnership Sub-Series incorporates activities undertaken in collaboration with NATO's Cooperation Partners, the countries of the CIS and Central and Eastern Europe, in Priority Areas of concern to those countries.

NATO-PCO-DATA BASE

The electronic index to the NATO ASI Series provides full bibliographical references (with keywords and/or abstracts) to more than 50000 contributions from international scientists published in all sections of the NATO ASI Series.
Access to the NATO-PCO-DATA BASE is possible in two ways:

– via online FILE 128 (NATO-PCO-DATA BASE) hosted by ESRIN,
Via Galileo Galilei, I-00044 Frascati, Italy.

– via CD-ROM "NATO-PCO-DATA BASE" with user-friendly retrieval software in English, French and German (© WTV GmbH and DATAWARE Technologies Inc. 1989).

The CD-ROM can be ordered through any member of the Board of Publishers or through NATO-PCO, Overijse, Belgium.

Series D: Behavioural and Social Sciences – Vol. 88

Psychopathy:
Theory, Research and
Implications for Society

edited by

David J. Cooke

Glasgow Caledonian University
and Douglas Inch Centre
Glasgow, U.K.

Adelle E. Forth

Carleton University,
Ottawa, Canada

and

Robert D. Hare

University of British Columbia
Vancouver, Canada

Kluwer Academic Publishers

Dordrecht / Boston / London

Published in cooperation with NATO Scientific Affairs Division

Proceedings of the NATO Advanced Study Institute on
Psychopathy: Theory, Research and Implications for Society
Alvor, Portugal
27 November – 7 December 1995

A C.I.P. Catalogue record for this book is available from the Library of Congress

ISBN 0-7923-4919-9

Published by Kluwer Academic Publishers,
P.O. Box 17, 3300 AA Dordrecht, The Netherlands.

Sold and distributed in the U.S.A. and Canada
by Kluwer Academic Publishers,
101 Philip Drive, Norwell, MA 02061, U.S.A.

In all other countries, sold and distributed
by Kluwer Academic Publishers,
P.O. Box 322, 3300 AH Dordrecht, The Netherlands.

Printed on acid-free paper

This volume is dedicated to the memory of Daisy Schalling, a dear friend and colleague, wonderfully warm and caring, widely respected and praised for her wisdom curiosity, and dedication to the pursuit of knowledge and excellence, and loved by all who knew her.

TABLE OF CONTENTS

There are many people to thank for making the conference and this book possible. Andra Smith, for the enormous amount of time and effort she put into the organization of the conference. Stephen Hart, for consultation and advice on the scientific program. Andrew Harris, Jim Hemphill and Michelle McBride for their help in ensuring that the conference ran smoothly. Tilo and Barbara Kester, for their advice and help with hotel and publication arrangements. The Scientific and Environmental Affairs Division of NATO, for its wisdom and foresight in developing the concept of the Advanced Study Institute, and for their generous financial support. The management and staff of the Hotel Dom Joao II, for making our stay enjoyable and memorable. Caroline Bruce, Rowena Cook and Lorraine Philip for their assistance in preparing the final manuscript.

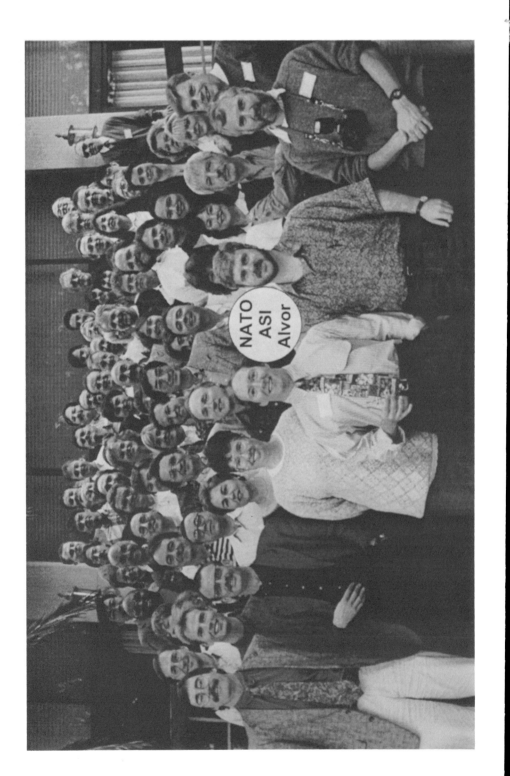

THE ALVOR ADVANCED STUDY INSTITUTE

ROBERT D. HARE
Department of Psychology
University of British Columbia
Vancouver, Canada.

INTRODUCTION

This book is based on a North Atlantic Treaty Organization (NATO) Advanced Study Institute (ASI) on psychopathy held in Alvor, Portugal from November 27 to December 7, 1995. Like the first ASI on psychopathy, organized by Daisy Schalling and me and held in Les Arcs, France in September, 1995 (Hare & Schalling, 1978), the Alvor meeting followed the format recommended by NATO for an ASI, described as high level teaching seminar in which *"lecturers"* and *"students"* meet in a relatively secluded location for an extended period of intensive instruction, discussion, and debate on a specific topic of international interest. However, the two ASIs differed dramatically in content and mood.

Les Arcs, 1975

As I've indicated elsewhere (Hare, 1996a), the participants at Les Arcs — psychologists, psychiatrists, sociologists, anthropologists, and criminologists — operated from a variety of conceptual frameworks and agendas, including some that seemed more ideological or political than scientific, and others that were concerned more with general theories of personality, or with criminality and social deviance, than with psychopathy. The result was a considerable amount of armchair speculation and uninformed debate, but few productive discussions about the nature of psychopathy. In some respects the Les Arcs ASI was like an invitational tennis tournament in which half the participants played ping pong or squash, but who either thought they were playing tennis or argued that it didn't really matter because everyone was hitting balls.

In an attempt to get everyone to agree on which game we were playing, or at least to use the same ball, one psychiatrist said that our difficulty in defining psychopathy was reminiscent of the parable of several blind men who each defined an elephant on the basis of the parts they happened to feel with their hands. A prominent psychologist replied that psychopathy was a *"white elephant that ought to be dumped into (nearby) Lake Annecy."* Another psychologist, during a heated debate, stated that my invitation for him to attend the ASI arrived at the *"last minute,"* indicating that I must be impulsive and lacking in planning ability, and he suggested — perhaps facetiously — that I could be a psychopath. The rest of the participants considered this unlikely, given that I apparently had not misappropriated the grant provided by NATO, but conscientiously was using it to pay for their travel and living expenses.

1

D.J. Cooke et al. (eds.), Psychopathy: Theory, Research and Implications for Society, 1–11.
© 1998 *Kluwer Academic Publishers. Printed in the Netherlands.*

,   In any case, the whole experience was very frustrating and, I thought, unproductive. However, with time the real value of the Les Arcs ASI became apparent. As envisaged by the Scientific Affairs Division of NATO, one of the purposes of an ASI is the fostering of international debate, cooperation, and collaboration on the topic of interest. In this respect, the Les Arcs meeting certainly was a success (see Hare & Schalling, 1978). For example, a major issue at the conference had been the lack of a generally acceptable operational definition for psychopathy. How do we study a construct if we can't agree on procedures for its measurement? Within five years several new methods for the assessment of psychopathy had emerged. One was represented by the diagnostic criteria for *antisocial personality disorder* listed in the third edition of the *Diagnostic and Statistical Manual of Mental Disorders* (DSM-III; American Psychiatric Association, 1980). Although I can't claim that the Les Arcs ASI was responsible for the use of these criteria, it is noteworthy that one of our lecturers was Lee Robins, a key figure in their formulation (Robins, 1978). It seems likely that her views on the need for objective diagnostic criteria for psychopathy at least were reinforced by her experiences at Les Arcs. My own experiences at the meeting motivated me and my students to develop a system for operationalizing the traditional features of psychopathy. The result was a 22-item research scale (Hare, 1980), the precursor of the Psychopathy Checklist (PCL) and its revision, the PCL-R (Hare, 1991).

Alvor, 1995

The Alvor ASI was much different from the previous one. Not only had the academic and clinical climates for psychopathy changed dramatically in the 20 years since Les Arcs, there now was a sizable number of international researchers and clinicians actively engaged in the study of the construct and its implications for society. The Organizing Committee (David Cooke, Adelle Forth, Joseph Newman) and I had little difficulty in putting together a stellar group of some 85 knowledgeable participants from 15 countries. As the contents of this volume attest, the presentations provided the participants with a wealth of information on current theory and research on psychopathy. In addition to the formal lectures and meetings, all of which were accompanied by lively interactions between speaker and audience, many of the participants presented their own research in paper and poster sessions. Abstracts of the presentations (35 in all) recently were published by the British Psychological Society (Cooke, Forth, Newman, & Hare, 1996).

A considerable amount of time was spent in informal discussions and in the establishment of new scientific and personal contacts, many of which will have a continuing impact on international research on psychopathy in particular, and personality disorders in general. Informal work groups were established to apply theory and research on psychopathy to practical issues, including the selection and training of law enforcement personnel, the training of hostage negotiators, and the establishment of educational programs for policy and decision makers, judges, lawyers, and parole, probation, and correctional personnel. The sense of common purpose that developed in Alvor was reflected in the *"reunion"* of 22 of the participants at the International Congress on the Disorders of Personality held in Vancouver in June, 1997.

An important aspect of the Alvor ASI was a working consensus on the assessment of psychopathy. International differences in terminology and conceptualization were discussed and, in most cases, resolved. Various ways of measuring the construct were examined, including the category, *dissocial personality disorder* listed in the 10th edition of the International Classification of Diseases (ICD-10; World Health Organization, 1990), the DSM-IV category of antisocial personality disorder (American Psychiatric Association, 1994), and several self-report inventories. However, the operational framework adopted for most of the presentations and discussions was the PCL-R, an instrument with established reliability and validity and known associations with other diagnostic systems (Hare, 1991; Fulero, S. M., 1995; Widiger et al, 1996). For this reason, the PCL-R is described briefly in the next section, followed by some comments about the DSM-IV category of antisocial personality disorder.

THE PCL-R

The PCL-R is firmly grounded in a clinical tradition that long has described psychopathy in terms of a constellation of affective, interpersonal, and behavioral characteristics (Cleckley, 1976; McCord & McCord, 1964; Millon, 1981). This traditional view of psychopathy cuts across a broad spectrum of groups, including psychiatrists, psychologists, criminal justice personnel, and experimental psychopathologists, as well as the lay public (see Hare, 1996a).

As indicated above, the PCL-R began as a research tool for operationalizing the construct of psychopathy (Hare, 1980). Later referred to as the Psychopathy Checklist (PCL), it was revised in 1985 and formally published several years later as the Hare PCL-R (Hare, 1991). The PCL-R is a 20-item clinical construct rating scale completed on the basis of a semi-structured interview and detailed collateral or file information. (see Table 1). Each item is scored on a 3-point scale according to specific criteria. The total score, which can range from 0 to 40, provides an estimate of the extent to which a given individual matches the prototypical psychopath, as exemplified, for example, in the work of Cleckley (1976). The PCL-R's psychometric properties are well established with male offenders and forensic patients (Cooke & Michie, 1997; Hare, 1991; Harpur, Hare, & Hakstian, 1989; Hart & Hare, 1989, in press; Heilbrun et al., in press). In this respect, Fulero (1995) described the PCL-R as the "*state of the art...both clinically and in research use*" (p. 454).

There also is increasing evidence of the reliability and validity of the PCL-R with female offenders and psychiatric patients (Cooke, 1995; Douglas, Ogloff, & Nicholls, 1997; Neary, 1990; Piotrowski, Tusel, Sees, Banys, & Hall, 1996; Rutherford, Cacciola, Alterman, & McKay, 1996; Salekin, Rogers, & Sewell, in press; Strachan & Hare, 1997). With only slight modifications (see Forth, Kosson, & Hare, in press), the PCL-R is proving as useful with adolescent offenders as with adult offenders (Chandler & Moran, 1990; Forth & Burke, this volume; Forth, Hart, & Hare, 1990; Gretton, McBride, O'Shaughnessy, & Hare, 1997; Toupin, Mercier, Dery, Cãte, & Hodgins, 1996; Trevethan & Walker, 1989).

TABLE 1. Items in the Hare
Psychopathy Checklist-Revised (PCL-R)

Factor 1: Interpersonal/affective	Factor 2: Social Deviance
1. Glibness/superficial charm	3. Need for stimulation/proneness to boredom
2. Grandiose sense of self worth	9. Parasitic lifestyle
4. Pathological lying	10. Poor behavioral controls
5. Conning/manipulative	12. Early behavioral problems
6. Lack of remorse or guilt	13. Lack of realistic, long-term goals
7. Shallow affect	14. Impulsivity
8. Callous/lack of empathy	15. Irresponsibility
16. Failure to accept responsibility	18. Juvenile delinquency
for own actions	19. Revocation of conditional release

Additional Items[1]

11. Promiscuous sexual behavior	20. Criminal versatility
17. Many short-term marital relationships	

Note: From Hare (1991). The rater uses specific criteria, interview and file
information to score each item on a 3-point scale (0, 1, 2).
[1] Items that do not load on either factor.

Indices of internal consistency (alpha coefficient, mean inter-item correlation) and interrater reliability generally are high, and evidence for all aspects of validity is substantial. Mean PCL-R scores in North American male and female offender populations typically range from about 22 to 24, with a standard deviation of from 6 to 8. Mean scores in North American forensic psychiatric populations are somewhat lower, at around 20, with about the same standard deviation. For research purposes, a score of 30 generally is considered indicative of psychopathy, although some investigators have obtained good results with cutoff scores as low as 25. Cross-cultural research by David Cooke and Christine Michie (see Cooke, this volume; Cooke, 1995; Cooke & Michie, 1997) attests to the generalizability of the construct of psychopathy and of the PCL-R as its operational measure. However, the metric equivalent of the scores obtained with North American samples may be somewhat lower in some European samples. An item-response theory (IRT) analysis of the PCL-R indicated that it showed that its performance in different settings and cultural groups: "*reveals remarkable consistency....There is no evidence detectable in these comparatively large samples that suggests that the test is biased due to race or presence of mental disorder*" (Cooke & Michie, 1997, p. 10).

The high internal consistency of the PCL and PCL-R indicates that they measure a unitary construct, yet factor analyses of each version consistently reveal a stable two-factor structure (Hare et al., 1990; Harpur et al., 1989). Factor 1 consists of items having to do with the affective/interpersonal features of psychopathy, such as egocentricity, manipulativeness, callousness, and lack of remorse, characteristics that many clinicians consider central to psychopathy. Factor 2 reflects those features of psychopathy associated with an impulsive, antisocial, and unstable lifestyle, or social deviance. The two factors are correlated about .5 but have different patterns of correlations with external variables. These patterns make theoretical and clinical sense. For example, Factor 1 is correlated positively with prototypicality ratings of narcissistic and histrionic personality disorder, self-report measures of narcissism and machiavellianism, risk for recidivism and violence, and unusual processing of affective material. It is correlated negatively with self-report measures of empathy and anxiety. Factor 2 is most strongly correlated with diagnoses of antisocial personality disorder, criminal and antisocial behaviors, substance abuse, and various self-report measures of psychopathy. It also is correlated negatively with socioeconomic level, education, and standard measures of intelligence. The PCL-R factors appear to measure two facets of a higher-order construct, namely psychopathy. However, IRT analyses conducted by Cooke & Michie (1997) indicate that Factor 1 items are more discriminating and provide more information about the construct than do Factor 2 items. Factor 1 items occur at high levels of the construct and in the most extreme cases, whereas Factor 2 items are present at low levels of the construct.

The PCL:SV

The PCL-R recently was supplemented by a 12-item screening version, the Hare PCL:SV (Hart, Cox, & Hare, 1995). The PCL:SV was developed at the request of John Monahan for use in the John D. and Catherine T. MacArthur Foundation project on the prediction of violence in the mentally disordered (see Hart, Hare, & Forth, 1993; Monahan & Steadman, 1993). It is conceptually and empirically related to the PCL-R, and can be used as a screen for psychopathy in forensic populations or as a stand-alone instrument for research with noncriminals, including civil psychiatric patients. It has the same factor structure as the PCL-R, with the affective/interpersonal and socially deviant components of psychopathy each being measured by six items. The Total score can range from 0 to 24, and a cutoff score of 18 is considered equivalent to a score of 30 on the PCL-R. There is rapidly accumulating evidence for the construct validity of the PCL:SV, including its ability to predict aggression and violence in offenders and forensic psychiatric patients (e.g., Douglas et al., 1997; Hill et al.,1996).

The PCL-R and DSM-IV

I noted above that the publication of DSM-III in 1980 marked an attempt to provide an objective means of diagnosing psychopathy, renamed antisocial personality disorder. Unfortunately, the result was a sharp departure from clinical tradition, and the subsequent source of considerable confusion about the nature and measurement of psychopathy. DSM-III defined antisocial personality disorder primarily in terms of persistent violations of social norms, including lying, stealing, truancy, inconsistent work behavior, and traffic arrests. Among the main reasons given for this dramatic shift away from the use of clinical inferences were that personality traits are difficult to measure reliably, and that it is easier to agree on the behaviors that typify a disorder than on the reasons why they occur. The result was a diagnostic category that had good reliability but that was quite different from the traditional construct it purported to measure. This *"construct drift"* was not intentional but rather the unforeseen result of reliance on a fixed set of behavioral indicators that simply did not provide adequate coverage of the construct they were designed to measure.

The problems with DSM-III and its 1987 revision (DSM-III-R) were extensively discussed in the clinical and research literature (see review by Widiger & Corbitt, 1995). Much of the debate concerned the absence of personality traits in the diagnosis of antisocial personality disorder, an omission that allowed antisocial individuals with completely different personalities, attitudes, and motivations to share the same diagnosis. Because of widespread dissatisfaction with the conceptualization and criteria for antisocial personality disorder, the American Psychiatric Association initiated a field trial in preparation for DSM-IV. The criteria sets evaluated in the field trial included (1) the 10 adult symptoms for antisocial personality disorder listed in DSM-III-R; (2) the ICD-10 criteria for dyssocial personality disorder; and (3) 10 items derived from the PCL-R and PCL:SV and referred to in the trial as the *psychopathic personality disorder* (PPD) criteria (Hare, Hart, Forth, Harpur, & Williamson, 1993; Hare, Hart, & Harpur, 1991; Widiger et al., 1996). The PPD set consisted of five items derived from Factor 1 of the PCL-R and PCL:SV (lacks remorse, lacks empathy, deceitful and manipulative, glib and superficial, inflated and arrogant self-appraisal) and five items from Factor 2 (early behavior problems, adult antisocial problems, poor behavioral controls, impulsive, and irresponsible). The results of the field trial were described in detail by Widiger et al. (1996).

The field trial clearly indicated that most of the ICD-10 and PPD personality traits that reflect the traditional symptoms of psychopathy were just as reliable as those of the more behaviorally-specific DSM-III-R items (Widiger et al, 1996). Thus, the original DSM-III premise for excluding personality from the diagnosis of psychopathy/antisocial personality disorder turned out to be untenable. There was now a firm empirical basis for increasing the content-related validity of the formal criteria for antisocial personality disorder without a reduction in reliability. Yet, this did not happen, for a variety of reasons discussed elsewhere (Hare, 1996a; Hare & Hart, 1995; Widiger et al.,1996). Instead, the DSM-IV adult criteria (age at least 15) now consist of 7 items. But these items actually were not evaluated in the field trial. They were derived from the 10-item DSM-III-R set (see above) used in the field trial. The derivation was logical rather than empirical.

Things become even more problematical when we consider that the DSM-IV *text* description of antisocial personality disorder (which it says is also known as psychopathy) contains many references to traditional features of psychopathy. However, the listed diagnostic criteria actually identify individuals who are persistently antisocial, most of whom are not psychopaths. The problem is compounded by the following statements in the DSM-IV text: *"deceit and manipulation are central features of Antisocial Personality Disorder" p. 645). "Individuals with Antisocial Personality Disorder frequently lack empathy....may have an inflated and arrogant self-appraisal....(and) may display a glib, superficial charm....Lack of empathy, inflated self-appraisal, and superficial charm are features that have commonly been included in traditional conceptions of psychopathy and may be particularly distinguishing of*

Antisocial Personality Disorder in prison or forensic settings where criminal, delinquent, or aggressive acts are likely to be nonspecific" (p. 647).

These DSM-IV text descriptions of antisocial personality disorder look suspiciously like inferred personality traits, and they bear a remarkable resemblance to the items contained in Factor 1 of the PCL-R and the PCL:SV, and to the PPD items used in the field trial (see above), although no mention is made of this fact.

In any case, it is now possible for one clinician or researcher to give a diagnosis of antisocial personality disorder to an offender or forensic patient who meets the formal criteria for the disorder (which includes exhibiting 3 of the 7 adult features), and for another clinician or researcher to withhold the diagnosis because the offender or patient does not also exhibit the personality traits for psychopathy listed in the DSM-IV text. Curiously, clinicians are left entirely on their own when it comes to whether, and how, to assess these traits; no guidelines are provided nor are clinicians referred to an instrument — such as the PCL-R — that does provide explicit criteria for each symptom.

THIS VOLUME

As the contents of this volume indicate (also see the Abstracts in Cooke et al., 1996), the presentations at the Alvor ASI covered most of the current issues surrounding the construct of psychopathy. Cross-cultural conceptualizations and measurement procedures were emphasized throughout the ASI (**Cooke**). There was remarkable international convergence on the implications of psychopathy for criminal behavior and violence (**Hart**; **Hemphill, Templeman, Wong, & Hare**), and the legal issues associated with the concept of psychopathy (**Ogloff & Lyon**) were considered. In most of the countries represented psychopathy was associated with high rates of crime and violence, and poor institutional adjustment. The poor response of psychopaths to treatment was discussed, and a program for their management was presented (**Lösel**). There was considerable debate about the comorbidity of psychopathy with other mental disorders, especially schizophrenia (**Hodgins Cote, & Toupin**; **Nedopil, Hollweg, Hartmann, & Jaser**). Several contributions focused on etiological, developmental, cognitive, and neurobiological aspects of psychopathy, including the role played by genetics (**Livesley**), biological factors (**af Klinteberg**), early precursors of psychopathy (**Frick**; **McBurnett & Pfiffner**), and pathways to adult psychopathy (**Forth & Burke**). Several presentations mapped psychopathy onto interpersonal theory and models of normal personality (**Blackburn**; **Widiger**). Experimental approaches to the disorder included research on information processing deficits (**Newman**) and on the processing and use of emotional material (**Hare**).

THE FUTURE

In a recent article (Hare, 1996a) I argued that psychopathy has long been a poor relative of experimental psychopathology, even though it has no equal in terms of the amount and degree of social, economic, physical, and emotional distress generated. The number of dedicated researchers is small and the research funding minuscule in comparison with schizophrenia, the affective disorders, and even antisocial personality disorder. The nature of psychopathy, though, provides just as much of a challenge as does any other clinical disorder. Of course, it is easier and more convenient to study psychiatric patients than psychopaths. The former manifestly are impaired and either seek or are sent for treatment, where they provide a steady pool of readily available research subjects for well-funded programs designed to understand and help them. Psychopaths, on the other hand, suffer little personal distress, seek treatment only when it is in their best interests to do so, such as when seeking probation or parole, and elicit little sympathy from those who study them. Furthermore, studying them in a prison environment is fraught with so many institutional and political problems, inmate boycotts, staff roadblocks, and red tape that many researchers simply give up after a few projects. Additionally, and unfortunately in my view, resources have been targeted primarily at programs and projects that eschew the politically incorrect idea that individual differences in personality are as important determinants of crime as are social forces.

Fortunately, the situation is changing rapidly. Even those opposed to the very idea of psychopathy cannot ignore its potent explanatory and predictive power, if not as a formal construct then as a static risk factor. In the next few years, indices of psychopathy almost certainly will become a routine part of the assessment batteries used to make decisions about competency, sentencing, diversion, placement, suitability for treatment, and risk for recidivism and violence. Because psychopaths with a history of violence are a poor risk for early release, more and more will be kept in prison for their full sentence, whereas many other offenders will be released early with little risk to society. However, unless we are content simply to warehouse high-risk offenders, we must develop innovative programs aimed at making their attitudes and behaviors less self-serving and more acceptable to the society in which most eventually must function.

For a variety of reasons — high base rates, adequate file information for a diagnosis, willingness to participate in research — almost all of the research on psychopathy is conducted with offenders and forensic psychiatric patients. However, many people are victimized by psychopaths who seldom, if ever, see the inside of a prison. The plight of these individuals raises an issue that urgently needs to be addressed and researched: the prevalence of psychopathy in the general population, and its expression in ways that are personally, socially, or economically damaging but that are not necessarily illegal or that do not result in criminal prosecution. We must find ways of studying psychopaths in the community if we are ever to provide some relief for their victims, which is to say, all of us.

Finally, we know a lot about the behavior of psychopaths but relatively little about their inner workings. However, there are some exciting developments emerging from interdisciplinary collaborations, particularly among psychology, psychiatry, developmental psychopathology, neurobiology, behavioral genetics, and cognitive neuroscience (see chapters in this volume by Hare, Newman, Livesley; also see Damasio, 1994; Mealey, 1995).

Clearly, I look forward to *"Alvor II."*

References

American Psychiatric Association. (1980). *Diagnostic and statistical manual of mental disorders* (3rd ed.). Washington, DC: Author.

American Psychiatric Association. (1987). *Diagnostic and statistical manual of mental disorders* (3rd ed., rev.). Washington, DC: Author.

American Psychiatric Association. (1994). *Diagnostic and statistical manual of mental disorders* (4th ed.). Washington, DC: Author.

Chandler, M., & Moran, T. (1990). Psychopathy and moral development: A comparative study of delinquent and nondelinquent youth. *Development and Psychopathology, 2,* 227-246.

Cleckley, H. (1976). *The mask of sanity,* 5th edition. St. Louis, MO: Mosby.

Cooke, D. J. (1995). Psychopathic disturbance in the Scottish prison population: Cross-cultural generalizability of the Hare Psychopathy Checklist. *Psychology, Crime, and Law, 2,* 101-118.

Cooke, D.J., Forth, A.E., Newman, J., & Hare, R.D. (Eds). (1996). International perspectives on psychopathy: Abstracts from the Alvor NATO ASI on psychopathy . In *Issues in Criminological and Legal Psychology No. 24,* Leicester, England: British Psychological Society.

Cooke, D. J., & Michie, C. (1997). An Item Response Theory analysis of the Hare Psychopathy Checklist. *Psychological Assessment, 9,* 3-13.

Damasio, A. (1994). *Descartes' Error: Emotion, Reason, and the Human Brain.* New York: Putnam & Sons.

Douglas, K.S., Ogloff, J.R.P., & Nicholls, T.L. (1997, June). *Personality disorders and violence in civil psychiatric patients.* Paper presented at the 5th International Congress on the Disorders of Personality, Vancouver, British Columbia.

Forth, A. E., Hart, S. D., & Hare, R. D. (1990). Assessment of psychopathy in male young offenders. *Psychological Assessment: A Journal of Consulting and Clinical Psychology, 2,* 342-344.

Forth, A.E., Kosson, D.S., & Hare, R.D. (in press). *The Hare Psychopathy Checklist: Youth Version.* Toronto, Ontario: Multi-Health Systems.

Fulero, S. M. (1995). Review of the Hare Psychopathy Checklist-Revised. In J. C. Conoley & J. C. Impara (Eds.), *Twelfth mental measurements yearbook* (pp. 453-454). Lincoln, NE: Buros Institute.

Gretton, H.M., McBride, H.L., O'Shaughnessy, R., & Hare, R.D. (1997, June). *Sex offender or generalized offender? Psychopathy as a risk marker for violence in adolescent offenders.* Paper presented at the 5th International Congress on the Disorders of Personality, Vancouver, British Columbia.

Hare, R. D. (1980). A research scale for the assessment of psychopathy in criminal populations. *Personality and Individual Differences, 1,* 111-119.

Hare, R.D. (1991). *The Hare Psychopathy Checklist-Revised.* Toronto, Ontario: Multi-Health Systems.

Hare, R. D. (1992). *A model program for offenders at high risk for violence.* Ottawa, Canada: Correctional Service of Canada.

Hare, R. D. (1993). *Without conscience: The disturbing world of the psychopaths among us.* New York: Simon & Schuster. (Paperback version published in 1995).

Hare, R. D. (1995). Psychopaths and their victims. *Harvard Mental Health Letter, 12,* 4-5.

Hare, R.D. (1996a). Psychopathy: A construct whose time has come. *Criminal Justice and Behavior. 23,* 25-54.

Hare, R. D. (1996b). Psychopathy and antisocial personality disorder: A case of diagnostic confusion. *Psychiatric Times, 13,* 39-40.

Hare, R. D., Harpur, T. J., Hakstian, A. R., Forth, A. E., Hart, S. D., & Newman, J. P. (1990). The Revised Psychopathy Checklist: Descriptive statistics, reliability, and factor structure. *Psychological Assessment, 2,* 338-341.

Hare, R. D., & Hart, S. D. (1995). Commentary on antisocial personality disorder: The DSM-IV field trial. In W.J. Livesley (Ed.), *The DSM-IV personality disorders* (pp. 127-134). New York: Guilford.

Hare, R. D., Hart, S. D., & Harpur, T. J. (1991). Psychopathy and the DSM-IV criteria for antisocial personality disorder. *Journal of Abnormal Psychology, 100*, 391-398.

Hare, R.D., and Schalling, D. (Eds.). (1978). *Psychopathic behavior: Approaches to research*. Chichester, England: Wiley.

Harpur, T. J., Hare, R. D., & Hakstian, R. (1989). A two-factor conceptualization of psychopathy: Construct validity and implications for assessment. *Psychological Assessment: A Journal of Consulting and Clinical Psychology, 1*, 6-17.

Hart, S. D., Cox, D. N., & Hare, R. D. (1995). *The Hare Psychopathy Checklist: Screening Version*. Toronto, Canada: Multi-Health Systems.

Hart, S. D., & Hare, R. D. (1989). Discriminant validity of the Psychopathy Checklist in a forensic psychiatric population. *Psychological Assessment: A Journal of Consulting and Clinical Psychology, 1*, 211-218.

Hart, S. D., & Hare, R. D. (in press). Psychopathy: Assessment and association with criminal conduct. In D. M. Stoff, J. Brieling, & J. Maser (Eds.), *Handbook of antisocial behavior*. New York: Wiley.

Hart, S. D., Hare, R. D., & Forth, A. E. (1993). Psychopathy as a risk marker for violence: Development and validation of a screening version of the Revised Psychopathy Checklist. In J. Monahan & H. Steadman (Eds.), *Violence and mental disorder: Developments in risk assessment* (pp. 81-98), Chicago: University of Chicago Press.

Heilbrun, K., Hart, S. D., Hare, R. D., Gustafson, D., Nunez, C., & White, A. (in press). Inpatient and post-discharge aggression in mentally disordered offenders: The role of psychopathy. *Journal of Interpersonal Violence*.

Hill, C. D., Rogers, R., & Bickford, M. E. (1996). Predicting aggressive and socially disruptive behavior in a maximum security forensic psychiatric hospital. *Journal of Forensic Sciences, 41*, 56-59.

McCord, W., & McCord, J. (1964). *The psychopath: An essay on the criminal mind*. Princeton, NJ: Van Nostrand.

Mealey, L. (1995). The sociobiology of sociopathy: An integrated evolutionary model. *Behavioral and Brain Sciences, 18*, 523-599.

Millon, T. (1981). *Disorders of personality: DSM-III Axis II*. New York: Wiley.

Monahan, J. & Steadman, H. (Eds.), *Violence and mental disorder: Developments in risk assessment*. Chicago: University of Chicago Press.

Neary, A. (1990). *DSM-III and Psychopathy Checklist assessment of antisocial personality disorder in Black and White female felons*. Unpublished doctoral dissertation, University of Missouri, St. Louis, MO.

Piotrowski, N., Tusel, D. J., Sees, K. L., Banys, P., & Hall, S. M. (1996). Psychopathy and antisocial personality disorder in men and women with primary opioid dependence. In D. J. Cooke, A. E. Forth, J. P. Newman, & R. D. Hare (Eds.), *Issues in Criminological and Legal Psychology: No. 24, International perspectives on psychopathy* (pp. 123-126). Leicester, UK: British Psychological Society.

Robins, L. N. (1978). Aetiological implications in studies of childhood histories relating to antisocial personality. In R. D. Hare & D. Schalling (Eds.), *Psychopathic behavior: Approaches to research* (pp. 255-271). Chichester, England: Wiley.

Rutherford, M. J., Cacciola, J. S., Alterman, A. I., & McKay, J. R. (1996). Reliability and validity of the Revised Psychopathy Checklist in women methadone patients. *Assessment, 3*, 43-54..

Salekin, R., Rogers, R., & Sewell, K. (in press). Construct validity of psychopathy in a female offender sample: A multitrait-multimethod evaluation. *Journal of Abnormal Psychology*.

Strachan, C., & Hare, R.D. (1997). *Assessment of psychopathy in female offenders.* Manuscript under review.

Toupin, J., Mercier, H., Dery, M., Cãte, G., & Hodgins, S. (1996). Validity of the PCL-R for adolescents. In D. J. Cooke, A. E. Forth, J. P. Newman, & R. D. Hare (Eds.), *Issues in Criminological and Legal Psychology: No. 24, International perspectives on psychopathy* (pp. 143-145). Leicester, UK: British Psychological Society.

Trevethan, S. D., & Walker, L. J. (1989). Hypothetical versus real-life moral reasoning among psychopathic and delinquent youth. *Development and Psychopathology, 1*, 91-103.

Widiger, T. A., Cadoret, R., Hare, R. D., Robins, L., Rutherford, M., Zanarini, M., Alterman, A., Apple, M., Corbitt, E., Forth, A. E., Hart, S. D., Kultermann, J., Woody, G., & Frances, A. (1996). DSM-IV antisocial personality disorder field trial. *Journal of Abnormal Psychology, 105*, 3-16.

World Health Organization (1990). *International classification of diseases and related health problems* (10th ed.). Geneva, Switzerland: Author.

Author's notes

Correspondence should be addressed to Robert D. Hare, Department of Psychology, University of British Columbia, Vancouver, B.C., Canada V6T 1Z4. Fax: (604) 822-6923; e-mail: rhare@unixg.ubc.ca.

PSYCHOPATHY ACROSS CULTURES

DAVID J COOKE
Department of Psychology
Glasgow Caledonian University
and Douglas Inch Centre
Glasgow, United Kingdom.

INTRODUCTION

Like the poor, psychopaths have always been with us (Cleckley, 1976; Rotenberg & Diamond, 1971); while they appear in all societies — no matter what the level of economic development — the prevalence of the disorder shows marked cross-cultural variation (Mealey, 1995). This chapter will examine what we know about the cross-cultural variation in the rate and nature of psychopathy. The overarching themes of the chapter are that a cross-cultural perspective is not only necessary if we are to apply the diagnosis in an ethical manner, but also, such a perspective can inform research both about the nature and the etiology of the disorder.

Diagnosis is not a culture free activity. Awareness of the impact of culture on diagnostic decisions is growing. This awareness is no more apparent than in the significant changes made to the most recent edition of the Diagnostic and Statistical Manual (DSM-IV) as compared with the previous edition (DSM-IIIR) (American Psychiatric Association, 1994, 1987; Kleinman, 1996). The new edition of the diagnostic system not only provides information about culture-bound syndromes but also issues explicit instruction to consider ethnic and cultural features when coming to a diagnosis.

All mental disorders vary across cultures: Kleinman (1996) indicated that even an ubiquitous disorder such as schizophrenia — contrary to conventional assumption — demonstrates substantial cross-cultural variation in both presentation and prevalence. He argued that there may be a ten-fold difference in the prevalence of the disorder between Western and non-Western societies: indeed, schizophrenia is unknown amongst certain preliterate hunter-gatherers and nomads. The ubiquity of schizophrenia has been used as an argument for biological etiology, yet even this most biological of disorders appears to be molded by cultural influence. It is likely that personality disorders will be substantially influenced by cultural effects. Draguns (1986) contended that personality disorders — such as psychopathy — are less likely to be as stable across cultures as compared with the major mental disorders such as depression and schizophrenia. He argued further that the diagnostic and descriptive systems developed in North America may not ensnare the cross-cultural diversity of the features that characterize personality disorders (Fiske, 1995; Lewis-Fernandez & Kleinman, 1994).

13

D.J. Cooke et al. (eds.), Psychopathy: Theory, Research and Implications for Society, 13–45.

In relation to psychopathy, in particular, it has been argued elsewhere that the Psychopathy Checklist-Revised (PCL-R) is the ideal tool with which to pursue the issue of cross-cultural variation in the presentation and prevalence of psychopathy (Cooke, 1997). However, this statement must be couched with the caveat that, as yet, the PCL-R has been standardized primarily on white, male prisoners in North America. If the PCL-R is used in other settings — and with other populations — the assumption that it will generalize to these groups is just that — an assumption.

THE STRUCTURE OF THE CHAPTER

Initially, this chapter considers what is known about the cross-cultural variation in the prevalence of psychopathy; anecdotal evidence is provided suggesting that the disorder can be identified across time and across culture. More systematic evidence is then considered and PCL-R data from a variety of European and North American samples are compared. Having considered the available data, the chapter then focuses on methodological issues. Any cross-cultural comparison raises many problems concerning the equivalence of the instruments that are used (Van de Vijver & Leung, 1997); the chapter describes psychometric explorations of apparent differences between Scotland and North America in the rate and expression of psychopathy. The initial focus is on using traditional psychometric methods before going on to describe the use of more modern psychometric techniques, in particular, Item Response Theory (IRT) techniques. Having established the likelihood of a difference in the prevalence of the disorder between Scotland and North America, possible explanations for the putative differences are then explored. Initially, it is argued that differential migration may lead to many Scottish psychopaths migrating to England and beyond. Other more general explanations are then explored: in particular, it is argued that the impact of cultural transmission, both through socialization and enculturation, may account for some of the apparent differences. The chapter closes by examining potential approaches for enhancing our understanding of this important disorder.

EVIDENCE FOR CROSS-CULTURAL VARIATION IN PSYCHOPATHY

Although the evidence is less extensive, the evidence available indicates that like schizophrenia, psychopathy and cognate disorders — e.g., sociopathy, dissocial and antisocial personality disorders — occur in most societies and at most points in historical time (Cleckley, 1976; Mealey, 1995; Robins, Tipp & Przybeck, 1991). Robins et al's., (1991) comment about antisocial personality disorder is apposite: *"it occurs and is recognized by every society, no matter what its economic system, and in all eras, showing that it is not purely an indication of a modern 'sick' society. Although its prevalence varies with time and place, the same can be said of almost every psychiatric and non-psychiatric disorder."* (p. 259).

In terms of historical times, Cleckley (1976) identified the Athenian general of the fifth century BC — Alcibiades — as a prototypical psychopath. He was charming and manipulative he repeated contravened the mores of his time; his early behavior was reckless, impulsive and violent. Murphy (1976), bolstered Robins et al's., (1991) contention that antisocial personality is not merely a product of *"modern 'sick' society"*, by providing intriguing accounts of psychopathy in two contrasting non-industrialized cultures. Murphy (1976) examined concepts of psychopathology among the Yorubas of rural Nigeria and the Inuit of North-West Alaska: she found that both these communities could identify and distinguish between schizophrenia and psychopathy. The Yorubas concept of Aranakan has clear parallels with Western constructs of psychopathy: *"a person who always goes his own way regardless of others, who is uncooperative, full of malice, and bullheaded."* (p. 1026). The same is true of the Eskimo concept of Kunlangeta: *"his mind knows what to do but he does not do it...This is an abstract term for the breaking of the many rules when awareness of the rules is not in question. It might be applied to a man who, for example, repeatedly lies and cheats and steals things and does not go hunting and, when the other men are out of the village, takes sexual advantage of many women — someone who does not pay attention to reprimands and who is always being brought to the elders for punishment."* (p. 1026)

Small close knit communities could cope with those suffering from schizophrenia, however, the Inuit management strategy for the Kunlangeta sufferer was to invite them to go hunting and, when no one was looking, push them off the ice (Murphy, 1976).

Systematic comparison of variation in the prevalence of psychopathy is hampered by a multitude of methodological difficulties; proper studies are not available, thus the available evidence can only provide hints (Cooke, 1995b). From the methodological perspective, the base rate of the disorder is so low in the general population that we must depend on prison studies — such dependence creates problems. There is little agreement about the prevalence of psychological disorders in prison settings; a recent review indicated that estimates ranged from 2% to 78% (Cooke, 1995b). This variation is probably underpinned as much by method variance as it is by true variance. Cooke (1995a) compared prevalence estimates for psychopathy in the United Kingdom and North America. Even taking into account variations in sampling frame, diagnostic criteria, approach to evaluating the prisoner and the point of historical time at which the studies took place, it appeared that a cross-cultural difference in the prevalence of psychopathy may exist between the United Kingdom and North America.

COMPARISONS BETWEEN NORTH AMERICA AND EUROPE USING THE PCL-R

The development of the PCL-R, with the extensive nomological network that testifies to its validity as a measure of the disorder, provides the opportunity to pursue questions of cross-cultural variation in both the presentation and prevalence of the disorder (Cooke, 1997; Hare, 1991; 1996). Within North America the use of the PCL-R has shown remarkable stability in the distributional and psychometric characteristics of scores across a variety of settings and samples. This is true even when the instrument has been used with groups other than the white adult male prisoners on which the instrument was standardized. Similar distributional and psychometric characteristics were found for samples of Native Indian Canadian prisoners (Wong, 1984), Black prisoners in the United States (Kosson, Smith & Newman, 1990) and French speaking Canadian prisoners (Hodgins, Cote & Ross, 1992).

Until fairly recently there was a paucity of studies outwith North America: there is now a growing number of studies — most as yet unpublished — from a variety of European countries, including the Scandinavian countries in the north, through Germany, Belgium, the United Kingdom to the Iberian peninsular. The nature of these samples and the characteristics of their PCL-R scores are presented in table one.

TABLE 1. Distribution of PCL-R scores in a selection of European samples compared to the Standardization samples

Researchers	Country	Subjects	N	Mean	SD
Haapasalo & Pulkinen (1992)[1]	Finland	Prisoners	92	17.6	8.8
Klinteberg et al (1992)[2]	Sweden	Criminals & Controls	199	8.7	10.9
Rasmussen & Levander (1995)[3]	Norway	Security patients	94	21.1	9.8
Anderson (1996)	Denmark	Prisoners	229	11.3	9.0
Pham	Belgium	Security patients	94	18.4	7.2
Pham	Belgium	Prisoners	103	18.8	9.3
Nedopil et al. (1995)	Germany	Security patients	131	18.1	6.4
Molto et al., 1996	Spain	Prisoners	117	22.4	7.5
Goncalves (1995)	Portugal	Prisoners	80	16.8	6.0
Raine (1985)[4]	England	Prisoners	136	16.2	8.6
Shine[5]	England	Prisoners	104	24.2	6.2
Clark[6]	England	Prisoners	174	15.3	8.1
Cooke (1989,1997)[7]	Scotland	Prisoners	36	27.0	4.3
Cooke (1995)[8]	Scotland	Prisoners	307	13.8	7.4
Cooke et al (1997)[9]	Scotland	Prisoners	142	15.3	9.0
Marshall & Cooke[10]	Scotland	Prisoners	105	20.5	9.2
All European samples			2143	16.2	8.4
Standardization sample (Hare, 1991)	North America	Prisoners	1192	23.6	7.9
Standardization sample (Hare, 1991)	North America	Forensic Patients	440	20.6	7.8
Standardization sample (Hare, 1991)	North America	All subjects	1632	22.8	7.9

[1] Sampled for high scorers, prorated from 17 items
[2] Prorated from 13 PCL items, included community controls
[3] Highly disordered group
[4] Prorated from 22 item PCL
[5] Referred for treatment of their personality disorder
[6] Systematic sample of prison population
[7] Prisoners in a 'Special Unit' for violence cohort collected over a 23 year period
[8] Representative sample of total population
[9] Case control study of violent men
[10] Case control study sampled for high scorers

Data from sixteen European samples are tabulated above: the combined samples contains 2143 subjects with a mean PCL-R score of 16.2. This mean appears to be substantially lower than the mean obtained in the North American standardization samples. Comparisons of this type, however, must be couched with caveats; sampling may affect the level of score observed. Nonetheless, the current comparison should not necessarily be dismissed as an artifact of sampling — sampling may not necessarily have a critical effect. On the one hand these samples include some community controls (e.g., Af Klinteberg, Humble & Schalling, 1992) but on the other hand they include both case-control samples, where subjects were selected for their high scores (e.g., Haapasalo & Pulkkinen, 1992) and prison samples where the subjects were assessed because they had been referred specifically for treatment of their personality disorder. The studies that are closest to representative samples of the prison populations tend to have relatively low means compared with North American samples. Comparing the overall means in the European and the standardization samples reveals a substantial difference ($t = 24.5$; $df = 3773$, $p<0.0001$); this difference represents a large effect size (Cohen's $d = 0.81$; Cohen, 1977). These results suggest that either there is a substantial difference in the prevalence of psychopathy between European and North American prisons and secure hospitals or that the presentation of psychopathy varies between Europe and North America. In order to pursue these alternative explanations detailed analysis of PCL-R data collected in Scotland was carried out.

Comparing Scottish and North American PCL-R scores using traditional psychometric methods

In 1989 the PCL-R was selected as part of the procedure in a study of the rate, nature and etiology of psychological disturbance within the Scottish prison system. The Scottish prison system, although comparatively small (i.e., average daily population of circa 5,500), has a per capita rate of imprisonment similar to the rate in Canada. The Scottish prison system holds all prisoners in Scotland — both those on remand and those who are sentenced — there is no distinction between provincial (state) and federal establishments — either on the basis of jurisdiction or length of sentence — equivalent to the North American distinctions.

A systematic sample of 310 prisoners, who were housed in 8 out of the 21 Scottish penal establishments, was subjected to detailed and lengthy interviews. These interviews were followed by a systematic file review (See Cooke, 1994; 1995b, for a detailed account of the study). The sentences that the prisoners were serving ranged from a few days to life imprisonment. In common with most prison populations, the Scottish prison population is young, unskilled, with a long history of criminal behavior; a significant proportion of the sample was living in unsettled conditions prior to incarceration, and their rate of psychiatric disturbance was high.

The prevalence of psychopathy

How prevalent was psychopathy in the Scottish sample? Hare (1991) indicated that a cut-off score of 30 on the PCL-R should be used in the classification of individuals as psychopathic. Individuals in the range 20-29 may be considered to have *'moderate'* levels of psychopathy, while those with a PCL-R score of less than 20 can be regarded as non-psychopathic. Hare (1991) presented data from a variety of North American adult male prisoner samples and indicated that the mean rate of psychopathy in these samples was 28.4% with approximately 43% of the prisoners falling in the *'moderate'* psychopathy group. These results are a sharp contrast to the results found in Scotland. Only 3% of Scottish adult male prisoners were classified as psychopathic, with 15% falling in the *'moderate'* category (Cooke, 1995a).

Statistical comparison of the mean score of adult males in North America (23.63) and those in Scotland (13.82) revealed a substantial difference ($t = 15.08$, $p < 0.001$). It might be hypothesized that this divergence reflects differences in the mean length of sentence being served in the different jurisdictions; the Scottish sample containing more short term prisoners. The evidence does not support this view. If only those Scottish prisoners who are serving sentences of 2 years or more are considered the divergence in means increases.

The substantial and significant difference in the prevalence of psychopathy between Scotland and North America may be explained by a range of processes. The most immediate explanations are, first, Scottish researchers are measuring different constructs as compared with North American researchers, second, Scottish raters are underrating PCL-R items as compared with their North American counterparts, and third, a genuine cross-cultural difference in the rate of psychopathy exists. Each of these possibilities will be considered in turn.

Are different constructs being measured?

There are always dangers inherent in taking an instrument developed in one country and applying it in a new country: this is true even when there is a common language, the dangers are even more profound when translation into a new language is required (Van de Vijver & Leung, 1997).

Fundamental to any cross-cultural comparison is the presence of a common measure of the construct of interest. Traditionally, the cross-cultural comparability of any psychometric instrument is assessed in three stages. First, through the evaluation of the extent to which the factor structures underpinning the instrument are similar in different settings. Second, by determining whether the scoring of specific items requires to be modified in the new setting. Third, by deciding whether a common set of unbiased items can be specified which will allow comparison of mean trait levels across cultures (Barrett & Eysenck, 1984; Arrindell et al., 1992). Kosson, Smith, & Newman (1990) used similar methods in their comparison of PCL scores obtained by White prisoners and scores obtained by Black prisoners.

The factor structure underpinning the PCL in a variety of North American samples (and Raine's 1985 English sample) has been examined in great detail (Harpur, Hare & Hakstian, 1989). They demonstrated that ratings on the PCL could best be described in terms of two distinct yet correlated factors. The first factor, which was characterized as representing the *'Selfish, callous and remorseless use of others'* was specified by interpersonal and affective characteristics including superficiality, habitual lying, manipulativeness and callousness, together with a lack of affect, guilt, remorse, and empathy. The second factor, which was characterized as *'Chronically unstable and antisocial life-style'*, was specified by behavioral characteristics including the need for stimulation, poor behavioral controls, lack of realistic long term goals, impulsivity and juvenile delinquency. The factor structures underpinning PCL-R ratings were essentially the same as those which underpinned the PCL (Hare, 1991; Hare et al., 1990; Templeman & Wong, 1994).

The comparison of factor solutions across cultures can be used as a method for determining whether the same constructs are being measured in these different contexts. Factor solutions may be compared by scrutinizing factor congruence, comparative factor strengths and internal consistency (Arrindell et al., 1992).

The congruence of factor solutions can be evaluated by estimating Tucker's coefficient of congruence; this coefficient ranges from -1.0 to +1.0, with a value of +1.0 indicating perfect similarity. Authorities differ on the value of Tucker's coefficient which may be regarded as representing similarity. Ten Berge (1986) argued that a coefficient of 0.80 or greater implies that the factors are equivalent, whereas Muliak (1972), rather more rigorously, argued that only when the coefficient reaches 0.90 can the factors be said to be identical. Arrindell et al. (1992) indicated that a further, but clearly related measure of factor similarity, is the comparability of factor strength as measured by the level of variance explained by the factors extracted. The level of internal consistency of the measure can be assessed in the conventional manner by assessing Cronbach's Alpha or by principal component analysis using the coefficient Theta (Armor, 1969).

Does the same factor structure underpin the PCL-R items in both the Scottish and the North American data? In order to compare the Scottish factor structures with the North American factor structures, a series of analyses was carried out on the full Scottish sample and four sub-samples, namely, on all males, all adult males, young males and all females. These analyses are described in detail elsewhere (Cooke, 1995a) thus, in this abbreviated account, I will merely describe the results pertaining to adult male prisoners ($n=158$) as this sample is most similar to the North American standardization samples.

The Scottish data were subjected to oblique factor analysis applying the same extraction and rotational criteria as Hare and his colleagues (Hare et al., 1990). The degree of congruence between the Scottish and North American samples for factor one was 0.92 and for factor two was 0.93. These values not only exceed the strict criterion proposed by Muliak (1972) but are also within the range of values found in comparisons of factor structures amongst North American samples (*range* 0.82 to 0.94, *mean* = 0.89; Hare et al., 1990).

The amount of variance explained by the two factors was also comparable across countries. The variance explained by factor one in Scotland and North America was 16.15% and 17.15% respectively, the variance explained by factor two was 19.30% and 15.00% respectively (Hare, 1991; common factor solution).

The levels of internal consistency as measured by Cronbach's Alpha were also comparable: for factor one in Scotland and North America, Chronbach's Alpha was 0.75 and 0.84 respectively, with the corresponding values for factor 2 being 0.80 and 0.79 (Cooke, 1995b; Hare et al., 1990).

It must be concluded, from this series of analyses, that the item ratings obtained for the Scottish sample load on the same theoretical constructs as item ratings obtained in the North American sample; the factor structures are congruent; the level of variance explained by corresponding factors are comparable; the level of internal reliability is equivalent and there is no evidence that the loadings of items change from one factor to another.

Although there is firm evidence for cross-national comparability of the overall factor structures, it may still be the case that individual items show cross-national bias. One method for examining bias across samples — the traditional method — is to examine differences in corrected item-to-total correlations and differences in the rank order of item means. If corrected item-to-total correlations are of comparable magnitude across samples then it may be argued that bias is absent (Arrindell et al., 1992; Ironson & Subkoviak, 1979). In the ideal case, the mean value of corresponding items in each sample should be the same, however, as Hulin (1987) pointed out this is an overly stringent requirement because variations in sampling will result in differences in the distribution of the trait across samples. Hulin (1987) argued that while the requirement for identity of means across samples is unreasonable, it is reasonable to expect that the means of equivalent items should retain the same rank orders across samples. The presence of item bias was explored by comparing the corrected PCL-R item-to-total correlations and the rank order of item means in the Scottish and North American samples. The corrected item-to-total correlations in the Scottish sample ranged from 0.30 to 0.71. These results indicate that all of the PCL-R items contribute significantly to the total PCL-R score within the Scottish samples. This replicates the findings in North America (Hare, 1991; Hare et al., 1990) but contrasts with those obtained by Haapasalo & Pulkkinen (1992) in Finland. Cross-national comparisons using Fisher's z indicated that five items differed in the magnitude of their corrected item-to-total correlations across the two samples, namely, Grandiosity, Lack of remorse or guilt, Parasitic life-style, Juvenile delinquency and Criminal versatility. All of the corrected item-to-total correlations, apart from that relating to Grandiosity, were stronger in the Scottish sample; this may reflect the greater heterogeneity of the Scottish sample.

Arrindell et al. (1992) indicated that item bias may be present when there is a significant difference in the rank order means of items across the different cultures or nations being considered. The mean item values for the Scottish adult males were significantly correlated with the mean item values for the North American subjects (Spearman rank order correlation 0.57, p<0.005). Closer inspection of the item means revealed that two items displayed substantial differences in their rank order positions in the two samples. The item pertaining to Juvenile Delinquency in the Scottish sample had a rank of 1 compared with a rank of 11.5 in the North American sample. Revocation of conditional release was ranked seventeenth in the North American sample and fifth in the Scottish sample. These substantial differences in the rank order may reflect, on the one hand, differences in the overall sample mean (e.g., Hulin, 1987) or, on the other hand, they may reflect differences in the recording of juvenile delinquency, or differences in the use of bail and parole, across the jurisdictions.

The overall pattern of results described above indicates that essentially the same constructs are being measured in the different settings. It is necessary, however, to be cautious in any attempt to compare means across samples. Item analysis suggests that there may be significant differences not only in the corrected item-to-total correlations across the samples, but also in the rank order of item means. A cautious and conservative approach to cross sample comparison of means requires the identification of a core set of items, that is, a set of items which behave in a uniform manner across cultural settings (Tarrier, Eysenck, & Eysenck, 1980; Eysenck, Kozeki, & Gellenne, 1980; Barrett and Eysenck, 1984; Arrindell et al., 1992).

The mean values for core set of items were calculated for the Scottish and North American samples; that is, mean scores were calculated using the 15 items that did not differ significantly in terms of their corrected item-to-total correlations (Cooke, 1995a). In an additional analysis Revocation of conditional release was also deleted because of its substantial difference in rank order position. It should be noted that the ratio of the means remains essentially the same irrespective of whether all the items or reduced sets of items are compared (Cooke, 1995a). It can be concluded, therefore, that the observed differences in sample means are unlikely to be the result of differences in the performance of items across samples.[11]

Are British raters under-rating?

The above analyses do not rule out the possibility that raters in the United Kingdom have an overall bias to under-detect or under-record characteristics of psychopathy as compared with their North American counterparts. Hare (personal communication) hypothesized that the low means found in British samples (i.e., Cooke, 1995a; Raine, 1985) might reflect a pervasive and generalized tendency to underrate. On the face of it, this is an unlikely explanation as the characteristics contained in the PCL-R come from such a wide range of domains — interpersonal, affective and behavioral — that the possibility of an underrating 'Halo' effect seems improbable. Fortunately, this hypothesis can be evaluated using the data considered above.

Clinical experience suggests, and examination of inter-rater reliability coefficients confirms, that there is considerable variation in the ease with which particular PCL-R items can be rated. Certain ratings are based on essentially 'soft' or impressionistic judgments, whereas other ratings are based on comparatively objective and 'hard' data.

This extract from the definition of Item 7, Shallow Affect illustrates that this item is based on comparatively 'soft' data; to score the item the rater requires to exercise considerable inference and judgment. "Item 7 describes an individual who appears unable to experience a normal emotional range and depth of emotion. At times, he may impress as cold and unemotional. Displays of emotion are generally dramatic, shallow and short-lived; they leave careful observers with the impression that he is play-acting and that little of real significance is going on below the surface. He may admit that he is unemotional or that he shams emotions." (Hare, 1991, p. 21).

By way of contrast, Item 19, Revocation of Conditional Release is based on comparatively 'hard' data; scoring is essentially a mechanical operation requiring little inference or judgment. "Item 19 describes an individual who, as an adult (aged 18 or

---

[11](Juvenile Delinquency the other item which displayed a substantial difference in rank order was deleted in the first analysis because of a cross-sample difference in corrected item-to-total correlation).

older), has violated a conditional release or escaped from an institution. Violations of conditional release include technical but non-criminal breaches (i.e., drinking alcohol while on parole), or new charges or convictions, while on parole, mandatory supervision, probation, bail, or restraining orders. Escapes from institutions include jail-breaking and violation of temporary absences." (Hare, 1991, p. 27).

It has been argued previously (Cooke, 1995b), that if under-rating is the explanation of the observed differences in overall sample means, then the Scottish ratings on *'soft'* items should be depressed compared with North American items whereas the ratings on *'hard'* items should be unaffected. The 20 PCL-R items were classified as *'soft'* and *'hard'* in terms of their inter-rater reliability coefficients (Hare, 1991). Those with inter-rater reliabilities of 0.60 or below were defined as *'soft'* items, whereas those of 0.61 and above were defined as *'hard'* indicators. This cut-off resulted in 9 *'hard'* indicators and 11 *'soft'* indicators.

While the mean values of the items were clearly different across the two samples, the ratio of the *'hard'* to the *'soft'* items was essentially the same: in the Scottish sample the ratio was 1:1 compared with a ratio of 1.08:1 in the North American sample (Cooke, 1995b). These results suggest the under-rating hypothesis does not explain the observed differences in mean PCL-R scores. The preceding discussion relied on the traditional psychometric methods that have been applied in cross-cultural studies; more modern psychometric approaches to the problem will now be explored.

USING ITEM RESPONSE THEORY METHODS TO MAKE CROSS-CULTURAL COMPARISONS

What are Item Response Theory Methods?

Item Response Theory (IRT) methods represent a revolution in psychometric methodology. This revolution was started by the seminal work of Lord and Noviak (1968) in which they introduced model-based measurement. More recently Steinberg and Thissen (1996) argued that that *"IRT provides a rich collection of statistical tools for item analysis and scale development and can often solve problems that are insurmountable using traditional approaches."* (p. 81). Indeed, in a recent special issue of Psychological Assessment it was demonstrated that many of the old rules of psychometrics — rules based on classical test theory — no longer apply (Embretson, 1996; Reckase, 1996). Embretson (1996) argued *"the new rules of measurement are fundamentally different from the old rules. Many old rules, in fact, must be revised, generalized, or even abandoned."* (p. 341).

From the perspective of cross-cultural comparisons, one of the critical *'rule changes'* is that it is not necessary to have representative samples in order to obtain unbiased estimates of item properties, unbiased estimates can be obtained from non-representative samples (Embretson, 1996).

IRT models examine the relationships between individual items and an underlying latent trait. IRT models use mathematical functions to specify the relation between item responses and the latent trait postulated to determine those responses. The relationships between item responses and the latent trait can be expressed graphically as Item Response Curves (IRCs) (Steinberg & Thissen, 1996).

The advantages of an IRT approach include the following: (1) IRCs are independent of the samples from which they are generated. In contrast, standard CTT indexes of reliability and validity, such as corrected item-to-total correlations and Cronbach's Alpha, are highly sensitive to variation across samples with respect to the range of observed scores. (2) IRT analyses provide information concerning the precision of a test's measurement at any value of the latent trait. CTT procedures merely estimate precision of measurement at the mean trait level of the sample. (3) IRT analyses can quantify the discriminative power of individual items and the overall test score at any value of the latent trait. If the test is diagnostic in nature — one of the uses of the PCL-R — then IRT analyses can be used to determine whether the majority of items provide maximum information at or around the diagnostic cut-off point. (4) IRT analyses permit direct comparison of the performance of parallel items, that is, different items purporting to measure the same domain in the same sample, or the same item in different samples. Thus, IRT is well suited for determining whether item and test scores are invariant across forms (e.g., original versus revision or translation; full versus short-form) and across respondents (e.g., men versus women, ethnic minority versus ethnic majority). For example, IRT analysis has been used to demonstrate that the Screening Version of the PCL-R (PCL:SV) measures the same underlying latent trait as the full version of the test (Cooke, Michie, Hart, & Hare, 1997).

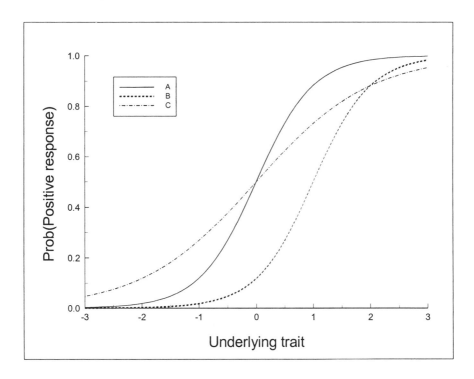

Figure 1. Three hypothetical item characteristic curves.

How can IRT models be interpreted? Perhaps the simplest way is through the examination of the IRCs of individual items. Three hypothetical IRCs are presented in figure 1 for the purposes of illustration. On the horizontal axis is the level of the hypothetical trait while on the vertical axis is the probability of a positive response on the item. Curves A and B are parallel — they are equally steep — thus they are equally good at discriminating between low and high levels of the latent trait. Although they are equally discriminating, they discriminate at different levels of the trait: item B discriminates at a higher level of the trait. Item C differs from the other curves in that it has a lower slope and therefore is less discriminating. A concrete example may assist the illustration.

If an IRT analysis was carried out on data collected using the Vocabulary Sub-test of the Wechsler Adult Intelligence Scale - Revised (WAIS-R; Wechsler, 1987) then a latent trait measuring general vocabulary skills should emerge. The IRC for simple word such as 'Ship' or 'Breakfast' might be represented by curve A whereas more complex words such as 'Matchless' or 'Tirade' might be represented by curve B — a curve which becomes positive at higher levels of the trait. Curve C may represent a word that is a specialist term used in a particular trade, profession or hobby; the ability to define it is not a good indicator of general vocabulary skills, it is merely an indicator of particular interests or experience.

It is through the examination of curves of this type that IRT analyses can assist in the development and refining of scales. If an item has an IRC curve such as curve C then this could be eliminated from the test because it does not provide useful information about the trait of interest. Perhaps of greater significance, in the context of cross-cultural differences, is that these curves can be used to identify item bias or, in the rather more neutral terminology of IRT — Differential Item Functioning (DIF). DIF occurs if, when groups are compared, differences emerge in the IRCs either in terms of differences in slopes or differences in extremity.

The advantages and disadvantages of IRT approaches over CTT approaches to the understanding of the functioning of the PCL-R are discussed in some detail elsewhere (Cooke & Michie, 1997a; 1997b; Cooke et al., 1997). In brief, there are two primary advantages of IRT over CTT in cross-cultural, or indeed in any cross-group, comparisons. Firstly, as noted above, the key concepts in CTT (including corrected item-to-total correlations, alpha reliability, and optimum cut-offs) are dependent on the sample from which they were derived. Whereas, by way of sharp contrast, the key indices in IRT analyses are independent of the samples from which they are derived (Hambleton, 1989; Mellenbergh, 1996; Nunnally & Bernstein, 1994).

Secondly — and of considerable practical and theoretical significance — IRT methods can be used to tackle the problem of so-called measurement invariance: no such methods exist for tackling this problem using CTT (Reise, Widaman, & Pugh, 1993; Hulin et al., 1983b). Clearly, in order to compare prevalence estimates of psychopathy in different settings, it is necessary to ensure that the trait is being measure on the same measurement scale in these settings (Reise, Widaman, & Pugh, 1993). If you were to compare levels of heat measured on the Centigrade scale in one setting and on the Fahrenheit scale in the other, then clearly this would be meaningless: these scales are different in the size of their intervals and the position of their zero points across these scales. Cross-group comparisons of the prevalence of psychopathy — be they across gender, ethnic, cultural or age groups — are essentially meaningless unless metric equivalence has been established. One particular strength of the IRT approach is that, even if some of the items on the scale show DIF across samples, it is still possible to derive a common metric on which the underlying latent trait can be measured to ensure valid comparisons (Reise, Widaman, & Pugh, 1993). Before considering the cross-cultural aspects of the PCL-R, basic findings from an IRT analysis of North American data will be outlined in order to demonstrate the value of the IRT approach.

An IRT analysis of the PCL-R in North America

The first important step that must be taken in carrying out any IRT analysis is the selection of the most appropriate mathematical function to describe the relationships between the item and the latent trait. The primary consideration is the nature of item scores: scores on the PCL-R fall into one of three ordered categories (0 = does not apply; 1 = applies to a certain extent or there is uncertainty that it applies; 2 = definitely applies). Given this pattern of item ratings, it is parsimonious to assume that as the underlying trait increases, the probability of being in Category 0 will decrease, the probability of being in Category 1 will increase and then decrease, finally, the probability of being Category 2 will increase as the underlying trait increases.

The so called two-parameter model (parameters a and b_i) provides the most appropriate mathematical expressions for describing the IRCs of individual PCL-R items. The a parameter is a measure of the slope of the IRC at the point of inflection and, therefore, is a measure of the discriminating power of the item (Hulin et al., 1983a). The b_i parameter specifies the point on the underlying latent trait where the trace line inflects; thus the b_i parameter is a measure of item difficulty or extremity. For example, the b_2 parameter marks the point at which the probability of receiving a score of 2 on the item crosses the 0.5 probability level. A model that is consistent with these assumptions is Samejima's graded model (Cooke & Michie, 1997a; Samejima, 1996; Thissen, 1991).

The data analysis

The data used in the standardization sample of the PCL-R (Hare, 1991) together with a sample of 991 prisoners from the United States kindly provided by Joe Newman (a total sample size of 2067) were examined using Multilog (Thissen, 1991). The fitted parameters for the items are displayed in table 2.

Examination of the a parameters reveals that the items Callous/lack of empathy, Shallow affect and Lack of remorse or guilt are the most discriminating items (i.e., they have the largest a parameters and thereby the steepest slopes) whereas Many short-term marital relationships, Juvenile delinquency and Revocation of conditional release are the least discriminating items (i.e., they have the smallest a parameters). This illustrates that some items are much better measures of the trait than others.

Examination of the b_1 and b_2 parameters for the items indicates that there is considerable variation in the level of the trait at which an item receives a 1 or 2 rating respectively. Variation of this type is valuable; it indicates that the PCL-R is a good measure of the underlying latent trait because, across the whole range of the trait, there are items which have discriminative power.

Table 2. Item parameters for the individual PCL-R items

ITEM	Item parameters		
	a	b_1	b_2
Glibness/Superficial charm	1.3	-0.2	1.6
Grandiose sense of self-worth	1.4	-0.5	1.2
Need for stimulation	1.5	-1.5	0.1
Pathological lying	1.4	-0.7	1.1
Conning/Manipulative	1.4	-0.6	1.1
Lack of remorse or guilt	1.6	-1.7	-0.1
Shallow affect	1.6	-1.0	0.7
Callous/Lack of empathy	1.9	-1.2	0.5
Parasitic lifestyle	0.9	-1.6	1.4
Promiscuous sexual behavior	0.7	-0.9	0.8
Poor behavioral controls	0.9	-1.4	0.6
Early behavior problems	0.9	-0.4	0.9
Lack of long term goals	1.2	-1.5	0.4
Impulsivity	1.4	-2.0	-0.2
Irresponsibility	1.3	-2.0	0.0
Failure to accept responsibility	1.0	-1.5	0.5
Short-term marital relationships	0.6	0.8	2.4
Juvenile delinquency	0.7	-0.8	0.5
Revocation of conditional release	0.7	-1.5	-0.2
Criminal versatility	0.8	-0.5	1.6

One of the strengths of IRT analysis is that the relationship between items and the underlying trait can be expressed in graphical terms. The IRCs for three PCL-R items are plotted in figure 2 for the purposes of illustration.

The IRCs for the item Glibness/superficial charm indicate that the item is moderately discriminating, with the item having discriminative power at high levels of the trait. By way of contrast, the IRCs for the item Irresponsibility, although equally discriminating, discriminate at lower levels of the trait. The IRCs for the item Callous/lack of empathy are very steep indicating that this item is a particularly discriminating item.

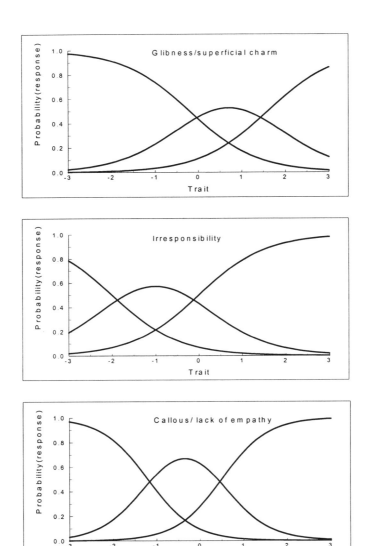

Figure 2. Item characteristic curves for three selected items

These results have practical relevance in that they confirm the discriminative utility of many of the PCL-R items. Perhaps of greater interest, from a theoretical perspective, is the nature of the items that have large b_2 parameters. As noted above, a number of factor analytic studies have demonstrated that the PCL-R can be described in terms of two underlying factors; *'The selfish, callous and remorseless use of others'* factor and the *'Chronically, unstable and antisocial lifestyle'* factor (Cooke, 1995a; Hare et al., 1990; Templeman & Wong, 1994). The first factor is more closely associated — both empirically and conceptually — with the traditional clinical concept of psychopathy, whereas the second factor is more closely associated with the concept of antisocial personality disorder (APD; American Psychiatric Association, 1994). The IRT analysis reveals that the threshold parameters for the first factor are significantly more extreme than the threshold parameters for the second factor (Cooke & Michie, 1997a). These results suggest that the emphasis on behavioral features in the diagnosis of APD may lead to the more salient features of the disorder being overlooked. This application of IRT to North American PCL-R data has added to our understanding of the instrument and the disorder: its application to cross-cultural comparisons will now be explored.

An IRT comparison of Scotland and North America

Multilog (Thissen, 1991) was used to compare the performance of PCL-R items in Scotland and North America. Maximum likelihood methods were used to estimate the item parameters. Generalized likelihood ratio testing (GLRT) methods were used to determine the equivalence of parameters across groups: in brief, this method works by comparing the goodness-of-fit of a constrained model with the goodness-of-fit of an unconstrained model. Essentially, two models are compared, one in which parameters are constrained to be equivalent across groups and one in which no such constraints are imposed; if GLRT reveals no significant difference between the models, then the parameters are deemed to be essentially equivalent across groups (Reise et al., 1993).

When the unconstrained model was compared with a model in which all the item parameters were constrained to be equal in Scotland and North America, GLRT revealed that the data could not be modeled adequately under this assumption of equal item parameters. However, it was found that when the **a** parameters alone where constrained to be equal then the model fitted well. This indicated that the a parameters were essentially equal and that the items discriminate as well in Scotland as they do in North America. However, the variation in the b_i parameters revealed that the level of the underlying trait at which the characteristics of the disorder — e.g., Glibness, Lack of remorse, Pathological lying — become apparent, differed in the two settings.

As noted above, differential item functioning (DIF) occurs when the IRCs are significantly different across settings; the presence of DIF indicates that the trait is being measured on different scales in the different settings. Metric inequivalence means that comparisons of prevalence figures are meaningless unless the metric inequivalence is taken into account. Fortunately, the presence of some DIF is not fatal to the endeavor of ensuring metric equivalence; if some items have similar item parameters in both settings then these items can be used as 'anchor' items to establish a common metric across the settings (See Reise, et al., 1993, for a detailed account of this method).

A final model was fitted with three 'anchor' items, namely, Pathological lying, Lack of realistic long term plans and Criminal versatility (Cooke & Michie, 1997b). There were substantial differences in the threshold parameters; the nature and magnitude of these differences may be best illustrated by examining the IRCs of two items: Glibness/superficial charm and Callous/lack of empathy (see figure 3).

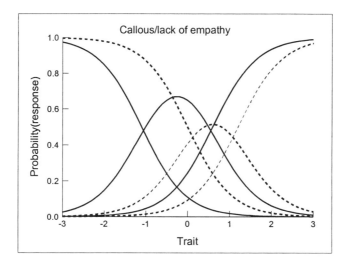

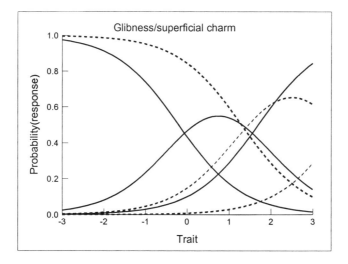

Figure 3. Item characteristic curves for Glibness/superficial charm and Callous/lack of empathy

In both North America and Scotland, Callous/lack of empathy was the most discriminating item; it had the largest **a** parameter. The **a** parameter is identical in both settings indicating that callousness and the absence of empathy have equal importance as a measure of psychopathy in both settings. By way of contrast, however, the b_i parameters vary such that individuals had to be higher on the underlying trait in Scotland before callousness became apparent.

A more dramatic difference was found when the IRCs for Glibness/superficial charm were examined. Only those at the highest level of the trait obtain a rating of 2 on this item in the Scottish sample; this is consistent with clinical experience which suggests that it is a rare characteristic of Scottish prisoners. The examination of individual items can suggest hypotheses about the processes leading to the observed differences; these will be explored in detail later in the chapter.

Comparing the prevalence of the disorder

My concern with the possibility of cross-cultural variation in psychopathy arose from the apparently dramatic differences in the prevalence of the disorder between Scotland and North America. Does a difference exist? Before valid comparisons of prevalence can be made across settings or across groups, it is necessary to ensure metric equivalence in the measurement of psychopathy. As noted above, the presence of a common metric was ensured by anchoring the traits together using the 3 *'anchor'* items; that is, with the items with similar parameters in Scotland and North America. Using regression procedures it was possible to demonstrate that the North American diagnostic cut-off score of 30 on the PCL-R North America is metrically equivalent to the diagnostic cut-off score of 25 in Scotland (Cooke & Michie, 1997b).[12] If the prevalence of psychopathy in Scottish prisons is re-estimated using a diagnostic cut-off of 25, the prevalence in Scotland increases, however, it remains substantially lower than in the North American samples (8% versus 29%; Cooke & Michie, 1997b).

Although the above sections contain some technical discussion, I hope it has highlighted issues which not only have theoretical relevance for our understanding of the nature of this disorder, but also, have practical relevance in relation to the use of the instrument in settings other than those in which it was first standardized. In the following sections possible explanations for the low prevalence of psychopathy in Scottish prisons will be explored. Two broad explanations are examined, the potential impact of migration and the potential impact of cultural transmission through socialization and enculturation.

WHERE ARE THE SCOTTISH PSYCHOPATHS?

The impact of migration

It has long been recognized that there is a link between migration and psychological disorder. Westermeyer (1987) argued that the migration of those who cope — and he gives the example of Ireland and Bavaria — may result in elevated rates of schizophrenia amongst those who remain. Mealey (1995), in her extensive discourse on the sociobiology of what she termed *'sociopathy'*, made the explicit prediction *"primary sociopaths emigrate."* (p. 541). This prediction is intriguing and merits further exploration. What are primary sociopaths? Mealey (1995) attempted to distinguish between primary and secondary sociopaths. Initially, she made the distinction in terms of the etiology of the disorder, arguing that primary sociopathy is underpinned primarily by biological factors whereas secondary sociopathy is more closely tied to the processes of socialization and enculturation. Later, in the same issue,

---

[12] In general, Scottish scores can be made equivalent to North American scores by adding 5.

Mealey shifted her definition and refers to the two factors extracted from the PCL-R (Cooke, 1995a; Harpur, Hare, & Hakstian, 1989; Templeman & Wong, 1994). She contended that primary sociopaths are those who score highly only on the factor that measures the *'Callous and remorseless use of others'* whereas secondary sociopaths are those who score highly only on the *'Chronically unstable and antisocial lifestyle'* factor. At first glance this is an appealing distinction, unfortunately, it is a distinction that cannot be sustained. Firstly, Mealey (1995) committed the common error of conflating factors and subjects; the fact that two factors underpin PCL-R scores does not imply that there are two types of people it merely implies that individuals can be said to vary along these two dimensions (Eysenck, 1970). Secondly, the empirical evidence from IRT analyses, referred to above, indicates that primary personality factors generally only occur in those who display the secondary antisocial lifestyle features.

Despite the short-comings of the distinction between primary and secondary sociopaths, Mealey's (1995) hypothesis that sociopaths emigrate is consistent with my clinical experience. Many of the more serious Scottish prisoners move to England, at some stage, during their criminal careers. In order to carry out a more systematic, albeit indirect, test of the hypothesis that psychopaths emigrate, data regarding reconviction data were collected for the sample of Scottish prisoners that was described in detail above (Cooke, 1995b; Cooke & Michie, 1997c).

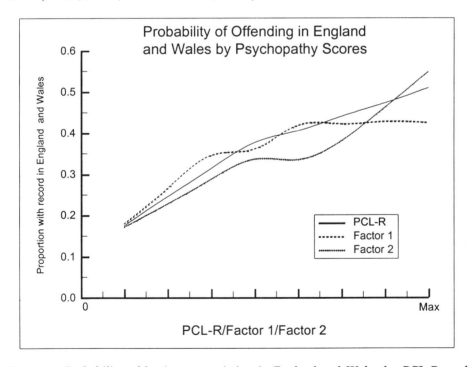

Figure 4. Probability of having a conviction in England and Wales by PCL-R total scores and factor one and factor two scores. Weighted least squares solution

Thirty three per cent of the sample had a conviction in England and Wales at some stage in their criminal careers: was there a link with psychopathy? The relationships between total PCL-R scores and factor one and factor two scores were calculated using weighted least squares and the regression lines are displayed in figure 4. These findings suggest a link between psychopathy and migrating to offend, however, there is no evidence to confirm the specificity of effect postulated by Mealey (1995), namely, that factor one rather than factor two would be most strongly associated with migration — if anything, the trend is in the opposite direction.

Why should psychopaths emigrate? There is converging thinking from a variety of theoretical frameworks that may explain these relationships. Wilson and Herrstein (1985), in their attempt to explain cross-cultural variation in crime in general (rather than cross-cultural variation in the crimes committed by psychopaths), argued that it is not the size of modern cities per se which is important in increasing the level of crime, but rather the tendency for modern cities to be populated by many transient individuals. The relationships between neighbors tend, therefore, to be superficial. Such conurbations provide densely packed targets for the predator; the predator is able to attack, extort or steal from individuals, with little danger of being recognized by his victims. Clearly, such an environment would be advantageous to the psychopath.

Using mathematical game-theoretic models Dugatkin (1992) and Dugatkin and Wilson (1991) emphasized that those who adopt a conning strategy in their interactions with co-operators can survive either in a low or a high frequency within a population dependent on the mode of cultural transmission which operates within and across groups. In this context, reputation is the critical form of cultural transmission. Wilson and Herrstein (1985) argued that there is a low prevalence of psychopaths in small close-knit communities because a reputation for cheating and conning is soon transmitted within the closed group. Harpending and Draper (1988) suggested that *"...the mobility of sociopaths in our contemporary complex society is an adaptation in the sense that the longer they stay in one place the more visible their fundamental failure to reciprocate and the lower their fitness."* (p. 304).

While the need to seek out new opportunities and victims to exploit may explain the tendency to migrate to some extent, other characteristics of the disorder may also play a significant role. The psychopaths' impulsivity and need for stimulation together with their lack of significant long-lasting relationships and their lack of realistic, long term goals may all contribute to the desire to migrate. These characteristics may contribute over and above the psychopath's desire to seek fresh targets to exploit.

Migration may have longer term impact on the prevalence of psychopathy in a population if there is differential migration of those who carry the biological predisposition for the disorder, given that such a predisposition appears to exist (Mealey, 1995; Livesley, this volume). Farley (1986) argued that one characteristic commonly associated with psychopathy — thrill seeking or type T personality characteristics — may be transmitted biologically and culturally and be more apparent in some populations than others: *"The type 'T' personality may be an American archetype. Those who manned the tossing barks searching for the New World, explored the American continent, opened up the West and carried the United States into world leadership on their creative, adventurous, energetic shoulders were probably Big T people. They, and the wave upon wave of Type T immigrants who built this nation, may have passed on the Type T personality genetically to subsequent generations. This heritage, combined with continuing immigration and our Type T influenced political and legal systems, may give our national character a strongly Type T flavor."* (Farley, 1986; p. 51).

Winchie and Carment (1988) provided some limited empirical support for the notion that those who chose to migrate from a population are not representative of that population in terms of their personality characteristics. They found that individuals who desired to migrate to Canada from India were more sensation-seeking than their compatriots who harbored no such desires.

THE VALUE OF THE CROSS-CULTURAL APPROACH

Given that a prima facie case can be made for the presence of a significant cross-cultural difference in the prevalence of psychopathy between Europe and North America, why should this be of interest? At a merely practical level, awareness of the value of the PCL-R in North American forensic practice has led to a dramatic increase in the use of the instrument in forensic practice in Europe. This has dangers: in many cases significant decisions about individual liberties can be made on the basis of a score on this instrument. Ethical considerations demand, therefore, that the validity of the instrument is established beyond the samples on which the instrument was standardized; namely samples of North American adult males.

Although, practical and ethical issues are important, it is perhaps at the level of theory that cross-cultural comparisons have the potential for the greatest impact. The development of the PCL-R has provided us with the methodology by which to examine the impact which culture may have on the expression of this important disorder. Given that the PCL-R has provided us with a useful diagnostic procedure, a procedure that allows the phenomena of interest to be described reliably, it is now important to go beyond mere classification towards a greater understanding of the etiology of the disorder. Many approaches may be adopted in the pursuit of greater understanding of etiology, however, the cross-cultural approach may offer particular benefits.

The etiological processes that underpin psychopathy are unlikely to be simple, it is likely that a concatenation of adverse risk factors must occur before an individual achieves a significant trait strength or, in particular, a trait strength within the diagnostic range. In his account of the appropriate models to apply to the etiology of personality disorders, Paris (1993) argued that it is necessary to eschew simplistic linear mono-causal systems and replace these with more complex multiplicative and non-linear models. He argued that complex interactive processes are likely to underpin the creation of personality disorders and that it is necessary, therefore, to consider variables from the biological, psychological, social and cultural domains if a comprehensive theoretical model of the etiology of personality disorders is to be achieved.

The impact of cultural factors

What cultural factors influence the prevalence of psychopathy? If discussion is restricted merely to the impact of broad cultural factors on the etiology of psychopathy, then it is necessary, at this early stage in the development of our understanding, to explore a wide range of disciplines: a range of disciplines which bring their own particular techniques and perceptions to the problem. A full account is outwith the scope of this chapter, however, evidence should, at a minimum, be sought from the fields of cross-cultural psychology and psychiatry, socio-biology, anthropology and sociology.

It was argued in the introduction to this chapter that there is growing awareness of the impact of culture on the form and presentation of psychological disorders. The idea that cultural processes can influence psychopathy is not new. As far back as 1835, Pritchard contended that *'moral insanity'* — a precursor to the diagnosis of psychopathy — was linked to socio-cultural processes; in particular, Pritchard argued that the disruptive impact of industrialization contributed to the etiology of *'moral insanity'* (Sanchez, 1986). This is consistent with the cross-cultural approach to psychology and psychiatry, an approach founded on the principle that while there may be certain psychological universals, the form and expression of the psychological processes will be molded by cultural transmission. The processes of cultural transmission parallel the processes of biological transmission; they all act to determine which features of a population are maintained over time and across generations (Berry et al., 1992). The primary mechanisms by which cultural transmission operates are through enculturation and socialization. Essentially, enculturation enables the individual to learn what is deemed to be important in that culture, through immersion and experience of that culture. The process of socialization is distinct from, but related to, enculturation, in that it is the process by which an individual learns about what is important in their culture directly — through tutelage — by parents, teachers, peers and other significant contacts.

Socialization has been cited as a central mechanism in the ontogenesis of psychopathy and related disorders (Mealey, 1995; Lykken, 1995). Lykken (1995), for example, has argued that socialization, specifically socialization by parents, is critical in the etiology of the syndrome that he calls sociopathy. Lykken's model is essentially an interactive model in which the interplay between the biological vulnerability for the disorder and the quality of parenting which the child experiences leads to the emergence of the disorder. Lykken argued that biologically based variations in temperament — in particular, variations in fearlessness and impulsivity — influence how the child responds to the milieu created for him or her by their parents. Impulsive and fearless children who are unfortunate enough to have incompetent parents will, he argued, be very likely to emerge as antisocial, whereas such children who are fortunate enough to have competent parents may emerge without significant antisocial traits. *"Inadequate or incompetent parenting leads to insecure attachment bonding that forecasts low levels of empathy, compliance, co-operation and self-control."* (Lykken, 1995; p. 199).

Lykken's model echoes that presented by Raine (1988). Raine emphasized the interplay between biological vulnerability and social milieu; he argued that because children in higher socio-economic groups are less likely to experience the environmental risk factors which underpin antisocial behavior than are the children of lower socio-economic status (Loeber, 1990), then there should be a greater biological contribution to the antisocial behavior of individuals of higher social economic individuals. One marker of biological risk for antisocial behavior is hypo-arousal (Raine & Venables, 1992). On reviewing the relevant literature Raine (1988) found that hypo-arousal was a common feature of delinquents from the middle and upper social economic groups, whereas delinquents from lower socio-economic groups were much less likely to display hypo-arousal.

There is cross-cultural evidence that supports the role of different approaches to socialization in the development of antisocial behavior. Ekblad (1988; 1990) argued that cultures vary in the degree to which parents will allow their children to express aggressive behavior. Homes in which a permissive regime applies are more likely to produce aggression, particularly amongst boys. In her cross-cultural comparison of Sweden and China, Ekblad (1990) found substantial differences in the rate of aggressive behavior emitted by young boys; the rate being significantly higher in Sweden. Ekblad argued that these differences could be attributed, to a significant degree, to differences in the methods adopted by parents to contain the aggressive behavior.

Aggressive behavior, which is a frequent concomitant of psychopathic personality disorder, also shows dramatic cross-cultural variation. This variation is unlikely to be merely a consequence of biological variation, but is more likely to be the consequence of variation in norms and values regarding the appropriate use of violence (Moghaddam, Taylor & Wright, 1992). Evidence from anthropology, for example, indicates that there are cultural groups that prefer to negotiate or withdrawal when faced with a dispute rather than resort to violence. Moghaddam et al., (1992) provided evidence to support this view indicating that the Inuit of the Arctic, the Blackfoot Nation of North America and the Pygmies of Africa eschew violence. Other social-cultural milieus appear to promote aggressive behavior. Perhaps the most striking example of this is the anthropological evidence regarding the behavior of the Yanomano of the upper Amazon; Chagnon (1974; 1996) described the constant warfare amongst villages, and within villages, perpetrated by this group: the status of Yanomano men is closely tied to their ability to be aggressive.

Within North America there is also considerable variation in the level of aggression. Robins (1995) recently remarked that in terms of violence the United States is an *"outlier amongst nations"* (p. 52): nonetheless, low levels of aggressive behavior can be observed amongst certain groups within the United States such as the Mennonites, the Amish and the Hutterites. Bandura and Walters (1963) argued that the low level of aggression displayed by these groups is a consequence of their strong norms against aggression. This evidence suggests that perhaps the most profound form of antisocial behavior — violence — is influenced by cultural pressure.

Individualism as a promoter of psychopathy

Within cross-cultural psychology, a major dimension for distinguishing amongst societies — and a major explanatory variable — is the individualistic-collectivistic dimension. Those societies that are extreme in terms of individualism will emphasize competitiveness and self-confidence; because independence from other members of the society is encouraged, temporary and short-lived relationships are frequent. Collectivistic societies subsume the individual's needs and desires for the good of the group; individuals are subservient to the cultural group, authority is accepted and stable long-term relationships are the norm. Generally, North American societies are regarded as being prototypically individualistic, whereas Chinese and other Eastern societies are regarded as being prototypically collectivist.

Is there an association between psychopathy and social structures? Certain sociological thinking contends that individualistic cultures are nurturing environments for the psychopath: *"The achievement ethic of American society demands that individuals seek out self-satisfaction and economic success while, to some extent, suspending concern with the feelings of others. Late capitalism has placed a heavy burden of achievement and conspicuous consumption on Americans. In this environment the psychopath is often a most successful performer"* (Sanchez, 1986; p. 90). Ehrenreich (1983), argued that extreme individualistic pressure leads to both a severing of responsibility amongst people and a concomitant tendency for behavior to be driven by impulse, desire and selfish need. Other aspects of the syndrome — the grandiosity and narcissism — may be enhanced by certain cultural pressures. Sanchez (1986) has argued that social processes within America have promoted narcissism; indeed, Lasch, (1979) has argued that individualistic cultures inevitably lead to *"A narcissistic preoccupation with the self. "* (p. 21).

From a socio-biological perspective authors such as Mealey (1995) have argued that individualistic societies may promote characteristics that are central to the syndrome of psychopathy. Within individualistic societies the processes of enculturation are likely to enhance grandiosity, glibness and superficiality; the absence of responsibility for others will result in promiscuity and multiple pseudo-marital relationships. Mealey (1995) contended that the competitiveness that is a central feature of individualistic societies has a central role in promoting psychopathic like characteristics. *"As a society gets larger and more competitive, both theoretical models and empirical research show that individuals become more anonymous and more Machiavellian, leading to reductions in altruism and increases in crime. Social stratification and segregation can also lead to feelings of inferiority, pessimism, and depression among the less privileged, which can in turn promote the use of alternative competitive strategies, including antisocial behavior. "* (Mealey, p. 539).

Cultural values — in this case individualistic values — can be maintained and transmitted by the popular culture of the society. A central theme in popular North American culture is the notion of moving on and thereby moving up, of leaving behind the old and the failed to discover the new and the successful. It is a society that consists of the descendants of those who severed ties of kith and kin — frequently severing themselves from obligations and responsibilities — in order to construct a new life. Hare (1993) contended that psychopathic traits may be emerging in North America as these traits are accepted and promoted both overtly and covertly within the society. North American society *"is moving in the direction of permitting, reinforcing, and in some instances actually valuing some of the traits listed in the Psychopathy Checklist — traits such as impulsivity, irresponsibility, lack of remorse, and so on"* . (p. 177).

Most of these views are speculation in need of data, however, there is some evidence to suggest that the impact of cultural pressure does affect the rate of a related disorder, namely antisocial personality disorder. As demonstrated above it appears that antisocial personality disorder can be construed as a lesser degree of the latent trait that underpins the characteristics defined on the PCL-R. Compton et al. (1991) carried out epidemiological research in both Taiwan and the United States of America. Using standard diagnostic criteria and standard sampling procedures, they demonstrated substantial differences in the prevalence of the disorder in these distinct cultures: one a prototypically individualistic culture, the other a prototypically collectivistic culture. It will be argued below that the magnitude of this difference may be influenced to some extent by variations in patterns of self-disclosure across cultures, nonetheless, the magnitude of the difference in prevalence suggests that a real difference may exist.

Further evidence of the impact of cultural pressure comes from the Epidemiological Catchment Area study within the United States. Robins et al. (1991) predicted that the lifetime prevalence of antisocial personality disorder would increase from 3.7% to 6.4% by the time that those in the youngest cohort were over 30 years of age. Millon (1993) and Paris (1993) have argued that such increases in the rate of the disorder could be attributed to the loss of stable relationships, together with the loss of other aspects of the social fabric which suppress traits such as impulsivity.

Culture, reproductive strategy and psychopathy

Socio-biological theorists have argued that there is an interplay between social-cultural factors and genetic processes; with this interplay, in certain circumstances, leading to behaviors that are consonant with psychopathic behavior. Mealey (1995) provided a detailed overview of this type of theorizing. In brief, socio-biologists are interested in the behaviors that maximize genetic fitness; genetic fitness being the individual's total genetic representation in the next genetic pool. Essentially there are two strategies that can be adopted to maximize genetic fitness. Under one strategy a large degree of parental effort is invested in a small number of children. By way of contrast, under the alternative strategy, a large amount of effort is expended on reproduction with comparatively little effort been directed towards parenting. To be successful with the second strategy, it is necessary for males to have multiple female partners; they will be more successful with this strategy if they are able to con their partners about their willingness and ability to be effective parents. Raine and Venables (1992) argued that such behavior is consistent with psychopathic personality disorder.

Theorizing about the interplay between cultural pressure and reproductive strategies is apparent in disciplines other than socio-biology. Anthropologists have argued that societies in which competition is high and where parental commitment is low are likely to promote antisocial personality traits. Harpending and Draper (1988) described the behavior of two non-industrialized groups who, subject to very different environmental pressures, have evolved very different parenting styles, and different rates of antisocial behavior. The !Kung Bushmen exist in inhospitable desert and survive through co-operative hunting and by foraging for the scarce food resources that are available. They have egalitarian relationships between males and females; they form nuclear families in which few children are produced but in whom parental investment is high and long-term. Harpending and Draper (1988) argued that *"In societies of this type the contexts for the anti-social traits are unfavorable. There will be no pay-offs for anti-social behavior and the bearer of the trait will be readily detected and ostracized."* (p. 297).

The Mundurucu, by way of contrast, live as swiddeners in a land of plenty. Male-female relationships among the Mundurucu are hostile and disdainful; there is limited contact between the sexes. Males live together in a large house together and only sleep within their family homes when they are unwell. Harpending and Draper (1988) indicated that most men spend their day gossiping, planning raids on other villages, and fighting amongst themselves. When they go hunting their spoils add little to the total calorific intake of the group; the spoils of hunting are frequently used to trade for sexual intercourse rather than to provide nutrition for their children. Their reproductive strategy can be regarded as having high reproductive effort and low parental effort, this strategy stands in stark contrast to that adopted by the !Kung Bushmen. Harpending and Draper (1988) contended that the type of environment experienced by the Mundurucu will favor those who display the antisocial characteristics that are part of the syndrome of psychopathy: *"A successful male would be brave, even fearless, skilled at fighting and raiding, but even more skilled at bluff and bravado that might obviate the necessity for real battle. He would be good at impersonal manipulation and status gamesmanship — manipulating other men in face-to-face dominance struggles and manipulating females as a seducer if not a rapist. "* (p. 298)

The above discussion speculates about explanations for the apparent cross-cultural variation in this disorder; speculation is insufficient. If we are to collect data to pursue the hypothesis that both the prevalence and the presentation of the disorder is moderated by cultural pressures, how may this be achieved? Various research strategies will now be considered.

CROSS-CULTURAL RESEARCH: HOW DO WE MOVE FORWARD?

As noted earlier in this chapter, the pursuit of a cross-cultural perspective can be justified both in pragmatic terms, to ensure uniformity in nosological practice, and in terms of theory, to increase our understanding of etiology. As yet, the only verdict on the proposition that a cross-cultural difference exists, must be *'not proven'*. More evidence is required. The PCL-R probably represents the most appropriate instrument to use, not only does it possess impressive convergent and concurrent validity, but also, its use is becoming widespread. Of the many avenues that could be pursued, perhaps the first avenue that should be pursued is the question of rater bias.

Assessing the effects of raters: the Scottish-Canadian NATO collaborative study

Exploratory data analysis within one sample, as carried out above with the Scottish sample, cannot be considered to be a strong method for testing the hypothesis that observed differences are due to rating bias. Epidemiological research is replete with examples of cross-cultural differences that vanish when proper sampling and rating controls are put in place (Cooper et al., 1972). While it must be admitted that assessing personality disorder can be difficult, there are no cogent reasons why cross-cultural consistency cannot be achieved with PCL-R ratings. Tyrer et al., (1984) demonstrated that good consistency can be achieved between North American and British raters who are assessing personality disorder — including antisocial personality disorder — from videotaped interviews.

A study is currently underway to explore the impact of interviewer and interviewee nationality on PCL-R scores. The North Atlantic Treaty Organization has provided funds to allow collaboration between Robert Hare, Stephen Hart and myself to carry out a study. Twelve Canadian raters and 12 Scottish raters — who have been trained by the same trainers — will rate 12 videotaped interviews — interviews of 6 Canadian prisoners and 6 Scottish prisoners. The resulting matrix of PCL-R scores will be analyzed using the principles of Generalizability Theory (Schroeder, Schroeder & Hare, 1985). These analyses will provide quantitative estimates of the effects of the raters nationality and the effects of the prisoners' nationality on their PCL-R scores. These results should cast light on whether the apparently low Scottish means, described above, can, in part, be attributed to underrating.

Assessing the effect of variation in self disclosure

The above will examine the behavior of raters, however, there may be significant cross-cultural variation in a facet of the interviewee's behavior — self-disclosure — which leads to observed differences in ratings. When ratings are made with the PCL-R, the rater is dependent, in part, on what the interviewee reports or has reported to others in the past. There is evidence available that suggests that PCL-R scores are dependent, to some extent, on the amount of information available to the rater; scores obtained with interview and collateral information were higher than those obtained with interview alone (Alterman, Cacciola, & Rutherford, 1993).

Levels of self-disclosure appear to vary across cultures. Chen (1995) demonstrated that American students disclosed more than Chinese students; Lewin (1948) found that Germans disclosed less than Americans; Barnlund, (1975; 1989) in a series of studies, demonstrated that Americans reveal significantly more about their financial affairs, their sexual adequacy and personal traits than do Japanese subjects; similar findings were obtained by Nakanishi (1987). Cultures value talkativeness and self-disclosure to differing degrees; Chen (1995) suggests that Chinese society devalues the talkative, viewing such people as shallow and even dangerous. He quotes Lao Tze in support of his contention *"He who knows does not speak, he who speaks does not know."* The cultural norm in Scotland and much of Northern Europe is against self-disclosure, and this may influence the ratings obtained. Systematic studies of self-disclosure across target countries, and evaluation of the relationships between self-disclosure and PCL-R ratings, may cast light on apparent cross-cultural differences.

A second group of approaches to determining the presence or otherwise of cross-cultural differences — either in overall prevalence rates or differences in the behavior of specific PCL-R items — entail additional analyses of data sets that have already been collected. This is clearly a cost-effective and time efficient approach.

Assessing the effect of sampling

The observed differences in prevalence of psychopathy between Scotland and North America may be influenced by differences in sampling procedures. While the Scottish sample was selected in order to obtain a representative sample of the Scottish prison population, this was not the case for the North American samples; they were procured for a variety of purposes, including scale development and experimental research.

Despite the fact that the distribution characteristics of the North American samples show a degree of uniformity, they may not be truly representative of the populations from which they were drawn. One approach to ruling out the possibility that sampling variation is responsible for the observed differences in prevalence is to generate samples of Scottish and North American prisoners matched on variables — including type of offense, age, socio-economic status and educational level — which are known to be associated with PCL-R scores (Hare, 1991). Bontempo (1993), the proponent of this strategy, argued that if differences in prevalence still persist after the matching process, then the researcher should move from the variables that describe individuals towards variables that describe differences in the target cultures. They propose that a multiple regression strategy should be adopted whereby the descriptors of culture are stepped into the model, until, in the ideal case, no differences persist.

Assessing the diagnostic cut-off

Prevalence estimates are dependent not only on qualities measured by a scale but also on the cut-off point adopted to distinguish a case from a non-case. There is inevitably an arbitrary element in the selection of a suitable cut-off point and this can lead to difficulties in any etiological analysis (Cooke, 1980). Evaluating cross-cultural comparability of cut-offs may be achieved by capitalizing on the extensive body of construct related evidence obtained for the PCL-R in North American settings. The detailed accounts of construct related evidence in this volume reveal that there are substantial and significant individual differences on a range of dimensions when those who obtain high scores on the PCL-R are compared with those who obtain low scores. Differences between those who obtain high scores compared with those who obtain low scores include their hand gestures, their use of language, the cerebral organization of their language processes, their autonomic responsivity, their ability to shift attentional focus, and their recidivism (See chapters this volume).

It is now common practice, with North American samples, to adopt a cut-off point of 30 or above to classify individuals as psychopathic. Hare (1991) indicated that not only does this cut-off provide the most efficient diagnostic distinction in relation to global clinical assessments of psychopathy and DSM-IIIR diagnoses of antisocial personality disorder, but also, it renders substantial and significant differences between psychopathic and non-psychopathic individuals in a variety of experimental tasks.

One approach to determine whether the scale maintains a consistent cut-off across cultures is to replicate the North American laboratory studies in other settings and determine whether the most efficient cut-off point is the same in the new cultural setting. In selecting which cultures in which to collect new data it would be more effective to be driven by theory rather than mere convenience. If it is hypothesized that differences between individualistic and collectivist cultures might be of potential importance, then data should be sought in collectivist cultures. Compton et al's. (1991) results pertaining to anti-social personality disorder in Taiwan and the United States of America implies that a PCL-R study in a Chinese setting may be productive.

In conclusion, it would appear that psychopathy, one of the most destructive of the personality disorders, varies both in prevalence and presentation across cultures. The PCL-R represents a powerful tool by which such variations can be explored; it is likely that such explorations will enhance our understanding of this disorder. The NATO Advanced Study Institute held in Alvor served to foster greater collaboration amongst the international community of researchers concerned with this problem; it is to be hoped that this collaboration will lead to greater understanding of this disorder.

References

Af Klinteberg, B., Humble, K., & Schalling, D. (1992). Personality and psychopathy of males with a history of early criminal behaviour. *European Journal of Personality, 6*, 245-266.

Alterman, A. I., Cacciola, J. S., & Rutherford, M. J. (1993). Reliability of the Revised Psychopathy Checklist in substance abuse patients. *Psychological Assessment, 5*, 442-448.

American Psychiatric Association. (1987). *Diagnostic and statistical manual of mental disorders.* (3 Revised ed.). Washington DC: American Psychiatric Association.

American Psychiatric Association. (1994). *Diagnostic and statistical manual of mental disorders.* (4th ed.). Washington: American Psychiatric Association.

Armor, D. J. (1969). Theta reliability and factor scaling. *Sociological Methodology, 2*, 17-50.

Arrindell, W. A., Perris, C., Eisemann, E., Granell de Aldaz, J., Van der Ende, D., Kong Sim Guan, J., Richter, J., Gaszner, P., Iwawaki, S., Baron, P., Joubert, N., & Prud'homme, L. (1992). Cross-national transferability of the two-factor model of parental rearing behaviour: A contrast of data from Canada, The Federal Republic of Germany, Hungary, Japan, Singapore and Venezuela with Dutch target ratings on the EMBU. *Personality and Individual Differences, 13*, 343-353.

Bandura, A., & Walters, R. (1963). *Social learning and personality development.* (1st ed.). New York: Holt, Rinehart and Winston.

Barnlund, D. C. (1975). *Public and private self in Japan and the United States.* (1st ed.). Tokyo: Simuli.

Barnlund, D. C. (1989). *Communicative styles of Japanese and Americans: images and realities.* (1st ed.). Belmont, CA: Wadsworth.

Barrett, P., & Eysenck, S. B. G. (1984). The assessment of personality factors across 25 countries. *Personality and Individual Differences, 5*, 615-632.

Berry, J. W., Poortinga, Y. H., Segall, M. H., & Dasen, P. R. (1992). *Cross-cultural psychology: research and applications.* (1st ed.). Cambridge: Cambridge University Press.

Bontempo, R. (1993). Translation fidelity of psychological scales: a item response theory analysis of an Individualism-Collectivism Scale. *Journal of Cross-cultural Psychology, 24*, 149-166.

Chagnon, N. A. (1974). *Studying the Yanomano.* (1st ed.). New York: Holt, Rinehart and Winston.

Chagnon, N. A. (1996). Chronic problems in understanding tribal violence and warfare. In G. R. Bock & J. A. Goode (Eds.), *Genetic of criminal and antisocial behaviour.* (pp. 202-236). Chichester: John Wiley.

Chen, G. (1995). Differences in self-disclosure patterns among American versus Chinese: A comparative study. *Journal of Cross-cultural Psychology, 26*, 84-91.

Cleckley, H. (1976). *The mask of sanity.* (5th ed.). St Louis: Mosby.

Cohen, J. (1977). *Statistical power analysis for the behavioral sciences.* New York: Academic press.

Compton, W. M., Helzer, J. E., Hwu, H. G., Yeh, E. K., McEvoy, L., Tipp, J. E., & Spitznagel, E. L. (1991). New methods in cross-cultural psychiatry: psychiatric illness in Taiwan and the United States. *American Journal of Psychiatry, 148*, 1697-1704.

Cooke, D. J. (1980). Causal models with contingency tables. *British Journal of Psychiatry, 137*, 582-584.

Cooke, D. J. (1994). *Psychological disturbance in the Scottish Prison System: prevalence, precipitants and policy.* Edinburgh: SHHD.

Cooke, D. J. (1995a). Psychopathic disturbance in the Scottish prison population: the cross-cultural generalizability of the Hare psychopathy checklist. *Psychology, Crime and Law, 2,* 101-108.

Cooke, D. J. (1995b). Psychological disturbance in the Scottish prison system: a preliminary account. In G. Davie, S. Lloyd-Bostock, M. McMurran, & C. Wilson (Eds.), *Psychology, law and criminal justice: international developments in research and practice.* Berlin: Walter de Grutyer.

Cooke, D. J. (1997). Psychopaths: oversexed, overplayed but not over here? *Criminal Behaviour and Mental Health, 7,* 3-11.

Cooke, D. J., & Michie, C. (1997a). An Item Response Theory evaluation of Hare's Psychopathy Checklist: *Psychological Assessment, 9,* 2-13.

Cooke, D. J., & Michie, C. (1997b). Psychopathy across cultures: an Item Response Theory comparison of Hare's Psychopathy Checklist-Revised. *Submitted for publication,*

Cooke, D. J., & Michie, C. (1997c). *Predicting recidivism in a Scottish prison sample.* Edinburgh: Scottish Office.

Cooke, D. J., Michie, C., Hart, S. D., & Hare, R. D. (1997). The functioning of the Clinical Version of the Psychopathy Checklist: an Item Response Theory analysis. *Submitted for publication,*

Cooper, J. E., Kendell, R. E., Gurland, B. J., Sharpe, L., Copeland, J. R. M., & Simon, R. (1972). *Psychiatric diagnosis in New York and London.* (1st ed.). Oxford: Oxford University Press.

Draguns, J. G. (1986). Culture and psychopathology: What is known about there relationship. *Australian Journal of Psychology, 38,* 329-338.

Dugatkin, L. A., & Wilson, D. S. (1991). Rover: a strategy for exploiting cooperators in a patchy environment. *The American Naturalist, 138*(3), 687-701.

Dugatkin, L. A. (1992). The evolution of the "Con Artist". *Ethology and Sociobiology, 13,* 3-18.

Ehrenreich, B. (1983). *The hearts of men: American dreams and the flight from commitment.* (1st ed.). New York: Anchor.

Ekblad, S. (1988). Influence of child-rearing on aggressive behavior in a transcultural perspective. *Acta Psychiatrica Scandanavica, 78,* 133-139.

Ekblad, S. (1990). The children's behaviour questionnaire for completion by parents and teachers in a Chinese sample. *Journal of Child Psychology and Psychiatry, 31,* 775-791.

Embretson, S. E. (1996). The new rules of measurement. *Psychological Assessment, 8*(4), 341-349.

Eysenck, H. J. (1970). The classification of depressive illness. *British Journal of Psychiatry, 117,* 241-250.

Eysenck, S. B. G., Kozeki, B., & Gellenne, M. K. (1980). Cross-cultural comparison of personality: Hungarian children and English children. *Personality and Individual Differences, 1,* 347-353.

Farley, F. (1986) The Big T in personality. *Psychology Today, May,* 45-52.

Fiske, A. P. (1995). The cultural dimensions of psychological research: method effects imply cultural mediation. In P. E. Shrout & S. T. Fiske (Eds.), *Personality research method and theory: a fesctschrift honoring Donald W Fiske.* (pp. 271-294). Hillsdale New Jersey: Lawrence Erlbaum.

Haapasalo, J., & Pulkkinen, L. (1992). The Psychopathy Checklist and non-violent offender groups. *Criminal Behaviour and Mental Health, 2,* 315-328.

Hambleton, R. K. (1989). Principles and selected applications of item response theory. In R. L. Linn (Ed.), *Educational measurement*. (pp. 147-200). London: Collier MacMillan.

Hare, R. D. (1991). *The Hare Psychopathy Checklist - Revised*. Toronto, Ontario: Multi-Health Systems.

Hare, R. D. (1993). *Without conscience: the disturbing world of the psychopaths among us*. (1st ed.). New York: Pocket Books.

Hare, R. D. (1996). Psychopathy: a clinical construct whose time has come. *Criminal Justice and Behavior, 23*, 25-34.

Hare, R. D., Harpur, T. J., Hakstian, A. R., Forth, A. E., Hart, S. D., & Newman, J. P. (1990). The Revised Psychopathy Checklist: descriptive statistics, reliability, and factor structure. *Psychological Assessment: A Journal of Consulting and Clinical Psychology, 2*, 238-341.

Hare, R. D., & Hart, S. D. (1992). Psychopathy, mental disorder, and crime. In S. Hodgins (Ed.), *Mental disorder and crime*. Newbury Park, California: Sage (in press).

Harpending, H., & Draper, P. (1988). Antisocial behavior and the other side of cultural evolution. In T. E. Moffitt & S. A. Mednick (Eds.), *Biological contributions to crime causation*. Boston: Matinun Nijhoff.

Harpur, T. J., Hare, R. D., & Hakstian, A. R. (1989). Two-factor conceptualization of psychopathy: construct validity and assessment implications. *Psychological Assessment: A Journal of Consulting and Clinical Psychology, 1*, 6-17.

Hodgins, S., Cote, G., & Ross, D. (1992). Predictive validity of the French version of Hare's Psychopathy Checklist (Abstract). *Canadian Psychology, 33*, 300

Hulin, C. L., Drasgow, F., & Parsons, C. K. (1983a). Item and test bias. In Anonymous, *Item Response Theory: application to psychological measurement*. (pp. 152-184). Illinois: Dow Jones-Irwin.

Hulin, C. L., Drasgow, F., & Parsons, C. K. (1983b). Applications of IRT to language translations. In Anonymous, *Item Response Theory: application to psychological measurement*. (pp. 185-209). Homewood, Illinois: Dow Jones-Irwin.

Hulin, C. L. (1987). A psychometric theory of evaluations of item and scale translation: fidelity across languages. *Journal of Cross-cultural Psychology, 18*, 115-142.

Ironson, G. H., & Subkoviak, M. J. (1979). A comparison of several methods of assessing item bias. *Journal of Educational Measurement, 16*, 209-225.

Kleinman, A. (1996). How is culture important for DSM-IV. In J. E. Mezzich, A. Kleinman, H. Fabrega, & D. L. Parron (Eds.), *Culture & psychiatric diagnosis: A DSM-IV perspective*. (pp. 15-25). Washington: American Psychiatric Association.

Kosson, D. S., Smith, S. S., & Newman, J. P. (1990). Evaluating the construct validity of psychopathy in Blank and White male inmates: three preliminary studies. *Journal of Abnormal Psychology, 99*, 250-259.

Lasch, C. (1979). *The culture of narcissism: American life in an age of diminishing expectations*. (1st ed.). New York: Warner.

Lewin, K. (1948). Some socio-psychological differences between the United States and Germany. In G. Lewin (Ed.), *Resolving social conflicts: selected papers on group dynamics*. (pp. 1935-1946). New York: Harper.

Lewis-Fernandez, R., & Kleinman, A. (1994). Culture, Personality and Psychopathology. *Journal of Abnormal Psychology, 103*, 67-71.

Loeber, R. (1990). Development and risk factors of juvenile antisocial behavior and delinquency. *Clinical Psychology Review, 10*, 1-42.

Lord, F. M., & Noviak, M. (1968). *Statistical theories of mental tests*. (1st ed.). New York: Addison-Wesley.

Lykken, D. T. (1995). *The antisocial personalities*. (1st ed.). Hillsdale: Lawrence Erlbaum.

Mealey, L. (1995). The sociobiology of sociopathy: an integrated evolutionary model. *Behavioral and Brain Science, 18*, 523-599.

Mellenbergh, G. J. (1996). Measurement precision in test score and item response models. *Psychological Methods, 1*(3), 293-299.

Mezzich, J. E., Kleinman, A., Fabrega, H., & Parron, D. L. (1996). *Culture & Psychiatric diagnosis: a DSM-IV perspective.* (1st ed.). Washington: American Psychiatric Association.

Millon, T. (1993). Borderline personality disorder: a psychosocial epidemic. In J. Paris (Ed.), *Borderline personality disorder: etiology and treatment.* Washington: American Psychiatric Press.

Moghaddam, F. M., Taylor, D. M., & Wright, S. C. (1992). *Social psychology in cross-cultural perspective.* New York: Freeman and Co.

Muliak, S. A. (1972). *The foundations of factor analysis.* (1st ed.). New York: McGraw-Hill.

Murphy, J. M. (1976). Psychiatric labelling in cross-cultural perspective: similar kinds of disturbed behaviour appear to be labelled abnormal in diverse cultures. *Science, 191*, 1019-1028.

Nakanishi, M. (1987). Perceptions of self-disclosure in inital interaction: a Japanese sample. *Human Communication Research, 13*, 167-190.

Nunnally, J. C., & Bernstein, I. H. (1994). *Psychometric theory.* (3rd ed.). McGraw-Hill Inc.

Paris, J. (1993). Personality disorders: a biopsychosocial model. *Journal of Personality Disorders, 7*, 255-264.

Raine, A. (1985). A psychometric assessment of Hare's checklist for psychopathy on an English prison population. *British Journal of Clinical Psychology, 24*, 247-258.

Raine, A. (1988). Antisocial behavior and psychophysiology. In H. L. Wagner (Ed.), *Social psychophysiology and emotion: theory and clinical applications.* New York: Wiley.

Raine, A., & Venables, P. H. (1992). Antisocial behaviour: evolution, genetics, neuropsychology, and psychophysiology. In A. Gale & M. W. Eysenck (Eds.), *Handbook of individual differences: biological perspectives.* Chichester: John Wiley.

Reckase, M. D. (1996). Test construction in the 1990: recent approaches every psychologists should know. *Psychological Assessment, 8*(4), 354-359.

Reise, S. P., Widaman, K. F., & Pugh, R. H. (1993). Confirmatory Factor Analysis and Item Response Theory: Two approaches for exploring measurement invariance. *Psychological Bulletin, 114*, 552-566.

Robins, L. N., Tipp, J., & Przybeck, T. (1991). Psychiatric disorders in America. In L. N. Robins & D. A. Regier (Eds.), *Antisocial Personality Disorder.* (pp. 258-290). Free Press.

Robins, L. N. (1995). The epidemiology of aggression. In E. Hollander & D. J. Stein (Eds.), *Impulsivity and aggression.* (pp. 43-55). London: John Wiley & Son.

Rotenberg, M., & Diamond, B. L. (1971). The biblical conception of the psychopath: The law of the stubborn and rebellious son. *Journal of History of Behavioral Sciences, 7*, 29-38.

Samejima, F. (1996). Graded response model. In W. J. Van der Linden & R. K. Hambleton (Eds.), *Handbook of modern item response theory.* (pp. 85-100). New York: Springer.

Sanchez, J. (1986). Social crises and psychopathy: towards a sociology of psychopathy. In W. H. Reid, D. Dorr, J. I. Walker, & J. W. Bonner (Eds.), *Unmasking the psychopath: Antisocial personality disorders and related syndromes.* (pp. 78-97). New York: Norton & CO.

Schroeder, M., Schroeder, K., & Hare, R. D. (1985). Generalizability of a checklist for the assessment of psychopathy. *Journal of Consulting and Clinical Psychology, 51*, 511-516.

Steinberg, L., & Thissen, D. (1996). Uses of Item Response Theory and the testlet concept in the measurement of psychopathology. *Psychological Measurement, 1*(1), 81-97.

Tarrier, N., Eysenck, S. B. G., & Eysenck, H. J. (1980). National differences in personality; Brazil and England. *Personality and Individual Differences, 1*, 164-171.

Ten Berge, J. M. F. (1986). Rotation to perfect congruence and cross-validation of component weights across populations. *Multivariate Behavioural Research, 21*, 41-64.

Templeman, R., & Wong, S. (1994). Determining the factor structure of the Psychopathy Checklist: a converging approach. *Multivariate Experimental Clinical Research, 10*, 157-166.

Thissen, D. (1991). *Multilog user's guide (version 6)*. (1st ed.). Mooresville, IN: Scientific Software.

Thissen, D., & Steinberg, L. (1988). Data analysis using item response theory. *Psychological Bulletin, 104*, 385-395.

Tyrer, P. J., Cicchetti, D. V., Casey, P. R., Fitzpatrick, K., Oliver, R., Balter, A., Giller, E., & Harkness, L. (1984). Cross-national reliability study of a schedule for assessing personality disorders. *Journal of Nervous and Mental Disease, 172*, 718-721.

Van de Vijver, F. J. R., & Leung, K. (1997). *Methods and data analysis for cross-cultural research*. Thousand Oaks: Sage.

Wechsler, D. (1987). *Wechsler Memory Scale - Revised Manual*. (1st ed.). San Antonio: The Psychological Corporation.

Westermeyer, J. (1987). Cultural factors in clinical assessment. *Journal of Consulting and Clinical Psychology, 55*, 471-478.

Westermeyer, J. (1989). Psychiatric epidemiology across cultures: current issues and trends. *Transcultural Psychiatric Research Review, 26*, 5-25.

Wilson, J. Q., & Herrnstein, R. J. (1985). *Crime and human nature*. (1st ed.). New York: Simon & Schuster.

Winchie, D. B., & Carment, D. W. (1988). Intention to migrate: A psychological analysis. *Journal of Applied Social Psychiatry, 18*(9), 727-736.

Wong, S. (1984). *Criminal and institutional behaviors of psychopaths*. (1st ed.). Ottawa, Ontario: Ministry of the Solicitor-General of Canada.

Author's note.

I would like to acknowledge the support and guidance of Robert Hare and Stephen Hart in my endeavors to understand the mystery of psychopathy as it is emerges across cultures. I would like to thank all those researchers who have kindly given me access to their data. The Scottish data were collected with grants from the Criminological and Legal Research Branch and the Chief Scientist's Office of the Scottish Office. Finally, I must express my gratitude to Christine Michie for the care with which she has carried out the IRT analyses.

PSYCHOPATHY AND NORMAL PERSONALITY

THOMAS A. WIDIGER
Department of Psychology
University of Kentucky
Kentucky, USA.

PSYCHOPATHY AND NORMAL PERSONALITY

The purpose of this chapter is to discuss the construct of psychopathy from the perspective of normal personality. It will be suggested that psychopathy can be understood as a maladaptive variant of common personality traits. The chapter will begin with a discussion of the constructs of mental and personality disorders, suggesting the absence of a discrete or qualitative point of demarcation between the presence versus absence of a personality disorder. Psychopathy, as a personality disorder, will then be considered from the perspective of a model of normal personality functioning. It will be suggested that the traits of psychopathy (and antisocial personality disorder) can be understood from the perspective of this model, but only the most prototypic cases would display all of the features. The complexity of the psychopathic personality profile and the variability in presentation is important to appreciate when attempting to understand individual cases of psychopathy, to explain variability in findings across different settings and populations, to identify the maladaptivity of the disorder within different social and environmental contexts, and to understand its etiology.

Mental and Personality Disorder

The construct of mental disorder has always been and continues to be controversial (Gorenstein, 1984; Lilienfeld & Marino, 1995; Wakefield, 1992b). The diagnoses of psychopathy and antisocial personality disorder have been particularly controversial, as some have argued that these diagnoses represent simply a *"confusion of deviant social mores with criminality"* (Wulach, 1983, p. 338).

The construct of a mental (or psychosocial) disorder, however, is as valid as the construct of a physical disorder. Its validity has been problematic in part because of the failure to recognize that mental health is not qualitatively distinct from mental disorder, nor is a personality disorder qualitatively distinct from normal personality functioning. A mental disorder is an *"involuntary organismic impairment in psychological functioning"* (Widiger & Trull, 1991, p. 112). This definition provides the concepts that are fundamental to the construct (Wakefield, 1992a). Two central features are dyscontrol (i.e., involuntary) and maladaptivity (i.e., impairment). Each will be discussed in turn, particularly as they relate to the distinction between the disorder of psychopathy and normal personality functioning.

D.J. Cooke et al. (eds.), Psychopathy: Theory, Research and Implications for Society, 47–68.

Dyscontrol

Mental disorders are *"involuntary"* in the sense that they are compelled, dyscontrolled behavior patterns. Persons who freely, voluntarily choose to engage in harmful or impairing behaviors would not be said to have a mental disorder. Persons can drink, gamble, shoot heroin, steal, cheat, rape, and assault without having a mental disorder. The occurrence of a harmful act does not, by itself, constitute a mental disorder (Gorenstein, 1984). It is only when the behavior is compelled or impelled by determinants beyond sufficient or adequate control of the person that he or she would be diagnosed with a mental disorder.

Dyscontrol is also fundamental to the construct of a personality disorder. *"Only when personality traits are inflexible . . . do they constitute Personality Disorders"* (American Psychiatric Association [APA], 1994, p. 630). However, there does not appear to be a discrete, distinct point at which one can distinguish the flexible from the inflexible personality trait. Inflexibility is inferred on the basis of observing a consistent manner of behaving across a range of situations. Likewise, the presence of any normal personality trait is inferred on the basis of observing a consistent manner of behaving across a range of situations (Revelle, 1995). Both normal and abnormal persons are compelled or disposed to act in a particular manner, as characteristically friendly or hostile, assured or insecure, altruistic or exploitative, or to any varying degree in-between these more extreme variants. The decision to become a college professor may not be any less determined than a decision to become a serial murderer.

Persons, however, may vary in their degree of flexibility, and for each person there may be variability with respect to their degree of control of different behavior patterns. It would not be surprising to find that persons who are provided personality disorder diagnoses are less flexible with respect to their characteristic manner of thinking, feeling, and/or relating to others than a random sample of persons from the entire population. However, this distinction will be more quantitative than qualitative. One is unlikely to find a group of persons who have virtually no control over their characteristic manner of thinking, feeling, and relating to others (i.e., inflexible), and all other, ostensibly normal persons being entirely in control (i.e., flexible).

Degree of control or flexibility is not simply an academic issue. It is at the heart of a number of very difficult social and clinical issues, such as the distinction between the mental disorder of psychopathy and volitional criminal behavior. Antisocial personality disorder (ASPD) is defined in the DSM-IV as a *"pervasive pattern of disregard for and violation of the rights of others"* (APA, 1994, p. 645) but this would be an apt description of most career criminals. Approximately half of male prison inmates will meet the DSM-IV diagnostic criteria for ASPD (Hare, 1985; Hart & Hare, 1989). This statistic is typically interpreted as indicating an overdiagnosis, but Robins, Tipp, and Przybeck (1991) suggest that it may in fact be an accurate estimate of the base rate of this personality disorder within prison settings.

It is stated in DSM-IV that *"Antisocial Personality Disorder must be distinguished from criminal behavior undertaken for gain that is not accompanied by the personality features characteristic of this disorder"* (APA, 1994, p. 649). This statement is rather ironic, given that the authors of the diagnostic criteria for ASPD have emphasized the importance of using overt behavioral indicators rather than personality traits in the diagnosis of the disorder (Spitzer, Endicott, & Robins, 1975). Hart and Hare (1989) suggest that the personality traits that discriminate the normal from the abnormal criminal include lack of empathy, callousness, superficial charm, lack of guilt, arrogance, and remorselessness, rather than overt acts of criminality. This is now acknowledged in the DSM-IV text discussion of ASPD. *"Lack of empathy, inflated self-appraisal, and superficial charm are features that have been commonly included in traditional concepts of psychopathy and may be particularly distinguishing of Antisocial Personality Disorder in prison or forensic settings where criminal, delinquent, or aggressive acts are likely to be nonspecific"* (APA, 1994, p. 647).

Nonetheless, it is difficult to imagine a person who has voluntarily chosen a life of crime failing to be significantly or excessively callous, remorseless, unempathic, or guiltless. The prototypic evil (or bad) person is often the prototypic psychopathic (disordered or ill) person (Hare, 1993). That which compels a person to become a career criminal (Wilson & Herrnstein, 1985) will overlap substantially with that which compels a person to develop a psychopathic and/or antisocial personality disorder (Lykken, 1995; Sutker, Bugg, & West, 1993). The distinction will again be more quantitative than qualitative (Livesley, Jang, Jackson, & Vernon, 1993; Patrick, 1994). Empathy, charm, remorse, callousness, and guilt are unlikely to be qualitative distinctions such that some persons (i.e., psychopaths) lack these traits whereas normal persons possess them. For example, empathy itself appears to be on a continuum (McCrae & Costa, 1990) with persons varying in the extent, depth, and breadth of their empathy (Marshall, Hudson, Jones, & Fernandez, 1995). There might be some persons with virtually no feelings of empathy for any person at any time, including their lover, mother, children, and close friends. Such persons would indeed be more psychopathic than a career criminal who displayed empathy for his wife and children while at the same time he exploited, brutalized, and perhaps even tortured various innocent victims. However, this person would still be said to have a significant degree of impairment in his capacity for empathy.

Maladaptivity

A second fundamental feature of a mental disorder is maladaptivity (Wakefield, 1992a; Widiger & Trull, 1991). *"Only when personality traits are . . . maladaptive and cause significant functional impairment or subjective distress do they constitute Personality Disorders"* (APA, 1994, p. 630). Maladaptivity is controversial with respect to the antisocial and psychopathic personality disorders, as many authors suggest that the behavior pattern is labeled a disorder only because it is harmful to others, not because it is harmful to the psychopath. Blackburn (1988), for example, argued that psychopathy *"is a moral judgment masquerading as a clinical diagnosis"* (p. 511).

Wakefield (1992b) acknowledged explicitly the place of value judgments in his definition of mental disorder as harmful dysfunction: *"A definition of disorder in terms of negative consequences or, more simply, harm has the disadvantage that negative and harmful are essentially value terms, introducing moral and social judgments and a degree of value relativity into what many feel should be a purely scientific concept"* (p.237). This acknowledgment, however, is often misunderstood, suggesting to some that the construct of mental disorder is invalid and scientifically meaningless. Kirmayer

(1994), for example, argues that mental disorders are simply *"culturally constituted and sanctioned idioms of distress"* (p. 7). Wulach (1983) likewise argued that *"terms such as moral insanity, constitutional psychopathic inferiority, psychopathy, and sociopathy have gradually been eliminated from standard diagnostic systems because of vague criteria, prejudicial labeling effects, and confusion of deviant social mores with criminality"* (p. 338). Blackburn (1988) suggested as well that *"given the lack of demonstrable or clinical utility of the concept [of psychopathy], it should be discarded"* (p. 511). Lilienfeld and Marino (1995) have argued more recently that *"controversies regarding the inclusion or exclusion of specific conditions in the DSM result . . . from a failure to recognize that the question of whether a given condition constitutes a mental disorder cannot be answered by means of scientific criteria"* (p. 417). They suggested that unless a mental disorder could be reduced to a specific biological distinction, it would remain *"a nonscientific concept lacking clearcut natural boundaries"* (Lilienfeld & Marino, 1995, p. 417).

However, the presence of a value judgment in this context does not mean or imply that the construct of psychopathy represents simply the whims or preferences of a particular person or culture. It means instead that the impairment is secondary or relative to the optimal psychosocial functioning of the individual within a group. *"The fact that all disorders are undesirable and harmful according to social values shows only that values are part of the concept of disorder, not that disorder is composed only of values"* (Wakefield, 1992a, p. 376).

The construct of a mental disorder is no more value-laden than the construct of a physical disorder, as the latter is equally arbitrary and relative to the optimal, ideal functioning of an individual organism. Sedgwick (1982) expressed it well:

> *'There are no illnesses or diseases in nature . . . . The fracture of a septuagenarian's femur has, within the world of nature, no more significance than the snapping of an autumn leaf from its twig; and the invasion of a human organism by cholera-germs carries with it no more the stamp of "illness" than does the souring of milk by other forms of bacteria . . . . Out of his anthropocentric self-interest, man has chosen to consider as "illnesses" or "diseases" those natural circumstances which precipitate . . . death (or the failure to function according to certain values)'.* (Sedgwick, 1982, p. 30)

A flu is a physical disorder only from the perspective of the host organism; from the perspective of the virus this host is a meal, and nature cares less who survives the struggle. The construct of physical disease is one's value judgment for the side one wants to win.

Mental disorders, similarly, are psychosocial impairments from the perspective of the individual functioning within a social group. The construct of a mental disorder would admittedly be much different for persons who lived independently of any social interactions or involvements, but this is comparable to (and as realistic as) an organism living within a biologically harmless environment. The construct of a physical disorder would also be much different in an environment that posed no demands, threats, or dangers to the physical functioning of the organism. The construct of a mental (psychosocial) disorder is no less arbitrary.

There are indeed a variety of costs in being psychopathic, including (but not limited to) loss of jobs, unemployment, injuries, impoverishment, lawsuits, arrests, incarceration, death, and failed relationships (Hare, 1991; Robins et al., 1991; Sutker et al., 1993). There are some advantages to having limited feelings of guilt, remorse, and conscience, but it is an overly romanticized view of psychopathy to suggest that these advantages outweigh the costs. However, the point at which the disadvantages, costs, and suffering are sufficiently maladaptive to warrant a diagnosis of a personality disorder is unclear (Widiger & Corbitt, 1994). *"The definition of mental disorder in the introduction to DSM-IV requires that there be clinically significant impairment"* (APA, 1994, p. 7) but nowhere in DSM-IV is a *"clinically significant"* impairment defined. It is only stated that this is an inherently difficult clinical judgment.

The threshold of impairment that is used by most persons who seek or are referred to treatment is not that point at which they have, or would receive a diagnosis of, a personality disorder. It is probably that point at which their personality traits become sufficiently distressing or troubling to themselves or to others. This is not to say that the point of demarcation is meaningless, or that no actual dysfunction or disorder exists. It is only to say that the particular point of demarcation is arbitrary and does not define or identify a qualitatively distinct difference in functioning.

A useful analogy is provided by the construct of intelligence. Intelligence is associated with a variety of indicators of adaptive and maladaptive functioning (Neisser et al., 1996). Optimal functioning is facilitated by increasing levels of intelligence, and decreasing levels of intelligence are associated with maladaptive functioning. However, there is no nonarbitrary, discrete, or qualitatively distinct point of demarcation for identifying when the mental disorder of mental retardation occurs. Current convention places this point of demarcation at an intelligence quotient (IQ) of approximately 70 (APA, 1994), but it is evident that persons with IQs of 75, 80, and even higher can and do experience (or suffer from) impairments in academic and occupational success secondary to their level of intelligence. An IQ of 70 does not identify a discrete point of demarcation between pathology and health. Low intelligence is a quantitative rather than a qualitative distinction (Popper & Steingard, 1994). This is not to say that the point of demarcation is meaningless, or that no actual dysfunction exists below any particular point. It is only to say that the particular point of demarcation is arbitrary and does not define or identify a qualitatively distinct difference in functioning.

Psychopathy as a Variant of Normal Personality Functioning

Having suggested that there may be no discrete point of demarcation between the presence versus absence of a personality disorder, one might then ask whether the personality disorder of psychopathy could be understood in terms of common personality traits. A compelling and predominant model of normal personality functioning is the five-factor model (FFM). The FFM consists of five broad dimensions of personality functioning: neuroticism (or negative affectivity); extraversion versus introversion (or positive affectivity); openness versus closedness to experience (or unconventionality); antagonism versus agreeableness; and conscientiousness (or constraint) (Digman, 1996; Goldberg, 1993; McCrae & Costa, 1990). Each of these five broad domains can be further differentiated into underlying facets. Table 1 presents a summary of the five factors and their facets, derived from Costa and McCrae (1995).

TABLE 1. Five-Factor Model of Personality: Domains and Facets[a]

Neuroticism (or Negative Affectivity)
Anxiousness (fearful, tense vs relaxed, calm)
Angry hostility (angry, bitter, hostile vs even-tempered)
Trait depression (pessimistic vs optimistic)
Self-Consciousness (timid, shy vs self-assured, smooth, self-confident)
Impulsivity (recklessness, hasty vs controlled)
Vulnerability (fragile, cautious, uncertain vs stalwart, brave, risky)
Extraversion (vs. introversion)
Warmth (affectionate, friendly vs cold, aloof, detached)
Gregariousness (sociable, outgoing vs withdrawn, isolated)
Assertiveness (forceful, assertive, enthusiastic vs unassuming)
Activity (active, energetic, determined vs passive, lethargic)
Excitement-Seeking (adventurous, adventurous, daring vs cautious)
Positive emotions (high-spirited vs unemotional, placid, anhedonic)
Openness to Experience (or Unconventionality)
Fantasy (imaginative, strange, dreamy vs practical)
Aesthetic (aesthetic, inventive vs anesthetic)
Feelings (emotionally responsive vs unresponsive)
Actions (novelty seeking, peculiar, odd vs conventional, set in ways)
Ideas (curious, inquisitive, original vs pragmatic, down-to-earth)
Values (broad-minded, unconventional vs dogmatic, conservative)
Agreeableness (vs. antagonism)
Mistrust (cynical, prejudicial, suspicious, paranoid vs gullible, trusting)
Low straightforwardness (deceptive, manipulative, shrewd vs honest)
Low altruism (selfish, egocentric, exploitative vs generous, sacrificial)
Low compliance (oppositional, argumentative, aggressive vs cooperative)
Low modesty (conceited, arrogant, denigrating vs self-effacing)
Tough-mindedness (tough, callous, cruel vs concerned, sympathetic, empathic)
Conscientiousness (vs. negligence)
Competence (efficient, skilled, competent vs confused)
Order (organized, methodical, punctual vs disorganized)
Dutifulness (dutiful, dependable vs lax, negligent, irresponsible)
Achievement striving (ambitious, workaholic vs aimless)
Self-Discipline (industrious vs hedonistic)
Deliberation (thorough, perfectionistic vs careless, neglectful)

---

[a](Costa & McCrae, 1995); illustrative trait adjectives associated with each facet are presented in parentheses.

Space limitations prohibit a summary of the empirical support for the FFM. However, this material is available elsewhere (Costa & McCrae, 1992; Digman, 1996; Goldberg, 1993; McCrae & Costa, 1990; Saucier & Golberg, 1996). A variety of studies, using different methods of assessment and sampling from different populations, have indicated a close association of the five-factor model of normal personality with models of personality disorder (e.g., Clark & Livesley, 1994; Clarkin, Hull, Cantor, & Sanderson, 1993; Costa & McCrae, 1990; Schroeder, Wormworth, & Livesley, 1992; Soldz, Budmam, Demby, & Merry, 1993; Trull, 1992; Trull, Useda, Costa, & McCrae, 1995; Wiggins & Pincus, 1989; Yeung, Lyons, Waternaux, Faraone, & Tsuang, 1993). Table 2 presents a conceptual summary of how each of the Psychopathy Checklist Revised (PCL-R) items would be understood from the perspective of the FFM. Three of the domains of the FFM (along with extraversion) appear to be particularly important in accounting for the features of psychopathy: neuroticism, antagonism, and conscientiousness. Each of the features of psychopathy will be discussed below in terms of a respective FFM domain and facet.

TABLE 2. FFM Representation of Revised Psychopathy Checklist[a] items

1. **Glibness/superficial charm**: Low self-consciousness
2. **Grandiose sense of self-worth**: Arrogance & Low vulnerability
3. **Need for stimulation/proneness to boredom**: Excitement-seeking
4. **Pathological lying**: Deception/manipulation
5. **Conning/manipulative**: Deception/manipulation
6. **Lack of remorse or guilt**: Tough-mindedness
7. **Shallow affect**: Low positive emotionality
8. **Callous/lack of empathy**: Tough-mindedness
9. **Parasitic lifestyle**: Egocentricity/exploitation, Low discipline, & Low achievement striving
10. **Poor behavioral controls**: Angry hostility & Impulsivity
11. **Promiscuous sexual behavior**: Egocentricity/exploitation & Low discipline
12. **Early behavior problems**: Egocentricy/exploitation & Oppositional/aggressive
13. **Lack of realistic, long-term goals**: Low vulnerability, Low deliberation, & Low achievement-striving
14. **Impulsivity**: Impulsivity
15. **Irresponsibility**: Low dutifulness, Low discipline, & Low deliberation
16. **Failure to accept responsibility for actions**: Low dutifulness and Low deliberation
17. **Many short-term marital relationships**: Egocentricity/exploitation, Low dutifulness, & Low self-discipline
18. **Juvenile delinquency**: Egocentricity/exploitation & Oppositional/aggressive
19. **Revocation of conditional release**: Egocentricity/exploitation & Oppositional/aggressive
20. **Criminal versatility**: Egocentricity/exploitation, Deception/manipulation, & Oppositional/aggressive

[a]Hare (1991)

Neuroticism

Neuroticism (identified as negative affectivity by others; Saucier & Goldberg, 1996) is a domain of personality functioning included in most theoretically derived models of personality (e.g., Eysenck, 1994). Costa and McCrae (1995) have differentiated neuroticism into six underlying facets of anxiousness, angry hostility, trait depression, self-consciousness, impulsivity, and vulnerability.

It is evident from Table 2 that neuroticism would be important in understanding psychopathy. Glib, superficial charm, the first item of the PCL-R, is related closely to low self-consciousness. The average person is characterized by a degree of self-consciousness and will be, to some extent, sensitive to ridicule, prone to embarrassment, socially anxious, awkward, or insecure (McCrae & Costa, 1990). Lykken (1995) suggests that most persons lack psychopathic charm because they are *"a little shy, a bit self-conscious, afraid to say the wrong thing, afraid to alienate, a little tongue-tied, inclined to get a bit rattled when it is your turn to say something"* (p. 136). Prototypic psychopathic persons, on the other hand, will be extremely low in self-consciousness. They tend to be smooth, engaging, charming, slick, and verbally facile (Hare, 1991). *"More than the average person, he is likely to seem free from social or emotional impediments, from the minor distortions, peculiarities, and awkwardness so common even among the successful"* (Cleckley, 1941, p. 205). Psychopathic persons will be very comfortable and relaxed with other persons, and can readily put them at ease. Regrettably, they will often use their engaging low self-consciousness to exploit others, commensurate with their high levels of antagonism (discussed below).

Psychopathy, as described by the PCL-R, also includes very low vulnerability. The average person has characteristic feelings of vulnerability to stress, conflict, risk, and danger. Feelings of vulnerability are helpful to adaptive functioning in anticipating and avoiding realistic threats and risks. However, *"individuals who score [very] high on this scale feel unable to cope with stress, becoming dependent, hopeless, or panicked when facing emergency situations"* (Costa & McCrae, 1992, p. 16). A number of the DSM-IV personality disorders involve excessive vulnerability, particularly the dependent and avoidant (Widiger, Trull, Clarkin, Sanderson, & Costa, 1994). Psychopathy, on the other hand, involves excessively low feelings of vulnerability, contributing to the tendency to engage in highly risky and reckless criminal, sexual, business, drug, and other activities. The prototypic psychopathic person will feel invulnerable to risk, failure, and danger. Lykken (1995) in fact suggests that fearlessness is the central, fundamental trait of psychopathy. Feelings of invulnerability are evident in the PCL-R items concerned with a grandiose sense of self-worth (e.g., self-assurance and insensitive to or concerned with legal problems) and lack of realistic, long-term goals (e.g., does not give serious thought to the future).

Excessively low anxiousness may also be characteristic of the prototypic psychopath. Cleckley (1941) had included an *"absence of 'nervousness' or psychoneurotic manifestations"* (p. 206) as one of his 16 characteristic features of psychopathy. *"The psychopath is nearly always free from minor reactions popularly regarded as 'neurotic' or as constituting 'nervousness'. . . . It is highly typical for him not only to escape the abnormal anxiety and tension . . . but also to show a relative immunity from such anxiety and worry as might be judged normal or appropriate"* (p. 206). *"He appears almost as incapable of anxiety as of profound remorse"* (Cleckley, 1941, p. 206). Patrick (1994) suggests that low neuroticism (or negative affectivity) is the fundamental pathology of psychopathy. *"The observed absence of startle potentiation in psychopaths . . . may reflect a temperamental deficit in the capacity for negative affect and could serve as a potential marker of the disorder"* (Patrick 1994, p. 325).

The potential importance of low neuroticism to psychopathy is intriguing in light of the fact that DSM-IV does not include any features of low neuroticism within its diagnostic criteria for ASPD (APA, 1994). There are no indicators of low self-consciousness, feelings of invulnerability, or low anxiousness. In fact, it is noted in the text discussion for ASPD that individuals with this disorder are prone to feelings of *"dysphoria, including complaints of tension"* (APA, 1994, p. 647) and will have associated anxiety disorders, such as generalized anxiety disorder, panic disorder, or perhaps even social phobia. This unusual description of ASPD is opposite to that of Cleckley (1941) and is perhaps due in part to psychiatric experience and research being confined largely to clinical settings. Psychiatric patients will often, if not invariably, have symptoms of anxiety and tension (Eysenck, 1994), and may then provide atypical cases of psychopathy. Prototypic psychopathy is more likely to be found and is perhaps better researched within other settings, such as a prison (Hare, Hart, & Harpur, 1991; Hart & Hare, 1989). Lilienfeld (1994) noted as well that *"a number of self-report measures of psychopathy appear to be heavily saturated with negative affectivity . . . or general maladjustment or neuroticism" (p. 30) and that "a substantial saturation with this dimension may compromise the ability of psychopathy measures to discriminate between psychopathy and other syndromes"* (p. 30).

However, prototypic psychopathy will include some facets of excessive neuroticism, such as impulsivity and angry hostility (see Table 2). These facets of neuroticism are evident in the PCL-R items of impulsivity and poor behavior controls, respectively. The control of impulses is problematic to some degree for most persons (McCrae & Costa, 1990), but the prototypic psychopathic person is especially *"impulsive, unpremeditated, and lacking in reflection or forethought"* (Hare, 1991, p. 25). PCL-R poor behavior controls involves primarily the tendency to be short-tempered and hot-headed, comparable to FFM angry hostility. Angry hostility is the disposition to feel angry, rageful, hostile, bitter, and frustrated (Costa & McCrae, 1992). As noted by Hare (1991), the psychopathic person *"takes offense easily and becomes angry and aggressive over trivialities; these behaviors will often seem inappropriate, given the context in which they occur"* (Hare, 1991, p. 23). The DSM-IV description of ASPD (APA, 1994) includes FFM impulsivity in its diagnostic criteria of impulsivity and recklessness, and FFM angry hostility in its irritability criterion.

Antagonism versus Agreeableness

Antagonism versus agreeableness is one of the fundamental dimensions of personality (Digman, 1996; Goldberg, 1993; Wiggins & Pincus, 1992). It involves primarily one's manner of relatedness to others (as does the dimension of extraversion versus introversion), and is related closely to the interpersonal circumplex (McCrae & Costa, 1989; Wiggins & Pincus, 1989). It is also the five-factor dimension with the greatest number of trait terms (Goldberg, 1992), suggesting that this domain of functioning is particularly important to persons in describing themselves and each other. It is evident from Table 2 that psychopathy (and DSM-IV ASPD) involve many of the facets of antagonism, including deception-manipulation (vs. straightforwardness), egocentricity-exploitation (vs. altruism), oppositionalism-aggression (vs. compliance), tough-mindedness (vs. tendermindedness), and arrogance (vs. modesty).

All persons vary in the extent to which they are characteristically straightforward versus deceptive (Costa & McCrae, 1995). Prototypic psychopathic persons occupy the most extreme variant of this facet of agreeableness versus antagonism, as they will be consistently dishonest, deceptive, and manipulative. These traits are represented in the PCL-R items of pathological lying and conning/manipulative, and in the DSM-IV diagnostic criterion of *"deceitfulness, as indicated by repeated lying, use of aliases, or conning others for personal profit or pleasure"* (APA, 1994, p. 650). Many psychopathic persons appear to lie simply for the sport or pleasure of deception and manipulation. *"Lying and deceit are a characteristic part of his interactions with others . . . . He often lies for obvious reasons, but deceiving others also appears to have some intrinsic value for him"* (Hare, 1991, p. 19). This personality trait will contribute to the criminal behaviors of cheating, conning, defrauding, and scamming others.

A closely related FFM facet of antagonism is egocentricity-exploitation (correlating .34 on the NEO-PI-R; Costa & McCrae, 1992). Persons with a dependent personality disorder tend to be excessively altruistic, sacrificing their own wishes, needs, and safety for the benefit of others. Psychopathic and antisocial persons are just the opposite. Their interests, wishes, and desires will come first, and they will even use, exploit, abuse, and victimize others for their desires, interests, and needs. Their egocentricity is evident in part in the PCL-R parasitic lifestyle item. *"Although able-bodied, he avoids steady, gainful employment; instead, he continually relies on family, relatives, or social assistance"* (Hare, 1991, p. 22). This behavior reflects not only an irresponsibility (i.e., low conscientiousness, discussed below) but also *"a persistent pattern of behavior in which others are called upon to support him and to cater to his needs, no matter what the economic and emotional cost to them"* (Hare, 1991, p. 22). Egocentricity is not included within the DSM-IV criteria for ASPD, although Robins (1966) had included a criterion of public financial care within her original set of 19 diagnostic criteria for sociopathic personality disorder (i.e., being *"totally or partially supported by relatives, friends, social agencies, or public institutions,"* p. 342).

Egocentricity, however, is evident in the DSM-III-R ASPD and PCL-R items that describe the many sexual and/or marital relationships. A successfully maintained relationship requires the ability to make a commitment, a concern for and interest in the needs of the other person, and a desire for a sustained involvement. Psychopathic and antisocial persons will instead have a history of many brief relationships, and these relationships will tend to be impersonal, casual, and trivial (Hare, 1991). The most extreme form of sexual egocentricity would to be to force one's own sexual desires and wishes onto another person, and a psychopathic person will indeed *"coerce others into sexual activity with him, and may have charges or convictions for sexual assault"* (Hare, 1991, p. 23).

Criminal activity is the most obvious and explicit manifestation of this facet of antagonism, and is represented well within the PCL-R items concerned with early behavior problems, juvenile delinquency, revocation of conditional release, and criminal versatility (Hare, 1991). The defining trait of DSM-IV ASPD is a *"disregard for, and violation of, the rights of others"* (APA, 1994, p. 645), and the first and most diagnostic criterion for ASPD is a *"failure to conform to social norms with respect to lawful behaviors as indicated by repeatedly performing acts that are grounds for arrest"* (APA, 1994, p. 649). Such criminal acts can concern other personality traits, such as impulsivity (e.g., driving while intoxicated), but most antisocial-psychopathic criminal behaviors will reflect the disposition to be exploitative.

Antagonistic aggression is also characteristic of the prototypic psychopath. Aggressive behavior will at times reflect the neuroticism facet of angry hostility. However, angry hostility, as a facet of negative affectivity, is the disposition to experience feelings of anger, frustration, annoyance, or bitterness. *"Whether the anger is expressed depends upon the individual's level of [antagonism]"* (Costa & McCrae, 1992, p. 16). This facet of antagonism includes the more calculated, dispassionate, and purposeful aggression that will be evident in prototypic psychopathy. Some of their acts of abuse, assault, and rape will not reflect an explosive anger, but will instead be more calculated, premeditated, and purposeful efforts to subjugate, humiliate, and/or harm others.

Tough-mindedness versus tender-mindedness is an additional facet of antagonism versus agreeableness that is important to the diagnosis of psychopathy. Tender-mindedness is the tendency to be sympathetic, concerned, and empathic (Costa & McCrae, 1995; McCrae & Costa, 1990). At the opposite pole of this dimension of personality is the tendency to be unconcerned, dispassionate, callous, unempathic, and perhaps even contemptuous, cruel, or vicious. The inclusion of a callous lack of empathy is one of the major distinctions of PCL-R psychopathy versus DSM-IV ASPD (Hare et al., 1991). A *"callous disregard for the feelings, rights, and welfare of others"* (Hare, 1991, p. 22) is clearly evident in the DSM-IV definition of ASPD as a *"disregard for . . . the rights of others"* (APA, 1994, p. 645) but the DSM-IV diagnostic criteria for ASPD emphasize the behavioral manifestations of violating the rights of others (i.e., criminality) rather than the attitudinal disregard for others.

This trait, however, is evident in the DSM-IV and PCL-R items involving a lack of remorse or guilt. Guilt is a negative affect that is often seen in persons with a depressive personality disorder (Widiger et al., 1994), but the absence of guilt in persons with psychopathy can reflect their antagonism rather than low negative affectivity. As noted by Hare (1991), lack of remorse or guilt *"describes an individual who shows a general lack of concern for the negative consequences that his actions, both criminal and non-criminal, have on others"* (p. 20). *"These individuals may blame the victims for being foolish, helpless, or deserving their fate; they may minimize the harmful consequences of their actions; or they may simply indicate complete indifference"* (APA, 1994, p. 646). Their callous antagonism will at times be so extreme that they may even experience significant enjoyment in an especially vicious brutality.

Arrogance versus modesty is an additional facet of antagonism versus agreeableness that is evident in psychopathic persons. Persons with a dependent personality disorder will be excessively self-effacing (Widiger et al., 1994) whereas the prototypic psychopathic person will display a grandiose sense of self-worth (Hare,

1991). The psychopathic person *"may impress as a braggart. He often appears self-assured, opinionated, and cocky"* (Hare, 1991, p. 18). Arrogance is an aspect of psychopathy not included within the DSM-IV diagnostic criteria for ASPD, due in part to a concern that its inclusion would complicate the differentiation of ASPD from the narcissistic personality disorder (Widiger & Corbitt, 1995). The failure to include these traits reflects in part the difficulty in providing descriptively accurate diagnostic categories that are also qualitatively distinct (Widiger, 1993). Arrogance, glib charm, and lack of empathy are all characteristic of psychopathy (Cleckley, 1941; Hare, 1991) but they have not been included within the criteria for ASPD in part because they are also characteristic of another personality disorder diagnosis that must be distinguished from ASPD (Widiger & Corbitt, 1995).

Conscientiousness

The third FFM domain of personality that appears to be important in psychopathy and ASPD is conscientiousness. FFM conscientiousness includes such traits as dutifulness, achievement-striving, order, competence, self-discipline, and deliberation (Costa & McCrae, 1995). Persons who are excessively conscientious might be diagnosed with a compulsive personality disorder (i.e., workaholism, perfectionism, and excessive emphasis upon organization, structure, and order), whereas persons who are excessively low in conscientiousness will present with antisocial, psychopathic, and other maladaptive personality traits. The facets of conscientiousness that appear to be especially involved in psychopathy and ASPD are excessively low dutifulness, self-discipline, achievement-striving, and deliberation. Such persons tend to be unreliable, undependable, irresponsible, lax, aimless, negligent, and careless (see Table 1).

Low conscientiousness is explicitly represented by the PCL-R item of irresponsibility. The psychopathic person *"has little or no sense of duty or loyalty to family, friends, employers, society, ideas, or causes"* (Hare, 1991, p. 25). DSM-IV ASPD also includes a comparable item of *"consistent irresponsibility, as indicated by repeated failure to sustain consistent work behavior or honor financial obligations"* (APA, 1994, p. 650).

Low conscientiousness, however, is also evident in additional PCL-R items, including parasitic lifestyle (e.g., avoidance of steady, gainful employment), lack of realistic, long-term goals (e.g., living day to day), failure to accept responsibility for own actions, and many short-term marital relationships. All of these behaviors involve, at least in part, the disposition to be negligent, undependable, lax, irresponsible, and aimless. Low conscientiousness is also evident in the ASPD criteria of *"reckless disregard for safety of self or others"* and *"failure to plan ahead"* (APA, 1994, p. 650).

Extraversion versus Introversion

Two of the PCL-R items appear to involve facets of extraversion versus introversion: need for stimulation or proneness to boredom, and shallow affect. PCL-R need for stimulation is almost synonymous with the extraversion facet of excitement-seeking. FFM excitement-seeking is the disposition to *"crave excitement and stimulation"* (Costa & McCrae, 1992, p. 17). Likewise, PCL-R need for stimulation concerns *"a strong interest in taking chances, 'living life in the fast lane' or 'on the edge', being 'where the action is', and in doing things that are exciting, risky, or challenging"* (Hare, 1991, p. 18).

Shallow affect is described in the PCL-R as being *"unable to experience a normal range and depth of emotion"* (Hare, 1991, p. 21), comparable to the introversion facet of low positive emotionality. The shallow affect of psychopathic persons contributes to the development of weak, if not nonexistent, emotional bonds. Psychopathic persons do not develop close, sustained, or deep relationships. *"He may impress as cold and unemotional"* (Hare, 1991, p. 21). A closely related facet of introversion is interpersonal coldness (see Table 1). However, psychopathic persons may not be withdrawn or isolated. They may in fact be very gregarious (a different facet of extraversion). As indicated in the first PCL-R item, prototypic psychopathic persons will be very charming and can be very engaging. They may have many *"friends,"* but one will find that these friendships lack much depth, intimacy, or emotional involvement. As noted in the assessment of this PCL-R item, *"if the individual expresses love for family or friends can he provide details about their current whereabouts, health, . . . and general well-being?"* (Hare, 1991, p. 21).

It should be noted, however, that psychopathy does not involve the most extreme form of low positive emotionality. A more extreme variant of shallow affect would be seen in the schizoid personality disorder. Schizoid persons display a more severe *"emotional coldness, detachment, or flattened affectivity"* (APA, 1994, p. 641). As suggested by Lykken (1995), *"I see no evidence that the psychopath cannot feel ecstatic or joyful or delighted"* (p. 141). Psychopathic persons will at times be very emotional. However, their *"displays of emotion generally are dramatic, shallow, short-lived; they leave careful observers with the impression that he is playacting . . . He may admit that he is unemotional or that he shams emotions"* (Hare, 1991, p. 21). Shallow affect may in this respect involve a degree of antagonism, particularly the facet of deception-manipulation (discussed earlier).

Empirical Support for the FFM Description of Psychopathy and ASPD

There have been a number of studies on the relationship of ASPD to the FFM but only two papers to date have reported data concerning the relationship of psychopathy to the FFM (Harpur, Hart, & Hare, 1994; Hart & Hare, 1994). Harpur et al. (1994) indicated that their research team *"has begun to administer the NEO-PI to inmates assessed on the PCL"* (p. 158) and provided preliminary findings in their chapter on the personality of the psychopath. They reported a significant correlation of PCL psychopathy with antagonism (r=.47, p<.05) but not with neuroticism or conscientiousness.

Hart and Hare (1994) subsequently rated PCL interviews for the FFM constructs using the Interpersonal Adjective Scales - Big Five (IASR-B5; Trapnell & Wiggins, 1991). They suggested that these observers' ratings of interviews with inmates are preferable to self-report questionnaires due to concerns regarding the validity of questionnaires within inmate settings. *"The tendency to lie and manipulate is an important symptom of psychopathy"* (Hart & Hare, 1994, p. 34), questioning the value of any self-report measure of personality in studies concerning psychopathy (Hare, 1985). Hart and Hare (1994) suggested that the dishonesty of psychopathic persons *"may well be responsible for the low magnitude of the correlations between the PCL-R and self-report personality measures reported in past research"* (p. 34). In their study with observer ratings, they obtained substantial correlations with conscientiousness (r = -.79) and neuroticism (r = -.41), and the IASR-B5 Love-Hate (r = -.64) and Dominance-Submission (r = .52) scales that relate closely to the FFM domains of agreeableness-antagonism and extraversion-introversion (McCrae & Costa, 1989; Wiggins & Pincus, 1989).

All but one of the FFM studies concerning ASPD have reported significant and usually substantial correlations with antagonism and conscientiousness (Costa & McCrae, 1990; Trull, 1992; Wiggins & Pincus, 1989; Yeung et al., 1993). The one exception was the study by Soldz et al. (1993) whose sample had excluded explicitly persons with an antisocial personality disorder. None of the above studies obtained significant correlations with extraversion but, as indicated below, this is consistent with the involvement of only two, opposing facets of extraversion. Only one study (Costa & McCrae, 1990) obtained a significant correlation with the FFM domain of openness, as expected.

The findings for neuroticism and ASPD have been inconsistent, but this is also to be expected. As noted earlier, the DSM (unlike the PCL-R) has not included any indicators of low neuroticism in its diagnostic criteria for ASPD (i.e., glib charm, fearlessness, invulnerability, and low anxiousness) and in fact suggests that ASPD is associated with tension, dysphoria, and anxiety disorders. It is interesting to note in this context that Costa and McCrae (1990) reported a significant negative correlation of neuroticism with ASPD (r= -.27, p<.001) when they used the first edition of the Millon Clinical Multiaxial Inventory (MCMI-I; Millon, 1983) but they obtained positive correlations with neuroticism when ASPD was assessed with the second edition of the MCMI (MCMI-II; Millon, 1987). The antisocial scale of the MCMI-I was based in part on Cleckley's (1941) original description rather than the more behavioral and sociological description by Robins (1966) that Millon (1981) had opposed for inclusion in DSM-III. However, the subsequent editions of the MCMI have been revised to be more closely coordinated with the DSM (Millon, 1987). Hare (1991) reported comparable findings, noting an increase from .26 to .51 in the correlation of the MCMI-I and MCMI-II ASPD scales with the second factor of the PCL (i.e., unstable and antisocial lifestyle), and a comparable decrease from .31 to .24 in their correlations with the first PCL factor (i.e., selfish, callous, and remorseless use of others).

A final note with respect to the above research is that none of the studies have considered the facets of antagonism and conscientiousness, and only a few studies have considered the facets of neuroticism and extraversion. As noted by Harpur et al. (1994), *"the specific traits [of psychopathy] . . . tend to be at a lower level of generality than are the broad dimensions that form the framework for the FFM"* (p. 156). It is of theoretical interest and importance to relate psychopathy to the broad domains of personality (Widiger & Costa, 1994) but clinical and forensic applications will not become apparent until the FFM is assessed at the level of the more specific facets (Harkness, 1992). In addition, the associations of psychopathy with the FFM may at times be masked at the level of the broad domains. For example, Harpur et al. (1994) reported an insignificant correlation of PCL psychopathy with the domain of extraversion (r = .07) but they did obtain a substantial correlation with the extraversion facet of excitement-seeking (r = .42, p<.05). They did not obtain a significant negative correlation with positive emotionality, but this may be due in part to the lack of a substantial correlation of shallow affect with the total PCL-R score. To the extent that shallow affect does not account for a substantial proportion of variance in total PCL-R scores, one would not expect to obtain a correlation of PCL-R psychopathy with introversion or even with the facet of positive emotionality.

Objections to FFM Description of Psychopathy

Empirical support for an understanding of psychopathy from the perspective of the FFM is limited, due largely to the absence of a substantial amount of research to date. Conceptually, however, all of the traits of psychopathy identified by Hare (1991) and all of the diagnostic criteria for DSM-IV ASPD (APA, 1994) do appear to be included in the FFM description of normal personality functioning (see Table 2). Harpur et al. (1994), however, raised compelling objections and concerns regarding the association of psychopathy with the FFM. Each will be discussed in turn.

Complexity of the FFM Description

Harpur et al. (1994) argued that *"the FFM profile of the psychopath is considerably more complex than that envisaged for several other personality disorders"* (p. 167), suggesting that the FFM is not as successful in accounting for psychopathy as it is for many of the DSM-IV personality disorders. The FFM description of psychopathy is indeed complex, with five of six facets from antagonism, three of six from conscientiousness, two opposing facets from extraversion, three facets of low neuroticism, and two facets of high neuroticism.

However, it is not the case that this description of psychopathy is any more complex than the FFM description of most of the DSM-IV personality disorders (see Widiger et al., 1994), nor does the complexity of the FFM profile suggest an inadequate description. The complexity of the FFM descriptions of the DSM-IV personality disorders is in fact an argument for the inadequacy of the DSM-IV categorical distinctions (Widiger, 1993). The DSM-IV diagnostic categories are unlikely to be successful as distinct clinical conditions in part because they involve heterogeneous, overlapping, and complex representations of a variety of facets from most to all of the FFM domains. The DSM-IV diagnostic categories do not appear to define distinct personality profiles, and their excessive comorbidity can be explained in part by the overlap among the FFM domains (e.g., the avoidant and schizoid personality disorders share many of the facets of introversion, whereas the avoidant and dependent personality disorders share many of the facets of neuroticism; Widiger et al., 1994).

Psychopathy is typically understood as a relatively distinct and homogenous clinical syndrome (Lilienfield, 1994; Lykken, 1995), and there is empirical support for this perspective, most recently by Harris, Rice, and Quinsey (1994). Harpur et al. (1994) noted that *"psychopathy as assessed by the PCL is perhaps the most reliable and well-validated diagnostic category in the field of personality disorders"* (p. 169). They suggest that it is then difficult to understand how it could involve such a collection of facets from different domains of personality functioning.

However, there are also reasons to doubt whether psychopathy is in fact a homogenous syndrome, qualitatively distinct from normal personality functioning (Blackburn, 1988; Lilienfeld & Marino, 1995). Clinical and research literature has recognized for sometime the presence of many different variants of psychopathy (Lykken, 1995). Levenson, Kiehl, and Fitzpatrick (1995) provided a recent empirical illustration. The PCL-R has itself been distinguished in terms of two factors (Harpur, Hare, & Hakstian, 1989) that appear to have quite different patterns of correlations with other variables (Hare, 1991).

The PCL-R diagnosis of psychopathy uses a cutoff point of 30 for its diagnosis but Hare (1991) acknowledges that *"dimensional ratings are more useful than categorical diagnoses in several respects: For example, they have superior psychometric properties, and they do not require that firm assumptions be made about whether or not the underlying construct is [dis]continuous"* (Hare, 1991, p. 17). The cutoff point of 30 on the PCL-R might not be demarcating the presence versus absence of a distinct clinical condition, indicating instead a useful point of demarcation along a continuum of psychopathic functioning. Those above the cutoff point have most of the traits of psychopathy, while persons below the cutoff point have significantly fewer of them. Many researchers in fact have recognized the value of different cutoff points within particular settings and populations (e.g., Harris, Rice, & Cormier, 1991; Serin, Peters, & Barbaree, 1990). Alterman, Cacciola, and Rutherford (1993) recommend a much lower cutoff point of 25 within substance abuse populations. Not as many traits of psychopathy will need to be present within a substance abuse treatment setting to indicate a clinically significant impairment than within an inmate prison setting. Even lower cutoff points might be useful (and perhaps necessary) within higher functioning populations, such as white collar business settings (e.g., Babiak, 1995) or college populations (e.g., Gustafson & Ritzer, 1995). Persons with scores of just 20 on the PCL-R might appear to be as distinctive and dysfunctional relative to their peers within these settings as persons with scores of 30 within an inmate prison population.

Prototypic cases of psychopathy do indeed present with relatively specific clinical syndromes, characterized by a particular profile of FFM domains and facets. The presence of the FFM facets of deceptiveness, exploitativeness, aggression, callousness, arrogance, self-assuredness, low self-consciousness, feelings of invulnerability, angry hostility, impulsivity, excitement-seeking, irresponsibility, aimlessness, and unreliability does provide a particularly problematic and volatile constellation of personality traits that would be prominent and vivid within any setting, including a prison setting wherein many of the persons will have at least some degree of antagonism and low conscientiousness.

However, an advantage of understanding psychopathy from the perspective of the FFM is its ability to characterize more precisely the individual, atypical, and nonprototypic cases. Harpur et al. (1994) lament that *"in the absence of, say, Dominance, Excitement Seeking, and Impulsivity . . . the syndrome fails to take on its distinctive form: one might see a shiftless authoritarian person but not a psychopath"* (p. 167). This is indeed true, but it may also be precisely the advantage of the FFM approach. Not all cases will be prototypic. Some persons will be characterized primarily by the facets of antagonism rather than low conscientiousness; others may have only some of the facets of antagonism (e.g., exploitation and arrogance) but not all of them (e.g., absence of significant levels of tough-mindedness, callousness, or aggression). These different variants will be important clinically and empirically to distinguish (Lykken, 1995). DSM-IV ASPD, for example, emphasizes low conscientiousness and the antagonism facets of exploitation, deception, and aggression, but not the facets of low neuroticism. It might then be fruitless to study Patrick's (1994) hypothesis of low negative affectivity with subjects diagnosed according to the DSM-IV ASPD criteria set.

On the other hand, excessive antagonism coupled with low neuroticism and high (rather than low) conscientiousness might be characteristic of the successful psychopath, a variant often discussed but rarely seen within prison, forensic, or general psychiatric settings (Lykken, 1995; Sutker et al., 1993; Widiger & Hicklin, 1995). Deceptive, exploitative, callous, charming, and engaging persons who are also well-organized, diligent, disciplined, and achievement-striving could be even more destructive and problematic, at least to others, than persons who are low in conscientiousness. The former persons may express their psychopathic traits of antagonism within more legitimate careers, or at least be much more successful in not getting arrested for their crimes than the prison psychopaths that are currently the focus of research. Psychopathy, as a distinct clinical syndrome, may appear to involve low conscientiousness in part because current research is confined largely to psychopaths who have been unsuccessful (legally or clinically) in their antagonistic exploitation, deception, and victimization.

Specific Etiology and/or Pathology

Harpur et al. (1994) suggest that *"psychopaths, as a group, [also] display a puzzling set of abnormalities in several basic cognitive functions involved in attention . . . impulse control . . . and the processing of affect and language"* (p. 170). Many of the personality traits of psychopathy might be distributed continuously within the general population, but the pathology of psychopathy is perhaps distinct and specific to those persons with the disorder. *"These may represent critical additional risk factors for the development of the disorder in addition to, or in combination with, the underlying personality structure"* (Harpur et al., 1994, p. 170). If there is a specific etiology for and pathology of psychopathy, then it might not be appropriate or valid to suggest that psychopathy is on a continuum with normal personality functioning. Psychopathy would then be something qualitatively different from the personality functioning that occurs within the rest of the population (Lilienfeld & Marino, 1995; Lykken, 1995).

The search for the unique pathology of psychopathy has been a major focus of research interest and attention (e.g., Fowles & Missel, 1994; Newman, Kosson, & Patterson, 1992; Williams, Harper, & Hare, 1991). However, the many alternative models for this pathology often fail to replicate across settings and populations or fail to maintain their empirical support over time (Lilienfeld, 1994). A more fruitful approach might be to investigate factors that are on a continuum with normal personality functioning (e.g., Livesley et al., 1993; Patrick, 1994). The constellation of personality traits that together characterize prototypic cases of psychopathy may have a complex, diverse, and multifactorial etiology.

Consider again the analogy of mental retardation. There are cases of mental retardation with a specific etiology and pathology. One such example would be mental retardation secondary to Down's syndrome. However, Down's syndrome is not mental retardation. Down's syndrome is a medical disorder that is one possible etiology, among many other possibilities, for the mental disorder of mental retardation. *"There are [in fact] more than 200 recognized biological syndromes involving mental retardation . . . entailing disruptions in virtually any sector of brain biochemical or physiological functioning"* (Popper & Steingard, 1994, p. 777). The number is much greater when one includes psychosocial etiologies and determinants of mental retardation. Approximately 40% of cases of mental retardation lack a known etiology in part because the determinants are complex, interactive, and multifactorial, reflecting normal genetic variation, fetal development, infant nutrition, early infant/child development, and socio/cultural deprivation (APA, 1994).

The same could be said for psychopathy. Specific etiologies for some cases of psychopathy may eventually be discovered, but psychopathy, like intelligence and other personality traits, might itself remain as a continuum of functioning with no discrete point at which the disorder of psychopathy is distinguished from normal personality functioning. Many, if not most, of the cases might be the result of a complex set of interacting biogenetic and environmental factors, such as an inherited temperament of low levels of distress-proneness and attentional self-regulation (Kochanska, 1991); coupled with modeling by parental figures and peers; excessively harsh, lenient, or erratic discipline (e.g., Luntz & Widom, 1994); and a tough, harsh environment in which feelings of empathy and warmth are discouraged (if not punished) and tough-mindedness, aggressiveness, and exploitation are encouraged (if not rewarded) (Dodge, 1993). Such complex pathways with multiple and interacting variables will result in an array of variants of personality traits that would be on a continuum with normal personality functioning.

CONCLUSIONS

In sum, it is the suggestion of this author that psychopathy can be understood in terms of the FFM, particularly when the analysis is conducted at the facet level. Psychopathy may indeed represent an extreme variant of common personality traits that are evident to varying degrees in all persons. A five-factor model understanding of psychopathy may also be helpful in clarifying different formulations of the disorder (e.g., PCL-R psychopathy versus DSM-IV ASPD) and in recognizing sub-threshold and nonprototypic cases.

It is also important to emphasize that the relationship between the PCL-R and the FFM models of psychopathy is complementary rather than contradictory, in the same manner in which the FFM and interpersonal circumplex models of personality provide a mutual, compatible, and complementary affirmation of the validity of these two models of interpersonal functioning (McCrae & Costa, 1989). The FFM and the PCL-R appear to mesh quite well. The PCL-R is more readily coordinated with the FFM than the DSM-IV ASPD diagnostic criteria, as the PCL-R and the FFM are largely at the same level of personality trait description. In addition, all of the traits of the PCL-R do appear to be contained within the FFM description of normal personality, enriching the understanding of the syndrome of prototypic psychopathy by placing it within the broader context of normal personality functioning and normal personality development. On the other hand, the PCL-R in turn provides a vivid description of an especially problematic and even volatile constellation of personality traits. Identifying this constellation with a single term, psychopathy, is then appropriate and very useful to clinical practice and empirical research.

References

Alterman, A.I., Cacciola, J.S., & Rutherford, M.J. (1993). Reliability of the revised Psychopathy Checklist. *Psychological Assessment, 5*, 442-448.

American Psychiatric Association. (1994). *Diagnostic and statistical manual of mental disorders* (4th ed.). Washington, DC: Author.

Babiak, P. (1995). When psychopaths go to work: A case study of an industrial psychopath. *Applied Psychology: An International Review, 44*, 171-188.

Blackburn, R. (1988). On moral judgments and personality disorders. The myth of psychopathic personality revisited. *British Journal of Psychiatry, 153*, 505-512.

Clark, L.A., & Livesley, W.J. (1994). Two approaches to identifying the dimensions of personality disorder: Convergence on the Five-Factor model. In P.T. Clarkin, J.F., Hull, J.W., Cantor, J., & Sanderson, C. (1993). Borderline personality disorder and personality traits: A comparison of SCID-II BPD and NEO-PI. *Psychological Assessment, 5*, 472-476.

Cleckley, H. (1941). *The mask of sanity.* St. Louis, MO: C.V. Mosby.

Costa. P.T. & Widiger, T.A (Eds.) (1993) *Personality disorders and the five-factor model of personality* (pp. 261-277). Washington, DC: American Psychological Association.

Costa, P.T., & McCrae, R.R. (1990). Personality disorders and the five-factor model of personality. *Journal of Personality Disorders, 4*, 362-371.

Costa, P.T., & McCrae, R.R. (1992). *Revised NEO Personality Inventory (NEO-PI-R) and NEO Five-Factor Inventory (NEO-FFI) professional manual.* Odessa, FL: Psychological Assessment Resources.

Costa, P.T., & McCrae, R.R. (1995). Domains and facets: Hierarchical personality assessment using the Revised NEO Personality Inventory. *Journal of Personality Assessment, 64*, 21-50.

Digman, J.M. (1996). The curious history of the five-factor model. In J.S. Wiggins (Ed.), *The five-factor model of personality. Theoretical perspectives* (pp. 1-20). NY: Guilford.

Dodge, K.A. (1993). Social-cognitive mechanisms in the development of conduct disorder and depression. *Annual Review of Psychology, 44*, 559-584.

Eysenck, H.J. (1994). Normality-abnormality and the three-factor model of personality. In S. Strack & M. Lorr (Eds.), *Differentiating normal and abnormal personality* (pp. 3-25). NY: Spring.

Fowles, D.C., & Missel, K.A. (1994). Electrodermal hyporeactivity, motivation, and psychopathy: Theoretical issues. In D.C. Fowles, P. Sutker, & S.H. Goodman (Eds.), *Experimental personality and psychopathology research* (Vol. 15, pp. 263-283). NY: Springer.

Goldberg, L.R. (1992). The development of markers of the Big Five factor structure. *Psychological Assessment, 4*, 26-42.

Goldberg, L.R. (1993). The structure of phenotypic personality traits. *American Psychologist, 48*, 26-34.

Gorenstein, E.E. (1984). Debating mental illness: Implications for science, medicine, and social policy. *American Psychologist, 39*, 50-56.

Gustafson, S.B., & Ritzer, D.R. (1995). The dark side of normal: A psychopathy-linked pattern called aberrant self-promotion. *European Journal of Personality, 9*, 147-183.

Hare, R.D. (1985). Comparison of procedures for the assessment of psychopathy. *Journal of Consulting and Clinical Psychology, 53*, 7-16.

Hare, R.D. (1991). *The Hare Psychopathy Checklist-Revised*. Toronto: Multi-Health Systems.

Hare, R.D. (1993). *Without conscience: The disturbing world of the psychopaths among us*. NY: Pocket Books.

Hare, R.D., Hart, S.D., & Harpur, T.J. (1991). Psychopathy and the DSM-IV criteria for antisocial personality disorder. *Journal of Abnormal Psychology, 100*, 391-398.

Harkness, A.R. (1992). Fundamental topics in the personality disorders: Candidate trait dimensions from lower regions of the hierarchy. *Psychological Assessment, 4*, 251-259.

Harpur, T.J., Hare, R.D., & Hakstian, A.R. (1989). Two-factor conceptualization of psychopathy: Construct validity and assessment implications. *Psychological Assessment, 1*, 6-17.

Harpur, T.J., Hart, S.D., & Hare, R.D. (1994). The personality of the psychopath. In P.T. Costa & T.A. Widiger (Eds.), *Personality disorders and the five-factor model of personality* (pp. 198-216). Washington, DC: American Psychological Association.

Harris, G.T., Rice, M.E., & Cormier, C. (1991). Psychopathy and violent recidivism. *Law and Human Behavior, 15*, 223-236.

Harris, G.T., Rice, M.E., & Quinsey, V.L. (1994). Psychopathy as a taxon: Evidence that psychopaths are a discrete class. *Journal of Consulting and Clinical Psychology, 62*, 387-397.

Hart, S.D., & Hare, R.D. (1989). Discriminant validity of the Psychopathy Checklist in a forensic psychiatric population. *Psychological Assessment, 1*, 211-218.

Hart, S.D., & Hare, R.D. (1994). Psychopathy and the big 5: Correlations between observers' ratings of normal and pathological personality. *Journal of Personality Disorders, 8*, 32-40.

Kirmayer, L.J. (1994). Is the concept of mental disorder culturally relative? In S.A. Kirk & S.D. Einbinder (Eds.), *Controversial issues in mental health* (pp. 2-9). Boston: Allyn & Bacon.

Kochanska, G. (1991). Socialization and temperament in the development of guilt and conscience. *Child Development, 62*, 1379-1392.

Levenson, M., Kiehl, K.A., & Fitzpatric, C.M. (1995). Assessing psychopathic attributes in a non-institutionalized population. *Journal of Personality and Social Psychology, 68*, 151-158.

Lilienfeld, S.O. (1994). Conceptual problems in the assessment of psychopathy. *Clinical Psychology Review, 14*, 17-38.

Lilienfeld, S.O., & Marino, L. (1995). Mental disorder as a Roschian concept: A critique of Wakefield's "harmful dysfunction" analysis. *Journal of Abnormal Psychology, 104*, 411-420.

Livesley, W.J., Jang, K.L., Jackson, D.N., & Vernon, P.A. (1993). Genetic and environmental contributions to dimensions of personality disorder. *American Journal of Psychiatry, 150*, 1826-1831.

Luntz, B.K., & Widom, C.S. (1994). Antisocial personality disorder in abused and neglected children grown up. *American Journal of Psychiatry, 151*, 670-674.

Lykken, D.T. (1995). *The antisocial personalities*. Hillsdale, NJ: Lawrence Erlbaum.

Marshall, W.L., Hudson, S.M., Jones, R., & Fernandez, Y.M. (1995). Empathy in sex offenders. *Clinical Psychology Review, 15*, 99-113.

McCrae, R.R., & Costa, P.T. (1989). The structure of interpersonal traits: Wiggins' circumplex and the Five-Factor Model. *Journal of Personality and Social Psychology, 56*, 586-595.

McCrae, R.R., & Costa, P.T. (1990). *Personality in adulthood*. NY: Guilford.

Millon, T. (1981). *Disorders of personality. DSM-III: axis II*. NY: Wiley.

Millon, T. (1983). *Millon Clinical Multiaxial Inventory manual* (2nd ed.). Minneapolis, MN: National Computer Systems.

Millon, T. (1987). *Manual for the MCMI-II* (3rd ed.). Minneapolis, MN: National Computer Systems.

Neisser, U., Boodoo, G., Bouchard, T.J., Boykin, A.W., Brody, N., Ceci, S., Halpern, D.F., Loehlin, J.C., Perloff, R., Sternberg, R.J., & Urbina, S. (1996). Intelligence: Knowns and unknowns. *American Psychologist, 51*, 77-101.

Newman, J.P., Kosson, D.S., & Patterson, C.M. (1992). Delay of gratification in psychopathic and non-psychopathic offenders. *Journal of Abnormal Psychology, 101*, 630-636.

Patrick, C.J. (1994). Emotion and psychopathy: Startling new insights. *Psychophysiology, 31*, 415-428.

Popper, C.W., & Steingard, R.J. (1994). Disorders usually first diagnosed in infancy, childhood, or adolescence. In R.E. Hales, S.C. Yudofsky, & J.A. Talbott (Eds.), *Textbook of psychiatry* (2nd ed., pp. 729-832). Washington, DC: American Psychiatric Press.

Revelle, W. (1995). Personality processes. *Annual Review of Psychology, 46*, 295-328.

Robins, L.N. (1966). *Deviant children grown up*. Baltimore, MD: Williams & Wilkins.

Robins, L.N., Tipp, J., & Przybeck, T. (1991). Antisocial personality. In L.N. Robins & D.A. Regier (Eds.), *Psychiatric disorders in America. The epidemiologic catchment area study* (pp. 258-290). NY: The Free Press.

Saucier, G., & Goldberg, L.R. (1996). The language of personality: Lexical perspectives on the five-factor model. In J.S. Wiggins (Ed.), *The five-factor model of personality. Theoretical perspectives* (pp. 21-50). NY: Guilford.

Sedgwick, P. (1982). *Psycho politics*. NY: Harper & Row.

Serin, R.C., Peters, R.D., & Barbaree, H.E. (1990). Predictors of psychopathy and release outcome in a criminal population. *Psychological Assessment, 2*, 419-422.

Schroeder, M.L., Wormworth, J.A., & Livesley, W.J. (1992). Dimensions of personality disorder and their relationships to the Big Five dimensions of personality. *Psychological Assessment, 4*, 47-53.

Soldz, S., Budman, S., Demby, A., & Merry, J. (1993). Representation of personality disorders in circumplex and Five-Factor space: Explorations with a clinical sample. *Psychological Assessment, 5*, 41-52.

Spitzer, R.L., Endicott, J., & Robins, E. (1975). Clinical criteria for psychiatric diagnosis and DSM-III. *American Journal of Psychiatry, 132*, 1187-1192.

Sutker, P.B., Bugg, F., & West, J.A. (1993). Antisocial personality disorder. In P.B. Sutker & H. Adams (Eds.), *Comprehensive handbook of psychopathology* (2nd ed., pp. 337-369). New York: Plenum.

Trapnell, P.D., & Wiggins, J.S. (1990). Extension of the Interpersonal Adjective Scales to include the Big Five dimensions of personality. *Journal of Personality and Social Psychology, 59*, 781-790.

Trull, T.J. (1992). DSM-III-R personality disorders and the Five Factor Model of personality: An empirical comparison. *Journal of Abnormal Psychology, 101*, 553-560.

Trull, T.J., Useda, J.D., Costa, P.T., & McCrae, R.R. (1995). Comparison of the MMPI-2 Personality Psychopathology Five (PSY-5), the NEO-PI, and the NEO-PI-R. *Psychological Assessment, 7*, 508-516.

Wakefield, J.C. (1992a). The concept of mental disorder. On the boundary between biological facts and social values. *American Psychologist, 47*, 373-388.

Wakefield, J.C. (1992b). Disorder as harmful dysfunction: A conceptual critique of DSM-III-R's definition of mental disorder. *Psychological Review, 99*, 232-247.

Widiger, T.A. (1993). The DSM-III-R categorical personality disorder diagnoses: A critique and an alternative. *Psychological Inquiry, 4*, 75-90.

Widiger, T.A., & Corbitt, E.M. (1994). Normal versus abnormal personality from the perspective of the DSM. In S. Strack & M. Lorr (Eds.), *Differentiating normal and abnormal personality* (pp. 158-175). NY: Springer.

Widiger, T.A., & Corbitt, E.M. (1995). Antisocial personality disorder. In W.J. Livesley (Ed.), *The DSM-IV personality disorders* (pp. 103-126). NY: Guilford.

Widiger, T.A., & Costa, P.T. (1994). Personality and personality disorders. *Journal of Abnormal Psychology, 103*, 78-91.

Widiger, T.A., & Hicklin, J. (1995). Antisocial personality disorder. In P. Wilner (Ed.), *Psychiatry* (Chapt. 23, pp. 1-13). Philadelphia, PA: J.B. Lippincott.

Widiger, T.A., & Trull, T.J. (1991). Diagnosis and clinical assessment. *Annual Review of Psychology, 42*, 109-133.

Widiger, T.A., Trull, T.J., Clarkin, J.F., Sanderson, C., & Costa, P.T. (1994). A description of the DSM-III-R and DSM-IV personality disorders with the five-factor model of personality. In P.T. Costa & T.A. Widiger (Eds.), *Personality disorders and the five-factor model of personality* (pp. 41-56). Washington, DC: American Psychological Association.

Wiggins, J.S., & Pincus, H.A. (1989). Conceptions of personality disorder and dimensions of personality. *Psychological Assessment, 1*, 305-316.

Wiggins, J.S., & Pincus, H.A. (1992). Personality: Structure and assessment. *Annual Review of Psychology, 43*, 473-504.

Wilson, J. Q., & Herrnstein, R. J. (1985). *Crime and human nature.* (1st ed.). New York: Simon & Schuster.

Williamson, S.W., Harpur, T.J., & Hare, R.D. (1991). Abnormal processing of affective words by psychopaths. *Psychophysiology, 28*, 260-273.

Wulach, J.S. (1983). Diagnosing the DSM-III antisocial personality disorder. *Professional Psychology: Research and Practice, 14*, 330-340.

Yeung, A.S., Lyons, M.J., Waternaux, C.M., Faraone, S.V., & Tsuang, M.T. (1993). The relationship between DSM-III personality disorders and the five-factor model of personality. *Comprehensive Psychiatry, 34*, 227-234.

THE PHENOTYPIC AND GENOTYPIC STRUCTURE OF PSYCHOPATHIC TRAITS

W. JOHN LIVESLEY
Department of Psychiatry
University of British Columbia
Vancouver, Canada.

INTRODUCTION

Considerable progress has been made in recent years in delineating the concept of psychopathy, the structure of psychopathic traits, and associated psychopathology. Psychopathy has also been shown to be a useful clinical and forensic concept. This progress owes much to the development of a reliable assessment procedure — the Psychopathy Checklist (PCL-R; Hare, 1991), that is easily administered in a variety of settings. The evidence also suggests that psychopathy as assessed using the PCL-R is not an homogeneous entity but consists of two components, an interpersonal component characterized by such traits as disregard for others, lack of empathy, and tendencies toward grandiosity, and a behavioral component involving antisocial behaviors (Harpur, Hakstian, & Hare, 1988).

There are two aspects to research on psychopathy that are especially interesting to psychiatric classification. First, the two component structure provides a different representation of the domain of antisocial and psychopathic psychopathology from that proposed by psychiatric classifications such as the DSM-IV. The concept of antisocial personality disorder in the DSM-IV makes greater reference to the interpersonal pathology described by the PCL-R than did the DSM-III-R (Widiger & Corbitt, 1995). Nevertheless, it is more oriented toward the behavioral component of the PCL-R. Consequently the two concepts overlap but they do not assess the same construct.

Second, the PCL-R and many of the studies contributing to the progress in understanding psychopathy, appear to be based on the assumption that psychopathy is a discrete category of psychopathology. This assumption justifies the typical research design used in many studies; the comparison of a group of psychopathic individuals with a group of normal subjects. Although this methodology has been productive, the approach conflicts with the conclusions of contemporary research on the structure of personality disorder. Almost without exception, investigations have failed to identify discrete categories of disorder, or a distinct boundary between normal and abnormal personality functioning (Livesley, Schroeder, Jackson, & Jang, 1994; Widiger, 1993). Instead, overlap among diagnoses of personality disorder is substantial (Widiger, Frances, Harris, Jacobsberg, Fyer, Manning, 1991) and personality disorder merges with normality. Difficulty in establishing discontinuity between diagnoses is not specific to personality disorders; it is also observed in many mental state disorders (Kendell, 1975; Kendell & Brocklington,1980).

D.J. Cooke et al. (eds.), Psychopathy: Theory, Research and Implications for Society, 69–79.
© 1998 *Kluwer Academic Publishers. Printed in the Netherlands.*

These conclusions raise questions about the generalizability of the two factor structure of psychopathic traits when these traits are measured using different methods of measurement and when they are assessed in the context of traits selected to assess all forms of personality disorder. They also raise questions about the extent to which differences between psychopathic and normal subjects are specific to psychopathy. The studies to be described address three questions related to these issues: (i) whether the two factor structure of psychopathy generalizes across different methods of measurement; (ii) whether psychopathy and the two component structure emerges when psychopathic traits are examined in the context of a comprehensive list of traits delineating all forms of personality disorder; and (iii) whether the phenotypic structure of psychopathy is associated with a similar genotypic structure.

These studies adopted a "bottom-up approach" to identifying the structure of personality disorder. A large pool of traits, selected to represent the overall domain of personality disorder, was reduced using successive multivariate statistical procedures to progressively fewer higher order factors. This contrasts with the "top-down" approach to studies of the structure of psychopathy. With this approach, a general definition of psychopathy based on Cleckley's (1941) formulations was used to define the specific traits that characterize the condition. The hypothetical structure to these traits was then confirmed statistically.

DELINEATING PERSONALITY DISORDER DIAGNOSES

The first step in this research was to develop systematic descriptions of the various forms of personality disorder, including psychopathy and antisocial personality disorder. A four stage process was used (Livesley, 1986, 1987): 1) identification of the descriptive features of each diagnosis listed in DSM-III through content analysis of the literature, 2) identification of the highly prototypical features of each diagnosis by using the judgments of random panels of psychiatrists, 3) development of definitions of each diagnosis based on highly prototypical features, and 4) preliminary confirmation of the resulting definitions by a further sampling of psychiatric opinion.

An extensive literature was content analyzed to ensure that the preliminary list of descriptive features included all important features. This resulted in a large pool of items with as many as fifty traits and trait terms used to describe a given diagnoses. Ratings of the prototypicality of these items by psychiatrists were highly reliable (Livesley, 1986). Items were reduced to fewer trait dimensions using a combination of expert judgement and rational judgements. A further sampling of expert opinion confirmed that the trait dimensions provided a reliable description of the features of personality disorder (Livesley, 1987). These procedures resulted in a list of 100 traits. Self report scales were developed to assess these traits (Livesley, Jackson, & Schroeder, 1989).

The next step was to evaluate the structure underlying these traits using multivariate statistical procedures. These were applied to subsets of the 100 traits describing individual diagnoses including antisocial personality disorder, to determine the structure of each diagnosis, and to all 100 traits to determine the structure underlying the overall domain.

The general strategy adopted in these studies was the to evaluate factorial structure in two samples, a clinical sample and a general population sample. The purpose for this procedure this was to evaluate factor stability. As Eysenck (1987) pointed out, evidence that the factor structure is similar in samples that differ with regard to the presence of personality disorder provides strong support as a dimensional as opposed to categorical representation of personality disorder.

PHENOTYPIC STRUCTURE

Phenotypic Structure of Psychopathic and Antisocial Traits

Content analysis of the clinical literature describing antisocial and psychopathic personality disorders yielded an extensive list of descriptive features that were organized on the basis of expert judgement and rational considerations into 13 trait and behavioral dimensions: juvenile antisocial behavior, egocentrism, exploitation, externalization, failure to follow social norms, impulsivity, interpersonality irresponsibility, interpersonality lability, lack of affect, remorselessness, sadism, unstable employment history, and contemptuousness. Self report scales developed to assess these traits were administered to general population and clinical samples (Livesley & Schroeder, 1991). The general population sample consisted of 274 volunteers (125 men, 149 women, mean age 29.7 years; SD, 11.2 years) from diverse groups, including hospital and university employees, university students, members of community organizations, and other members of the general population. The clinical sample consisted of 133 patients (49 men, 84 women; mean age 33.6 years; SD, 7.7 years) with a primary diagnosis of personality disorder. Patients who met the criteria for a major Axis I disorder, such as schizophrenia, major mood disorder, delusional disorder, or organic disorder were excluded.

Data from the two groups were examined separately using unweighed least squares factor analysis with varimax rotation. Factor analysis of the 13x13 correlation matrix yielded two eigenvalues greater than unity in both the general population and clinical samples, accounting for 52.7% and 44.7% of the variance respectively. Similarity of factor structure in the two samples was determined by computing congruence coefficient. A value of .97 was obtained for factor 1 and .91 for factor 2. These values indicate that the factors obtained from the two samples are very similar.

The results of these analyses are shown in Table 1. Scales salient on the first factor describe tendencies to show little empathy for other people, to be unconcerned about the welfare of others, to be contemptuous of others, and to show little regret about the effect the harm done to others. The factor was labelled callousness to describe the general tendency to disregard others. This pattern shows a closer general resemblance to the concept of psychopathy than to antisocial personality disorder and it is remarkably similarity to the interpersonal factor 1 extracted by Hare and colleagues from PCL-R ratings (Harpur et al, 1988).

The second factor was labeled conduct problems to describe the lack of social conformity as indicated by the angry, impulsive, and antisocial behaviors that formed the salient loadings. The factor appears to correspond to the second factor described by Hare and colleagues.

TABLE 1. Factor loadings for thirteen behavioral dimensions

	Factor 1		Factor 2	
Dimension	General Population Sample	Clinical Sample	General Population Sample	Clinical Sample
Lack of Empathy	76	63	8	14
Contemptuousness	73	78	37	32
Interpersonal irresponsibility	71	57	18	21
Egocentrism	69	57	34	31
Exploitation	68	67	49	28
Sadism	65	65	37	41
Remorselessness	59	70	22	17
Externalization	56	36	36	38
Impulsivity	14	17	66	57
Juvenile antisocial	16	30	63	41
Unstable employment history	26	11	60	59
Failure to adopt social norms	45	54	58	44
Interpersonal lability	51	31	51	65
Percentage of total variance	32.4%	28.2%	20.3%	16.5%

Phenotypic Structure Underlying the Domain of Personality Disorder

Having identified a two component structure to psychopathic and antisocial traits that converges with the two-factor structure underlying the Psychopathy Checklist, the next step was to evaluate the stability of this structure when the traits delineating psychopathy are examined in the context of traits describing all forms of personality disorder. The same procedure was used, namely administration of self report scales to assess all 100 traits to general population and clinical samples (Livesley, Jackson, & Schroeder, 1992). The general population sample was the same as that used in the previous analysis (N = 274). A larger clinical sample of 158 subjects was used (95 women, 63 men; age mean = 32.4 years; SD = 7.9). As in the previous study, patients had a primary diagnosis of personality disorder based on clinical interviews. All DSM-III-R Axis II diagnoses were represented in the sample.

Data analysis began by examining the descriptive properties of the 100 scales in the two samples. Inspection of t-tests comparing the group means revealed, not surprisingly, a large number of statistically significant differences. The distribution of scores on all scales were examined for evidence of discontinuity. On all scales considerable overlap was observed in the distribution of the two samples. Evidence of bimodality was not obtained.

A question of interest was whether the clinical and general population samples yielded important differences in structure in the principle component loadings and whether the two features of psychopathy are identified within the larger correlational matrix. Separate analyses were performed for the clinical and non-clinical samples. Decisions about the number of factors to retain for rotation and inspection were based upon several criteria, including inspection of eigenvalues, the Scree test, simple structure properties, and interpretability of the rotated solution. In both samples, a 15 component solution was evaluated, accounting for 74.4% and 75.1% of the variance in the clinical and general population data, respectively. Similarity in the two component patterns was determined by treating the varimax rotated solution of the clinical data as the target for an orthogonal Procrustes rotation (Schonemann, 1966). The general population pattern matrix was rotated to this target. Similarity of the rotated components was evaluated by computing factor congruence coefficients. The results indicated substantial similarity between the two solutions.

Because of the degree of similarity observed between the clinical and general population factor structures, the data from the two samples were combined and evaluated by factor analysis. Again, 15 components were retained for rotation and inspection. These accounted for 71.6% of the variance. Of particular interest, with regard to the structure of psychopathy, was the fact that specific factors were identified that resemble the two components of the PCL-R. The labels callousness and conduct problems were retained. Scales with salient loadings on callousness were: Lack of Empathy, 0.61; Interpersonal Responsibility, 0.61; and Compulsive Care-Giving, -0.76. The component labeled conduct problems was defined by the following scales: Juvenile Antisocial Behavior, 0.77; Addictive Behaviors, 0.67; Low School Achievement, 0.55; Failure to Adopt Social Norms, 0.45; Interpersonal Violence, 0.42; and Self Damaging Acts, 0.41.

Additional factors were identified describing other behaviors associated with psychopathy and antisocial behavior, namely stimulus seeking and narcissism. Thus, the two factor structure of psychopathy is sufficiently robust to emerge from a matrix of correlations among all traits delineating personality disorder. Given the size of the data matrix, this degree of convergence with previous structure is remarkable and lends considerable support to the two component description of psychopathy.

The results of these analyses were used to define 18 basic dimensions of personality disorder. A self report inventory, the Dimensional Assessment of Personality Pathology (DAPP-BQ), was developed to assess these 18 traits (Livesley & Jackson, in press). The traits assessed using this instrument are: Affective Lability, Anxiousness, Callousness, Cognitive Distortion, Compulsivity, Conduct Problems, Identity Problems, Intimacy Problems, Narcissism, Oppositionality, Rejection, Suspiciousness, Social Avoidance, and Submissiveness.

Higher Order Phenotypic Structure

The higher order structure underlying the 18 dimensions was evaluated in a two new samples: a general population sample of 942 subjects and a clinical sample of 650 patients with a primary diagnosis of personality disorders (Livesley, Jang, & Vernon, 1995). The same data analytic strategy was used as previously. Data from the two samples were examined separately using principal components analysis. In both cases, a four factor solution was optimal. This accounted for 68.8% and 66.7% of the variance in the clinical and general population samples, respectively. Examination of the pattern matrices indicated high similarity in the factor structure in both samples. The four factors were labeled: Affective Reactivity, Antagonism, Inhibition, and Compulsivity.

The first factor was defined by a large number of scales:

TABLE 2. Component loadings on first component

	Clinical	General Population
Anxiousness	85	89
Identity Problems	81	78
Submissiveness	78	79
Social Avoidance	76	71
Affective Instability	69	76
Cognitive Distortion	69	77
Insecure Attachment	69	75
Oppositionality	66	66
Self-Harm	46	54
Suspiciousness	57	52
Narcissism	45	57

This factor appears to be a general factor of personality pathology that underlies many of the categorical diagnoses of DSM-IV. The existence of this factor presumably accounts for the substantial overlap noted among categories of personality disorder. The second component shows remarkable similarity to psychopathy. We labeled it Antagonism to avoid premature conclusions of identity between the two structures. Nevertheless, salient loadings are similar to the construct described by Cleckley and measured by the PCL-R:

TABLE 3. Component loadings traits on second component

	Clinical	General Population
Callousness	78	76
Rejection	76	81
Stimulus Seeking	74	72
Conduct Problems	73	73
Narcissism	49	51
Suspiciousness	47	57
Affective Lability	41	--

The third component showed some similarity to the general domain of introversion. The term Inhibition was adopted to capture the quality of being unable to express feelings or tolerate closeness and intimacy. The scales with salient loadings were: restricted expression, intimacy problems, and social avoidance. The fourth component had a single salient loading, compulsivity, in both samples. It is interesting to note the loadings of stimulus seeking and narcissism on Antagonism. Stimulus seeking includes: impulsivity and sensation seeking. The pattern of salient loadings show remarkable convergence with the content of the PCL-R.

GENOTYPIC STRUCTURE

The final question addressed in these studies was whether the phenotypic structure of psychopathy is matched by a corresponding genotypic structure. This question was addressed by examining the genetic and environmental etiology of psychopathic traits using a twin study approach. This involved administering the DAPP-BQ to a sample of 483 twin pairs consisting of 236 MZ twin pairs (165 sister pairs and 71 brother pairs; mean age 30.3 years, SD = 11.5 years, range = 16-84 years) and 247 DZ twin pairs (131 sister pairs, 37 brother pairs, 79 sister-brother pairs; mean age = 30.4 years, SD = 10.6 years, range = 16-68 years) (Jang, Livesley, Vernon, & Jackson, in press). This was a volunteer sample obtained by advertising widely throughout the lower mainland of British Columbia. Zygosity was determined through a questionnaire designed by Nicholls and Bilbro (1966). This method has a reported accuracy of 95% when compared to the results of zygosity determined by red blood cell polymorphism (Kasriel & Eaves, 1976).

Prior to conducting behavior genetic analyses, the data were transformed were necessary to obtain adequate symmetry. The possible biasing effects of age and gender were corrected by computing the standardized residual scores from the simultaneous multiple regression of each of the 18 dimensions on age and gender as suggested by McGue and Bouchard (1984). A simple additive genetic model was used to estimate the proportion of variance of each DAPP dimension attributable to additive genetic factors, shared environmental factors, and unique environmental factors.

Heritability estimates for the DAPP-BQ scales related to psychopathy were as follows: Callousness, 0.56; Conduct Problems, 0.56; Narcissism, 0.53; Rejection, 0.35; Stimulus Seeking, 0.40; and Suspiciousness, 0.40.

These results are similar to those obtained for the other DAPP dimensions. They are also consistent with the heritability estimates of normal personality traits which are typically in the 40-60% range, and with other reports on the genetic factors associated with antisocial behaviors (Cloninger & Gottesman, 1987). Environmental affects were largely confined to unique factors, that is, factors that are specific to one twin, such as differential treatment by parents, teachers, or peers. Common environmental effects contributed little variance. These effects describe factors that are common to both twins in a given family, for example, social class or family income. Again these results are similar to those reported for normal personality traits.

The next step was to determine the genetic structure underlying the 18 dimensions using genetic factor analysis. Genetic (as opposed to phenotypic) correlations were computed according to the method described by Crawford & Defries, (1978). Principal components analysis on the resulting matrix yielded a four factor structure that bears strong correspondence to the high order phenotypic structure.

TABLE 4. Loadings on factor one and factor two

Factor I	
Anxiousness	92
Identity Problems	74
Self-Harm	74
Affective Instability	73
Oppositionality	73
Cognitive Distortion	68
Insecure Attachment	62
Narcissism	57
Social Avoidance	58
Conduct Problems	40
Factor II	
Callousness	82
Rejection	82
Stimulus Seeking	73
Suspiciousness	57
Narcissism	52
Conduct Problems	49

The third and fourth factors also resemble those extracted from the phenotypic data. These results suggest that the traits delineating personality disorder are organized similarly at phenotypic and genotypic levels. They also indicate a clear genetic factor of antagonism or psychopathy that is distinct from other components of personality disorder.

Together, the analyses of phenotypic and genotypic structure of personality disorders provides additional support for a dimensional model. The possibility remains, however, that the etiology of normal range and extreme range scores indicative of psychopathy is different. Evidence of genetic discontinuity would be indicated if the heritability of extreme range scores was significantly different from the heritability of scores in the normal range. This possibility can be investigated using a multiple regression technique developed by DeFries & Fulker (1985, 1988; Plomin, 1991). The method uses continuously distributed data from general population twin studies to test the magnitude of genetic influence of scores in the extreme range. The approach involves identifying a sample of monozygotic (MZ) and dizygotic (DZ) twins from a general population twin sample in which one member of each pair has an extreme score on a continuous measure and the unaffected co-twin has a score in the normal range. If the extreme scores have a heritable basis, the mean score of the unaffected MZ co-twins will be more extreme than the mean score of the unaffected DZ co-twins. The DeFries-Fulkner method uses a multiple regression approach to estimate of the heritability of extreme scores, referred to as group heritability (h^2_g).

For this study a sample of twins with at least one member of each pair having an extreme score on a DAPP-BQ scale was selected from a general population volunteer sample of 692 twin pairs (Jang, Livesley, & Vernon, 1996). The mean score on each DAPP scale from an independent sample of patients with a primary diagnosis of personality disorder attending psychiatric outpatient clinics (males = 235, females = 416) was used to define the extreme scores. The patient means typically fall about 1 to 1.5 standard deviations above the means for the general population. The results showed that no significant genetic etiology was found for extreme scores on: Submissiveness, Cognitive Distortion, Stimulus Seeking, Restricted Expression, Oppositionality, Conduct Problems, Social Avoidance, and Self-Harm. For these dimensions, extreme scores are clearly caused largely by environmental influences. For the other scales, including Callousness, the results were less conclusive.

DISCUSSION

The observed convergence between the structure underlying the PCL-R and that emerging from these studies is especially striking because the two instruments used different measurement methods, and they were developed independently using very different ways. This degree of convergence across methods and studies testifies to the robustness of the concept of psychopathy. The structure of antisocial or psychopathic personality emerging from both approaches incorporates the interpersonal component that is part of traditional descriptions of psychopathy and antisocial behaviors that form the major component of DSM-III-R and DSM-IV criteria sets. Given these results, and the well documented differences in the network of relationships of the two components, it is difficult to justify the emphasis on antisocial behaviors in the DSM-IV criteria set.

Although supporting the component structure of psychopathy these results do not lend strong support to the concept of psychopathy as a discrete category of psychopathology. The stability of factor structure across clinical and non-clinical samples is also a robust finding that is consistent with a dimensional model. The genetic analyses were less conclusive. Evidence of genetic discontinuity was not observed for the Conduct Problems component of psychopathy but the results were less clear for Callousness. Other studies using a different methodology have, however, reported evidence of discontinuity. Harris, Rice, and Quinsey (1994) applied taxometric analyses to variables assessed by the PCL-R and variables reflecting antisocial childhood behaviors, adult criminality, and criminal recidivism and found evidence of discontinuity. Thus, the important issue of the status of psychopathy as a taxon remains unclear.

References

Cleckley H. (1941) *The Mask of Sanity*. St. Louis, MO: Mosby, 1941.

Cloninger, C.R., & Gottesman, I.L. (1987) Genetic and environmental factors in antisocial behaviors. In: Mednick, S.A., Moffit, T.E., Stack, S.A. (eds). *The Causes of Crime: New Biological Approaches*. New York: Cambridge University Press.

DeFries, J.C., & Fulker, D.W. (1985) Multiple regression analysis of twin data. *Behavior Genetics*, *15*: 467-473.

Crawford, C.B., & DeFries, J.C. (1978) Factor analysis of genetic and environmental correlation matrices. *Multivariate Behavioral Research,13*, 297-318.

DeFries, J.C., & Fulker, D.W. (1988) Multiple regression analysis of twin data: Etiology of deviant scores versus individual differences. *Acta Geneticae Medicae et Gemellologiae, 37,* 205-216.

Eysenck, H.J. (1987) The definition of personality disorders and the criteria appropriate to their definition. *Journal of Personality Disorders, 1,* 211-219.

Hare, R.D. (1991) *Manual for the Hare Psychopathy Checklist -- Revised.* Toronto; MultiHealth Systems.

Harpur, T.J., Hakstian, A.R., & Hare, R.D. (1988) Factor structure of the Psychopathy Checklist. *Journal of Consulting and Clinical Psychology, 56,* 741-747.

Harris, G.T., Rice, M.E., & Quinsey, V.L. (1994) Psychopathy as a taxon: Evidence that psychopaths are a discrete class. *Journal of Consulting and Clinical Psychology, 62,* 387-397.

Jang, K.L., Livesley, W.J., & Vernon, A.P. (1996) *The interface of normal and abnormal behavior: A DF analysis of personality.* Paper presented at the Eighth European Congress on Personality, Ghent.

Kasriel, J., & Eaves, L.J., (1976) The zygosity of twins: further evidence on the agreement between diagnosis by blood groups and written questionnaires. *J Biosocial Science 8,* 263-266.

Kendell, R.E. (1975) *The Role of Diagnosis in Psychiatry.* Oxford: Blackwell.

Kendell, R.E., & Brocklington, I.F. (1980) The identification of disease entities and the relationship between schizophrenia and affective psychoses. *British Journal of Psychiatry, 137,* 324-331.

Livesley, W.J., (1986) Trait and behavioral prototypes of personality disorder. *American Journal of Psychiatry, 143,* 728-732.

Livesley, W.J., (1987) A systematic approach to the delineation of personality disorders. *American Journal of Psychiatry, 144,* 772-777.

Livesley, W.J. & Jackson, D.N. (in press) *Dimensional assessment of personality disorder (DAPP-BQ).* Port Huron, Michigan: Sigma Publications.

Livesley, W.J., Jackson, D.N., & Schroeder, M.L. (1989) A study factorial structure of personality pathology. *Journal of Personality Disorders, 3,* 292-306.

Livesley, W.J., Jackson, D.N., & Schroeder, M.L., (1992) Factorial structure of traits delineating personality disorders in clinical and general population samples. *Journal of Abnormal Psychology, 101,* 432-440.

Livesley, W.J., Jang, K.L., & Vernon, P.A., (1995) *The phenotypic and genotypic structure of personality disorder.* Paper presented at the International Conference on Personality and Individual Differences, Warsaw.

Livesley, W.J., Jang, K.L., Vernon, P.A., & Jackson, D.N., (in press) The heritability of personality disorder traits: A twin study. *Acta Psychiatrica Scandinavica.*

Livesley, W.J., Schroeder, M.L., (1991) Dimensions of personality disorder; The DSM-III-R cluster B diagnosis. *Journal of Nervous and Mental Disease, 179,* 320-328.

Livesley, W.J., Schroeder, M.L., Jackson, D.N., & Jang, K.L., (1994) Categorical distinctions in the study of personality disorder: Implications for classification. *Journal of Abnormal Psychology 103,* 617.

McGue, M., & Bouchard, T.J.Jr., (1984) Adjustment of twin data for the effects of age and sex. *Behavior Genetics, 14,* 325-343.

Nichols, R.C., & Bilbro, W.C.Jr. (1966) The diagnosis of twin zygosity. *Acta Geneticae Medicae et Gemellologiae (Roma), 16,* 265-275.

Plomin, R. (1991) Genetic risk and psychosocial disorders: Links between the normal and abnormal. In: Rutter, M. & Cesaer, P. (eds). *Biological Risk Factors for Psychosocial Disorders.* London: Cambridge.

Schonemann, P.H., (1966) A generalized solution of the orthogonal Procrustes problem. *Psychometrika, 31*, 1-10.

Widiger, T.A. (1993) The DSM-III-R categorical personality disorder diagnoses: The critique and an alternative. *Psychological Inquiry, 4*, 75-90.

Widiger, T.A., & Corbitt, E.M., (1995) Antisocial personality disorder. In: Livesley, W.J. (ed). *The DSM-IV personality disorders*. New York, Guilford.

Widiger, T.A., Frances, A.J., Harris, M., Jacobsberg, L., Fyer, M., & Manning, D., (1991) Comorbidity among Axis II disorders. In: Oldham J (ed). *Personality Disorders: New Perspectives on Diagnostic Validity* (page 163-194). Washington, DC; American Psychiatric Press.

PSYCHOPATHIC BEHAVIOR: AN INFORMATION PROCESSING PERSPECTIVE

JOSEPH P. NEWMAN
Department of Psychology
University of Wisconsin
Madison, USA.

In contrast to syndromes such as schizophrenia, depression, and the various anxiety disorders in which the contribution of some disordered psychological process is taken for granted, there is considerable skepticism regarding the existence of psychopathology in psychopaths. When a person has difficulty regulating thoughts or feelings we find it natural to attribute the problem to psychopathology but, when it is a person's behavior that is poorly regulated, we are more inclined to attribute the problem to inadequate motivation or maliciousness. In other words, we find it plausible that thoughts and feelings may escape voluntary control, but we seem to have trouble thinking about behavior in the same way.

I believe that our disinclination to conceptualize psychopathy as a psychological deficit as opposed to an inherently antisocial condition is a major factor impeding progress in the understanding and treatment of this disorder. In this vein, it is important to recognize that psychopaths not only engage in antisocial behavior that is hurtful to others, much of their behavior is self-defeating and results in considerable personal suffering. Though it may be difficult to evoke sympathy for adult psychopaths with a long history of callous, exploitative behavior, a developmental perspective suggests an alternative view. If, as I believe, children at risk for psychopathy suffer from an information processing deficit that interferes with effective self-regulation, then our failure to appreciate the existence of this problem and our consequent reactions to the child's behavior are likely to be compounding their risk.

The principal goal of this chapter is to articulate an information processing deficiency that might plausibly account for the psychopath's chronic failures of self-regulation. Specifically, I propose that psychopaths have a cognitive processing deficiency that hampers their ability to accommodate the meaning of contextual cues while they are engaged in the active organization and implementation of goal-directed behavior. To advance this hypothesis, I will (a) briefly discuss the relation between psychopathy and cognitive processing deficiencies; (b) examine clinical portrayals of the psychopath that support the plausibility of an information processing deficiency; (c) present experimental evidence that substantiates and clarifies the nature of the deficiency; and (d) examine the relation between the proposed information processing deficit and other relevant hypotheses and evidence concerning psychopaths' failure to make use of contextual cues.

D.J. Cooke et al. (eds.), Psychopathy: Theory, Research and Implications for Society, 81–104.
© *1998 Kluwer Academic Publishers. Printed in the Netherlands.*

BACKGROUND

Historically, the term *"psychopathy"* has been used to describe individuals who display adequate intellectual functioning but who appear to have a profound affective or inhibitory defect that impairs their ability to conduct themselves properly. Pritchard, for instance stated that in psychopaths *"the power of self-government is lost or greatly impaired"* (see Millon, 1981). In his classic book *"The Mask of Sanity"* which provides the foundation for the current concept of psychopathy, Cleckley (1976) clearly de-emphasized antisocial motivation. According to Cleckley, psychopaths are not especially disposed to violence or other strong urges but, given an urge to respond, psychopaths are especially unlikely to restrain it. Whereas antisocial behavior may be the most salient and clinically meaningful characteristic of psychopathy, the psychopath's lack of restraint may be the most integral. Before discussing the evidence for a cognitive processing deficiency in psychopathy, I want to clarify my use of this expression. Kendall and Dobson's (1993) draw a distinction between cognitive deficiencies and distortions: *"**Deficiencies** refer to the lack of certain forms of thinking (e.g., the absence of information processing where it would be beneficial), whereas **distortions** refer to active but dysfunctional thinking processes"* (p. 10).

The focus of this chapter is on cognitive deficiencies rather than cognitive distortions. Readers are referred to Millon (1981), Serin and Kuriychuk (1994) and Widom (1976) for information on cognitive distortions in psychopaths. To date, investigators have paid relatively little attention to cognitive deficits in psychopathy. It seems likely that the neglect of cognitive factors relates, in part, to early descriptions of psychopathy which de-emphasized and even ruled out thought disorder. Indeed, Pinel (1801) used the term ***Manie sans delire*** to highlight this group's intact reasoning. Cleckley (1976) concluded that in the psychopath:

"logical thought processes may be seen in perfect operation no matter how they are stimulated or treated under experimental conditions... All judgments of value and emotional appraisals are sane and appropriate when the psychopath is tested in verbal examinations" (p. 369).

In lieu of cognitive explanations, researchers focused on the concept *"arousal"* and motivational explanations for psychopathy. In retrospect, however, it is interesting to contemplate the extent to which this emphasis on motivational as opposed to cognitive explanations was driven by the nature of psychopathy versus the theoretical concepts and laboratory techniques that were available to researchers at the time the theories were proposed. For example, in his classic paper setting out the *"low-fear hypothesis"*, Lykken (1957) labeled Cleckley's characterization of the psychopath too *"subjective and unreliable"* to be useful and recommended instead *"expressing this putative defect...in terms of the anxiety construct of experimental psychology"* (p. 6). Lykken's decision to substitute low fear/anxiety for Cleckley's more abstruse characterization of the problem proved to be a fruitful one which, as he predicted, stimulated a good deal of research. An important consequence of this decision, however, was that Lykken (1995) and others attributed the symptoms of psychopathy to insufficient motivation as opposed to the cognitive-affective deficiency proposed by Cleckley (1976).

Of course, a lot has changed in the 40 years since Lykken first offered his timely observation. The field of psychology has been transformed by a *"cognitive revolution"*

(Posner, 1989) and there has been a resurgence of interest in the psychology of emotions (Ekman & Davidson, 1994). Both movements have given rise to new and more sophisticated techniques for measuring cognitive and emotional processing in a reliable fashion. In light of these developments, it is reasonable to ask whether psychopaths are truly free of cognitive processing deficits or whether we simply lacked the tools for assessing them. As demonstrated in the following sections, both clinical description and laboratory evidence support the possibility that psychopaths do, indeed, suffer from information processing deficiencies.

CLINICAL EVIDENCE

In spite of Cleckley's (1976) remarks regarding the quality of psychopaths' thought processes in abstract (i.e., verbal) tests, he recognized the profound problem that psychopaths have using their good intelligence in the process of living. He stated: "*Only when the subject sets out to conduct his life can we get evidence of how little this good theoretical understanding means to him... What we take as evidence of his sanity will not significantly or consistently influence his behavior.*" (p. 385).

This mismatch between psychopaths' verbal awareness and actual behavior prompted Cleckley (1976) to hypothesize that they have "*a serious and subtle abnormality or defect at deep levels disturbing the integration and normal appreciation of experience...*" (p. 388). To clarify the nature of this deficiency, Cleckley (1976) related psychopathy to "*semantic aphasia*". People with a semantic aphasia are capable of generating perfect speech sounds, sentences, and grammar but their "*language does not represent or express anything meaningful...Like real speech, it appears to represent the inner human intention, thought, or feeling, but actually it is an artifact*" (p. 379). Just as this severe language disorder is "*masked by the mechanical production of a well-constructed but counterfeit speech*" (p. 379), Cleckley believed that the psychopath's inability to appreciate the affective accompaniments of experience was masked by their otherwise adequate intellectual abilities.

Clearly, Cleckley's (1976) characterization of the psychopath emphasized affective experience. He wrote: "*My concept of the psychopath's functioning postulates a selective defect or elimination which prevents important components of normal experience from being integrated into the whole human reaction, particularly an elimination or attenuation of those strong affective components that ordinarily arise in major personal and social issues*" (p. 374). However, evidence of psychopaths' defective emotional response appears to depend on what they are doing. "*In complex matters of judgment involving ethical, emotional, and other evaluational factors...(the psychopath) shows no evidence of a defect. So long as the test is verbal or otherwise abstract, **so long as he is not a direct participant** (emphasis added), he shows that he know his way about...When the test of action comes to him we soon find ample evidence of his deficiency*" (p. 346).

In light of such observations, it is worth considering the possibility that psychopaths have the capacity for sound judgment and genuine affect but that a cognitive deficiency interferes with their ability to integrate the products of these faculties with ongoing behavior.

Such speculation is consistent with Shapiro's characterization of psychopaths' deficit. According to Shapiro (1965), the psychopath is characterized by "*an insufficiency of active integrative processes...*" which causes him to remain "*oblivious to the drawbacks or complications that would give another person pause and might otherwise give him pause as well.*" (p. 149). According to Shapiro (1965), the cognitive/affective process by which a passing thought or whim normally accrues interest and emotional support owing to its association with preexisting aims and interests is "*short-circuited*" in psychopaths.

Regarding the nature of this process, Shapiro wrote "*In the normal person, the whim or the half-formed inclination to do something is the beginning of a complex process, although, if all is well, it is a smooth and **automatic** one*" (p. 140).
The "*automatic*" generation of meaningful associations, in turn, lends context to one's goals, relationships, and decisions. To the extent that we are cognizant of the relation between present circumstances and future goals, our ability to tolerate frustration and exercise restraint in the present is enhanced. To the extent that our feelings for and commitments to another person are represented in awareness, we are more likely to behave in an empathic and responsible manner because awareness of future interactions enhances accountability. Of course, sound judgment also relies on accessing past experiences and future considerations. To the extent that past experiences are automatically primed by similar circumstances, it is possible to benefit from them. Indeed, Shapiro's (1965) insightful chapter provides a cogent argument for linking this integrative process with the development of sustained goals, affective depth, lasting affections, self-restraint, sound judgment, and what is often referred to as "*conscience*" (see also Newman & Wallace, 1993).

Although Cleckley (1976) and Shapiro (1965) appeared to have similar perceptions of the psychopathic deficit, Shapiro's view is more explicitly cognitive: "*The cognition of impulsive people is characterized by an insufficiency of integrative processes that is comparable to the insufficiency of integrative processes on the affective side...*" (p. 299). Indeed, the clinical literature on psychopathy provides numerous examples of this problem: "*I always know damn well I shouldn't do these things, that they're the same as what brought me to grief before. I haven't forgotten anything. It's just that when the time comes I don't think of anything else. I don't think of anything but what I want now.*" (Grant, 1977, p. 60). Referring to a similar example, Shapiro (1965) noted: It is "*not pertinent information that was lacking or unavailable to this man but rather the active, searching attention and organizing process that normally puts such information to use.*" (p. 149).

These classic descriptions of the psychopath provide a relatively specific characterization of the psychopathic deficit. In particular, the descriptions suggest that psychopaths are deficient in the ability *to realize* and *be guided by* the "*meaning*" of their actions. Thus, psychopaths appear to be characterized by a subtle, but crucial and pervasive problem placing their actions in perspective. Whereas most people automatically anticipate the consequences of their actions, automatically feel shame for unkind deeds, automatically understand why they should persist in the face of frustration, automatically distrust propositions that seem too good to be true, and are automatically aware of their commitments to others, psychopaths may only become aware of such factors with effort.

This emphasis on automatic versus effortful processing[1] is consistent with Shapiro's (1965) portrayal of the psychopath's cognitive deficiency and suggests an explanation for Cleckley's (1976) observation that psychopaths' difficulty understanding the implications of their behavior is specific to circumstances in which they are behaving as opposed to discussing their actions. Whereas psychopaths may use their excellent intellectual faculties to provide thoughtful answers in response to verbal questions, they must rely on relatively automatic processes to guide their actions while devoting their intellectual capacity to achieving immediate goals. This does not mean that psychopaths are incapable of regulating behavior, only that self-regulation will be more effortful (i.e., capacity demanding) for psychopaths. Consequently, their self-regulation will be especially vulnerable to disruption when circumstances reduce available capacity, as when their attention is committed to goal-direct behavior, when they are reacting emotionally to a situation, or when they have been using drugs that reduce attentional capacity. Furthermore, owing to this deficiency, it might be especially easy for psychopaths to ignore the "*affective components of experience*" when it suits them to do so.

EXPERIMENTAL EVIDENCE

Paralleling these clinical accounts of psychopathy, my colleagues and I have proposed a laboratory-based model that focuses on the psychopath's failure to accommodate potentially significant, contextual cues while engaged in goal-directed behavior. Though based on a physiological model involving the consequences of septal lesions in animals (Gorenstein & Newman, 1980), our theorizing about psychopathy has focused on psychological (i.e., perceptual, learning, motivational, attentional, and affective) processes contributing to disinhibited behavior (see Patterson & Newman, 1993). The key concept in this model is response modulation. Response modulation involves suspending a dominant response set in order to accommodate feedback from the environment. In animal studies, deficient response modulation typically involves response perseveration or a tendency to continue some goal-directed behavior (e.g., running down the arm of a maze) despite punishment or frustrative nonreward (i.e., extinction). The focus of such studies is on the consequences of deficient response modulation (i.e., the failure to make use of potentially relevant information to adjust responding) rather than on information processing per se.

In applying the concept to people, we have found it useful to define response modulation in attentional terms. Specifically, we define response modulation as a brief and relatively automatic shift of attention from the organization and implementation of goal-directed action to its evaluation. Defined in this manner, the concept of response modulation is quite general and may apply whenever a person has to modify ongoing behavior in accord with environmental or proprioceptive feedback. If behavior is deemed appropriate it continues, if slight modification is necessary then adjustments are made, and

---

[1] I realize that the word *"automaticity"* has been used in diverse ways by different investigators and is therefore problematic (see Logan, 1988). My use of the term is most similar to Schneider, Dumais, & Shiffrin's (1984) who emphasize the ability of potentially significant stimuli to attract attention and prime related associations in a relatively fast, effortless, and autonomous fashion.

if the behavior is viewed as inappropriate it is likely to be inhibited and replaced with another response strategy. Despite the fact that response modulation involves a relatively primitive and largely automatic process, it subserves more elaborate cognitive and affective processing which, in turn, provides a meaningful context for evaluating one's behavior and exercising adaptive self-regulation (see Patterson & Newman, 1993, for more details).

The hypothesis derived from the septal model is that psychopaths have a cognitive processing deficiency that hampers their ability to accommodate the meaning of contextual cues while they are engaged in the active organization and implementation of goal-directed behavior (i.e., a response modulation deficit); and secondarily, that their poor self-regulation represents a situation-specific failure to suspend ongoing behavior and reallocate attention.

Over the years, our research on the response modulation hypothesis has shifted as the most pressing questions have changed. Our first concern was determining whether psychopaths do, in fact, have difficulty altering an ongoing *"response set"* (i.e., way of perceiving and responding to the environment). Similar to the research with animals, these early investigations examined the consequences of deficient response modulation. Next, we explored the circumstances that produce deficient response modulation in psychopaths to evaluate the generality of their information processing deficiency and specify the circumstances that give rise to it. To the extent that psychopaths' information processing deficiency is situation specific, the circumstances engendering the problem may be informative about the nature of the problem. In the third and fourth phases of the research program, we have tried to be more specific in our measurement of the response modulation process. In the third phase, we attempted to assess our subjects' tendency to stop and evaluate the consequences of their behavior (i.e., reflectivity) and the implications of reflectivity for self-regulation. In the fourth stage, we have been investigating the extent to which psychopaths' failure to accommodate contextual cues is associated with *"automatic"* (i.e., involuntary) as opposed to *"effortful"* (i.e., voluntary, deliberate) processes.

The participants in these studies were 18 to 40 year old male inmates from a minimum security prison in southern Wisconsin who had 4th grade or better reading skills, had no history of psychosis, and were not taking psychoactive medications. In all cases, interview and file information were used to diagnose psychopathy using the Psychopathy Checklist (Hare, 1980) or Psychopathy Checklist-Revised (PCL-R; Hare, 1991). Subjects earning 32 or greater on the PCL or 30 or greater on the PCL-R were classified as psychopaths and those scoring 20 or less on the PCL or 22 or less on the PCL-R were classified as nonpsychopathic controls. The PCL and PCL-R have proven to be highly reliable and valid measures of psychopathy (Hare, 1991; Hare, Harpur, Hakstian, Forth, Hart, Newman, 1990; Kosson, Smith & Newman, 1990; Serin, 1992).

With the exception of our earliest studies, psychopathic and nonpsychopathic groups were subdivided into high- and low- anxious subgroups using the Welsh Anxiety Scale (Welsh, 1956). The rationale for this procedure is three-fold: (1) Historically, investigators have distinguished between primary and secondary psychopathy in an effort to distinguish offenders whose predisposition to antisocial behavior is *"primary"* rather than a *"secondary"* consequence of negative emotionality (i.e., neuroticism); (2)

Laboratory research on psychopaths suggests that poor passive avoidance (i.e., failure to inhibit punished responses) is relatively specific to low-anxious as opposed to high-anxious psychopaths; and (3) By comparing groups of psychopaths and controls with comparable levels of anxiety investigators may examine and rule out the potentially confounding effects of anxiety on performance (see Newman & Brinkley, in press). Like others, we had hoped that the PCL-R would obviate the need for such supplementary measures, but investigations of passive avoidance learning and other performance indices often yield significant psychopathy by anxiety interactions (see Newman & Wallace, 1993). Such findings support the continued use of measures like the Welsh anxiety scale to assess the extent to which anxiety/neuroticism is moderating the effects of psychopathy on performance.

PHASE I: DO PSYCHOPATHS HAVE DIFFICULTY ALTERING AN ONGOING "RESPONSE SET" FOR REWARD?

Before investigating the factors contributing to deficient self-regulation, it was necessary to ascertain whether psychopaths would, in fact, be deficient in modulating dominant response sets. It is worth noting that most laboratory studies differentiating psychopaths and controls do not address performance *deficits*. For instance, group differences in psychophysiological responding to aversive and nonaversive stimuli have been commonly observed (see Fowles, 1980; Hare, 1978) but because such differences are of no consequence to subjects, they do not necessarily reflect a processing limitation. Alternatively, a number of studies have shown that psychopaths display poorer passive avoidance of electric shocks than controls but such differences are commonly attributed to a motivational deficit as opposed to a cognitive processing limitation because psychopaths appear to be less fearful than controls. According to Lykken (1995), for example, *"the psychopath is perfectly capable of learning to avoid what he really wants to avoid but he is likely not to bother to avoid eventualities to which he is indifferent"* (p. 149).

Given the dearth of evidence documenting *"consequential"* performance deficits in psychopaths, it seemed essential to investigate whether psychopaths would display a response modulation deficit despite monetary consequences for poor self-regulation. Toward this end, we developed a measure of self-regulation which, like the paradigms used in animal research, promoted a dominant response set for reward that eventually had to be modified (Newman, Patterson, & Kosson, 1987). The study involved a computerized card game in which the probability of playing a face card (i.e., jack, queen, king, ace) was high (90%) initially but decreased steadily as the game progressed. Subjects earned 5 cents each time that a face card was played and lost 5 cents each time that a number (i.e., 2-10) card was played. The primary dependent measure was the number of cards that a subject played before terminating the game. To perform optimally on this task, subjects had to play cards initially but then suspend their dominant response set for reward, evaluate the changing circumstances, and passively avoid the increasing punishments by quitting the game when the probability of losing grew greater than the probability of winning. The response modulation hypothesis predicts that psychopaths will find this more difficult than controls. Consistent with this prediction, psychopaths played significantly more cards and lost significantly more money than nonpsychopathic controls. Given the use of monetary incentives, psychopaths' poor performance on this task appears more consistent with an information processing than with a motivational deficit (see also Siegel, 1978). Thus, it seemed reasonable to investigate the psychological factors contributing to psychopaths' poor self-regulation.

PHASE II: UNDER WHAT CIRCUMSTANCES DO PSYCHOPATHS DISPLAY DEFICIENT PASSIVE AVOIDANCE?

According to the response modulation hypothesis, the psychopath's poor passive avoidance learning derives from their difficulty suspending and evaluating ongoing, goal-directed behavior (i.e., modulating dominant response sets) as opposed to a general intellectual, motivational, or inhibitory deficit. Thus, psychopaths' deficient passive avoidance learning should be relatively specific to situations requiring them to alter a dominant response set for reward (see Patterson & Newman, 1993).

This aspect of the response modulation hypothesis has been evaluated using a go/no-go discrimination (passive avoidance) task with monetary incentives to motivate performance. The basic task involves eight, two-digit numbers (e.g., 68, 23) which are presented one at a time on a computer monitor. Each of the eight numbers appears 10 times during the task and subjects must learn, by trial and error, to use the numbers to know when to press a button and when not to press a button. In the basic reward-punishment (R+P) condition, subjects win 10 cents for responding to *"go"* numbers and lose 10 cents for responding to *"no-go"* numbers. In a punishment-only (PUN) control condition, subjects lose 10 cents for responding to no-go numbers and also lose 10 cents when they fail to respond to go numbers. In both conditions, incorrect responses to no-go stimuli represent a failure to inhibit a punished response and thus provide a measure of passive avoidance. To the extent that psychopaths are characterized by a general intellectual, motivational or inhibitory deficit in passive avoidance learning, they would perform more poorly than controls in both conditions. To the extent that their poor passive avoidance involves difficulty suspending a dominant response set for reward to process the cues for punishment, psychopaths and controls should differ in Condition R+P only.

Consistent with the more specific prediction derived from the response modulation hypothesis, psychopaths committed more passive avoidance errors than controls in Condition R+P but did not differ from controls in Condition PUN. Although both groups had more difficulty in Condition PUN than in Condition R+P, evidence for deficient passive avoidance learning in psychopaths was specific to the condition requiring subjects to alter a dominant response set for reward (Newman & Kosson, 1986; see also Thornquist & Zuckerman, 1995).

In addition to Condition PUN, we have employed a number of other control conditions to assess psychopaths' passive avoidance when demands for response modulation are minimized. In one condition, for instance, the task design forced subjects to process both reward and punishment contingencies from the outset — a procedure which theoretically prevents the reward contingency from predominating and, thus, eliminates the need to alter a dominant response set during the task (Newman, Patterson, Howland, & Nichols, 1990). Other studies have used relatively long intertrial intervals which reduce the demand for *efficient* response modulation by providing subjects with ample time to process response feedback and revise their response strategy (Arnett, Howland, Smith, & Newman, 1993; Newman et al., 1987). Supporting the specificity of the response modulation hypothesis, our measures of passive avoidance and behavioral inhibition did not differentiate the performance of psychopaths and controls under these conditions (i.e., when demands for response modulation were minimized; see Newman & Wallace, 1993 for a review).

PHASE III: DO PSYCHOPATHS STOP AND EVALUATE THEIR GOAL-DIRECTED BEHAVIOR WHEN CONFRONTED WITH NEGATIVE RESPONSE FEEDBACK?

Whereas the tasks discussed in Phases I and II require response modulation to avoid losing money, they assess the consequences of response modulation (i.e., passive avoidance) as opposed to the response modulation process *per se*. To assess response modulation more directly, we began recording response times after correct (i.e., reward) and incorrect (i.e., punished) responses to observe the extent to which subjects paused to process response feedback following mistakes (i.e., passive avoidance errors). More specifically, the computer administering the task was programmed to record how long subjects *paused* following correct and incorrect responses as the response feedback was being displayed. By subtracting subjects' response times after reward from their response times following punishment, it is possible to estimate how long subjects suspend their goal-directed behavior to process unexpected, negative feedback (i.e., response modulation). Based on the response modulation hypothesis, we predicted that low-anxious psychopaths would pause less than low-anxious controls.

As predicted, low-anxious psychopaths paused less following punishment than did low-anxious controls. Moreover, consistent with regarding this difference in response times as a measure of reflectivity (i.e., pausing to evaluate one's behavior), there was a significant relationship between pausing after punishment and passive avoidance learning: The longer that subjects paused after punishment relative to pausing after reward, the fewer passive avoidance errors they made. Finally, consistent with the observed relationship between pausing after punishment and passive avoidance learning and consistent with earlier research, low-anxious psychopaths committed significantly more passive avoidance errors than low-anxious controls. There was no evidence that these group differences were related to speed-accuracy tradeoffs or overall response speed (Newman et al., 1990).

Similar findings have also been observed using other performance measures. One study examined performance on a computerized version of the Wisconsin Card Sorting Task that involved monetary incentives. Subjects were instructed to *"place"* cards (i.e., four-symbol displays) into one of four piles (i.e., by pressing one of four buttons) based on the features of the display (i.e., color, shape, & number of symbols). After each 10 consecutive correct responses, the sorting rule was changed (e.g., from color to shape) without warning and subjects therefore had to use the negative feedback from incorrect responses to interrupt and revise an established sorting strategy. Unfortunately, chance differences in intelligence complicated interpretation of the main findings and convinced us not to publish the study[2]. Nevertheless, low-anxious controls displayed pronounced inhibition after rule changes as predicted whereas low-anxious psychopaths did not. In fact, psychopaths actually responded more quickly following the first rule change when controls displayed the greatest behavioral inhibition (i.e., reflectivity). This significant group difference was not related to intelligence or altered by matching psychopaths and controls based on intelligence scores (Newman & Howland, 1987).

Another related finding was recently reported by Arnett, Smith, and Newman (in press) who used a continuous motor task. Subjects sat at a small table-top apparatus which had five buttons arranged in a semi-circle and a sixth button placed in the center, equidistant from the others. In addition, there were two small lamps (i.e., domed lights; one green and one red) placed above each of the outer buttons and two larger lamps placed above the center button. At the beginning of the task, the center green lamp was lit indicating the reward-only phase of the task was in effect. After one minute, however, the center red lamp was also lit indicating that subjects might be required to inhibit reward-seeking to avoid a relatively large punishment (i.e., the equivalent of 10 rewards) and, thus, needed to be more cautious. Relative to nonpsychopathic controls, low-anxious psychopaths displayed significantly less response modulation following the onset of the center red light. As in the Wisconsin Card Sorting Task, this group difference was greatest on the first trial.

PHASE IV: IS THE PSYCHOPATH'S FAILURE TO ACCOMMODATE PERIPHERAL CUES SPECIFIC TO PUNISHMENT STIMULI?

As already noted, in comparison to theories positing low fear or a general insensitivity to punishment cues, the response modulation hypothesis postulates a more circumscribed insensitivity to punishment stimuli. It predicts that psychopaths are less sensitive to punishment cues to the extent that processing such stimuli relies on automatic processing or, in other words, when they are engaged in the organization and implementation of goal-directed behavior so that their effortful processing resources are being allocated elsewhere. As noted above, the evidence on passive avoidance learning appears to support the situational specificity of psychopaths' insensitivity to punishment stimuli: When punishment contingencies are *"latent"* (e.g., Lykken, 1957) or otherwise peripheral to a participant's dominant response set (see Newman & Wallace, 1993), psychopaths appear relatively insensitive to punishment stimuli. Conversely, when the requirement to attend to punishment is salient and/or explicit from the outset, before subjects have established an alternative response set, then psychopaths appear to perform as well as controls.

Equally important, however, the response modulation hypothesis may be distinguished from other prominent theories of psychopathy by the greater *generality* of its predictions. The response modulation hypothesis predicts that psychopaths will be less influenced by the meaning of affectively-neutral stimuli as well as by the meaning of

---

[2] Psychopaths earned higher intelligence scores in one condition and lower intelligence scores in another condition. Although they were similar to controls across conditions, random assignment to condition apparently resulted in the group differences that compromised the validity of the study.

affectively-significant stimuli, provided that such information is peripheral to their ongoing goal-directed behavior. We recently evaluated this prediction using a task developed by Gernsbacher and Faust (1991). The task is ideally suited to measuring the extent to which the meaning of peripheral or *"contextual"* cues (i.e., pictures or words) automatically interrupt the dominant response set of psychopathic and nonpsychopathic offenders (Newman, Schmitt, & Voss, 1996).

The task involves 160 trials during which subjects must determine if two pictures or two words are conceptually related. Subjects press one button to indicate that the two stimuli are related and another button to indicate that they are unrelated. This is subjects' primary task and they win money according to the speed and accuracy of their responses. The first stimulus or *"context display"* always involves the simultaneous presentation of a picture and a word. On picture trials, the word in the context display is irrelevant (i.e., to-be-ignored) whereas on word trials, the picture in the context display is irrelevant. Each trial begins with the presentation of a *"P"* or a *"W"* so that participants know to focus on the picture or word component of the context display. Importantly, the to-be-ignored contextual cues may also be either conceptually related or unrelated to the subsequent *"test"* display. Although the relation of the contextual cues to the test display is irrelevant for correct responding, this relationship has a significant bearing on performance. Specifically, when the primary task stimuli are unrelated, subjects respond significantly more slowly when the contextual cue is related to the test display than when it is not (Gernsbacher & Faust, 1991). In light of the fact that contextual cues are irrelevant and subjects are instructed to ignore them, it is reasonable to assume that interference by the contextual cues is relatively automatic.

Because the response modulation hypothesis holds that processing the meaning of contextual cues is less automatic for psychopaths than for controls while they are engaged in effortful goal-directed behavior, we predicted that the contextual cues would produce less interference in low-anxious psychopaths than in controls. Similar to other *"normal samples"* (e.g., Gernsbacher & Faust, 1991), low-anxious controls responded approximately 60 ms slower on interference trials than when the to-be-ignored stimuli were unrelated to the test display. Low-anxious psychopaths, on the other hand, displayed *no interference*. Psychopaths responded just as quickly when the contextual cues were related to the test stimuli as when they were unrelated (see Figure 1). The results of this experiment provide differential support for the response modulation hypothesis: Psychopaths' lack of responsiveness to *affectively-neutral* contextual cues while actively engaged in an alternative task, is consistent with the response modulation hypothesis but is not easily explained by the low-fear hypothesis or related models which attribute psychopaths' lack of responsiveness to fear stimuli to inadequate motivation.

Combined, the results from these four phases of research suggest that while they are engaged in reward seeking, psychopaths are (a) less likely to reflect on relevant feedback that would help them benefit from experience (phase 3); (b) less likely to process the meaning of contextual cues (phase 4); and (c) less likely to revise a response strategy when changing circumstances make continuation of the response set maladaptive (phase 1). On the other hand, psychopaths appear to perform as well as nonpsychopaths when they are not expected to process peripheral cues or otherwise alter a dominant response set for reward (Phase 2).

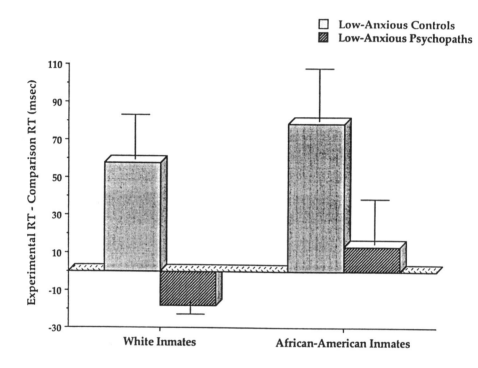

Figure 1. Differences in reaction times for low anxious psychopaths and controls

Thus, psychopaths appear to be characterized by an information processing deficiency that hampers their awareness of potentially relevant contextual information and interferes with their ability to regulate dominant response inclinations. Although further research is needed to replicate these findings and rule out alternative interpretations, a number of the findings are already supported by related evidence (e.g., Newman et al., 1990; Siegel, 1978; Thornquist & Zuckerman, 1995).

RELATED PROPOSALS

As already noted, the main purpose of this chapter is to demonstrate the plausibility and potential utility of an information processing perspective on psychopathy. Paralleling Cleckley's (1976) and Shapiro's (1965) clinical observations, our laboratory investigations of response modulation in psychopaths highlights a subtle but potentially consequential deficit that interferes with the psychopath's ability to use contextual cues to enhance self-regulation. Moreover, as noted by these clinicians, the problem does not appear to involve lack of information or lack of ability to manipulate information when doing so is the focus of attention. Rather, the psychopath's deficiency appears to involve comprehending the potential significance of contextual cues when processing them relies on relatively automatic shifts of attention.

Though I have emphasized deficient information processing in characterizing the psychopath's inadequate self-regulation, it is important to note that the present proposal is not necessarily at odds with proposals involving low fear, neuropsychological deficits, or other processing anomalies which diminish the influence of affectively significant stimuli on behavior. Indeed, there is considerable overlap between the response modulation hypothesis (see also Newman & Wallace, 1993; Patterson & Newman, 1993) and a number of these alternative perspectives. Although space limitations preclude a rigorous comparison of these alternative perspectives, I believe that even a brief analysis of the similarities and differences is worthwhile because it will (a) reinforce the plausibility of some (i.e., affective or cognitive) processing deficiency and (b) suggest a number of hypotheses that are worthy of investigation.

The low-fear hypothesis

According to the low-fear hypothesis, *"the primary psychopath has an attenuated experience, not of all emotional states, but specifically of anxiety or fear"* (Lykken, 1995, p. 118). Owing to their *"below average endowment of innate fearfulness"* (Lykken, 1995, p. 154), psychopaths are more difficult to socialize using typical parenting methods which rely on a child's being motivated to avoid punishment.

Of course, most of the evidence regarding poor passive avoidance learning in psychopaths is consistent with the low-fear hypothesis as well as with the response modulation hypothesis. Indeed, Lykken's (1957) classic investigation of psychopathy used a measure of passive avoidance learning to evaluate the low-fear hypothesis, though it may be significant that he used a *latent* avoidance learning task. Lykken (1957) used the term *"latent"* to describe the fact that subjects were not told that shocks were contingent on responses (i.e., could be avoided). Although the publication does not describe the procedure, subjects were apparently told that they would receive shocks from time to time to facilitate performance on the primary task, which involved learning a complex sequence of responses to traverse a *"mental maze"*. Using a similar task, Schmauk (1970) replicated Lykken's finding using electric shocks but observed adequate passive avoidance learning in a condition involving loss of money.

The difference between the low-fear and response modulation hypotheses relates to situation factors (i.e., controlling variables) which served to differentiate psychopaths and controls. Unlike the low-fear hypothesis which asserts that psychopaths are less motivated to perform the secondary avoidance contingencies, the response modulation hypothesis holds that psychopaths have greater difficulty recognizing the significance of secondary/nondominant information while engaged in goal-directed behavior. The findings reported by Schmauk (1970) appear to be more consistent with the low-fear hypothesis than with the response modulation hypothesis because although the avoidance contingency was *"latent"* in both conditions, group differences were only observed in the condition involving electric shocks (i.e., fear). However, the procedure that Schmauk (1970) used to deliver monetary punishments was quite likely to make it more conspicuous than the shock contingency. Specifically, he used an elaborate video set-up showing a stack of 40 quarters which was present from the outset of the experiment. Combined with the absence of monetary incentives on the primary task, this procedure must have made the avoidance contingency quite salient (i.e., not latent) from the beginning. Indeed, across groups, subjects displayed superior avoidance learning in the monetary condition relative the shock condition. To the extent that the avoidance contingency was a primary focus of attention from the outset, group differences in response modulation would be irrelevant.

As already noted, recent evidence employing monetary rewards and punishments indicates that psychopaths commit more passive avoidance errors than controls even when the consequences of passive avoidance errors involve loss of money (e.g., Newman & Kosson, 1986; Newman et al., 1987; 1990; Siegel, 1978). Although such findings are not easily explained by the low-fear hypothesis, they are predicted by the response modulation hypothesis. Moreover, the fact that psychopaths performed as well as controls in avoiding monetary punishments when these were the only incentives (cf. Schmauk, 1970) suggests that psychopaths' difficulty modulating a response set for reward in Condition R+P was instrumental in determining their poor avoidance learning. Finally, the fact that psychopaths were also less sensitive than controls to affectively-neutral contextual cues (e.g., Newman et al., 1996a) is predicted by the response modulation hypothesis but is not easily explained by the low-fear hypothesis.

With regard to psychopaths' use of peripheral stimuli to inform goal-directed behavior, the response modulation hypothesis yields predictions that are, at once, more specific and more far reaching. On the other hand, the low-fear hypothesis predicts weaker skin conductance responses (SCRs) to threatening stimuli — a prediction that has received substantial research support. Although this prediction is less straight-forward for the response modulation hypothesis, a *post-hoc* interpretation of such findings is that SCRs reflect a subject's registration of the significance of particular stimuli and that this encoding of stimulus significance is less automatic for psychopaths than controls under certain conditions (Arnett et al., in press; Newman & Brinkley, in press; see Newman & Wallace, 1993 for a more detailed discussion of the low-fear hypothesis).

The weak BIS hypothesis

Another perspective meriting consideration concerns Fowles' (1980) proposal relating Gray's (1987) *Behavioral Inhibition System* (BIS) construct to psychopathy. The weak BIS hypothesis has much in common with the low-fear hypothesis (see Lykken, 1995) as well as with the response modulation hypothesis (see Patterson & Newman, 1993). The BIS is a hypothetical construct which characterizes the psychological processes of the septo-hippocampal system. The BIS is activated by cues for punishment, nonreward, and novel stimuli and, once activated, serves to increase nonspecific arousal, interrupt ongoing goal-directed behavior, and direct attention to relevant environmental stimuli (Gray, 1982). Gray (1982; 1987; 1991) often characterizes inputs to the BIS as *"mismatches"* to indicate that stimuli which activate the BIS are unexpected (i.e., represent a mismatch between a person's expectations and actual events). Such mismatches, in turn, normally trigger an automatic attention response that enables individuals to examine the unexpected feedback, evaluate their response strategy, and revise expectancies concerning the consequences of their behavior (see Gray, 1987).

The weak BIS and response modulation hypotheses have much, in common. Indeed, both hypotheses are modelled on the function of the septo-hippocampal system and, thus, involve a number of overlapping propositions. For instance, both hypotheses involve the relatively automatic interruption of behavior and reallocation of attention in response to potentially significant cues. Because the BIS is a general construct with multiple functions, it is broad enough to subsume most predictions and findings generated by the response modulation hypothesis. In its most general form, the weak BIS hypothesis holds that psychopaths are deficient in every aspect of BIS functioning. That is, they are less responsive to punishment cues, less likely to inhibit responding in the presence of cues for punishment, and less likely to process (i.e., allocate attention to) environmental stimuli associated with punishment. Such a proposal is obviously encompassing, but may lack specificity. For this reason, we have advocated using Gray's model as a general framework for conceptualizing multiple pathways to behavioral dysregulation (e.g., Newman, in press; Newman & Wallace, 1993b).

Without specifying which component of BIS functioning is dysfunctional in psychopaths, it is difficult to contrast the weak BIS hypothesis with other proposals, including the response modulation hypothesis. Most discussions of the weak BIS hypothesis (e.g., Fowles, 1980; Lykken, 1995), however, focus on psychopaths' relative insensitivity to punishment cues. If psychopaths are less sensitive to punishment cues, the cues would produce less BIS activation and weaken all of its other functions. To the extent that the weak BIS hypothesis is characterized this way, it is, as suggested by Lykken (1995), basically an elaboration of the low-fear hypothesis. In which case, our discussion contrasting the low-fear and response modulation hypotheses is relevant to the weak BIS hypothesis as well (see Newman, in press and Patterson & Newman, 1993 for a more detailed comparison of these hypotheses).

However, the BIS subserves a variety of other processes that might contribute to the psychopath's deficit in self-regulation. Thus, investigators may also conceptualize the BIS as a fundamental psychological mechanism that enables people to commit attentional and cognitive processing resources to a particular task while *"automatically"* monitoring contextual cues so that they may shift the focus of attention and alter their behavior when circumstances demand it (e.g., Newman, in press; Newman et al., 1996b). Because the BIS is activated by cues for punishment, nonreward, and novel stimuli, it would be well-equipped to serve this function. Once activated, it would initiate an automatic *"call for processing"* and, in turn, more detailed processing of the unexpected or, otherwise, potentially significant information. Conceptualized in this manner, the weak BIS hypothesis would be quite similar to the response modulation hypothesis.

At present, the weak BIS hypothesis seems broad enough to be consistent with both the low-fear and the response modulation hypotheses. Differentiating these proposals will require greater specificity regarding which aspects of BIS functioning are hypothesized to differentiate psychopaths and how (see Newman, in press).

Damasio's neuropsychological model

Another theoretical perspective that overlaps with the current proposal is Damasio's (1994) *"somatic marker"* hypothesis (see also, Gorenstein, 1991). The primary focus of Damasio's work involves the consequences of ventromedial frontal lesions in humans, but he has repeatedly compared the resulting syndrome to psychopathy (e.g., Damasio, Tranel, & Damasio, 1990). The concept of somatic markers refers to affect-related associations that come to be associated with (i.e., mark) particular stimuli and responses. According to Damasio (1994), somatic markers are *"created in our brains during the process of education and socialization, by connecting specific classes of stimuli with specific classes of somatic state"* (p. 177). Once formed, somatic markers facilitate decision making and behavior regulation by calling to mind the positively or negatively valanced outcomes that have been associated with particular situations or followed particular responses. Referring to their role in avoidance learning, Damasio (1994) wrote that a somatic marker *"functions as an automated alarm signal which says: Beware of danger ahead..."* (p. 173).

To illustrate the consequences of a deficit in applying somatic markers, Bechara, Damasio, Damasio, and Anderson (1994) developed a card game that resembles the one used by Siegel (1978) and Newman et al. (1987) with psychopathic offenders. The game involves four piles of playing cards. Playing cards from either of two decks yields relatively large rewards but will occasionally result in relatively large losses as well. Playing cards from the other two piles results in smaller rewards but also entails much smaller losses. Although participants initially prefer the high payoff decks, they tend to shift to the safer choices after experiencing the large losses. Contrary to the typical pattern, patients with ventromedial frontal damage continue to prefer the high payoff deck and ultimately lose more money than controls owing to the large and unpredictable loses that they encounter. In describing this study, Damasio (1994) suggests that appropriate responding relies on *"a nonconscious process gradually formulating a prediction for the outcome of each move, and gradually telling the mindful player, at first softly but then ever louder, that punishment or reward is about to strike if a certain move is indeed carried out"* (p. 214). Damasio further suggests that patients with ventromedial frontal lesions, and psychopaths, are deficient in this process. Notably, Damasio (1994) does not attribute this failure to benefit from such *"predictions"* to a motivational defect. With regard his patients, he argues that *"they are still sensitive to punishment and reward but neither punishment nor reward contributes to the automated marking or maintained deployment of predictions of future outcomes..."* (p. 216). Whereas the somatic marker hypothesis is similar to the low-fear and weak BIS hypotheses in emphasizing the failure of punishment cues to influence behavior, it resembles the response modulation hypothesis in relating psychopaths' poor self-regulation to their difficulty processing meaningful associations that are normally primed by proprioceptive and environmental stimuli with learned associations to relevant outcomes (i.e., conditioned stimuli).

In contrast to the response modulation hypothesis, the somatic marker hypothesis appears to be specific to affective markers whereas the response modulation hypothesis applies to affectively-neutral as well as affectively-significant, contextual cues. Moreover, Damasio's hypothesis appears to target a generalized deficit in the formation and/or utilization of affective associations whereas the response modulation hypothesis posits a more situation-specific deficiency involving the ability to accommodate such associations while controlled processing resources are allocated elsewhere. Damasio, for example, notes that his patients have difficulty making decisions regarding personal preferences because the affective valence associated with the options are less available to them (Damasio, 1994, p. 193-4). Though psychopaths do not appear to be impaired in this way, their ability to form and/or access somatic markers may be impaired to a lesser degree than patients with frontal lesions (see also Hart, Forth, & Hare, 1990; Smith, Arnett, & Newman, 1992) or their impairment may involve a different component of the neuropsychological mechanism responsible for effective use of somatic markers.

Affective processing deficits

Although I have characterized the current proposal as an information processing deficiency, in actuality it is difficult to dissociate a deficit accommodating meaningful associations generated by contextual cues from one involving the experience of affect in conjunction with affect-eliciting stimuli. Even Shapiro (1965), in setting out the perspective that guided our proposal, expressed doubts about the feasibility of dissociating the cognitive and affective components of the psychopath's deficit. He noted that "*both areas of functioning and the modes that respectively characterize them exist together, each is hardly imaginable without the other, and, in all likelihood, they develop together*" (p. 154-155). Similarly, Newman and Wallace (1993) noted that the same problem which hampers psychopaths' ability to exercise sound judgment (i.e., evaluate the wisdom of their behavior) "*apparently interferes with their ability to appreciate the emotional and moral significance of events...*" (p. 300).

Thus, the current proposal also connects with recent proposals positing affective processing deficits in psychopathic offenders (e.g., Hare, Williamson, & Harpur, 1988; Patrick, 1994). Following up on Cleckley's (1976) characterization of the psychopath, Williamson, Harpur, and Hare (1991) noted that the "*inability to experience or appreciate the emotional significance of everyday life events*" (p. 260) appears to be a fundamental problem for psychopaths. Based on prior research with lexical decision (i.e., designating a string of letters as a word or nonword) tasks which shows that subjects identify words with affective significance more quickly than "*neutral*" words, Williamson et al. (1991) predicted that this effect would be less apparent in psychopaths than in controls. As predicted, psychopaths showed less behavioral and electrocortical differentiation between the affective and neutral words. In another, more recent study which presented psychopathic and nonpsychopathic offenders with "*emotional*" and neutral slides, psychopaths were less likely than controls to show the typical "*narrowing of attention with negative emotion*" that leads to enhanced memory for central as opposed to peripheral features of a slide (Christianson, Forth, Hare, Strachan, Lidberg, & Thorell, 1996).

Further evidence suggesting that psychopaths process affective stimuli differently than controls is provided by Patrick and his colleagues (e.g., Patrick, Bradley, & Lang, 1993). Based on the impressive literature demonstrating that the magnitude of a startle response is potentiated when people are processing aversive stimuli and inhibited while they are processing positive stimuli relative to neutral stimuli, Patrick and colleagues predicted that affective context would play a less significant role in modulating startle magnitude in psychopaths. As predicted, nonpsychopathic controls displayed the typical pattern (i.e., greater startle magnitude during negative than during neutral slides plus greater startle magnitude during neutral than during positive slides). Psychopaths, however, failed to display this linear trend, as their startle magnitude was smaller during negative slides than during neutral slides.

The response modulation hypothesis resembles these proposals regarding deficient processing of affective stimuli in proposing that psychopaths are less affected by the meaning of affectively significant stimuli. In contrast to Williamson et al. (1991), however, we do not believe that psychopaths' failure to process contextual cues is specific to affective stimuli. Patrick's (1994) emphasis on deficient processing of negative affect is even more specific and, thus, more at odds with the current proposal.

Further research is needed to investigate the extent to which psychopaths' information processing deficiency is specific to affectively significant stimuli using well matched, affectively-neutral control conditions. Our findings on the picture-word task appear to show that psychopaths are less affected by the meaning of affectively-neutral cues and are, thus, more consistent with a general deficiency in information processing. Conversely, the fact that the psychopaths in Patrick et al.'s (1993) study did not show the expected potentiation of startle during negative versus neutral slides appears more consistent with a specific processing deficit involving negative affect. Because the Williamson et al. (1991) lexical decision study found less facilitation in psychopaths in response to positively as well as negatively valanced stimuli and the Christianson et al. (1996) study assessed the effects of negative affect only, these studies do not clearly support one position or another.

After discussing research by Cook, Stevenson, and Hawk (1993) which showed "*dramatic startle potentiation during unpleasant imagery whereas low negative emotionality subjects showed no such effect.*" (p. 324), Patrick (1994) noted that "*the observed absence of startle potentiation in psychopaths (Patrick et al., 1993) may reflect a temperamental deficit in the capacity for negative affect...*" (p. 325). The fact that Patrick's findings have been relatively specific to the emotional detachment factor (i.e., factor 1) as opposed to antisocial behavior factor (i.e., factor 2) of the PCL also supports this contention because trait measures of neuroticism/negative emotionality are negatively related to factor 1 and positively related to factor 2 (-.23 and +.31, respectively in Patrick's study). The relation between neuroticism and startle magnitude, however, also raises a complex interpretive issue. Owing to its significance in predicting a subject's reaction to punishment cues, we have argued that investigators should control for neuroticism when comparing psychopaths and nonpsychopaths on measures of "*sensitivity to punishment*" (Newman & Brinkley, in press). Without controlling for neuroticism, it is difficult to determine whether group differences in response to punishment stimuli are related to neuroticism or psychopathy. Similarly, it will be important to examine the extent to which group differences in startle potentiation during aversive slides is related to psychopathy and/or neuroticism.

In judging the conclusiveness of the evidence from the startle magnitude paradigm, it is also worth noting that psychopaths and controls did not differ significantly in their startle magnitude during negative stimuli. The effects of affect on startle magnitude are analyzed by comparing the within group linear trends (i.e., from positive to neutral to negative affect). Moreover, because these data are standardized, a group's startle response during negative slides is not independent of their reaction to positive and neutral slides. Thus, localizing the nature of any group difference can be quite complex.

Attentional anomalies

Not surprisingly, the information processing perspective presented in this chapter also overlaps with earlier proposals regarding modulation of attention in psychopaths. Both Hare (e.g., 1978) and Lykken (e.g., 1995) have proposed that psychopaths have a propensity to *"gate out"* aversive stimulation. In particular, these authors have interpreted the combination of heart rate acceleration and low EDA in anticipation of aversive stimuli as evidence for a reflex-like coping strategy that reduces the impact of aversive stimulation. Of immediate relevance to the current proposal, Hare (1978) noted that while this reaction may serve to reduce fear, it may also prevent psychopaths from processing information that would facilitate avoidance learning.

Kosson and Harpur (in press) have provided an excellent summary of research on attentional processes in psychopaths. Based on the review, they tentatively rule out problems in sustained attention (i.e., vigilance), excessive exogenous shifts of attention (i.e. excessive reactivity to environmental changes); and inhibition of return (disinclination to return to previously attended stimuli). Instead, they conclude that (a) *"psychopaths may be overly responsive to cues inducing endogenous shifts of attention in some situations..."*; (b) *"such overresponsiveness may also be affected by the allocation of left hemisphere resources or right-handed responses"*; (c) psychopaths appear to be characterized by *"excessively narrow attention in situations involving multiple contingencies and multi-dimensional stimuli"*; and (d) psychopaths' reduced breadth of attention may help to explain observed deficits in passive avoidance and inter-level shifts of attention" (p. 29-30).

As evidence for *"reduced breadth of attention"*, Kosson (in press) cites evidence indicating that psychopaths commit more commission errors than nonpsychopaths when a secondary feature of a stimulus display indicates that subjects should not respond to that display (i.e., it is a distractor rather than a target stimulus). Such secondary features may involve the orientation of the frame surrounding the stimulus (i.e., horizontal or vertical), the overall pitch of a tone sequence (high versus low), or the color of a visual character string (red versus blue). In each case, the secondary stimuli are peripheral to subjects' primary task which requires them to (a) locate and respond to specific target letters, (b) discriminate among letter-only, number-only, or mixed character strings, or (c) discriminate among ascending, descending, or steady tone sequences. Thus, Kosson's (in press) proposal regarding breadth of attention is quite consistent with the current proposal: In both cases, psychopaths are said to be less influenced by peripheral stimuli while they are devoting effortful processing resources to a primary task involving the organization and implementation of goal-directed behavior (i.e., response readiness). Moreover, the psychopaths' difficulty processing the secondary characteristics of stimulus displays appears consistent with a deficiency in automatically accommodating the meaning of nondominant cues.

Kosson (in press) contrasts the breadth of attention hypothesis with an *"interference hypothesis"*, noting that the former predicts weaker processing of peripheral components of a single display (e.g., a frame around a target stimulus), whereas the latter relates to shifting attention from one display to another. The evidence from his program of research with psychopathic offenders provides differential support for the reduced breadth of attention explanation. Although both the interference and breadth of attention hypotheses appear to involve shifting attention, the demand to shift attention is more salient in his tests of the interference hypothesis than in his tests of the breadth of attention hypothesis. When a second stimulus is presented as it is in the tests of the interference hypothesis, the demand to shift attention is explicit. Conversely, in the single display used to assess the breadth of attention hypothesis, subjects must (a) automatically accommodate the significance of this contextual cue in order to label it a *"distractor"* and inhibit their dominant response set; or (b) deliberately (i.e., using effortful as opposed to automatic processing) remember to check the peripheral elements of the display before enacting their dominant response set.

The response modulation and breadth of attention hypotheses appear to yield similar predictions with regard to processing the *"distractor"* status of displays in Kosson's research. A more discriminating test of the breadth of attention hypothesis would seem to involve assessing psychopaths's processing of central and peripheral components of a display where neither component is accorded *a priori* significance. The response modulation hypothesis would predict adequate processing of peripheral cues under such circumstances because there is no demand to alter a dominant response set. The breadth of attention hypothesis would seem to predict weaker processing of peripheral cues. The latter prediction appears inconsistent with the recent report by Christianson et al. (1996) which examined processing of central and peripheral aspects of visual slides and found no overall differences.

SUMMARY AND CONCLUSIONS

Despite an historical precedent to the contrary, the clinical and experimental literatures on psychopathy provide numerous indications that the psychopath's inability to achieve a stable, prosocial adjustment may, indeed, involve information processing deficits.

Moreover, even allowing for the selectivity of this brief review, the literature provides a relatively consistent characterization of the psychopaths' deficiencies. Relative to nonpsychopaths, psychopaths appear to be less adept at allocating processing resources to secondary tasks while engaged in goal-directed behavior. Such secondary tasks may include (a) the major components of self-regulation (i.e., self-monitoring, self-evaluation, and self-control; see Kanfer & Gaelick, 1986), (b) linking immediate actions and environment stimuli with past experiences, and (c) decoding the cognitive and affective significance of contextual cues.

There is not yet good agreement concerning the circumstances that give rise to the psychopath's deficient processing of secondary information. Cleckley (1976) noted that their deficiency becomes apparent *"when the test of action comes to him"* (p. 346) as opposed to abstract discussions about behavior. Similarly, my colleagues and I have proposed a situation-specific deficit in information processing that occurs when relevant information is peripheral to the psychopaths' dominant response set (Newman & Wallace, 1993; Patterson & Newman, 1993). Kosson and Harpur (in press) proposed that psychopaths' information processing anomalies may relate to their *"difficulty interrupting left hemisphere-based attentional allocations"* (p. 27). Reports by Hare and his colleagues most often (though not always) indicate that psychopaths' deficient information processing is specific to aversive or other affective stimuli (e.g., Hare, 1978; Williamson et al., 1991). More research is needed to clarify the circumstances which differentiate psychopaths and controls. Such research should be given high priority because, in addition to differentiating among the proposals reviewed in this chapter, identifying the circumstances that engender psychopaths' performance deficits will almost certainly clarify the nature of the information processing limitation.

Research is also needed to investigate the extent to which psychopaths' apparent insensitivity to peripheral information reflects low fear, a dysfunction in some aspect of BIS functioning, or some neuropsychological, affective, or attentional deficit. As already noted, these proposals are not mutually exclusive but do have important implications for conceptualizing the psychopathic deficit and mobilizing interventions to counteract it. In most cases, these proposals are specific enough to generate differential predictions. As investigators begin to conduct studies contrasting predictions from the alterative perspectives (e.g., Arnett et al., in press; Kosson, in press; Newman & Kosson, 1986), we can expect the proposals to become more differentiated and better developed.

The purpose of this chapter was not to generate strong conclusions regarding the nature of psychopaths' deficient self-regulation. Rather, my goal was to encourage greater breadth of theory and hypothesis testing. Motivational (e.g, low fear) theories have dominated research and theory on psychopathy for forty years. Though this perspective has generated many significant findings over the years, we believe that it also has important limitations which commend consideration of alternative perspectives (Newman, in press; Newman & Brinkley, in press; Newman & Kosson, 1986; Newman & Wallace, 1993; Patterson & Newman, 1993). I hope that this chapter has convinced the reader regarding the plausibility of such alternatives.

References

Arnett, P. A., Howland, E. W., Smith, S. S., & Newman, J. P. (1993). Autonomic responsivity during passive avoidance in incarcerated psychopaths. *Personality and Individual Differences*, 14, 173-185.

Arnett, P. A., Smith, S. S. & Newman, J. P. (in press). Approach and avoidance motivation in incarcerated psychopaths during passive avoidance. *Journal of Personality and Social Psychology*.

Bechara, A., Damasio, A. R., Damasio, H., & Anderson, S. (1994). Insensitivity to future consequences following damage to human prefrontal cortex, *Cognition, 50*, 7-12.

Cleckley, H. (1976). *The Mask of Sanity* (5th Ed.). St. Louis, MO: Mosby.

Christianson, S., Forth, A. E., Hare, R. D., Strachan, C., Lidberg L., & Thorell, L. (1996). Remembering details of emotional events: A comparison between psychopathic and nonpsychopathic offenders. *Personality and Individual Differences, 20*, 437-444.

Cook, E. W., Stevenson, V. E., & Hawk, L. W. (1993, October). *Enhanced startle modulation and negative affectivity*. Paper presented at the Annual Meeting of the Society for Research in Psychopathology, Chicago, IL.

Damasio, A. R. (1994). *Descartes' Error: Emotion, Reason and the Human Brain*, New York: Putnam (Grosset Books).

Damasio, A. R., Tranel, D., & Damasio, H. (1990). Individuals with sociopathic behavior caused by frontal damage fail to respond autonomically to social stimuli. *Behavioral Brain Research, 41*, 81-94.

Ekman, P., & Davidson, R. J. (1994). *The nature of emotion: fundamental questions,* New York : Oxford University Press.

Fowles, D. C. (1980). The three arousal model: Implications of Gray's two-factor learning theory for heart rate, electrodermal activity, and psychopathy. *Psychophysiology, 17,* 87-104.

Gernsbacher, M. A., & Faust, M. E. (1991). The mechanism of suppression: A component of general comprehension skill. *Journal of Experimental Psychology: Learning, Memory, and Cognition, 17,* 245-262.

Gorenstein, E. E. (1991). A cognitive perspective on antisocial personality. In P. A. Magaro (Ed.), *Annual Review of Psychopathology: Cognitive bases of mental disorders,* (Vol. 1, pp. 100-133).

Gorenstein, E. E., & Newman, J. P. (1980). Disinhibitory psychopathology: A new perspective and a model for research. *Psychological Review, 87,* 301-315.

Gray, J. A. (1982). *The neuropsychology of anxiety.* New York: Oxford University Press.

Gray, J. A. (1987). *The psychology of fear and stress.* New York: Cambridge University Press.

Gray, J. A. (1991). Neural systems, emotion and personality. In John Madden IV (Ed.), *Neurobiology of learning, emotion, and affect* (pp. 273-396). New York: Raven Press, Ltd.

Hare, R. D. (1978). Electrodermal and cardiovascular correlates of psychopathy. In R. D. Hare & D. Schalling (Eds.), *Psychopathic behavior: Approaches to research* (pp. 107-143). Chichester, England: Wiley.

Hare, R. D. (1980). A research scale for the assessment of psychopathy in criminal populations. *Personality and Individual Differences, 1,* 111-119.

Hare, R. D. (1991). *The Hare Psychopathy Checklist-Revised.* Toronto: Multi-Health Systems.

Hare, R. D., & Harpur, T. J., (1986). Weak data, strong conclusions - Some comments on Howard, Bailey, and Newman's use of the psychopathy checklist. *Personality and Individual Differences, 7,* 147-151.

Hare, R. D., Harpur, T. J., Hakstian, A. R., Forth, A. E., Hart, S. D., Newman, J. P. (1990). The revised psychopathy checklist: Descriptive statistics, reliability, and factor structure. *Journal of Consulting and Clinical Psychology: Psychological Assessment, 2,* 338-341.

Hare, R. D., Williamson, S. E., & Harpur, T. J. (1988). Psychopathy and Language. In T. E. Moffitt and S. A. Mednick (Eds.), *Biological Contributions to Crime Causation.* Dordrecht, Netherlands: Nijhoff Martinus.

Hart, S. D., Forth, A. H., & Hare, R. D. (1990). Performance of criminal psychopaths on selected neuropsychological tests. *Journal of Abnormal Psychology, 99,* 374-379.

Kanfer, F. H. & Gaelick, L. (1986). Self-Management Methods. In F. H. Kanfer & A. P. Goldstein (Eds.), *Helping People Change: A Textbook of Methods.* (3rd Edition). Elmsford, NY: Pergamon Press Inc.

Kendall, P. C., & Dobson, K. S. (1993). On the nature of cognition. In P. C. Kendall & K. S. Dobson (Eds.), *Psychopathology and Cognition,* New York: Academic Press, Inc. (pp. 3-17).

Kosson, D. S., Smith, S. S., & Newman, J. P. (1990). Evaluating the construct validity of psychopathy in Black and White male inmates: Three preliminary studies. *Journal of Abnormal Psychology, 99,* 250-259.

Kosson, D. S. (in press). Psychopathy and dual-task performance under focusing conditions. *Journal of Abnormal Psychology.*

Kosson, D. S., & Harpur, T. J. (in press). Attentional functioning of psychopathic individuals: Current evidence and developmental implications. In J. A. Burack & J. Enns (Eds)., *Attention, Development, and Psychopathology.*

Lykken, D. T. (1957). A study of anxiety in the sociopathic personality. *Journal of Abnormal and Social Psychology, 55,* 6-10.

Lykken, D. T. (1995). *The Antisocial Personalities.* Hillsdale: New Jersey.

Millon, T. (1981). *Disorders of Personality: DSM-III Axis II.* New York: Wiley, (pp. 181-215).

Logan, G. D. (1988). Toward an instance theory of automatization. *Psychological Review, 95*, 492-527.

Millon, T. (1981). *Disorders of Personality: DSM-III Axis II.* New York: Wiley, (pp. 181-215).

Newman, J. P. (in press). Conceptual nervous system models of antisocial behavior. In D. Stoff, J. Breiling, & J. Maser (Eds.). *Handbook of Antisocial Behavior*, New York: Wiley & Sons.

Newman, J. P., & Brinkley, C. A. (in press). Reconsidering the low-fear explanation for primary psychopathy. *Psychological Inquiry.*

Newman, J. P., & Howland, E. W. (1987). *The effect of incentives on Wisconsin Card Sorting Task performance in psychopaths.* Unpublished manuscript.

Newman, J. P., & Kosson, D. S. (1986). Passive avoidance learning in psychopathic and nonpsychopathic offenders. *Journal of Abnormal Psychology, 95*, 257-263.

Newman, J. P., Kosson, D. S., & Patterson, C. M. (1992). Delay of gratification in psychopathic and nonpsychopathic offenders. *Journal of Abnormal Psychology, 101*, 630-636.

Newman, J. P., Patterson, C. M., Howland, E. W., & Nichols, S. L. (1990). Passive avoidance in psychopaths: The effects of reward. *Personality and Individual Differences, 11*, 1101-1114.

Newman, J. P., Patterson, C. M., & Kosson, D. S. (1987). Response perseveration in psychopaths. *Journal of Abnormal Psychology, 96*, 145-148.

Newman, J. P., Schmitt, W., & Voss, W. (in press). Processing of contextual cues in psychopathic and nonpsychopathic offenders. *Journal of Abnormal Psychology.*

Newman, J. P., Schmitt, W., & Voss, W. (1996b). *Processing of contextual cues in psychopathic and nonpsychopathic offenders*, submitted.

Newman, J. P., Wallace, J. F., Schmitt, W. A., & Arnett, P. A. (1996a). *Behavioral inhibition system functioning in anxious, impulsive, and psychopathic individuals*, submitted.

Newman, J. P., & Wallace, J. F. (1993). Psychopathy and cognition. In P. C. Kendall & K. S. Dobson (Eds.), *Psychopathology and Cognition*, New York: Academic Press, Inc. (pp. 293-349).

Newman, J. P., & Wallace, J. F. (1993b). Diverse pathways to deficient self-regulation: Implications for disinhibitory psychopathology in children. *Clinical Psychology Review, 13*, 690-720.

Newman, J. P., Widom, C. S., & Nathan, S. (1985). Passive-avoidance in syndromes of disinhibition: Psychopathy and extraversion. *Journal of Personality and Social Psychology, 48*, 1316-1327.

Patrick, C. J. (1994). Emotion and psychopathy: Startling new insights. *Psychophysiology, 31*, 319-330.

Patrick, C. J., Bradley, M. M., & Lang, P. J. (1993). Emotion in the criminal psychopath: Startle reflex modulation. *Journal of Abnormal Psychology, 102*, 82-92.

Patterson, C. M., & Newman, J. P. (1993). Reflectivity and learning from aversive events: Toward a psychological mechanism for the syndromes of disinhibition. *Psychological Review, 100*, 716-736.

Pinel, P. (1801). *Traite medico-philosophique sur l'alienation mentale.* Paris: Richard, Cailleet Ravier.

Posner, M. (1989). *Foundations of cognitive science.* Cambridge, Mass.: MIT Press.

Schmauk, F. J. (1970). Punishment, arousal, and avoidance learning in sociopaths. *Journal of Abnormal Psychology, 76*, 325-335.

Schneider, W., Dumais, S. T., & Shiffrin, R. M (1984). Automatic and control processing and attention. In R. Parasuraman & D. R. Davies (Eds.), Varieties of attention (pp. 1-27). New York: Academic Press.

Serin, R.C., (1992). The Clinical Application of the Psychopathy Checklist - Revised (PCL-R) in a prison population. *Journal of Clinical Psychology, 48*, 637-642

Serin, R. C., & Amos, N. C. (1995). The role of psychopathy in the assessment of dangerousness. *International Journal of Law and Psychiatry, 18*, 231-238.

Serin, R. C., & Kuriychuk, M. (1994). Social and cognitive processing deficits in violent offenders: Implications for treatment. *International Journal of Law and Psychiatry, 17*, 431-441.

Shapiro, D. (1965). *Neurotic styles*. New York: Basic Books.

Siegel, R. A. (1978). Probability of punishment and suppression of behavior in psychopathic and nonpsychopathic offenders. *Journal of Abnormal Psychology, 87*, 514-522.

Smith, S. S., Arnett, P. A., & Newman, J. P. (1992). Neuropsychological differentiation of psychopathic and nonpsychopathic criminal offenders. *Personality and Individual Differences, 13*, 1233-1245.

Thornquist, M. H., & M. Zuckerman, M. (1995). Psychopathy, passive-avoidance learning and basic dimensions of personality. *Personality and Individuals Differences, 19*, 525-534.

Welsh, G. (1956). Factor dimensions A and R. In G. S. Welsh & W. G. Dahlstrom (Eds.), *Basic readings on the MMPI in psychology and medicine* (pp. 264-281). Minneapolis: University of Minnesota Press.

Widom, C. S. (1976). Interpersonal and personal construct systems in psychopaths. *Journal of Consulting and Clinical Psychology, 44*, 614-623.

Williamson, S., Harpur, T. J., & Hare, R. D. (1991). Abnormal processing of affective words by psychopaths. *Psychophysiology, 28*, 260-273.

Author's notes

Preparation of this chapter was supported by a grant from the National Institute of Mental Health. I wish to thank Chad Brinkley and Bill Schmitt for their comments on earlier versions of the chapter.

PSYCHOPATHY, AFFECT AND BEHAVIOR

ROBERT D. HARE
Department of Psychology
University of British Columbia
Vancouver, Canada.

INTRODUCTION

Psychopathy is a socially devastating personality disorder defined by a constellation of affective, interpersonal, and behavioral characteristics, including egocentricity, manipulativeness, deceitfulness, lack of empathy, guilt or remorse, and a propensity to violate social and legal expectations and norms (Cleckley, 1976; Hare, 1995, 1996). In this chapter I selectively review recent research on the role played by emotional processes in the disorder. Because some of the most illuminating insights into the emotional life of psychopaths are provided by close scrutiny of their psycholinguistic processes, I emphasize work that has implications for understanding the complex interplay of the psychopath's language, affect, and predatory behavior.

Clinicians and researchers often are stunned by the apparent ease with which psychopaths engage in cold-blooded, instrumental behavior. They also are puzzled by the apparently candid — yet superficial and mechanical — manner in which many of these individuals describe their actions, their feelings about what they have done, and the impact their behavior might have had on others. Their expressions of remorse are unconvincing to astute observers, and their use of emotional words and phrases seem like mere mimicry.

Some psychopaths are perfectly frank about their inability to understand or experience what others describe as intense emotional feelings. *"There are emotions — a whole spectrum of them — that I know only through words, through reading and in my immature imagination. I can imagine I feel these emotions but I do not,"* wrote convicted killer Jack Abbott (1981). With the help of several prominent people, including writer Norman Mailer, Abbott secured his release from prison and promptly stabbed to death an unarmed waiter. The depth of Abbott's emotional concern for the man he killed, an aspiring actor, is apparent from the following remarks, *"There was no pain, it was a clean wound....He had no future as an actor — chances are he would have gone into another line of work"* (see Hare, 1993, pp. 42-43). Here we have an otherwise intelligent man who describes a killing in a dispassionate, matter-of-fact manner, and who cannot comprehend what the fuss is all about. To say that there is something unusual about people like Abbott is an understatement. While the cognitions and interpersonal interactions of most members of our species are heavily laden with emotion (Damasio, 1994), the inner life, experiences, and behaviors of psychopaths seem shallow and emotionally barren.

D.J. Cooke et al. (eds.), Psychopathy: Theory, Research and Implications for Society, 105–137.
© 1998 *Kluwer Academic Publishers. Printed in the Netherlands.*

The biological and environmental factors responsible for development and maintenance of psychopathy are not well understood, although recent theory and research in behavioral genetics (see Livelsey, this volume) and developmental psychopathology (see chapters by af Klinteberg; Frick; McBurnett & Pfiffner) offer some promising leads. One thing is clear: most conceptualizations of psychopathy place certain affect-related personality traits and dispositions at the core of the syndrome. These traits and dispositions are operationalized in the Hare Psychopathy Checklist-Revised (PCL-R; Hare, 1991). The 20 items in the PCL-R fall into two correlated clusters, or factors (see Table 1). Factor 1 consists of items that measure a cluster of affective/interpersonal features of psychopathy, while Factor 2 consists of items that describe an impulsive, antisocial, and unstable lifestyle, or social deviance. Although it has been argued (Harpur, Hare, & Hakstian, 1989) that the two factors are sufficient and necessary for an adequate conceptualization of psychopathy, Cooke and Michie (1997) have used item-response theory to argue that Factor 1 items are more discriminating at *"higher levels"* of the construct than are Factor 2 items.

TABLE 1. Items in the Hare Psychopathy Checklist-Revised (PCL-R)

Factor 1: Interpersonal/affective	Factor 2: Social Deviance
1. Glibness/superficial charm	3. Need for stimulation/proneness to boredom
2. Grandiose sense of self worth	9. Parasitic lifestyle
4. Pathological lying	10. Poor behavioral controls
5. Conning/manipulative	12. Early behavioral problems
6. Lack of remorse or guilt	13. Lack of realistic, long-term goals
7. Shallow affect	14. Impulsivity
8. Callous/lack of empathy	15. Irresponsibility
16. Failure to accept responsibility	18. Juvenile delinquency
for own actions	19. Revocation of conditional release

Additional Items [1]

11. Promiscuous sexual behavior	20. Criminal versatility
17. Many short-term marital relationships	

Note: From Hare (1991). The rater uses specific criteria, interview and file information to score each item on a 3-point scale (0, 1, 2). [1] Items that do not load on either factor.

Clinicians, researchers, and the public often see some of the features that define psychopathy in themselves and people they know (as well as in narcissistic, histrionic, and borderline personality disorders), and they assume that we are all more or less psychopathic. Indeed, some researchers and theorists argue that psychopathy is best represented by a multi-dimensional model or as a maladaptive variant of common personality traits found in everyone (see chapters by Blackburn; Livelsey; Widiger). However, although the PCL-R provides a dimensional score, the construct that it measures in fact may be a distinct clinical category or taxon (Harris, Rice, & Quinsey,

1994). That is, psychopathy might be an emergent entity formed by particular numbers and combinations of traits, dispositions, and behaviors that, by themselves and in different degrees and combinations, occur in many individuals or clinical conditions. To use a simple analogy, musical notes by themselves are just sounds, but when the same notes are put together in different ways they emerge as readily distinguishable melodies.

Before outlining some recent research on semantic and affective processes in psychopaths, I offer some comments on autonomic studies of psychopathy. I also describe a curious electrodermal response observed in psychopaths many years ago but never before reported, and briefly refer to recent research on nonverbal studies of affect in psychopaths.

NONVERBAL STUDIES OF AFFECT

Autonomic Studies

Much of the early laboratory research on psychopathy focused on classical and instrumental conditioning, including the role of fear and anxiety in passive avoidance learning. A study by Lykken (1957) formed the basis for much of this research. He found that psychopaths had difficulty in acquiring conditioned fear responses (as measured by anticipatory electrodermal activity) and in avoiding punishment in a passive avoidance learning paradigm. Conditioned anticipatory fear was an essential element in Mowrer's (1960) two-stage theory of passive avoidance learning, and the failure of psychopaths to exhibit such fear was consistent with clinical accounts of their relative failure to avoid punishment. I was impressed by Lykken's successful attempt to coordinate an emotional event with a behavioral one, and some of my early work on psychopathy sought to extend his findings (Hare, 1965, 1970, 1978). At least one part of Lykken's study, poor electrodermal conditioning in psychopaths, has been replicated conceptually many times by different investigators (see reviews by Hare, 1978; Lykken, 1995; Newman & Wallace, 1993). These findings generally are taken to mean that, consistent with clinical impressions, psychopaths show little fear in anticipation of an unpleasant or painful event.

Although I do not dispute the essentials of this interpretation, I should point out that poor fear or anxiety arousability provides a reasonable explanation for only some aspects of psychopathy (see Lykken, 1995, for a different view). As we will see below, psychopaths have difficulty in experiencing and discriminating among a variety of important emotions. As well, psychopathy appears to be related to several neurobiological anomalies that are not specific to fear and anxiety.

An Active Coping Mechanism?

As recorded in the laboratory, an exosomatic electrodermal response reflects a transitory increase in the secretion of eccrine sweat glands and, consequently, a decrease in the electrical resistance (or an increase in its reciprocal, conductance) between two electrodes, typically placed on the fingers. Unlike heart rate, which is controlled by the joint effect of the sympathetic and parasympathetic branches of the autonomic nervous system (and therefore rapidly can increase or decrease), electrodermal responses result from a brief increase in sympathetic arousal following some form of external or internal stimulation. The response begins within a few seconds of stimulus onset, reaches a peak in several more seconds, and then gradually returns to the prestimulus baseline. The response itself is nonspecific and unidirectional; that is, it is elicited by any relevant stimulus, consists of a transitory decrease in skin resistance (increase in skin conductance), and must be interpreted in terms of the context in which it occurs.

Because Lykken's (1957) study, as well as several of my own, used a painful electric shock as an unconditioned stimulus and as a punishment, it is reasonable to assume that the failure of psychopaths to exhibit normal electrodermal responses in anticipation of the shock reflected a relative lack of fear. However, I often have wondered what the impact on the research community would have been had Lykken used cardiovascular activity, including heart rate, as his measure of fear arousal. Presumably, he would have found, as my colleagues and I later found, that psychopaths exhibited normal or relatively large increases in heart rate in anticipation of a noxious stimulus (Hare & Quinn, 1971; Hare & Craigen, 1974; Hare, Frazelle, & Cox, 1978). At the time these studies were conducted it was not uncommon to associate heart rate acceleration with emotional arousal, and it would have been difficult not to conclude that psychopaths exhibited more fear arousal in anticipation of the noxious stimulus than did normal individuals. This conclusion would have been at odds with clinical wisdom and might have stifled subsequent laboratory research on emotion in psychopaths.

In the early 1970s my colleagues and I began a series of studies in which we recorded both electrodermal and cardiovascular activity in a *"countdown"* paradigm in which offenders awaited delivery of an electric shock or a loud tone (see review by Hare, 1978). We consistently found that nonpsychopaths exhibited large increases in skin conductance and moderate decreases in heart rate, whereas psychopaths exhibited small increases in skin conductance and large increases in heart rate. These apparently incongruous findings actually made psychophysiological sense, given what was known at the time about the autonomic components of orienting and defensive responses (Hare, 1973; Lacey, 1967). Thus, novel, interesting, or important events elicit an orienting response, which includes an increase in skin conductance and a decrease in heart rate, while unpleasant or threatening events elicit a defensive response, which includes an increase in both skin conductance and heart rate. I argued that these autonomic patterns indicated that the nonpsychopaths focused attention on the impending noxious stimulus and experienced an increase in fear, whereas the psychopaths *"tuned out"* the impending stimulus with little or no increase in fear (Hare, 1978). That is, rather than being incapable of experiencing anticipatory fear, psychopaths appeared to have ready access to a dynamic protective mechanism that attenuated the psychological/emotional impact of cues associated with impending pain or punishment. This mechanism apparently operated whether the pain was about to be experienced by themselves or by others (Hare & Craigen, 1974). Perhaps this is why, unpleasant, psychopaths find it easy to say such things as, *"I just put it out of my mind,"* or, *"I think positively."*

Although we did not explore these issues further, other researchers have replicated and extended our findings (Larbig, Veit, Rau, Schlottke, & Birbaumer, 1992; Ogloff & Wong, 1990). Besides skin conductance and heart rate, Larbig et al. (1992)

recorded slow cortical potentials (related to attentional processes) while their subjects (flagrant traffic violators in Germany assessed with the PCL-R) awaited delivery of a loud noise. The psychopaths gave much smaller cortical responses than did the other subjects, leading the authors to conclude that the former failed to focus attention on the impending noise.

A Curious Electrodermal Response

My hypothesis that psychopaths are somehow capable of actively coping with threatening and unpleasant stimuli may help to explain some curious findings obtained many years ago, then filed away and all but forgotten. In the early 1970s (before the establishment of the Ethics Committee at my University) Michael Quinn and I came across several psychopathic offenders who gave strange electrodermal responses in a classical conditioning paradigm that involved very strong and painful electric shock.

In this study (Hare & Quinn, 1971) we recorded palmar skin resistance and heart rate while the inmate listened to a random sequence of three different tones, each 10 sec long. One tone was followed by a strong electric shock, another by a slide of a nude female, and the third by nothing. We found that the anticipatory electrodermal responses (decreases in skin resistance) of the psychopaths were much smaller than those of the nonpsychopaths, particularly prior to shock, but that their heart rate responses were similar to those of the nonpsychopaths. But we omitted from analysis and did not report odd electrodermal responses exhibited by several psychopaths, primarily because at the time the responses seemed inexplicable. Formally depicted here for the first time, these responses may represent an interesting example of the putative coping mechanism referred to above.

Figure 1 provides a basis for appreciating the difference between these responses and those typically given by nonpsychopaths and psychopaths. The upper tracing (A) depicts the skin resistance of a nonpsychopath in the Hare & Quinn (1971) classical conditioning study. (In those days the pen linkage of our polygraph made curvilinear ink tracings, with the result that electrodermal responses that are large and that recover quickly appear to swing backward to a small degree). The pattern of activity is a *"textbook"* illustration of the conditioned anticipatory response that occurs prior to presentation of an unconditioned stimulus, in this case, an electric shock. Also clearly shown is the skin resistance response to the shock.

The second tracing (B) depicts the electrodermal activity of a psychopath in the study. Typical of the rest of the other psychopaths, he showed little electrodermal activity in anticipation of the shock, but a more or less normal response to the shock itself. However, two psychopaths (not part of the 18 in the study) exhibited some decidedly odd electrodermal responses to the shock, but not to the slides of nude females. During the early trials their skin resistance responses to shock were quite normal — a decrease in skin resistance — but after a few more trials (tracings C and D) they consisted primarily of a large — and anomalous — increase in skin resistance. At the same time, their heart rate increased sharply following delivery of the shock.The responses of another psychopath, a pilot subject for the Hare & Quinn (1971) study, were equally strange, but primarily with respect to anticipatory activity. His electrodermal responses on early trials were much like those of the psychopaths in the study (i.e., similar to tracing B). On later trials, however, the shock was preceded by a sharp increase in skin resistance and by a negligible response to the shock (Figure 1, tracing E). For this psychopath, the anticipatory electrodermal response was just the opposite of what is normally expected. At the same time, his heart rate increased considerably in anticipation of the shock.

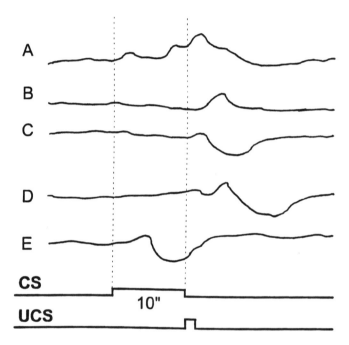

Figure 1. Tracings A and B depict, respectively, typical palmar skin resistance responses of a nonpsychopath and a psychopath in a classical conditioning paradigm in which a 10 second warning tone (the conditioned stimulus; CS) is followed by a strong electric shock (the unconditioned stimulus; UCS). A decrease in skin resistance (an increase in sympathetic innervation) is depicted by an upward deflection in the tracing. Tracings C, D, and E are odd skin resistance responses of three psychopaths. Rather than a decrease in skin resistance in response to the electric shock, two psychopaths (tracings C and D) exhibited a sharp increase in skin resistance. A third psychopath (tracing E) showed an increase in skin resistance prior to the shock. Unpublished data from Hare & Quinn (1991).

For several years after obtaining these data I showed them to various members of the Society For Psychophysiological Research. The responses were as perplexing to them as they were to me, and explanations included, *"I've seen that before but thought it was an equipment problem," "not possible," "a large skin potential response,"* and *"a dramatic example of active sweat reabsorption."* The latter explanation seemed most plausible, in light of Edelberg's (e.g., 1970) work on the mechanisms responsible for the recovery limb (return to baseline) of the electrodermal response. According to Edelberg, the sweat secreted by the eccrine glands is reabsorbed into the gland and the adjoining tissue. But it is clear from inspection of Figure 1 that something more must have been involved; skin resistance did not simply return to baseline but rapidly fell well below the prestimulus level. Perhaps the presentation of the electric shock was accompanied by a sudden decrease in sympathetic arousal, causing marked relaxation of the myoepithelial fibers responsible for *"squeezing"* the sweat out of the gland. Whether this was part of a protective response — or what Lykken (1968) referred to as *"negative preception"* — that served to reduce the impact of the shock, or whether there is some other, more prosaic explanation, is unknown. At the very least, it is clear that simple conditioning models, though important, do not provide complete explanations of the disorder (see chapter by Newman for a discussion of psychopathy as a cognitive/affective deficit).

Other Nonverbal Studies of Affect

Besides classical conditioning and *"countdown"* studies, there is other evidence that the difficulties psychopaths have in processing emotional information are not confined to language. For example, Patrick and his colleagues have conducted an intriguing series of experiments in which psychopaths failed to show normal modulation of the blink startle response during induced emotional states (Levenston, Patrick, Bradley, & Lang, 1996; Patrick, 1994; Patrick, Bradley, & Lang, 1993). The startle responses of nonpsychopaths typically are large when they view unpleasant slides, and small when they view pleasant slides (in each case, relative to when they view neutral slides). Psychopaths, on the other hand, give smaller responses when they view unpleasant and pleasant slides than when they view neutral slides, suggesting that the emotional valence of the stimuli have little differential effect on them. These group differences in startle modulation are related primarily to Factor 1 of the PCL-R, the affective/interpersonal components of psychopathy. After investigating the blink startle as a function of the content of the pleasant slides (erotica, thrill scenes) and the unpleasant slides (mutilations, assault, and threat), Levenston et al. (1996) suggested that *"psychopathy involves (a) normal or perhaps enhanced appetitive reactivity, and (b), defensive reactivity that is weak but not wholly absent."*

A typical finding with noncriminals is that emotional arousal is associated with a focus of attention to the central details of an event, at the expense of peripheral details. Christianson, Forth, Hare, Strachan, Lidberg, & Thorell (1996) presented a series of slides to psychopaths and nonpsychopaths, and asked them to report the details of a slide embedded midway in the sequence; the slide was designed to be emotionally arousing for half the subjects and neutral for the other subjects. The nonpsychopaths performed as expected; they recalled more central, and less peripheral, details of the emotional slide than of the neutral slide. Psychopaths, on the other hand, did not show this narrowing of attention to the central details of the emotional slide.

Imagery and Emotion

When I was a graduate student in the early 1960s my supervisor, Allan Paivio, was just beginning his ground breaking work on imagery (see Paivio, 1986). At the time, behaviorism was still a potent force in psychology, and I found myself more interested in mechanistic explanations of behavior than I was in inferences about fuzzy mental processes. Although I didn't participate directly in Paivio's research, his work influenced my later thinking about psychopathy, and made it easier for me to gradually bring cognition into the picture.

In a recent book (Hare, 1993) I discussed the role of *"inner speech"* and imagery in the development and operation of conscience. *"It is the emotionally charged thoughts, images, and internal dialogue that give the `bite' to conscience, account for its powerful control over behavior, and generate guilt and remorse for transgressions. This is something that psychopaths cannot understand. For them, conscience is little more than an intellectual awareness of rules others make up — empty words."* p. 132). I also wrote that the mental world of the psychopath was a bleak and barren landscape, devoid of rich, emotion-laden imagery. These certainly are not behavioristic statements, but, to a large extent, they were based more on the experiences and inferences of clinicians than on empirical research.

A study by Patrick, Cuthbert, & Lang (1994) adds empirical support to the proposition that the imaginal processes of psychopaths are emotionally flat. Prison inmates memorized and repeated aloud a series of sentences with either neutral or emotional content. They were then instructed to imagine the content of each sentence for six seconds. Inmates with low PCL-R scores showed greater increases in skin conductance, heart rate, and electromyographic (EMG) activity in facial muscles while imagining emotional content than when imagining neutral content. Those with high PCL-R scores, on the other hand, failed to show autonomic or EMG differentiation between emotional and neutral content.

LANGUAGE AND AFFECT

Clinicians have long been aware that psychopaths seem to know the dictionary meanings of words but fail to understand or appreciate their emotional significance. As Cleckley (1976) put it, the psychopath *"can learn to use ordinary words...(and) will also learn to reproduce appropriately all the pantomime of feeling...but the feeling itself does not come to pass."* Similarly, Johnson (1946) wrote that the psychopath *"exhibits a facility with words that mean little to him, form without substance... His seemingly good judgment and social sense are only word deep".* These clinical impressions are supported by the remarkable convergence of conclusions from a variety of laboratory studies, as illustrated below.

Before outlining this research, it is important to note that psychopathy is not readily interpreted in terms of traditional conceptions of damage to the frontal lobes. Standard neuropsychological tests fail to reveal any indications of brain damage, frontal or otherwise, in well-defined groups of psychopaths (Hare, 1991; Hart, Forth, & Hare,

1990; Smith, Arnett, & Newman, 1992). This does not necessarily mean that a brain abnormality model is untenable, only that the abnormality may be subtle and perhaps more functional than structural. Rather than standard neuropsychological tests that look for structural brain damage it would be more fruitful to employ the sorts of information-processing tasks used in cognitive neuroscience, particularly in conjunction with psychophysiological procedures and neuroimaging technology. Such an approach would allow us to investigate the manner in which psychopaths might differ from others in the use of cognitive strategies, and in the structural and functional mechanisms and circuits that underlie their cognitions, language, affect, and behavior.

Event-related Potentials

Williamson, Harpur, and Hare (1991) recorded reaction times and event-related potentials (ERPs) in a lexical decision task that required subjects (psychopaths and nonpsychopaths defined by the PCL-R) to press a button as quickly and accurately as possible if a letter-string formed a word. The letter-strings were presented on a computer screen for 176 milliseconds (msec), and consisted of neutral and emotional words and pronounceable pseudowords that appeared in a vertical orientation in either the left or the right visual field. Lexical decision studies with noncriminals indicate that responses to both positive words and negative words are more accurate and faster than are those to neutral words (Graves, Landis, & Goodglass, 1981; Strauss, 1983). Further, over central and parietal sites the early and late components of the ERP are larger in response to affective words than to neutral words (Begleiter, Gross, & Kissin, 1967; Kiehl, Mangun and Hare, 1995). Modulations of the early ERP components have been interpreted as a reflection of enhanced attentional processing of emotional words (e.g., Mangun, 1995), while the late components are thought to be indicative of enhanced elaborative processing of emotional words (Rugg, 1985).

We found that, like noncriminals, nonpsychopathic criminals were sensitive to the affective manipulations of the lexical decision task. They responded faster to emotional words than to neutral words, and showed the expected ERP differentiation between the two word types. Psychopaths, on the other hand, failed to show any reaction time or ERP differences between neutral and emotional words. Further, the morphology of their ERPs was strikingly different from that of the nonpsychopaths. One of these differences involved a positive slow wave. This wave generally was relatively small and brief in psychopaths, perhaps because they processed the information in a cursory, shallow manner and did little more than make a lexical decision, whereas the nonpsychopaths continued to process and mentally activate or *"elaborate"* the semantic and affective associations or networks of the word they had just seen.

Neuroimaging

Conceptually, this suggestion is consistent with the results of the first study to use brain imaging technology with a well-defined group of psychopaths (Intrator et al., 1993; 1997). Plans for the study were conceived in 1989 when Joanne Intrator and I began to correspond about psychopaths and their language. She had taken a position in the Psychiatry Service of the Bronx Veterans Affairs (VA) Medical Center in New York, and had access to the single photon computed tomography (SPECT) facilities. She suggested that we combine resources to do a SPECT study of psychopathy, and following a meeting at a scientific conference in San Diego in 1990 we developed a viable research protocol. The facilities and resources needed to conduct the study were provided by the Bronx VA Hospital, the Mount Sinai School of Medicine, and the New York State Psychiatric Institute, but the keys to its success clearly were Joanne Intrator and her remarkable ability to enlist and coordinate the talents and experience of experts in imaging technology. The results of the study were extensive and complex, and understandably led to some discussion about how best to interpret and present them. I'll come back to this issue after I briefly describe the study. Complete procedural and technical details are available in Intrator et al. (1997).

The premise of the study was that in normal subjects the cognitive demands imposed by a lexical decision task are associated with increases in activity in several parts of the brain, particularly prefrontal, temporal, and occipital cortex. However, the results of the Williamson et al. study (1991) suggested that psychopaths generate relatively few semantic/affective associations during lexical decisions, and we therefore expected that they would show less widespread activation than would normal subjects. Further, we expected that psychopaths and nonpsychopaths would differ in the pattern of cortical and subcortical activation associated with processing neutral and emotional information. Activation was defined in terms of relative cerebral blood flow (rCBF), as measured by SPECT.

The subjects were two groups of male inpatients of a substance abuse program (defined as psychopaths and nonpsychopaths on the basis of their PCL-R scores) and a comparison group of community volunteers. The patient groups were carefully matched for age, education, and alcohol, heroin, and cocaine use. All subjects had English as their native language, were strongly right-handed, and were free of potentially confounding neurological, medical, or psychiatric disease.

Because rCBF data are blended over several minutes of recording, rather than determined trial-by-trial, it was necessary to modify the lexical decision task used by Williamson et al. (1991). Although these modifications made it unlikely that we would obtain reliable group or condition (word-type) differences in decision times, they were consistent with our primary goal: to assess rCBF during the processing of neutral and emotional information. We constructed two blocks of stimuli, one neutral and the other emotional in content. The neutral block consisted of 96 words such as carpet, coach, and ounce, randomly interspersed with 96 pronounceable nonwords such as kinner, sepper, and harbage. The emotional block consisted of 96 words such as corpse, maggot, and torture, interspersed with 96 pronounceable nonwords. Each subject was tested in two sessions, one week apart. In one session he was presented with the neutral block of stimuli and in the other with the emotional block. The order in which the blocks were presented was counterbalanced across subjects. In each session the subject sat in front of a computer screen and was instructed to focus on a central fixation point which was replaced periodically by the stimulus, a letter-string. Exposure time was 183 msec. The subject's task was to press a button with the index finger of his right hand as quickly as possible whenever the stimulus was a real word.

Ninety seconds into a session 185 MBq (5mCi) 99mTc-hexamehtylpropylenamine oxime (99mTc-HMPAO) was injected via a heparin lock. The subject continued to perform the task for another five minutes. He was then moved to the SPECT scanner and positioned with the orbitomeatal line (OML) perpendicular to the axis of rotation.

The scanner provided five 18 mm-thick contiguous axial slices, acquired over a ten minute period. However, in an attempt to control the Type I error rate (wrongly concluding that a difference exists) Group (psychopath, nonpsychopath, control) X Condition (neutral, emotional) analyses of variance (ANOVAs) were performed on regions of interest in the slice that best reflected the cortical and subcortical regions likely to be activated by the lexical decision task. This was a mid-ventricular slice that encompassed prefrontal, anterior temporal, posterior temporal, temporal-parietal, and occipital cortex, as well as the basal ganglia and medial aspects of the frontal lobes. Significant Group X Condition interactions were obtained in right and left frontal-temporal cortical regions and in the contiguous right and left subcortical regions. In each case, psychopaths showed greater relative activation in the emotional than in the neutral condition, whereas the two nonpsychopathic groups showed just the opposite pattern. These results surprised us, but they made (after the fact) sense, given evidence that metabolic demands (and rCBF) decrease as the cognitive operations associated with performance of a task become deeply embedded or overlearned (Gur, 1992). In many tasks, including linguistic ones of the sort used in the present study, these operations include efficient (automatic?) extraction and use of affective information. The ability to evaluate things as good or bad, as safe or dangerous, clearly has implications for our survival and well-being. This obviously requires the integration of several cognitive and affective processes. With respect to linguistic stimuli, for example, the individual presumably must determine the physical characteristics of the word, match this information with a stored (and retrieved) lexicon, extract and use the word's denotative and connotative/affective meanings, integrate these meanings with other percepts and stored experiences, and prepare to make a motor response. Several areas of the brain appear to be actively involved in the process, including extrastriate cortex, anterior regions responsible for semantic processing and response preparation, and — most important for our purposes — medial frontal-temporal regions that have strong afferent and efferent connections to the amygdala and that play an important role in elaborating the emotional significance of the stimulus (Damasio, 1994; Peterson et al., 1990). In normal individuals the neurophysiological processes involved in decoding the affective information contained in words no doubt are so overlearned and efficient that metabolic requirements are minimal.

Psychopaths, on the other hand, seem to have difficulty in fully understanding and using words that for normal people refer to ordinary emotional events and feelings. Instead, they process and use them primarily in terms of denotative, dictionary meanings. It is as if emotion is a second language for psychopaths, a language that requires a considerable amount of mental transformation and cognitive effort on their part. It is possible that lexical decisions involving emotional words placed heavy demands on the psychopaths, and that the cortical and subcortical regions ordinarily involved in adding affect to language were very active (as reflected in increased rCBF) but relatively inefficient (Squire, 1987).

Other Findings

The decision by Intrator et al. (1997) to consider only Group X Condition interactions in the mid-ventricular slice reflected a desire to adopt a cautious, conservative approach, and was defensible on statistical grounds. However, at this early stage of neuroimaging research on psychopathy Type II errors (wrongly concluding that a group difference does not exist) can be as important as Type I errors (wrongly concluding that a group difference does exist). The concern with minimizing the Type I error rate meant that an interesting group effect (presented at a scientific meeting; Intrator et al., 1993) was not reported by Intrator et al. (1997).

These effects had to do with significant group differences in anterior and posterior activation. Unlike the interactions described above, these group effects were not unexpected. In fact, they were conceptually congruent with Williamson et al's. (1991) finding that the ERPs of psychopaths rapidly returned to prestimulus baseline following a lexical decision, and with the associated suggestion that cerebral activation during performance of cognitive tasks is less widespread in psychopaths than in other individuals. With Joanne Intrator's permission (personal communication, August, 1996) I briefly describe these findings here, primarily as a potential clue in the search for a neurobiolgical basis for psychopathy.

The findings in question were these: Psychopaths exhibited less anterior (frontal) activation, and more posterior (occipital) activation, during processing of the neutral and emotional tasks than did nonpsychopaths; and activation in the psychopaths was less widespread than was that in nonpsychopaths. For the psychopaths, the greatest activation was in occipital cortex, with considerably less activation in frontal, temporal, and parietal areas, particularly when they performed the neutral portion of the task. Of course, stimulus input for the task was visual and therefore initial processing occurred in occipital cortex, but it is clear that in the comparison subject a great deal of additional processing occurred in more anterior regions of the brain. Although it may be tempting to conclude that the psychopaths were not fully engaged in the task, perhaps because of drowsiness or boredom, there were no significant group differences in performance of the lexical decision task or in the speed-accuracy tradeoff. It is unlikely, therefore, that the SPECT results were related to group differences in level of alertness or motivation, at least to the extent that these factors are related to task performance. Similarly, all subjects had been screened for potentially confounding neurological, medical, and psychiatric disorders, suggesting that the relative lack of frontal activation in the psychopaths was not the result of palpable brain damage. However, the psychopaths differed less from the other patient group than from the comparison group, suggesting that at least part of the pattern of activation of the psychopaths was related to substance abuse.

In interpreting these results we can refer to brain-imaging studies of single-word processing which indicate that discrimination between visually presented words and pseudowords occurs early in visual processing, at the level of extrastriate cortex, and that anterior regions are involved in higher level processing of the words and their meanings (Peterson et al., 1990). Presumably the anterior activation exhibited by the nonpsychopaths reflected the increased metabolic demands associated with these higher level mental operations. In contrast, the psychopaths showed less anterior and more posterior activation than did the other subjects, suggesting that the former devoted considerable resources to the early identification and processing of the stimuli but relatively few resources to their cognitive elaboration. To put it another way, the psychopaths discriminated between words and nonwords — and even between neutral and affective words — but that may have been the extent of their cognitive effort. The normal subjects, on the other hand, continued to mentally *"work"* on the words. This interpretation of the rCBF findings is consistent with the ERP data obtained by Williamson et al. (1991), described above, as well as with clinical descriptions of the superficiality of psychopathic language (Cleckley, 1976). The deep meanings and subtle semantic and emotional nuances that form such an important part of language apparently are lost to psychopaths.

Brain Mechanisms and Circuits

Above, I briefly alluded to the possibility that psychopathy is associated with anomalies in cortical/subcortical structures and functional circuits responsible for the integration of cognition, affect, and behavior. These anomalies need not necessarily be the result of brain damage, impaired neural or biochemical development, or abnormal brain structure or function. It is possible that psychopathy and its neurobiological mechanisms represent variations on a normal theme. Sociobiologists, for example, argue that psychopathy can be understood as an adaptive cheating strategy for mating and reproduction (see Harpending & Sobus, 1987; MacMillan & Kofoed, 1984; Mealey, 1995). Similarly, psychopaths may use cognitive and behaviorial strategies that strike others as unusual but that do not emerge necessarily from neurobiological disorder or dysfunction. For example, an evolutionary game-theory model of antisocial personality disorder/psychopathy recently proposed by Coleman & Wilson (1997) predicts that the prevalence of the disorder will be much the same when the evolutionary mechanisms are social as when they are biological in nature.

　　　Recent developments in the coordination of cognitive science and neuroimaging techniques will no doubt go a long way toward resolving these issues. We should pay particular attention to structure and function of ventromedial prefrontal cortex, anterior temporal cortex, anterior cingulate cortex, and amygdala. These regions have rich afferent and efferent with each other and with other regions important in the processing and integration of semantic and affective information, planning, impulsivity, and the initiation and inhibition of behavior (Benes, 1993; Devinsky, Devinsky, Morrell, & Vogt, 1995). As Damasio (1994) put it, *"there is a region of the human brain, the ventromedial prefrontal cortices, whose damage consistently compromises, in as pure a fashion as one is likely to find, both reasoning decision making, and emotion/feeling, especially in the personal and social domain. One might say, metaphorically, that reason and emotion `intersect' in the ventromedial frontal cortices, and that they also intersect in the amygdala (p. 70)."* He went on to say, *"I would like to propose that there is a particular region in the human brain where the systems concerned with emotion/feeling, attention, and working memory intersect so intimately* *that they constitute the energy source of both external action (movement) and internal action (thought, animation, reasoning), This fountainhead region is the anterior cingulate cortex, another piece of the limbic system (p. 71)."*

Some recent findings are relevant here. Lapierre, Braun, & Hodgins (1995) found that psychopaths, defined by the PCL-R, were able to identify different odors but had difficulty in making fine discriminations among similar odors. Olfactory discrimination is a function of ventromedial frontal cortex, and the authors concluded that psychopathy is associated with dysfunction in this region of the brain. Behavioral and neuroimaging studies indicate that damage to this and related regions can produce a dissociation of the logical/cognitive and affective components of thought (Damasio, Grabowski, Frank, Galaburda, & Damasio, 1994), or even what Damasio, Tranel, and Damasio (1987) refer to as *"acquired sociopathy."* Interestingly, Tranel & Damasio (1994) found that patients with ventromedial prefrontal damage showed much the same pattern of classically conditioned electrodermal activity as that found with psychopaths: normal responses to unconditioned stimuli, such as loud noises, but little or no electrodermal activity in anticipation of the noxious stimulus. The significance of these parallel findings is that ventromedial prefrontal cortex plays a central role in the cognitive control of electrodermal activity (Damasio et al., 1994). Anticipatory electrodermal responses depend on the active involvement of this part of the brain, and the fact that such responses are greatly attenuated in psychopaths suggests that the integrity of their ventromedial prefrontal cortex (or its connections to other regions) might be compromised.

I might note here that Damasio (1994, p. 178) distinguishes between *"developmental psychopathy"* and *"acquired psychopathy;"* the former is the disorder described in this paper, whereas the latter is the result of brain damage. This is a long-standing distinction. Many clinicians and researchers have noted that some behaviors of frontal patients (e.g., impulsivity, recklessness, irresponsibility) are common in psychopaths, but the differences between these patients, sometimes referred to as *"pseudopsychopathic,"* and psychopaths typically are as important as the similarities (Hare, 1984). Damasio (1994) makes the same point, stating that, *"I use the term 'acquired sociopath' as qualified shorthand, to describe a part of the behaviors of such patients, although my patients and developmental sociopaths are different in several respects...(p. 178). "* Nevertheless, it is clear that the study of brain damaged patients can provide important clues to the neurobiology of psychopathy (Gorenstein & Newman, 1980; Newman & Wallace, 1993).

Similarly, the study of behaviors that imply dysfunction in particular brain mechanisms and circuits are extremely useful in helping us to understand psychopathy, particularly behavioral components such as impulsivity and disinhibition (Newman & Wallace, 1993). These components are reflected in several of the diagnostic criteria listed in the PCL-R: Impulsivity, Poor Behavioral Controls, Need For Stimulation/Boredom Susceptibility, Lack of Realistic Long-term Goals, and Irresponsibility.

Joseph Newman and his colleagues have conducted a series of laboratory studies — impressive in their conceptual and methodological rigor — that confirm and elucidate the view that psychopathy is a form of disinhibitory psychopathology that includes difficulty in passive avoidance learning (Newman and Kosson, 1986; Newman, Patterson, Howland, & Nichols, 1991; Newman, Widom, & Nathan, 1985), inhibition of well established dominant responses (Howland, Kosson, Patterson, & Newman., 1993), and poor response modulation (Newman, Patterson, & Kosson, 1987). The brain mechanisms that underlie these disinhibitory behaviors include ventromedial frontal cortex and anterior cingulate cortex (Damasio, Grabowski, Frank, Galaburda, & Damasio, 1994; Levin and Duchowny, 1991).

Confusion of Emotional Polarity?

There is considerable survival value in the ability to make rapid and accurate discriminations between things that are good or bad, safe or dangerous, pleasant or unpleasant. Discriminations of this sort are based on cognitive and emotional experiences and information. Psychopaths have difficulty in processing and evaluating affective information, and they should be relatively insensitive to the emotional polarity of events. As indicated above, they have difficulty in making behavioral and ERP discriminations between neutral and emotional words (Williamson et al., 1991). But there also is evidence that psychopaths also may treat positive and negative material and events as if they are affectively similar.

We investigated this *"confusion of emotional polarity"* in three experiments (Hare, Williamson, & Harpur, 1988; also see Williamson, Harpur, & Hare, 1990). In the first experiment we presented psychopathic and nonpsychopathic criminals with 56 word triads formed from different combinations of eight words: foolish, hateful, shallow, cold, warm, loving, deep, wise. For example, one triad was warm, loving, wise; another was foolish, shallow, deep. Their task was to select from each triad the two words that best went together. The task, adapted from Brownell, Potter, & Michelow (1984), was scored for six types of word groupings: Antonym (e.g., deep-shallow); Domain (e.g., loving-foolish; both are relevant to the domain of humans); Metaphor (e.g., wise-deep); Polarity (e.g., foolish-shallow; both have a negative connotation); Domain and Polarity (e.g., loving-wise; both are positively-toned and pertain to humans); and No Relation (e.g., warm-foolish). Compared with nonpsychopaths, psychopaths made little use of emotional polarity; they appeared to base their judgments more on learned associations between the words than on their emotional significance. For example, there were more likely to pair foolish with loving than with shallow.

Though the results of this word triad task were informative, the pairing of words could have been as much the result of familiarity with stock phrases or clichés as with an ability to perceive or understand semantic and emotional relationships. In a second, linguistically more complex, experiment (adapted from Cicone, Wapner, & Gardner, 1980), we presented criminals with a series of 14 emotional target phrases. Each target phrase (e.g., *"A man thrown overboard from a sinking ship"*) was accompanied by four test phrases of the following types: (1) Different descriptive features but the same emotional tone as the target phrase (e.g., *"A man running from a monster"*); (2) Similar descriptive characteristics and different emotional tone (e.g., *"A man surfing on a large wave"*); (3) Similar descriptive characteristics and neutral emotional tone (e.g., *"A woman standing on a yacht"*); and (4) Different descriptive characteristics and neutral tone (e.g., *"A boy carrying a lamp into his room"*). The subject was shown a target phrase and asked to select from the set of four test phrases, the one that most closely matched the emotional tone of the target phrase. Nonpsychopathic criminals had little difficulty in matching the emotional polarity of the target phrase in this affective phrases task. Psychopaths, however, frequently made an *"opposite polarity error;"* that is, they chose a test phrase (alternative 2 in the above example) that was opposite in emotional polarity to the target phrase. Interestingly, the psychopaths recognized that *"A man running from a monster"* and *"A man surfing on a large wave"* each had emotional connotations (one fear, the other exhilaration or excitement), but they saw them as being similar in polarity. Presumably, psychopaths readily identify events or experiences as more or less arousing, but find it more difficult to order them along a good-bad continuum. Alternatively, at least in this study, the psychopaths may have been more influenced by surface or semantic similarities between phrases than were the nonpsychopaths.

In the third experiment we presented the subjects with pictorial representations of the phrases used in the previous experiment. There were no significant differences between the psychopaths and nonpsychopaths in performance of this affective pictures task, but the task appeared to be too obvious for most subjects. It is possible that a pictorial task that relied on the ability to appreciate more subtle emotional connotations would have revealed performance differences between the psychopaths and the other offenders. In any case, other research clearly indicates that the insensitivity of psychopaths to emotional polarity is not confined to verbal contexts. As indicated above, Patrick (1994) found that the blink responses of psychopaths to startle stimuli were modulated in much the same way, regardless of whether the induced emotional state was positive or negative.

Nevertheless, it is apparent that the way in which psychopaths process and use language can provide us with important insights into their emotional experiences and capacities. Particularly helpful are paradigms that test the ability of psychopaths to understand and make use of the emotional nuances of complex verbal material, such as metaphors. Metaphor is a fundamental, ubiquitous part of language. It makes communication more vivid and comprehensible, and conveys subtle shades of meaning and emotion that are difficult to capture with literal language. Metaphor adds richness, color, and depth to language, and greatly increases one's ability to persuade, impress, and move others, as speech-writers and charismatic leaders are well aware (Beck, 1987, p. 14). Psychopaths often use metaphoric, figurative, and florid language to dazzle, obscure, impress, and manipulate others (Hare, 1993). But do they have a deep semantic and affective appreciation of what they say, or is what they say merely *"a matter of words?"*

To address this issue we tested psychopaths and others for their comprehension of the literal and the emotional aspects of metaphor (Hayes & Hare, 1997). We developed a set of 60 metaphorical statements, each rated for direction (30 were negative, 30 were positive) and degree (very negative to very positive) of emotional polarity. Psychopathic and nonpsychopathic criminals and a group of noncriminals differed little in their ability to interpret the literal meaning of the metaphors. They were then asked to perform a Q-sort of the metaphors; that is, they ranked them along a 6-

point scale (six bins) from -3 (very negative) to +3 (very positive), with the requirement that the number of statements put in each bin had to be as follows: -3 (2); -2 (9); -1 (19); +1 (19); +2 (9); +3 (2).

The psychopaths differed dramatically from the other groups in performance of this Metaphor Q-sort task. Thus, noncriminals and nonpsychopathic criminals had little difficulty in sorting the metaphors according to direction and degree of polarity. Psychopaths, on the other hand, made frequent sorting errors, both in terms of direction and degree of polarity. For example, metaphors rated by others as very positive (+3) were sometimes placed at the very negative (-3) end of the continuum, and vice versa. One psychopath considered *"Man is a worm that lives on the corpse of the earth"* to be strongly positive in connotation, whereas another psychopath considered *"Love is an antidote for the world's ills"* to be strongly negative in connotation.

One psychopath in the study wrote, just before his arrest, of an idyllic life with his wife. *"With her love I became a citizen of the celestial empire."* Following his arrest he was convinced that he and his wife were now closer than ever. He wrote, *"The crack in the wall that shielded us began to widen."* His use of flowery metaphors notwithstanding, he had not lived with his wife for two years before his arrest. His arrest was for burning down her house, appearing at her place of employment, and shooting two employees.

The ability of the psychopaths in this study to understand the literal meaning of metaphorical statements, but not the polarity of their emotional connotations, was striking. After all, these were not intellectually dull individuals; some had a college degree and all were of at least average intelligence. Clearly, the ability of most individuals to experience and comprehend a wide range of emotions is not shared by psychopaths.

Further evidence that psychopaths misinterpret the emotional significance of events was provided by Blair, Sellars, Strickland, Clark, Smith, & Jones (1995). They constructed nine emotional stories designed to elicit attributions of happiness, sadness, embarrassment and guilt. The subject's task was to describe how the person in each story would feel in that situation. Psychopaths and nonpsychopaths did not differ in the attributed emotional response for the happy, sad and embarrassed stories. However, the guilt stories yielded significant group differences in attribution. Nonpsychopaths attributed guilt appropriately, whereas psychopaths attributed little guilt to others; indeed, they frequently attributed indifference or a positive emotional state to the individuals in the guilt stories, particularly for the story in which intentional harm was inflicted. Further, psychopaths were significantly more likely than others to attribute happiness to an individual who had committed intentional harm. Psychopaths apparently have difficulty in attributing the correct emotions to individuals causing harm to others.

Speech and Affect

Most of the research described above involved the processing of linguistic input by psychopaths. However, equally important for understanding these individuals is their use of language. Relatively few empirical data are available, but what we do have suggests that psychopaths differ from others in the way they use language, as well as in the role played by emotion in their language. Their loquaciousness and ability to manipulate and deceive, and the often remarkable discrepancy between what they say and what they do, are of course well known (see Hare, 1995; Hare, Hart & Forth, 1989). Less known, and rarely studied, is the frequency with which the speech of psychopaths contains statements that appear to be conceptually inconsistent with one another and relatively devoid of substantive content. Eichler (1965), for example, reported that psychopaths used more retractions (putting two incongruent statements together) while speaking than did nonpsychopaths. Similarly, our videotapes of interviews with psychopaths indicate that they use a lot of jargon and short, poorly integrated phrases, and sometimes seem to have difficulty in developing and adhering to a logical train of thought.

A study of the narratives of psychopaths (Williamson, 1991) confirmed these impressions. She found that psychopaths made many contradictory and logically inconsistent statements, and frequently *"derailed,"* skipping from topic to topic and often giving roundabout, convoluted, and disjointed answers to apparently straightforward questions. This was not necessarily part of an intentional strategy to deceive and confuse the listener. Rather, it was almost as if the thoughts and concepts underlying their speech were poorly integrated or inefficiently connected to one another, making it difficult for them to detect the incongruencies in their own speech, particularly where emotional words were involved (see Hare, 1993). Moreover, the psychopaths seemed less *"tuned in"* to the cognitive and affective state of the listener than were nonpsychopaths. These results and their interpretation are consistent with the view (Newman, this volume) that psychopaths exhibit information processing deficits that result in poor self-regulation, difficulties in linking of current actions and stimuli to past experiences, and decoding of the significance of cognitive and affective contextual cues.

Physical Attributes of Speech

The acoustical aspects of speech are important part of conversation. Indeed, Feldstein and Welkowitz (1987) noted that conversation patterns are frequently used *"as a form of interpersonal contact in which participants attend primarily to the sound of each others' voices and minimally to the words that are uttered"* (p.452). This may be particularly true when psychopaths are doing the talking. We often describe psychopaths as charming, manipulative, and deceptive while seeming to be sincere. Like politicians and high-powered salesmen, psychopaths rely on listeners to pay more attention to how things are said than to what is said (see Hare, Hart & Forth, 1989 for a discussion of the psychopath as prototypical liar). Their lack of emotional investment in what they say frees psychopaths to talk glibly about themes of love and trust, pulling words from their overcoat pocket (cf., Hare, 1993, p.124).

In a recent study (Louth, Williamson, Alpert, Pouget, & Hare, in press) we investigated several acoustical characteristics of psychopathic speech. Acoustic analysis has been successfully used to isolate the blunted speech of schizophrenics (Alpert and Anderson, 1977), and the rapid production of syllables and words by manics (Meriwether and Alpert, 1990). We used a wide variety of verbal material in order to gauge the effect of dyadic, conversational-style speech; monologue; and negative, positive, and neutral material. We were interested in the loudness and rate of speech, on the assumption that they change with the emotional significance of the words spoken. The tasks included a semi-structured interview during which interviewer and inmate discussed a variety of bland topics; monologues by the offender on his most positive and most negative experiences; and reading a series of sentences, some containing a negative word and some a positive word. We used a computer system developed by Alpert et al. (1986) to measure variations in amplitude and speech rate. Psychopaths generally spoke more rapidly and more quietly than did nonpsychopaths. They also used less inflection than did the other offenders; the latter spoke more loudly when the words were emotional than when they were neutral, whereas the psychopaths did not, treating words of affective significance as if they were neutral in connotation.

Hand Gestures

As part of an attempt to understand the processes that underlie the speech of psychopaths, we conducted several analyses of their use of language-related hand gestures. The rationale for this research is the suggestion that hand gestures and speech may stem from the same internal processes, and that gestures provide an external representation of these processes (McNeill, 1985; Rime & Schiaratura, 1990). Rime, Bouvy, Leborgne, & Rouillon (1978) had reported that during an interview psychopaths used more hand gestures, and made more eye contact, than did nonpsychopaths. However, they were primarily interested in gestures as part of a general class of nonverbal behavior, and they did not distinguish between the various types of gestures.

In a study of videotaped interviews we replicated the Rime et al. (1978) finding that psychopaths used more hand gestures than did nonpsychopaths during narrations about their crimes and about their early family life (Gillstrom & Hare, 1988). But there are several classes of hand gestures, each with different psycholinguistic implications. We coded gestures into several major classes, including *"iconic"* gestures and *"beats."* Iconic gestures are related to the content of speech in a direct way. They appear to be intentional and serve to complement or add information to what is being said. For example, an individual may use his hands to depict a spatial relationship, point to a concrete object or a person present, paint a picture, or reenact human movement. Beats are small, rapid hand movements that occur only during speech or pauses in speech, but are unrelated to the propositional content of the narrative. They are not part of the story-line, do not appear to be intentional, and may occur at significant points of discontinuity in the structure of the narrative. Because beats are intimately phased with speech, Freedman, Blass, Rifkin, & Quinton (1973) refer to them as speech-primacy movements. McNeill & Levy (1982) have argued that beats may index the demarcation of discourse into functionally discrete units. McNeill (1985) has also suggested that beats mark meta-linguistic points in the breakdown of the speech process, and that they may reflect attempts to reinstate speech flow. The view that beats may reflect encoding difficulties is supported by evidence of increased use of beats in aphasics (Cicone, Wapner, Foldi, Zurif, & Gardner, 1979) and in bilingual individuals speaking their second language (Marcos, 1979).

We found that psychopaths differed significantly from others in the use of beats, but not in the use of iconic gestures. There was a tendency for this group difference in beats to be more pronounced during narrations about early family life than during narrations about crimes committed. Given theories about the functional significance of beats, we argued that psychopaths might have difficulty in conceptualizing and encoding verbal material. However, the study was an exploratory one, with a relatively small number of subjects. We therefore conducted a second study with larger groups of subjects (Hare & Gillstrom, 1997). Again, there were no group differences in the use of gestures related to the semantic content of the narrative. But, as in the previous study, psychopaths made significantly greater use of beats than did the other offenders. Moreover, the group differences were significant during narrations about family life but not during narrations about crimes, suggesting that psychopaths are more likely to experience speech encoding difficulties with abstract or affective material than with concrete or emotionally neutral material. Their frequent use of beats in the family segment of the interview may have reflected difficulty in processing, encoding, and verbalizing concepts for which they had only a superficial understanding (cf., Cleckley, 1976). It has been our experience, for example, that psychopaths are less likely than other people to describe their relations with their parents and siblings in terms of affective and interpersonal concepts, phrases, and words. Something more than a conscious attempt to avoid talking about feelings seems to be involved here. Rather, psychopaths may find it difficult to discuss issues of this sort because of a fundamental inability to understand the concepts in anything other than a literal or intellectual way. In some respects, the language of psychopaths may be analogous to a bilingual's second or nondominant language. Compared with words and concepts in the dominant language, those in the nondominant language have less *"ingrained"* meaning, are less easily encoded, and are associated with greater use of beats. We might argue that emotional/interpersonal words and concepts constitute the psychopath's nondominant language, and that he finds it difficult to speak this language without a great deal of cognitive effort. By way of contrast, talking about his crimes would present little difficulty to the psychopath because the concepts and words involved are likely to have experiential meaning for him.

We must also consider the possibility that psychopaths used a lot of beat gestures when talking about family life because of difficulty in conceptualizing and encoding abstract material in general, of which affective concepts are a subclass. There is little doubt that many of the key words used in the family segment were more abstract than those in the crime segment. Unfortunately, the present results do not permit us to determine whether beat gestures by psychopaths are related to the abstractness of the concepts in general, or specifically to affective concepts.

Cerebral Asymmetry

The neurobiological basis for the difficulties psychopaths appear to have with affective and deep semantic processes are unknown, but may involve anomalies in the integration of activities within and between hemispheres. Of particular interest here is the growing evidence that the two cerebral hemispheres are differentially specialized for the expression of certain positive and negative emotions (Boles, 1991; Davidson, 1984, 1987, 1993; Geschwind and Galaburda, 1987). Davidson and his colleagues (Davidson, 1984, 1987; Sutton, Davidson, & Rogers, 1996) has proposed that the left anterior region is associated with an approach system and the right anterior region with a withdrawal system. They also proposed that approach and withdrawal components are associated with different emotions. For example, fear and disgust have been associated with behavioral components of withdrawal (Plutchik, 1980), whereas happiness has been associated with approach. Some emotions (e.g. sadness) involve both approach and withdrawal components (Fox & Davidson, 1988).

Most research involving cerebral asymmetry in psychopaths has examined the processing and organization of verbal material. In normal right-handed males the left frontal, temporal and parietal lobes appear to be actively involved in the processing of verbal material, whereas the right hemisphere is more involved in the processing of the emotionality of language (Strauss, 1983). For example, as the emotional value of words increases, accuracy in discriminating words presented to the left visual field (right hemisphere) improves (Graves et al., 1981), and latencies decrease (Brownell, Potter, & Michelow, 1984).

This pattern of language processing is far less clear in psychopaths. In an early study (Hare and McPherson, 1984) we examined cerebral asymmetry with a verbal dichotic listening task, in which the subjects heard sets of one-syllable words, delivered through earphones. Each set was made up of three pairs of words (one member of each pair presented in each ear), and subjects were instructed to recall as many words as possible. Psychopaths showed a smaller right-ear advantage than did nonpsychopaths, but did not differ from them in overall performance. This led us to speculate that some language processes are not as lateralized in psychopaths as they are in nonpsychopaths. More recently, Raine, O'Brien, Smiley, Scerbo, & Chan (1990) replicated these findings with psychopathic and nonpsychopathic adolescents.

Other studies provide further evidence that the brains of psychopaths are lateralized in an unusual way, at least for linguistic processing. Jutai and Hare (1983) found that nonpsychopathic criminals exhibited a consistent left-hemisphere superiority on verbal tasks involving either simple recognition or semantic categorization of visually presented words. Psychopathic criminals also showed left-hemisphere superiority when the task involved simple recognition of the verbal stimuli, but an unexpected right hemisphere superiority when the task involved categorization into a semantic class. It appeared that words were categorized more efficiently by the left hemisphere in nonpsychopaths, and by the right hemisphere in psychopaths. A subsequent study (Hare and Jutai, 1988) found that as language tasks increased in complexity, nonpsychopaths relied more and more on the left hemisphere to process the information, while psychopaths relied more on the right hemisphere.

There is some evidence that the unusual cerebral asymmetry found in psychopaths is not confined to the processing of language. Mills (1995) recorded behavioral responses and ERPs while offenders performed a battery of seven verbal and nonverbal lateralized information processing tasks. One task, adapted from Nachshon (1988), involved the dichotic presentation of pairs of tones. The subject was instructed to attend to the tone presented in a given ear, following which he heard a test series of tones (including the ones he had already heard) in both ears. He was instructed to listen to the test tones and to indicate which of the tones previously had been heard in the designated ear. This dichotic *"memory for tones"* task draws heavily on left hemisphere resources. Mills found that nonpsychopathic offenders exhibited the expected right ear advantage (correctly identified more tones that had been presented in the right ear than those that had been presented in the left ear), but that psychopathic offenders showed a slight left ear advantage. The magnitude of the right ear advantage (REA) was computed as a laterality coefficient, defined as (R-L/R+L). The laterality coefficient was significantly correlated with PCL-R Total scores ($r = .41$) and with Factor 1 scores ($r = -.43$), but not with Factor 2 scores ($r = -.28$). The performance of the psychopaths was less lateralized in favor of the right ear than was that of the nonpsychopaths.

There have been several studies of lateralized emotional processing of words by psychopaths. In a divided visual field (DVF) study, Day and Wong (1996) found that right-handed psychopaths and nonpsychopaths differed in the way in which they processed negative-neutral pairs of words, one member of the pair presented in the left visual field and the other simultaneously in the right visual field. The task was to determine the side in which the emotional word appeared. Nonpsychopaths performed better (fewer errors, faster reaction times) when negatively-toned words were presented in the left visual field (directed to the right hemisphere) than when they were presented in the right visual field (directed to the left hemisphere). This result was consistent with evidence that the right hemisphere is specialized for processing the emotional significance of linguistic stimuli (Borod, Andelman, Obler, Tweedy, & Welkowitz, 1992). Psychopaths, on the other hand, showed a nonsignificant tendency for a RVF advantage for performance of the task. In interpreting their results, Day & Wong (1996) referred to evidence (Heilman, Schwartz, & Watson, 1978; Safer, 1981; Siberman & Weingartner, 1986) that the right hemisphere normally decodes emotional information *"by actual felt emotional reactions to the stimuli, that is, by a form of empathic responding"* (p. 651), and that it is specialized for modulating responses of the autonomic nervous system. They concluded that the right hemisphere of psychopaths may be relatively insensitive to the emotional qualities of a linguistic stimulus. This interpretation is weakened by other evidence that normal right-handed males process words presented in the RVF more quickly and accurately than words presented in the LVF, regardless of emotional valence (Eviator & Zaidel, 1991; Graves et al., 1981; Strauss, 1983). Thus, in the Day & Wong (1996) study it is not clear who was more abnormal, the psychopaths or the nonpsychopaths.

One of the tasks used in the study by Mills (1995), described above, was similar to the neutral-emotional word discrimination procedure used by Day & Wong (1996). The procedures differed primarily in terms of the degree of precision with which stimuli were presented and the responses scored. Day & Wong used a tachistoscope, whereas Mills used more tightly controlled computer presentation and scoring. Mills found no significant differences between psychopaths and nonpsychopaths in accuracy or reaction time, thereby failing to replicate the results reported by Day & Wong. However, she did find that the groups differed in the pattern of hemispheric activation in frontal cortex, as measured by amplitude of the P300. That is, when an emotional word appeared in the LVF nonpsychopaths showed greater right than left frontal activation, whereas psychopaths showed greater left than right frontal activation. Presumably, emotional information directed to the right hemisphere of nonpsychopaths differentially activated that hemisphere, but similar information directed to the right hemisphere of psychopaths differentially activated the left hemisphere.

Both Day & Wong (1996) and Mills (1995) included a facial emotional task in their DVF studies. The inmates were presented with bilateral pairs of faces (neutral-emotional) chosen from Ekman & Friesen's (1975) photographs of faces that differed in emotional expression. The task was to determine which visual field contained the face with the emotional expression. Consistent with evidence that the right hemisphere plays an important role in processing facial expressions of emotion (Bowers & Heilman, 1981; Safer, 1981), reaction times in both studies were significantly faster when the emotional face appeared in the LVF than when they appeared in the RVF. In the Day & Wong (1996) study the differences between groups in cerebral asymmetry were very small, and the authors suggested that psychopaths have difficulty in processing emotional information only when they are linguistic in nature. However, in Mills' (1995) study, the LVF superiority was largely due to the nonpsychopaths; the psychopaths showed little cerebral asymmetry. She concluded that nonpsychopaths identified the emotional faces relatively quickly when they appeared in the LVF because the information directly reached the hemisphere most efficient at processing this information, namely, the right hemisphere. She suggested that in psychopaths both hemispheres are able to access the neural structures necessary to process the information. This interpretation is consistent with data from other information processing tasks (see above) in which the performance of psychopaths was less lateralized in favor of a given hemisphere than was that of nonpsychopaths.

The emotional faces task used by Mills (1995) also produced some interesting ERP results. The latency and amplitude of the P300 response associated with processing the facial information may, among other things, provide an index of, respectively, the time taken for a particular region of the brain to become engaged in the task, and the degree of task involvement (Donchin, Karis, Bashore, Coles, & Gratton, 1986). In frontal (midline) cortex, the latency of P300 to emotional faces presented in the LVF was longer, and the amplitude smaller, in psychopaths than in nonpsychopaths; the groups did not differ in P300 latency of emotional faces presented in the RVF. In temporal cortex (right and left hemispheres) there were no group differences in the latency of P300 latency in response to emotional faces presented in the LVF, but the amplitude of the P300 was smaller in psychopaths than in nonpsychopaths. In Parietal cortex (left and right hemispheres) the latency of P300 latency to faces presented in the LVF was shorter, and the amplitude larger, in psychopaths than in nonpsychopaths. In interpreting these findings, Mills (1995) speculated that the nonpsychopaths made more use of anterior brain resources to process the task than did the psychopaths. For the latter, the task was primarily a perceptual task rather than a complex emotion discrimination task.

Mills (1995) also presented her offenders with a task in which they had to mentally rotate visually presented material. This mental rotation task is nonemotional and taps parietal resources in the right hemisphere. Psychopaths and nonpsychopaths performed the task equally well. However, analysis of the ERP data yielded a strange finding. In the nonpsychopaths the task drew primarily on right parietal resources, but in the psychopaths it was the frontal cortex that was most heavily engaged in performing this perceptual task. Clearly, anomalies abound in the organization of the psychopath's cerebral resources.

I have discussed only four of the seven tasks used by Mills (1995). The results of the entire study were complex and too extensive to present here. However, several general conclusions drawn by Mills are relevant here. The overall pattern of results suggested that the psychopaths did not suffer from localized brain damage, but rather used different areas of the brain than did other offenders to perform a given task. The brains of the psychopaths appeared to be more diffusely organized than those of the nonpsychopaths.

With respect to asymmetry, the pattern was inconsistent. In some cases there was reduced asymmetry for a given function (both sides of the brain were more active and involved than expected), in others there was increased asymmetry or reversed asymmetry (unexpected areas of the brain were involved). In some cases these cortical anomalies were associated with relatively inefficient information processing. *"Emotional tasks seem to be processed in merely perceptual, unelaborated ways (by psychopaths). The most conservative suggestion is that...(the brains) of psychopaths and nonpsychopaths are far more alike than different, (but that) the cortex of the psychopaths is organized in a somewhat more diffuse manner, with odd inter-and intra-hemispheric communication"* (Mills, 1995, p. 110). In addition, Mills obtained electrocortical evidence consistent with the hypothesis, described above, that psychopaths differ from other individuals in the anterior-posterior gradient or cortical activation. That is, she found that psychopaths were less likely than nonpsychopaths to use frontal and temporal regions of the brain while they performed verbal and emotional tasks.

Clearly, the issue of psychopathy, brain organization, cerebral asymmetry, and information processing is complex and poorly understood. Moreover, the psychological and behavioral implications of the unusual brain organization found in psychopaths are unclear. However, Geschwind & Galaburda (1987), among others, have argued that cognitive functions are most efficient when strongly lateralized. And Damasio (1994) and others have shown that anterior regions of the brain are crucial for the integration and elaboration of cognitive/affective processes. Psychopathy appears to be related to inefficient inter- and intra-hemispheric distribution of the cognitive and affective resources that control behavior (Hare, 1993).

Predatory Behavior

Unlike the case with other personality disorders, laboratory findings and neurobiological speculations merge seamlessly with the more salient behavioral aspects of psychopathy, particularly predatory behavior, to which I now turn.

Elsewhere (Hare, 1996) I argued that conceptualizing psychopaths as remorseless predators helped me to make sense of what often appears to be senseless behavior. These are individuals who, lacking in conscience and feelings for others, find it easy to use charm, manipulation, intimidation, and violence to control others and to satisfy their own selfish needs. They cold-bloodedly take what they want and do as they please, violating social norms and expectations without the slightest sense of guilt or regret. Their depredations affect virtually everyone at one time or another, because they form a significant proportion of persistent criminals, drug dealers, spouse and child abusers, swindlers and con men, mercenaries, corrupt politicians, unethical lawyers, terrorists, cult leaders, black marketeers, gang members, and radical political activists. They are well represented in the business and corporate world, particularly during chaotic restructuring, where the rules and their enforcement are lax and accountability is difficult to determine (Babiak, 1995). Many psychopaths emerge as *"patriots"* and *"saviors"* in societies experiencing social, economic, and political upheaval (e.g., Rwanda, the former Yugoslavia, and the former Soviet Union). They wrap themselves in the flag, and enrich themselves by callously exploiting ethnic, cultural, or racial tensions and grievances.

Space does not permit an extensive discussion of the psychopath as predator, and only a few illustrations are provided here.

Instrumental Violence

The ease with which psychopaths can engage in cold-blooded, casual violence has very real significance for society in general and for law enforcement personnel in particular. For example, a recent study by the Federal Bureau of Investigation (1992) found that almost half of the law enforcement officers who died in the line of duty were killed by individuals who closely matched the personality profile of the psychopath. More generally, psychopaths, as measured by the PCL-R, are far more likely to engage in violent and aggressive behavior, and to repeat such behavior following release from prison, than are other offenders (Hart & Hare, in press; also see a meta-analytic review by Salekin, Rogers, & Sewell, 1996).

Psychopaths not only engage in more violence than do nonpsychopaths, they also seem to engage in different types of violence. In one study (Williamson, Hare, and Wong, 1987) we examined police reports concerning the violent offenses of a random sample of adult male inmates. About two-thirds of the victims of psychopaths were male strangers, whereas two-thirds of the victims of nonpsychopaths were female family members or acquaintances. Furthermore, the violence of psychopaths apparently was motivated primarily by revenge or retribution, whereas most nonpschopaths committed acts of violence while in a state of extreme emotional arousal.

Researchers (e.g., Cornell et al., 1996) have identified two primary categories of aggression: reactive, emotional aggression that is elicited by frustration, provocation, or perceived threat; and instrumental aggression that is self-initiated, purposeful, goal-directed, and predatory. Cornell et al. (1996) argued that instrumental aggression is more stable (trait-like) than is reactive aggression. Using the Aggression Incident Coding Sheet (AICS; Cornell et al., 1996), they examined aggression in two samples of offenders. Almost all of the 106 violent male offenders in one sample had a history of reactive violence, but a minority also had a history of instrumental violence. The latter offenders had high PCL-R scores, their crimes were planned and goal-directed, and their victims were primarily strangers.

Cornell et al. (1996) replicated these results in a second sample of violent offenders (43 males and 7 females) referred for pretrial forensic examination and assessed with the Hare Psychopathy Checklist: Screening Version (Hart, Cox, & Hare, 1995). They concluded that offenders who used instrumental violence were more psychopathic — more dishonest, manipulative, superficial, impulsive, irresponsible, and lacking in feelings — than were other offenders. They also suggested that instrumental aggression was so strongly associated with psychopathy that it might be a defining feature of the disorder.

Dempster, Lyon, Sullivan, and Hart (1996) replicated these findings in a sample of 75 male offenders who had completed a program for violent offenders. In addition, they found that Factors 1 and 2 of the PCL-R had different patterns of correlations with the AICS. The results suggested that a high score on Factor 1 (interpersonal/affective features of psychopathy) increases the likelihood that an individual will choose to use violence, while a high score on Factor 2 (impulsive, social deviance features) influence the manner in which the violent act is executed. They concluded that violence of psychopaths is goal-directed, planned — *"impulsively instrumental."*

An interesting example of the predatory nature of the psychopath's violence is provided by male spousal abusers. Newlove, Hart, & Dutton (1992) found that about 25% of men taking part in a court-mandated treatment program for wife assaulters were psychopaths, defined by the PCL-R. Needless to say, programs of this sort do very little to change the behavior of psychopathic abusers who, like all psychopaths, see nothing wrong with their behavior (Hare, 1993).

The instrumental, predatory quality of these individuals is well illustrated in a study by Jacobson (1993) of the interactions between abusive men and their wives. He videotaped and recorded heart rate in the men while 60 couples tried to resolve conflicts in their marriage and engaged in heated arguments. During the conflicts most men became highly aroused, as reflected in behavioral agitation and increases in heart rate. But 20% of the men, though obviously extremely angry and aggressive, showed decreases in heart rate. As Jacobson put it, they *"became calm internally despite their emotionally aggressive behavior."* He suggested that these men were "sociopaths" and that their decrease in heart rate during conflict was *"associated with focused attention and successful attempts to control and contain arousal...After watching videotapes of these guys the metaphor that came to mind was that of a python, focusing attention on one's prey, waiting to strike."*

The metaphor is apt, given that heart rate deceleration is a component of the orienting response elicited by stimuli that are novel, interesting, or of particular significance to the individual. Presumably, the aggression exhibited by Jacobson's sociopaths/psychopaths was tightly controlled, focused, instrumental, and dispassionate. These individuals were watching the effect their intimidating behavior had on their wives.

The *"predatory gaze"* of the psychopath has been described by Meloy (1988) and Hare (1993). Perhaps the most vivid descriptions are by true-crime writers, who report that the intense, empty, riveting stare of the psychopath leaves most people feeling intimidated, uncomfortable, frightened and confused, the way potential prey must feel in the presence of a predator.

CONCLUSIONS

Our current knowledge of the etiological and neurobiological bases of psychopathy is still rather rudimentary. Nevertheless, it is clear that clinical impressions and insights, behavioral manifestations, and laboratory findings concerning psychopathy are remarkably convergent. Together, they form a reasonably coherent conceptual/empirical package that helps us to understand how and why psychopaths differ from others in the processing and use of semantic and affective information, and in their capacity for callous, predatory behavior. A great deal remains to be done, but the adoption of standardized assessments and the increasing application of paradigms and procedures from cognitive and clinical neuroscience will almost certainly lead to new levels of understanding of this complex condition. For example, we currently are using functional magnetic resonance imaging (fMRI) to investigate the neurophysiology of semantic and affective processing in psychopaths. The protocols will provide us with information about activity in key cortical and subcortical regions, including ventromedial frontal cortex, anterior cingulate cortex, temporal cortex, and amygdala, while psychopaths and others perform a variety of linguistic, nonlinguistic, and affective tasks.

Virtually all of the research on psychopathy, language, and affect has been conducted with male offenders. There is some evidence that the behavioral and personality correlates of psychopathy found with male offenders are much the same as those found with female offenders (Strachan & Hare, 1997), adolescent offenders (Forth, Hart, & Hare,1990; Gretton, McBride, O'Shaughnessy, & Hare, 1994; Gretton, O'Shaughnessy, & Hare, 1997) and noncriminals (Forth, Brown, Hart, & Hare, 1996). However, until the relevant research is done, we do not know the extent to which the findings and conclusions described above will generalize to female and adolescent offenders and to noncriminals.

References

Abbott, J. (1981). *In the Belly of the Beast: Letters From Prison*. New York: Random House.

Alpert, M., & Anderson, L.T. (1977). Imagery mediation of vocal emphasis in flat affect. *Archives of General Psychiatry, 8*, 362-365.

Alpert, M., Meriwhether, F., Homel, P., Martz, J., & Lomask, M (1986). VOXCOM: A system for analyzing natural speech in real time. *Behavior Research Methods, Instruments, and Computers. 18*, 267-272.

Babiak, P. (1995). When psychopaths go to work. *International Journal of Applied Psychology, 44*, 171-188.

Begleiter, H., Gross, M.M., & Kissin, B. (1967). Evoked cortical responses to affective visual stimuli. *Psychophysiology, 3*, 336-344.

Benes, F.M. (1993) Neurobiological investigations in cingulate cortex of schizophrenic brain (Review). *Schizophrenia Bulletin, 19*, 537-549.

Blair, R.J.R., Sellars, C., Strickland, I., Clark, F., Smith, M., & Jones, L. (1995). Emotional attributions in the psychopath. *Personality and Individual Differences, 19*, 431-437.

Boles, D. (1991). Factor analysis and the cerebral hemispheres: Pilot study and parietal functions. *Neuropsychologia, 29*, 59-91.

Borod, J.C., Andelman, F., Obler, L.K., Tweedy, J.R., & Welkowitz, J. (1992). Right hemisphere specialization for identification of emotional words and sentences: Evidence from stroke patients. *Neuropsychologia, 30*, 827-844.

Brownell, H.H., Potter, H.H., & Michelow, D. (1984). Sensitivity to denotation and connotation in brain-damaged patients: A double disassociation? *Brain and Language, 22*, 253-265.

Cicone, M., Wapner, W., & Gardner, H. (1980). Sensitivity to emotional expressions and situations in organic patients. *Cortex, 16*, 145-158.

Christianson, S.A., Forth, A.E., Hare, R.D., Strachan, C.E., Lidberg, L., & Thorell, L.H. (1996). Remembering details of emotional events: A comparison between psychopathic and nonpsychopathic offenders. *Personality and Individual Differences, 20*, 437-446.

Cleckley, H. (1976). *The Mask of Sanity*. St. Louis, MO: Mosby.

Coleman, A.M., & Wilson, J.C. (1997). Antisocial personality disorder: An evolutionary game theory analysis. *Legal and Criminological Psychology, 2*, 23-34.

Cooke, D.J., & Michie, C. (1997). An item response theory evaluation of Hare's Psychopathy Checklist. *Psychological Assessment, 9, 3-14*.

Cornell, D., Warren, J., Hawk, G., Stafford, E., Oram, G., & Pine, D. (1996). Psychopathy in instrumental and reactive offenders. *Journal of Consulting and Clinical Psychology, 64*, 783-790.

Damasio, A. (1994). *Descartes' Error: Emotion, Reason, and the Human Brain*. New York: Putnam & Sons.

Damasio, H., Grabowski, T., Frank, R., Galaburda, A. M., & Damasio, A. R. (1994). The return of Phineas Gage: Clues about the brain from the skull of a famous patient. *Science, 264*, 1102-1105.

Damasio, A., Tranel, D., & Damasio, H. (1987). Individuals with sociopathic behavior caused by frontal damage fail to respond autonomically to social stimuli. *Behavioral Brain Research, 41*, 81-94.

Day, R., & Wong, S. (1996). Anomalous perceptual asymmetries for negative emotional stimuli in the psychopath. *Journal of Abnormal Psychology, 105*, 648-652.

Davidson, R.J. (1984). Hemisphere asymmetry and emotion. In K. Scherer & P. Ekman (eds.), *Approaches to Emotion*, Hillsdale, NJ: Erlbaum.

Davidson, R.J. (1987). Cerebral asymmetry and the nature of emotion: Implications for the study of individual differences and psychopathology (pp. 71-83), In R. Takahashi, P. Flor-Henry, J. Gruzelier, & S. Niwa (eds.), *Cerebral dynamics, laterality, and psychopathology*, New York: Elsevier.

Davidson, R. (1993). Cerebral asymmetry and emotion: Conceptual and methodological conundrums. *Cognition and Emotion, 7*, 115-138.

Dempster, R. J., Lyon, D. R., Sullivan, L. E., Hart, S. D., Smiley, W. C., & Mulloy, R. (1996, August). *Psychopathy and instrumental aggression in violent offenders*. Paper presented at the Annual Meeting of the American Psychological Association, Toronto, Ontario.

Devinsky, O., Morrell, M.J. and Vogt, B.A. (1995). Contributions of anterior cingulate cortex to behavior. *Brain, 118*, 279-306.

Donchin, E., Karis, D., Bashore, T.R., Coles, M.G.H., & Gratton, G. (1986). Cognitive psychophysiology and information processing. In M.H.H. Coles, E. Donchin, & S.W. Porges (eds). *Psychophysiology: Systems, processes, & applications* (pp. 244-267). New York: Guilford.

Edelberg, R. (1970). The information content of the recovery limb of the electrodermal response. *Psychophysiology, 6*. 527-539.

Eichler, M. (1965). The application of verbal behavior analysis to the study of psychological defense mechanisms: speech patterns associated with sociopathic behavior. *Journal of Nervous and Mental Disease, 141*, 658-673.

Eviator, Z., & Zaidel, E. (1991). The effects of word length and emotionality on hemispheric contribution to lexical decisions. *Neuropsychologia, 29*, 415-428.

Federal Bureau of Investigation. (1992) *Killed in the Line of Duty*. Washington, DC: United States Department of Justice.

Feldstein, S., & Welkowitz, J. (1987). A chronography of conversation: In defense of an objective approach. In A. Siegman and S. Feldstein (eds), *Nonverbal Behavior and Communication*. Hillsdale: Laurence Erlbaum Associates.

Forth, A.E., Brown, S.L., Hart, S.D., & Hare, R.D. (1996). The assessment of psychopathy in male and female noncriminals: Reliability and validity. *Personality and Individual Differences, 20*, 531-543.

Forth, A., E., Hart, S. D., & Hare, R. D. (1990). Assessment of psychopathy in male young offenders. *Psychological Assessment: A Journal of Consulting and Clinical Psychology, 2*, 342-344.

Fox, N., & Davidson, R.J. (1988). Patterns of brain electrical activity during facial signs of emotion in 10-month-old infants. *Developmental Psychology, 24*, 230-236.

Geschwind, N. and Galaburda, A. (1987). *Cerebral Lateralization: Biological Mechanisms, Associations, and Pathology*. Cambridge: MIT Press.

Gillstrom, B., & Hare, R. D. (1988). Language-related hand gestures in psychopaths. *Journal of Personality Disorders, 2*, 21-27.

Gorenstein, E.E. & Newman, J.P. (1980). Disinhibitory psychopathology: A new perspective and a model for research. *Psychological Review, 87*, 301-315.

Graves, R., Landis, T., & Goodglass, H. (1981). Laterality and sex differences for visual recognition of emotional and non-emotional words. *Neuropsychologia, 19*, 95-102.

Gretton, H., McBride, M., O'Shaughnessy, R., & Hare, R.D. (1994, March). Patterns of violence and victimization in psychopathic adolescent sex offenders. Meeting of the American Psychology and Law Society, Sante Fe, New Mexico, March, 1994.

Gretton, H., O'Shaughnessy, R., & Hare, R.D. (1997). Psychopathy and recidivism in adolescent sex offenders. Manuscript in preparation.

Hare, R.D. (1965). Temporal gradient of fear arousal in psychopaths. *Journal of Abnormal Psychology, 70*, 442-445.

Hare, R.D. (1968). Psychopathy, autonomic functioning, and the orienting response. *Journal of Abnormal Psychology, 73*, Monograph Supplement, No. 3, Part 2, 1-24.

Hare, R.D. (1970). *Psychopathy: Theory and Research*. New York: Wiley.

Hare, R.D. (1973). Orienting and defensive responses to visual stimuli. *Psychophysiology, 10*, 453-464.

Hare, R.D. (1978). Electrodermal and cardiovascular correlates of psychopathy (pp. 107-144), In R.D. Hare and D. Schalling (eds.), *Psychopathic Behavior: Approaches to Research*, Chichester, England: Wiley.

Hare, R.D. (1984). Performance of psychopaths on cognitive tasks related to frontal lobe functions. *Journal of Abnormal Psychology, 93*, 133-140.

Hare, R.D. (1991). *The Hare Psychopathy Checklist-Revised*. Toronto, Ontario: Multi-Health Systems.

Hare, R.D. (1993). *Without Conscience: The Disturbing World of the Psychopaths Among Us*. New York: Pocket Books. (Paperback edition, 1995).

Hare, R.D. (1996). Psychopathy: A construct whose time has come. *Criminal Justice and Behavior, 23*, 25-54.

Hare, R. D., and Craigen, D. (1974). Psychopathy and physiological activity in a mixed-motive game situation. *Psychophysiology, 11*, 197-206.

Hare, R.D., Frazelle, J., and Cox, D.N. (1978). Psychopathy and physiological responses to threat of aversive stimulation. *Psychophysiology, 15*, 165-172.

Hare, R.D., & Gillstrom, B. (1997). Hand gestures and speech encoding difficulties in psychopaths. Manuscript in preparation.

Hare, R. D., Hart, S., & Forth, A. E. (1989). The psychopath as clinical prototype for lying and deception. In J. Yuille (ed.), *Credibility Assessment*. Dordrecht, The Netherlands: Martinus Nijhoff.

Hare, R.D., and Jutai, J.W. (1988). Psychopathy and cerebral asymmetry in semantic processing. *Personality and Individual Differences, 9*, 329-337.

Hare, R.D., and Quinn, M. (1971). Psychopathy and autonomic conditioning. *Journal of Abnormal Psychology, 77*, 223-235.

Hare, R.D., Williamson, S.E., & Harpur, T.J. (1988). Psychopathy and language. In T. E. Moffitt & S. A. Mednick (Eds.), *Biological contributions to crime causation* (pp. 68-92). Dordrecht, The Netherlands: Martinus Nijhoff.

Harpending, H., & Sobus, J. (1987). Sociopathy as an adaption. *Ethology and Sociobiology, 8*, 63-72.

Harpur, T.J., Hare, R.D., & Hakstian, A.R. (1989). Two-factor conceptualization of psychopathy: Construct validity and assessment implications. *Journal of Consulting and Clinical Psychology, 1*, 6-17.

Harris, G. T., Rice, M. E., & Quinsey, V.L. (1994). Psychopathy as a taxon: Evidence that psychopaths are a discrete class. *Journal of Consulting and Clinical Psychology, 62*, 387-397.

Hart, S.D., Cox, D.N., & Hare, R.D. (1995). *The Hare Psychopathy Checklist: Screening Version*. Toronto: Multi-Health Systems.

Hart, S. D., Forth, A. E., & Hare, R. D. (1990). Neuropsychological assessment of criminal psychopaths. *Journal of Abnormal Psychology, 99*, 374-379.

Hart, S.D., & Hare, R.D. (in press). Psychopathy: Assessment and association with criminal conduct. In D. Stoff, J.Breiling, & J. Maser (eds.). *Handbook of antisocial behavior*. New York: Wiley.

Hayes, J., & Hare, R.D. (1997) Psychopathy and confusion of emotional polarity during processing of metaphorical statements. Manuscript in preparation.

Heilman, K., Swartz, H.D., & Watson, R.T. (1978). Hypoarousal in patients with the neglect syndrome and emotional indifference. *Neurology, 28*, 229-232.

Howland, E.W., Kosson, D.S., Patterson, C.M. and Newman, J.P. (1993) Altering a dominant response: Performance of psychopaths and low-socialization college students on a cued reaction time task. *Journal of Abnormal Psychology, 102*, 379-387.

Intrator, J., Hare, R.D., Stritzke, P., Brichtswein, K., Dorfman, D., Harpur, T., Bernstein, D., Handelsman, L., Keilp, J., Rosen, J., & Machac, J. (1997). A brain imaging (SPECT) study of semantic and affective processing in psychopaths. *Biological Psychiatry, 42*, 96-103.

Intrator, J., Keilp, J., Dorfman, D., Bernstein, D., Schaefer, C., Wakeman, J., Harpur, T., Hare, R., Handelsman, L., & Stritske, P. (1993, September). Cerebral activation of emotion words in psychopaths. Third International Congress of the International Society for the Study of Personality Disorders, Cambridge, MA, September 8-11, 1993.

Johns, J.H., & Quay, H.C. (1962). The effect of social reward on verbal conditioning in psychopaths and neurotic military offenders. *Journal of Consulting Psychology, 26*, 217-220.

Johnson, W. (1946). *People in Quandaries: The Semantics of Personal Adjustment*. New York: Harper & Brothers.

Jutai, J., and Hare, R.D. (1983). Psychopathy and selective attention during performance of a complex perceptual-motor task. *Psychophysiology, 20*, 146-151.

Kiehl, K.A., Mangun, G.R., & Hare,R.D. (1995, March) Hemispheric processing of affective language: An ERP study. Poster presented at the Cognitive Neuroscience Society Annual Conference. San Francisco.

Lacey, J. I. (1967). Somatic response patterning and stress: Some revisions of activation theory. In M.H. Appley & R. Trumbell (eds), *Psychological Stress: Issues in Research*, New York: Appleton-Century-Crofts.

Lapierre, D., Braun, M. J., & Hodgins, S. (1995). Ventral frontal deficits in psychopathy: Neuropsychological test findings. *Neuropsychologia, 11*, 139-151.

Larbig, W., Veit, R., Rau, H., Schlottke, P., & Birbaumer, N. (1992, October). Cerebral and peripheral correlates in psychopaths during anticipation of aversive stimulation. Paper presented at Annual Meeting of the Society for Psychophysiological Research, San Diego.

Levenston, G.K., Patrick, C.J., Bradley, M.M., & Lang, P.J. (1996, October). Psychopathy and startle modulation during affective picture processing: A replication and extension. Annual meeting of the Society for Psychophysiological Research, Vancouver, Canada, October 16-20, 1996.

Levin, B. and Duchowny, M. (1991). Childhood obsessive-compulsive disorder and cingulate epilepsy. *Biological Psychiatry, 30*, 1049-1055.

Lindner, R. (1944). *Rebel Without a Cause.* New York, NY: Grune & Stratton.

Louth, S.M., Williamson, S.E., Alpert, M., Pouget, E.R., & Hare, R.D. (in press). Acoustic distinctions in the speech of psychopaths. Journal of Psycholinguistic Research.

Lykken, D.T. (1957). A study of anxiety in the sociopathic personality. *Journal of Abnormal and Social Psychology, 55*, 6-10.

Lykken, D.T. (1968). Neuropsychology and neurophysiology in personality research ((pp. 413-509), In E. Borgotta & W. Lambert (eds.), *Handbook of Personality Theory and Research*, New York: Rand McNally.

Lykken, D.T. (1995). *The Antisocial Personalities*, Hillsdale, NJ: Lawrence Erlbaum.

MacMillan, J., & Kofoed, L. (1984). Sociobiology and the antisocial personality: An alternative perspective. *The Journal of Nervous and Mental Diseases, 172*, 448-457.

Mangun, G.R. (1995), Neural mechanisms of visual selective attention. *Psychophysiology, 32*, 4-18.

Marcos, L. R. (1979). Nonverbal behavior and thought processing. *Archives of General Psychiatry, 36*, 940-943.

Mealey L. (1995). The sociobiology of sociopathy: An integrated evolutionary model. *Behavioral and Brain Sciences, 18*, 523-599.

Meloy, J. R. (1995). Antisocial personality disorder. In G. Gabbard (Ed.), *Treatment of psychiatric disorders* (2nd ed.) (pp. 2273-2290). Washington, DC: American Psychiatric Press.

Merewether, F.C., & Alpert, M. (1990). The components and neuroanatomic bases of prosody. *Journal of Communication Disorders, 23*, 325-336.

McNeill, D. (1985) So you think gestures are nonverbal. *Psychology Review, 91*, 332-350.

McNeill, D., and Levy, E. (1982). Conceptual representations in language activity and gesture. In R. J. Jarvella and W. Klein (eds), *Speech, Place and Action: Studies in Deixis and Related Topics.* Chichester, England: Wiley.

Mills, B. (1995). Cerebral asymmetry in psychopaths: A behavioral and electrocortical investigation. Unpublished doctoral dissertation, University of British Columbia, Vancouver, Canada.

Mowrer, O.H. (1960). *Learning theory and the symbolic processes.* New York: Wiley.

Newlove, T., Hart, S.D., & Dutton, D. (1992). Psychopathy and family violence. Unpublished manuscript, Department of Psychology, University of British Columbia, Vancouver, Canada.

Newman, J.P. and Kosson, D.S. (1986). Passive avoidance learning in psychopathic and nonpsychopathic offenders. *Journal of Abnormal Psychology, 95*, 252-256.

Newman, J.P., Patterson, C.M., Howland, E.W. and Nichols, S.L. (1990). Passive avoidance in psychopaths: The effects of reward. *Personality and Individual Differences, 11,* 1101-1114.

Newman, J. P., Patterson, C. M., & Kosson, D. S. (1987). Response perseveration in psychopaths. *Journal of Abnormal Psychology, 96,* 145-148.

Newman, J. P., & Wallace, J. F. (1993). Diverse pathways to deficient self-regulation: Implications for disinhibitory psychopathology in children. *Clinical Psychology Review, 13,* 699-720.

Newman, J.P., Widom, C.S. and Nathan, S. (1985). Passive avoidance in syndromes of disinhibition: Psychopathy and extroversion. *Journal of Personality and Social Psychology, 48,* 1316-1327.

Ogloff, J. R., & Wong, S. (1990). Electrodermal and cardiovascular evidence of a coping response in psychopaths. *Criminal Justice and Behavior, 17,* 231-245.

Paivio, A. (1986). *Mental Representations: A Dual Coding Approach.* London: Oxford University Press.

Patrick, C.J. (1994). Emotion and psychopathy: Startling new insights. *Psychophysiology, 31,* 319-330.

Patrick, C.J., Bradley, M.M., & Lang, P.J. (1993). Emotion in the criminal psychopath: Startle reflex modulation. *Journal of Abnormal Psychology, 102,* 82-92.

Patrick, C. J., Cuthbert, B. N., & Lang, P. J. (1994). Emotion in the criminal psychopath: Fear image processing. *Journal of Abnormal Psychology, 103,* 523-534.

Peterson, S.E., Fox, P.T., Snyder, A.Z., & Raichle, M.E. (1990). Activation of extrastriate and frontal cortical areas by visual words and word-like stimuli. *Science, 249,* 1041-1044.

Pfefferbaum, A., Wenegrat, B.G., Ford, J.M., Roth, W.T., & Kopell, B.S. (1984). Clinical applications of the P3 component of event-related potentials. II. Dementia, depression and schizophrenia. *Electroencephalography and Clinical Neurophysiology, Supplement, 59,* 104-124.

Plutchik, R. (1980). *Emotion: A Psychoevoluntionary Synthesis.* New York: Harper and Row.

Raine, A., O'Brien, M., Smiley, N., Scerbo, A., & Chan, C. (1990). Reduced lateralization in verbal dichotic listening in adolescent population. *Journal of Abnormal Psychology, 99,* 272-277.

Rime, B., Bouvy, H., Leborgne, B., & Rouillon, F. (1978). Psychopathy and nonverbal behavior in an interpersonal situation. *Journal of Abnormal Psychology, 87,* 636-643.

Rime, B., & Schiaratura, L. (1990). Gesture and speech. In R. Feldman & B. Rime (Eds.). *Fundamentals of Nonverbal Behavior.* New York: Cambridge University Press.

Rugg, M.D. (1985). The effects of semantic priming and word repetition on event-related potentials. *Psychophysiology, 22,* 642-647.

Safer, M.A. (1981). Sex and hemisphere differences in access to codes for processing emotional expressions and faces. *Journal of Experimental Psychology: General, 110,* 86-110.

Salekin, R.T., Rogers, R., & Sewell, K.W. (1996). A review and meta-analysis of the Psychopathy Checklist-Revised: Predictive validity of dangerousness. *Clinical Psychology: Science and Practice, 3,* 203-214.

Silberman, E.K., & Weingartner, H.W. (1986). Hemispheric lateralization of functions related to emotion. *Brain and Cognition, 5,* 322-353.

Smith, S.S., Arnett, P.A., & Newman, J.P. (1992). Neuropsychological differentiation of psychopathic and nonpsychopathic criminal offenders. *Personality and Individual Differences, 13,* 1233-1243.

Squire, L.R. (1987). Memory: Neural organization and behavior. In F. Plum (ed.), *Handbook of Physiology. The Nervous System.* Bethesda, MD: American Physiological Society.

Strachan, C.E., & Hare, R.D. (1997). Assessment of psychopathy in female offenders. Manuscript under review.

Strauss, E. (1983). Perception of emotional words. *Neuropsychologia, 21,* 99-103.

Sutton, S.K., Davidson, R.J., & Rogers, G.M. (1996, October). Resting anterior asymmetry predicts affect-related information processing. Annual meeting of the Society for Psychophysiological Research, Vancouver, Canada, October 16-20, 1996.

Tranel, D., & Damasio, H. (1994). Neuroanatomical correlates of electrodermal skin conductance responses. *Psychophysiology, 31*, 427-438.

Williamson, S.E. (1991). Cohesion and coherence in the speech of psychopathic criminals. Unpublished doctoral dissertation. University of British Columbia, Vancouver.

Williamson, S. E., Hare, R. D., & Wong, S. (1987). Violence: Criminal psychopaths and their victims. *Canadian Journal of Behavioral Science, 19*, 454-462.

Williamson, S.E., Harpur, T.J., & Hare, R.D. (1990, August). Sensitivity to emotional polarity in psychopaths. Paper presented at American Psychological Association Meeting, Boston, MA, August, 1990.

Williamson, S.E., Harpur, T.J., and Hare, R.D. (1991). Abnormal processing of affective words by psychopaths. *Psychophysiology, 28*, 260-273.

Author's notes

Preparation of this chapter and some of the research reported herein were supported by grants from the British Columbia Health Research Foundation, the British Columbia Medical Services Foundation, and the Medical Research Council of Canada. The cooperation of staff and inmates of the Correctional Service of Canada, and the assistance of Andra Smith and Kent Keihl in the preparation of this chapter, are greatly appreciated. Correspondence about this article should be addressed to Robert D. Hare, Department of Psychology, 2136 West Mall, University of British Columbia, Vancouver, Canada, V6T 1Z4. E-mail: rhare@unixg.ubc.ca.

BIOLOGY AND PERSONALITY: FINDINGS FROM A LONGITUDINAL PROJECT

BRITT AF KLINTEBERG
Department of Psychology
Stockholm University
Stockholm, Sweden.

INTRODUCTION

The activity of the enzyme monoamine oxidase (MAO) in blood platelets, which is assumed to reflect central serotonergic function (for a review, see Oreland, 1993), has been found to be of particular interest in understanding the biological bases for antisocial behavior and psychosocial disorders. Platelet MAO activity has recently been found to be related to persistent criminal behavior over the life span in a group of males with a history of early criminal behavior (Alm et al., 1994). This finding is of interest, since impulsivity-related personality traits, associated with platelet MAO activity (for a review, see Schalling, 1993) have, in turn, been shown to be useful as intermediates between biological 'vulnerability' and psychosocial disturbances, such as criminal behavior, alcohol problems and other forms of psychosocial disorders and disinhibitory syndromes (Barratt & Patton, 1983; af Klinteberg, Humble & Schalling, 1992; White et al., 1994). It has been proposed that only some aspects of the impulsivity concept, like those more related to disinhibitory tendencies, might be critical for the association with indications of dysfunctioning central serotonergic turnover (af Klinteberg et al., 1992). Of special interest for the present issue is violent behavior. High impulsivity indicates a vulnerability to act in a destructive way in stressful situations, often combined with a weak ability to foresee consequences of one's own behavior (Gorenstein & Newman, 1980; Shapiro, 1965).

In the following discussions, aspects of psychobiological functioning in a group of normal male and female subjects within a longitudinal program have been described. The main issue concerned risk factors within the area of the development of personality and antisocial behavior. The focus was on testing an interactive psychobiological vulnerability model, examining associations between psychological and biological indicators of vulnerability for psychosocial disturbances, particularly psychopathy.

When testing a vulnerability model, psychopathic personality is considered a dimension, in contrast to a category, as it is regarded in clinical work. The present research is based on the assumption that there are differences among normal subjects as to their vulnerability to externalizing disturbances, antisocial behavior, and psychopathy-related personality traits (see Figure 1). Certain of the components in these disorders, whether genetically influenced or due to early environmental causes, are manifested early in life as more subtle disturbances than those seen in clinical disorders. Among childhood disturbances found to be precursors of adult psychosocial

D.J. Cooke et al. (eds.), Psychopathy: Theory, Research and Implications for Society, 139–160.

disturbances and psychopathy are hyperactive behaviors - motor restlessness, impulsivity, and concentration difficulties (Satterfield, 1987; Taylor, 1988). Although aggressiveness has sometimes been included in this behavior syndrome, there are arguments for regarding aggressiveness as a separate dimension (McBurnett et al., 1993; McGee, Williams & Silva, 1985; af Klinteberg, Magnusson & Schalling, 1989; af Klinteberg .& Oreland, 1995). In these behavior precursors, as well as in adult psychopathy, signs of disturbances in neurochemical functions related to serotonergic activity in the central nervous system (CNS) and also in endocrine functions, e.g., adrenal-medullary activity/reactivity, have been reported (Kruesi et al., 1992; Lidberg, Modin, Oreland, Tuck & Gillner, 1985; Satterfield, 1987; Zahn, Kruesi, Leonard & Rapaport, 1994).

CATEGORICAL   **DIMENSIONAL**

The Diagnostic and Statistical Manual of Mental Disorders DSM III (Axis II)	Cleckley Hare	Personality syndrome Vulnerability model
Antisocial Personality Disorder (APD)	**Psychopathy**	**Psychopathic personality**
APD Criteria	PCL (Psychopathy Checklist)	EPQI, KSP Neuropsychological tasks
Behavior. criminal acts and lack of remorse	Behavior and personality	Personality traits and Cognitive style
Conduct Disorder (CD)	Attention Deficit Hyperactivity Disorder (ADHD)?	Hyperactive behavior Aggressiveness. Impulsiveness

Figure 1. Categorical and dimensional approaches in the study of antisocial and psychopathic personality. (From 'The psychopathic personality in a longitudinal perspective', by B. af Klinteberg, 1996, European Child and Adolescent Psychiatry, in press. Reprinted by permission.)

The studies to be reported here were performed on a group of normal male and female subjects (about 10 years of age, n = 541 and n = 551, respectively, up to adult age) within the Swedish project 'Individual Development and Adjustment' (IDA). The specific investigation group, representative of the total sample, which was employed in the biological analyses, consisted of boys and girls from whom the following data were collected: behavioral data at the age of 10 and 13 years; physiological measures at age 13; normbreaking behaviors at age 15; and personality and biological measures at age 26-27 years. Thus, the same individuals were followed over time from age ten to early adult life. The 'biological investigation' was completed on 82 male and 87 female subjects. Data concerning alcohol problems and criminality were obtained from police records during the age period of 15-25 and 15-40 years of age, respectively. There was no attrition (for detailed reports of the group and of the various measures, see Magnusson, 1988; af Klinteberg, 1996).

PERSONALITY CORRELATES OF BIOCHEMICAL CHARACTERISTICS AT ADULT AGE: RELATIONSHIPS WITH EARLY BEHAVIORS

In view of the above described hypothesis of vulnerability, the longitudinal prospective data on this non-clinical sample offered the opportunity to investigate the predictive influence of childhood behaviors on adult personality, reflecting the dimension adjustment-maladjustment. A dimensional description of personality syndromes was performed, separately for male and female subjects. The resulting syndromes were examined in relation to childhood behaviors assumed to be differentially reflecting vulnerability to externalizing and internalizing psychosocial disturbances. The personality dimensions were then related to biochemical factors in the representative sample of young male and female subjects within the project. Subsequently, childhood behaviors and personality scale scores were studied in relation to biochemical patterns at adult age.

A dimensional description of personality and relationships with childhood behaviors

For a dimensional description of the Karolinska Scales of Personality (KSP) self-report inventory at adult age, factor analyses were performed (af Klinteberg, Schalling & Magnusson, 1986). Scales included in the inventory were designed for the definition of certain vulnerability traits, the construct of which are derived from theories of biologically based temperament dimensions underlying psychiatric disorders. A description of extreme scorers on these scales is given in Schalling and co-workers (Schalling, Åsberg, Edman, & Oreland, 1987). The 15 KSP scales are classified on the basis of rational-theoretical considerations into four broad constructs: (1) introversion-extraversion related scales: impulsiveness, monotony avoidance and detachment (reversed); (2) conformity-nonconformity scales: socialization and social desirability; (3) anxiety-related scales: somatic anxiety, psychic anxiety, muscular tension, psychasthenia and inhibition of aggression; and (4) aggressivity-related scales: (a) aggression scales: indirect aggression, verbal aggression and irritability, and (b) hostility scales: suspicion and guilt (for more information about the scales, see af Klinteberg et al., 1990).

In the male group, a broad psychopathy-related factor, two anxiety factors (denoted as 'cognitive-social anxiety' and 'nervous tension and distress'), and an aggressive nonconformity factor were obtained. Low socialization was associated with high impulsivity and monotony avoidance. In females, the factors obtained were congruent with the Eysenckian personality structure (Eysenck & Eysenck, 1975), yielding one broad anxiety factor denoted as 'negative emotionality', one aggressive nonconformity factor, and one extraversion factor that included three aspects of extraversion — impulsivity, sensation seeking, and sociability.

It is noteworthy that, in males, maladjustment in general was associated with high extraversion and psychopathy-related traits, whereas in females it was associated with low extraversion, with 'dysthymic' vulnerability and with anxiety traits. An investigation of the relationships between the personality factors and vulnerability indicators from teacher ratings of behavior at age 13 was then undertaken (af Klinteberg, Schalling & Magnusson, 1990). The main findings for males were: (1) a significant positive relationship between childhood 'externalizing' (hyperactive-aggressive) behavior and the adult personality factor defined by the psychopathy-related scales, assumed to reflect impulsivity, sensation seeking, and low socialization (p<.01), and (2) a significant positive relationship between childhood timidity/shyness and the adult anxiety factors (p<.05). Among females, there were mixed relationships between early behavior and adult personality: motor restlessness correlated significantly and positively (p<.01), whereas aggressiveness tended to show a positive relationship over time with the extraversion factor. The findings on these normal subjects were consistent with clinical studies, suggesting that there is a high continuity of antisocial, 'externalizing' problems over time, especially among males.

Integrating biology

Considering the character of the present personality scales as assumed indicators of different kinds of vulnerability, it might be possible to link the relative stability of psychopathy-related early behaviors and corresponding personality scales to underlying biochemical bases. Several studies suggest the involvement of neurochemical systems in hyperactive and psychopathy-related behaviors and traits (for reviews, see Hare & Schalling, 1978; Zuckerman, 1991). Although impulsive-aggressive and disinhibited behaviors have been associated with low serotonergic activity in the CNS (Virkkunen & Linnoila, 1993), platelet MAO activity is a more accessible biological indicator. The possible mechanisms behind the correspondence between platelet MAO activity and processes in the CNS are reviewed in Oreland and Hallman (1995). It is noteworthy that in a non-linear examination of college students that related personality traits to MAO activity in groups of normals (af Klinteberg, Schalling, Edman, Oreland & Åsberg, 1987), low MAO activity was strongly associated with high scores in impulsivity related scales for both male and female subjects. Furthermore, in congruence with earlier findings (Murphy et al., 1976), males were found to have significantly lower platelet MAO activity than female subjects.

Other biochemical measures of interest in connection with externalizing disturbances and antisocial behaviors are thyroid activity and cortisol and testosterone levels. A generalized resistance to thyroid hormones was recently reported to be associated with Attention-Deficit Hyperactivity Disorder (ADHD) (Hauser et al., 1993), whereas an excess of thyroid functioning has been found to be related to a decrease in sympathetic activity in groups of male subjects with different forms of psychosocial deviancy (Moss, Guthrie & Linnoila, 1986; Whybrow & Prange, 1981). In a study within a longitudinal project on young lawbreakers, preliminary results indicated that thyroid levels were positively connected to persistent criminal behavior (Alm et al., 1996). Levels of plasma cortisol have been inversely related to high impulsivity in healthy volunteers (King, Jones, Scheuer, Curtis & Zarcone, 1990), and low levels of urinary cortisol have been found in groups of young offenders (Levander, Mattson, Schalling & Dalteg, 1987), in subjects suffering from lack of fear or anxiety, and in individuals showing disinhibitory tendencies (Schalling, 1993). Since steroid hormones are reported to be related to personality and to certain aspects of human behavior (Dabbs, Hopper & Jurkovic, 1990; Olweus, 1986), estimates of plasma levels of the androgens testosterone and dehydroepiandrosterone sulfate (DHEAS), as well as of estradiol, were included in the present study. Finally, prolactin was included for exploratory reasons concerning assumed hormonal influences on psychological development (Gray, Jackson & McKinlay, 1991).

Personality dimensions as related to biochemical factors

Correlation coefficients (product-moment) were calculated between the described personality dimensions and biochemical factors based on the biochemical variables included in the study, separately for male and female subjects (af Klinteberg & Magnusson, 1996). Among males, there were strong positive relationships between the adult psychopathy-related personality dimension and (1) a biochemical factor defined by positive loadings on dopamine and on the testosterone-related measure DHEAS (denoted the DA-DHEAS factor) ($p<.01$) and (2) a factor defined by positive loadings on testosterone and negative loadings on cortisol (denoted the TESTO-CORT-related factor) ($p<.001$). Furthermore, there was a trend toward a negative association between this psychopathy-related personality dimension and a biochemical factor defined by positive loadings on serum noradrenaline, adrenaline, prolactin and cortisol (denoted the NA-ADR-PRO-CORT factor) ($p<.10$). No significant relationships were observed between the other personality dimensions and biochemical factors.

For female subjects, there was a trend toward a relation between the extraversion personality dimension and a biochemical factor denoted by negative loadings on dopamine and positive loadings on noradrenaline and DHEAS (denoted the DA-NA-DHEAS-related factor) ($p<.10$). Taken together, these results indicate relationships between personality and biochemical factors in groups of normals only concerning psychopathy- and extraversion-related personality dimensions.

Childhood behaviors and adult personality as related to biochemical patterns at adult age

In the next step of the research, subjects were grouped/clustered on the basis of their factor scores (transformed into z-scores) on the obtained biochemical factors, separately for male and female subjects, according to a hierarchical method (WARD), using squared Euclidean distance (af Klinteberg & Magnusson, 1996). Preliminary results indicated the following: For the male subjects, a solution of five clusters differing in the biochemical factors was chosen. A cluster characterized by low scores (mean z-score: -1.5) on a biochemical factor with positive loadings on the two platelet MAO substrates (denoted the MAO factor), combined with high scores (mean z-score: 1.1) on the TESTO-CORT-related factor, was associated with higher childhood concentration difficulties ($p<.02$), aggressiveness ($p<.05$), stable hyperactive and aggressive behaviors ($p<.10$), disharmony ($p<.02$), being bored of school ($p<.01$); and with lower adult socialization ($p<.02$), and higher somatic anxiety ($p<.10$) as compared to the other clusters. A second cluster, characterized by high scores (mean z-score: 1.2) on the NA-ADR-PRO-CORT factor and scores close to mean on the MAO factor, displayed lower childhood problem behaviors, in terms of concentration difficulties, hyperactive behavior, aggressiveness ($p<.05$), being bored of school, and disharmony ($p<.001$); and higher adult socialization ($p<.10$) combined with lower somatic anxiety indications ($p<.05$) as compared to the former male cluster.

For females, in a solution of four clusters differing in the biochemical factors, one cluster, characterized by low scores (mean z-score: -1.2) on a biochemical factor defined by positive loadings on the two platelet MAO substrates and on thyroid-stimulating hormone (TSH) (denoted the MAO-TSH factor), and high scores (mean z-score: 1.0) on the DA-NA-DHEAS-related factor, was associated with a tendency to higher childhood concentration difficulties, lower school aspiration; and higher adult suspicion as compared to the other female clusters. In comparison to a normative female cluster, characterized by scores within one standard deviation above the mean scores in all three biochemical factors, the first cluster females displayed significantly lower adult socialization ($p<.01$). A third female cluster, characterized by high scores (mean z-score: 1.0) on a factor defined by positive loadings on serum testosterone, estrogen, and adrenaline (denoted the TESTO-OEST-ADR factor), combined with low scores (mean z-score: -1.5) on the DA-NA-DHEAS-related factor, displayed lower scores on childhood concentration difficulties, motor restlessness, stable hyperactive behavior ($p<.05$); and a tendency to lower adult impulsiveness scores than was observed among the first cluster females.

Concluding remarks

The results were discussed in terms of certain imbalances in biochemical patterns as possible risk factors for developing psychosocial disturbances as indicated by early behaviors. In the male group, associations between externalizing childhood behaviors and psychopathy-related personality traits and between internalizing childhood behavior and anxiety traits were found over a time period of 14 years. For female subjects, there was a paucity of relationships although motor restlessness was related over the life span with an extraversion dimension (impulsiveness, monotony avoidance, and sociability). It was suggested that females might be more susceptible to life changes, thus attenuating the prospective influence of childhood behavior. Moreover, personality factors of adult personality indicated that low socialization was related to high scores on impulsiveness and monotony avoidance scales in the male group, whereas among the female subjects it was associated with high scores on anxiety-related scales (af Klinteberg et al., 1990).

Finally, in this sample it was found that biochemical patterns grouped individuals who differed in childhood behavior and adult personality vulnerability indicators of psychosocial disturbances, both among males (as indicated by low socialization and high somatic anxiety) and more weakly among females (nonconformity, hostility, and impulsivity). It is noteworthy that low platelet MAO activity characterized one each of the male and female individual-related groups/clusters. This finding is consistent with the assumption that platelet MAO activity constitutes a vulnerability factor present in normal subjects as well as in relatives of patients. In the presence of other risk factors, such 'vulnerable' subjects might be more dependent than their less vulnerable counterparts on the quality of environmental support during the developmental process. The role of differential socialization processes in male and female subjects has been discussed (Caspi, Lynam, Moffitt & Silva, 1993; Stattin & Magnusson, 1990), and the importance of using measures of greater sensitivity to differences in socialization between the sexes has been emphasized (McCord, 1993).

BIOLOGY, NORMBREAKING BEHAVIOR, AND PERSONALITY

In a further study (af Klinteberg, 1995), it was hypothesized (1) that a pattern of externalizing disturbances in childhood and high normbreaking during adolescence behavior are related to subsequent criminal behavior (violent and/or non-violent) and (2) that adolescent normbreaking and adult criminal behaviors are associated with adult psychopathy-related personality traits, which among female subjects are coupled with anxiety-related traits and with a pattern of neurochemical vulnerability to psychosocial deviance. To examine these relationships, the analyses were applied to prospective longitudinal data. Since most research in this domain has been focused on the study of males, special interest was devoted to the data obtained for the female subjects. Criminal offending (violent and non-violent for the male subjects) was studied in relation to childhood vulnerability indicators (i.e., Table 1) and adult personality, as well as to biochemical variables. Because there were few criminally active female subjects, the strategy was to highlight the characteristics of males and females who were possibly prone to criminal activity. Thus, subgroups based on levels of normbreaking behavior in adolescence were studied in relation to personality and biochemical measures at adult age.

Childhood behavior as related to subsequent criminal offending

Behavior ratings assumed to reflect externalizing disturbances in childhood differed clearly among male criminal groups, with motor restlessness separating the criminals (violent and non-violent) from non-criminals (see Table 1). For female subjects, the indicators of externalizing disturbances also differentiated the criminal groups from the non-criminals, with concentration difficulties being the key differentiating characteristic. Timidity, which had been assumed to reflect internalizing disturbances, did not differentiate either the male or the female groups.

TABLE 1. Differences of sub-groups of males — violent crime (VC, n = 40), non-violent crime (NVC, n = 163) and no crime (NC, n = 338) — in behavior ratings at age 13 years

	Group VC		Group NVC		Group NC				
	M	SD	M	SD	M	SD	F	p<	post-hoc
Indicators of 'externalizing disturbances'									
Aggressiveness	5.2	1.6	4.2	1.6	3.5	1.5	29.85	.0001	VCvsNC; VCvsNVC; NVCvcNC
Motor restlessness	5.2	1.4	4.6	1.7	3.5	1.7	37.99	.0001	VCvsNC; NVCvsNC
Concentration difficulties	.5.3	1.4	4.6	1.5	3.6	1.6	39.83	.0001	VCvsNC; VCvsNVC; NVCvsNC
Indicators of 'internalizing disturbances'									
Timidity	3.7	1.6	3.9	1.4	3.9	1.5	0.56	ns	

Note. One-way ANOVAs (df 2, 538) with behavior ratings as dependent and groups as independent variable, and significant post-hoc testing (Scheffé) between subgroups (p<0.05).

Personality as related to criminal offending

Among males, the criminals (whether violent or non-violent) differed from the non-criminals in having higher scores on the psychopathy-related impulsiveness (p<.001) and monotony avoidance (p<.01) scales, and lower scores on socialization (p<.001) and social desirability (p<.01). Moreover, the criminal male subjects had higher somatic anxiety in terms of muscular tension scores; they also displayed lower inhibition of aggression and higher scores on verbal aggression and on the hostility scale of suspicion (p<.05), as compared to the non-criminal male subjects who displayed scores close to normal means (T = 50). When comparing violent with non-violent subjects (non-violent criminals and non-criminals), an interesting pattern emerged for the violent group (see Figure 2), similar to that of criminal males but more extreme in certain dimensions. The pattern was characterized by high scores on the impulsiveness (T = 64; p<.01) and irritability scales (T = 57; p<.05) and low scores on socialization (T = 37; p<.001) and inhibition of aggression (T = 42; p<.05). Among female subjects, criminals tended to differ from non-criminals by displaying higher scores on the psychasthenia scale (reflecting cognitive-social anxiety: T = 59) and lower scores on the hostility scale of guilt (T = 43).

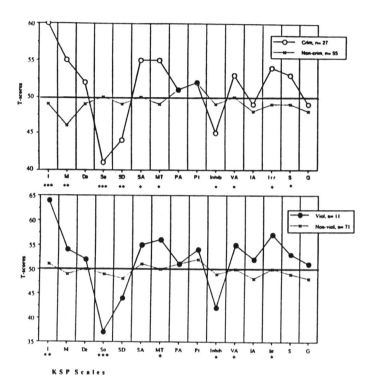

Figure 2. Comparison of mean personality scale scores, transformed into T scores, in a group of males (n = 82) at age 27, divided into subgroups with (a) criminal (crim, n = 27) and non-criminal (non-crim, n = 55) subjects; and with (b) violent (viol, n = 11) and non-violent criminal/non-criminal (non-viol, n = 71) subjects.

Note. Results of one-way ANOVAs are indicated by significance level (+p<.10; *p<.05; **p<.01; ***p<.001) and significant t (5 per cent) for subgroup comparisons (Scheffé); I = Impulsiveness; M = Monotony avoidance; De = Detachment; So = Socialization; SD = Social desirability; SA = Somatic anxiety; MT = Muscular tension; PA = Psychic anxiety; Pt = Psychasthenia; Inhib = Inhibition of aggression; VA = Verbal aggression; IA = Indirect aggression; Irr = Irritability; S = Suspicion; and G = Guilt.

Biochemical measures as related to criminal offending

What associations were then found between the biochemical indicators and criminal behavior? The results of one-way ANOVAs indicated differences between crime groups in platelet MAO activity for both male and female subjects. Among male subjects, the non-violent criminals exhibited the lower and the violent criminals the higher mean levels, with the non-criminals showing a mean z-score level close to the normal mean (F(2,68) = 3.48, p<.04). Among females, the criminal group displayed lower mean platelet MAO activity than did the non-criminal group (F(1,70) = 5.85, p<.02). None of the other biochemical measures indicated significant differences between crime groups for the males or the females.

Adult personality and biochemical measures in the light of adolescent normbreaking behavior

In adolescence, for male subjects, normbreaking behavior in terms of *'truancy'* and *'being drunk'* differentiated the criminal groups (violent and non-violent) from non-criminals, as indicated by higher scores (p<.0001). Normbreaking behaviors such as *'being out late without permission'* and *'shoplifting'* differed strongly among criminal behavior groups (p<.0001; post-hoc tests significant), with violent criminals displaying most frequent normbreaking behavior, non-criminals the less frequent and non-violent criminals exhibiting scores in between. For female subjects, all normbreaking items except *'cheating'* significantly differentiated criminals from non-criminals (see Table 2). These findings indicated some validity for the use of adolescent normbreaking scores to predict groups prone to criminal activity.

TABLE 2.   Normbreaking behavior at age 15 years. Violent/nonviolent crime sub-group (VC/NVC, n = 548) compared with no crime sub-group (NC, n = 502)

	VC/NVC	VC/NVC	NC	NC		
	M	SD	M	SD	F	P<
Normbreaking behaviors						
Obstinary defiance of parents	2.50	1.22	1.94	0.98	13.08	.0005
Being out late without permission	2.70	1.35	2.00	1.01	18.97	.0001
Drifting around in the city	2.35	1.08	1.93	1.10	6.08	.02
Shoplifting	2.09	1.28	1.63	0.99	8.54	.005
Truancy	2.91	1.50	1.94	1.17	27.74	.0001
Cheating	2.48	1.19	2.07	0.98	7.11	.01
Being drunk	2.80	1.60	1.88	1.24	22.03	.0001
Tried drugs	1.26	0.80	1.04	0.27	16.98	.0001
Sum of Normbreaking behaviors	19.1	7.50	14.4	5.3	30.59	.0001

Note.   One-way ANOVAs (df 1,546) with normbreaking behavior as dependent and group as independent variable.

Statistical analyses of the males indicated positive correlation coefficients between adolescent normbreaking behavior and both externalizing childhood behaviors (p<.001) and adult psychopathy-related personality traits (p<.05 - p<.001), and a negative correlation between normbreaking behavior and the biochemical indicator of psychosocial deviance - platelet MAO activity (p<.05 - p<.01). In the female group, there were no relations involving childhood behaviors; however, adolescent normbreaking behavior was associated with low adult socialization (p<.01) and with low platelet MAO activity (p<.01 - p< 001, see af Klinteberg, 1996).

In view of the difficulty of finding sufficiently large samples of females with criminal behavior, the alternative of using normbreaking behavior scores, to investigate antisocial personality patterns and biochemical profiles, was applied. Thus, the interest was focused on analyzing differences in personality scale scores and biochemical measures at adult age, between subgroups of subjects with different levels (low, intermediate, and high) of normbreaking behavior during adolescence, separately for male and female subjects.

The results of the analyses with respect to personality indicated, for the male subjects, differences on the impulsiveness (p<.01) and socialization scales (p<.05), with the high normbreaking group and the intermediate group being higher on impulsiveness than the low normbreaking group; the high normbreaking group lower on socialization than the low normbreaking group, and the intermediate group showing scores in between. Among females, there were differences between normgroups on the impulsiveness (p<.001) and socialization (p<.01) scales and a tendency to differ on the sensation-seeking related monotony avoidance scale and verbal aggression (p<.10); the high normbreaking group displayed a pattern of high impulsiveness and monotony avoidance, low socialization, and high indirect aggression.

Finally, the results of the analyses concerning the biochemical measures, transformed into z-scores indicated the following: Among male subjects, a pattern of differences between normgroups was found in platelet MAO activity (F(2,59) = 3.63, p<.05) and serum noradrenaline (F(2,58) = 3.76, p<.05), and a tendency to difference in serum TSH; the high normbreaking group displayed the lower levels in platelet MAO activity, noradrenaline, and TSH, as compared to low normbreaking male subjects. Among females, the only biochemical measure found to differ between normgroups was platelet MAO activity (F(2,66) = 4.28, p<.02); the high normbreaking group showed lower mean MAO activity level in comparison to the low normbreaking females (see af Klinteberg, 1996).

Concluding remarks

In the present study of normal groups, criminal behavior over the life span was associated with childhood externalizing and adolescent normbreaking behaviors in both male and female subjects. Furthermore, in the male group, criminal offending was found to be associated with adult psychopathy-related personality traits (high impulsiveness and monotony avoidance, and low socialization) and to the indirect indicator of disturbances in the serotonergic system, platelet MAO activity, in line with earlier findings on criminal and clinical groups (Alm et al., 1994; Schalling, 1993). Low and also high platelet MAO activity levels, as found in the present study among violent criminals, have in earlier research been associated with hostile and schizoid traits (Schalling, Åsberg, Edman & Oreland, 1987), which, in concurrence with psychopathy-related traits, were recently reported to be associated with serious violent behavior (Gacono & Meloy, 1994). Among female subjects, criminal offenders were characterized by higher scores in the anxiety-related scale psychasthenia and lower scores on the hostility scale guilt, which is partly consistent with findings by Caspi and collaborators (Caspi et al., 1994); this result suggests that negative emotionality accompanied by deficient impulse control might be more readily linked to antisocial acts in groups of females than in groups of males. Indications of a higher susceptibility to contextual variation in female subjects have also been discussed elsewhere (Caspi et al., 1993; Robins, 1986). However, in the Caspi study, the same tendency was also found in male subjects. Interestingly, in the present study, high normbreaking behavior in adolescence was associated with adult high impulsivity, low conformity, and signs of low platelet MAO activity, considered a biological marker of vulnerability for disinhibition in terms of impulsivity, impulsive cognitive style, and motor disinhibition, and for psychosocial deviances (Oreland, 1993).

Neuroendocrine responses to psychosocial environment are assumed to reflect the environment's emotional impact on and the situational involvement of the individual (Frankenhaeuser, 1983; Mason, 1975; Tucker & Williamsson, 1984). Children showing indications of externalizing problem behaviors seem to have limited abilities to perceive situational demands and thus diminished capabilities of interacting effectively with the environment (Douglas, 1984). Furthermore, there is evidence indicating that persistent offenders as a group have a more dysfunctional CNS than do control groups of non-offenders (Buikhuisen, 1987). It was assumed that unrecognized cognitive dysfunctions will interfere with the development of the socialization process, and the importance of identifying these cognitive dysfunctions at an early age was underscored. This line of research is noteworthy, in view of the present results of (1) strong associations between adolescent normbreaking behavior and indications of externalizing disturbances during childhood among male subjects; (2) the marked relations between adult criminal activity and childhood vulnerability indicators and adolescent normbreaking behavior among both males and females; and (3) the low MAO activity associated with criminal and high adolescent normbreaking behavior, in both male and female subjects.

Studies on groups of young offenders and healthy controls have indicated low levels of urinary cortisol in subjects with low fear or anxiety. However, in the present study of biochemical measures, no association was found between level of plasma cortisol and criminal and/or high adolescent normbreaking behavior. Concerning noradrenergic activity, it has been assumed that noradrenergic hyperactivity is associated with aspects of human anxiety states and that drugs with anti-anxiety effects reduce central noradrenergic function. It is notable, though caution is required, that the present results demonstrated (1) low levels of plasma noradrenaline for the high normbreaking male group and (2) a personality pattern including disinhibitory tendencies as reflected in high impulsivity scale scores and low socialization for high normbreaking male and female subjects. High impulsivity and relatively low cognitive-social anxiety, together with low socialization, are characteristics of theoretical interest, since they are in accordance with the psychopathic personality concept (Hare, 1991).

CO-EXISTING BEHAVIORAL MALADJUSTMENT PROBLEMS IN EARLY ADULT LIFE

Childhood hyperactivity and subsequent antisocial behavior have been related in previous studies (Loeber, 1990; Satterfield, 1987; Thorley, 1984), as have childhood hyperactivity and later alcohol abuse. Explanations of the origins of antisocial behavior and alcohol problems have focused either on the importance of psychosocial influences or on genetic-biological factors. When studying individual development from an interactional view on individual functioning, these two lines of theoretical approaches are regarded as complementary. This approach is illustrated in Figure 3, which shows measurable indicators in the interactional process that are assumed to reflect individual differences in resources for managing environmental demands. Psychosocial behavior problems often occur in the same subjects over time as empirically demonstrated in longitudinal studies. There are suggestions that early hyperactive behavior, antisocial behavior and alcohol problems have some common underlying mechanism, especially concerning the personality trait impulsivity and its associated biological indicators (af Klinteberg & Oreland, 1995; Oreland & Hallman, 1995; Anthenelli et al., 1995).

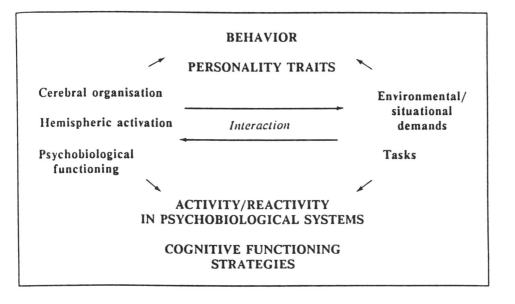

Figure 3. Measurable indicators, assumed to reflect individual differences in resources for managing environmental demands. (From 'Studies on sex-related psychological and biological indicators of psychosocial vulnerability: A developmental perspective', by af Klinteberg, 1988, Thesis. Reprinted by permission.)

Hyperactive behavior, later alcohol problems and violent offending possibly mediated by impulsivity?

In an earlier study within the present project, hyperactive behavior in childhood was found to be highly related to adult impulsivity (af Klinteberg et al., 1989). There is also empirical evidence for relationships between impulsivity, on the one hand, and alcohol problems and antisocial behavior, on the other (af Klinteberg et al., 1992; von Knorring, von Knorring, Smigan, Lindberg & Edholm, 1987). With regard to antisocial behavior, biological linkages are primarily attributable to aggressive, violent behavior (Brennan, Mednick & Mednick, 1993; Kruesi et al., 1992).

Previous findings suggest that normal children and adolescents with extreme platelet MAO activities, especially in the low end of the MAO distribution, are more impulsive on tests designed as indices of the dimension 'reflection - impulsivity' than are subjects with platelet MAO activity values in the middle range (af Klinteberg, Levander, Oreland, Åsberg & Schalling, 1987; Shekim et al., 1984). Associations have also been found between low MAO activity and alcohol abuse, hyperactivity, criminality, and psychopathy theoretically including high impulsivity (Hare, 1991; Lewis, 1991; Lidberg et al., 1985; Shekim et al., 1982; von Knorring, Oreland & von Knorring, 1987), see Figure 4.

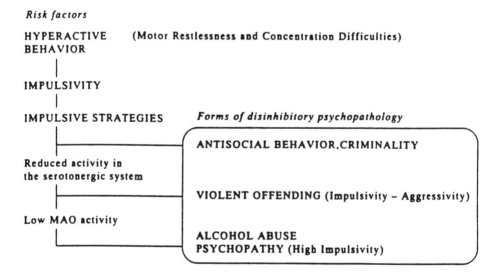

Figure 4. Illustration of a theoretical assumption that childhood hyperactive behavior, alcohol problems, and violent offending are linked to an underlying vulnerability of high impulsivity. (From 'Hyperactive behavior in childhood as related to subsequent alcohol problems and violent offending: A longitudinal study of male subjects, by af Klinteberg, Andersson, Magnusson, & Stattin, 1993, Personality and Individual Differences, 15, 381-388. Reprinted by permission.)

In the light of the above, the present interest was focused on the relationships between childhood hyperactive behavior, later alcohol problems, and violent offending.

It was hypothesized that hyperactive behavior in childhood is closely linked to later alcohol problems and to violent offending in the same individuals (af Klinteberg, Andersson, Magnusson & Stattin, 1993), hence constituting a subgroup among hyperactive children. To elucidate the existence of the three problem behaviors occurring in the same persons, a configural frequency analysis (CFA) (von Eye, 1990) was applied to test the existence of syndromes. The CFA compares the observed frequencies of all possible behavior combinations according to a chance model. A pattern that occurs more often than could be expected by chance is considered, according to the model, a significant configurational *'type'*; a pattern that occurs less often than could be expected by chance is denoted *'antitype'*. In such a person approach, individual functioning is the central interest and individuals are grouped on the basis of their characteristical patterns of level on behavioral variables relevant to the problem. In this case the behaviors were based on results of variable approach analyses.

Here, the critical pattern to be investigated was that of *'high'* hyperactive behavior, alcohol problems and violent offending. The *'hyperactive behavior'* indicator in the present examination was used as follows: the hyperactive group (subjects classified as high on both motor restlessness and concentration difficulties) was coded as *'high'*, and the other three groups (the non-hyperactive group and the groups with subjects low on either one of the components of hyperactive behavior) were coded as *'low'*. The maladjustment variables were coded as referring to having/not having a record for alcohol problem and/or violent offending. In line with the expectations, a significant overrepresentation of cell frequencies was found for a pattern indicating the co-occurrence of *'high'* childhood hyperactivity, subsequent alcohol problems, and violent offending in the same individuals (*'type'*, p<.0001); another significant pattern was defined by the co-occurrence of *'low'* hyperactive behavior in childhood, no subsequent alcohol problems, and no violent offending (*'type'*, p<.005). Furthermore, significant *'antitypes'* were found, implying that having only alcohol problems or having only been sentenced for violent offending, without exhibiting the other maladjustment indicators, occurred less often than expected according to a random model (see Table 3).

It is of interest to note that in the present study comprising a group of normal male subjects, violent offending appeared together with alcohol problems and childhood hyperactive behavior, in the same subjects, ten times more often than could be expected by chance. Conversely, a pattern of violent offending without alcohol problems and without early hyperactive behavior occurred about three times less often than could be expected by chance, thus supporting the prevalence of the former pattern. In contrast, in a large follow-up study of hyperactive children (Weiss, Hechtman, Milroy & Perlman, 1985), no clear relations between childhood hyperactive behavior and later alcohol problems were found. However, alcohol abuse has been discussed in terms of different types (von Knorring, Hallman, von Knorring & Oreland, 1991), one of which is assumed to have a strong genetic influence (Type II), showing an early onset and characterized by psychopathy-related personality traits (von Knorring et al., 1987). Age at onset has been discussed as a key criterion in the subclassification of alcoholism (von Knorring & Oreland, 1996).

TABLE 3. Configurations of dichotomized Hyperactive Behavior variable at 13, and presence-no presence of alcohol problems and violent offending up to age 25-26 for a group of normal males Ss (n = 540)

Pattern			Size			
Hyperactive behavior	Alcohol Problems	Violent offending	Obtained	Expected	Adjusted Significance	Type/ antitype
Low	No	No	344	306.7	<0.005	T
High	No	No	90	109.4	NS	
Low	Yes	No	41	65.5	<0.005	AT
High	Yes	No	30	23.4	NS	
Low	No	Yes	6	21.3	<0.005	AT
High	No	Yes	5	7.6	NS	
Low	Yes	Yes	7	4.5	NS	
High	Yes	Yes	17	1.6	<0.0001	T

Note. The adjusted level of significance was obtained by multiplying the nominal significance level by 8 (the number of possible variable combinations in the present design). From 'Hyperactive behavior in childhood as related to subsequent alcohol problems and violent offending: A longitudinal study of male subjects', by af Klinteberg, Anderson, Magnusson, & Stattin, 1993, Personality and Individual Differences, 15, 381-388. Reprinted by permission).

Moreover, the above-mentioned genetically influenced type of alcohol abuse has shown associations with low platelet MAO activity (von Knorring et al., 1991) and is only found in male subjects (von Knorring et al., 1987). Because, in the present study, the alcohol data covered the age range up to age 25, only early onset subjects were involved, perhaps accounting for the observed relation between hyperactive behavior and alcohol problems.

Childhood hyperactive and aggressive behaviors as related to low platelet MAO activity at adult age

The majority of the hyperactive behavior boys at age 13 were also rated high on aggressiveness (20/25). Earlier studies, within the present longitudinal project, on the specific contribution of hyperactive behavior and aggressiveness, respectively, to their significant associations with (1) level of sympathetic-adrenal activity in normal and stressful situations; and (2) adult impulsivity, indicated the following: Hyperactive behavior significantly contributed to the associations, whereas aggressiveness did not (af Klinteberg & Magnusson, 1989; af Klinteberg et al., 1989).

In a subsequent study of childhood externalizing behaviors and their linkage to possible underlying mechanisms, measures of adult platelet MAO activity were examined in relation to the persistence of relevant childhood behaviors. Behavior ratings pooled across the two age levels of 10 and 13 years were combined to yield an indicator of persistence for the variables hyperactive behavior and aggressiveness. A final solution of loglinear modeling, including two interactions, indicated that hyperactive behavior was negatively associated with MAO activity (p<.05); aggressiveness was strongly positively related to hyperactive behavior (p<.001), but not to platelet MAO activity per se (af Klinteberg & Oreland, 1995). In a configuration frequency analysis, both these interactions contributed positive effects to the statistical overrepresentation of individuals characterized by the pattern of 'high' persistent hyperactive behavior, 'high' persistent aggressiveness, and 'low' adult platelet MAO activity ('type', p<.005). The non-significant interaction between aggressiveness and the biochemical indicator examined here suggest a more peripheral importance of aggressiveness to an underlying mechanism and might support earlier assumptions of aggressiveness being more situation-dependent than hyperactive behavior, which appears to be more related to cognitive deficits (McGee et al., 1985).

Concluding remarks

The analyses in the present studies, examining relationships between childhood behaviors and sympathetic activity/reactivity and the assumed indirect indicator of central serotonergic turnover - platelet MAO activity - suggested a possible underlying biological indicator of vulnerability to psychosocial disturbances connected with childhood problem behaviors such as hyperactive and aggressive behaviors in the same individuals, prominently the hyperactive behavior component.

GENERAL DISCUSSION

The results presented support the assumption of underlying psychobiological mechanisms of the maladjustment problems discussed, indicating the possibility of (1) diminished capabilities for the individual to interact effectively with the environment in the socialization process and (2) a less mature CNS functioning in terms of subtle frontal dysfunctions, as indicated in disinhibited and impulsive behaviors. An underlying condition of abnormally low arousal and inhibitory levels in the CNS has been proposed as being common in disinhibitory syndromes (Gorenstein & Newman, 1980). Taken together, the results presented above underscore the possible importance of individual traits in the development of such disinhibitory psychosocial disorders. The present results specified psychopathy-related personality traits associated with biochemical levels, especially with low platelet MAO activity, among a group of normal subjects. The results are consistent with findings from clinical groups (Virkkunen & Linnoila, 1993).

However, the predominant risk indicator (low MAO activity), characterizing the form of psychosocial disorder evidenced in early onset (Type II) alcoholic males might, among a subgroup of low MAO activity female subjects, result in internalizing symptoms evidenced in somatizing tendencies, as suggested in a study on clinical groups (von Knorring et al., 1986). This suggestion is in accordance with the present findings of low socialization being associated with high extraversion and psychopathy-related traits in the normal male subjects, and with low extraversion, dysthymic vulnerability and anxiety traits in normal females. Type II alcoholic abuse has been found to be strongly associated with impulsive violent offending under the influence of alcohol (Virkkunen & Linnoila, 1993) and with mixed drug abuse (von Knorring et al., 1987).

The results of early childhood externalizing behaviors, alcohol problems, and violent offending in the same subjects in the present group of normal males, along with the associations between psychopathy-related traits and low platelet MAO activity in the same subjects, are congruent with the assumptions of genetically induced disinhibitory psychopathology (Oreland, 1993). Furthermore, signs of internalizing syndromes in subgroups of females with low socialization and/or low MAO activity are consistent with assumptions of somatizing problems in groups of female psychopaths (Lilienfeld, 1992), findings of a high rate of adult somatization disorders among female subjects characterized by childhood externalizing disturbances (Robins, 1986), and recently reported results of deficient serotonergic functioning in patients with anorexia nervosa (Brewerton & Jimerson, 1996).

In conclusion, the results presented here carry serious theoretical and strategy implications for this area of research: In the development of antisocial behavior, psychosocial influences and biological factors act together in the continuously ongoing process between the individual and his/her environment. From a theoretical point of view it is of crucial importance to follow groups of normal subjects, over time, to consider individual and sex-related differences, and to interpret the developmental process within a framework of interactional psychology.

References

Alm, P. O., af Klinteberg, B., Humble, K., Leppert, J., Sörensen, S., Tegelman, R., Thorell, L.-H., & Lidberg, L. (1996). Criminality and psychopathy as related to thyroid activity in juvenile delinquents grown up. Acta Psychiatrica Scandinavica, in press.

Alm, P. O., Alm, M., Humble, K., Leppert, J., Sörensen, S., Lidberg, L., & Oreland, L. (1994). Criminality and platelet monoamine oxidase activity in former juvenile delinquents as adults. *Acta Psychiatrica Scandinavica, 89*, 41-45.

Anthenelli, R. M., Smith, T. L., Craig, C. E., Tabakoff, B., & Schuckit, M. A. (1995). Platelet monoamine oxidase activity levels in subgroups of alcoholics: Diagnostic, temporal, and clinical correlates. *Biological Psychiatry, 38*, 361-368.

Barratt, E. S., & Patton, J. H. (1983). Impulsivity: Cognitive, behavioral, and psychophysiological correlates. In M. Zuckerman (Ed.), *Biological Bases of Sensation Seeking, Impulsivity and Anxiety*, (pp. 77-122). Hillsdale, NJ: Erlbaum.

Brennan, P. A., Mednick, B. R., & Mednick, S. A. (1993). Parental psychopathology, congenital factors and violence. In S. Hodgins (Ed.), *Mental Disorder and Crime*, (pp. in press). Newbury Park, Ca: Sage.

Brewerton, T. D. & Jimerson, D. C. (1996). Studies of serotonin function in anorexia nervosa. *Psychiatry Research, 62*, 31-42.

Buikhuisen, W. (1987). Cerebral dysfunctions and juvenile crime. In S. A. Mednick, T. E. Moffitt, & S. A. Stack (Eds.), *The Causes of Crime. New Biological Approaches*, (pp. 168-184). Cambridge: Cambridge University Press.

Caspi, A., Lynam, D., Moffitt, T. E., & Silva, P. A. (1993). Unraveling girls' delinquency: Biological, dispositional, and contextual contributions to adolescent misbehavior. *Developmental Psychology, 29(1)*, 19-30.

Caspi, A., Moffitt, T. E., Silva, P. A., Stouthamer-Loeber, M., Krueger, R. F., & Schmutte, P. S. (1994). Are some people crime-prone? Replications of the personality-crime relationship across countries, genders, races and methods. *Criminology, 32*, 163-195.

Dabbs, J. M., Hopper, C. H., & Jurkovic, G. J. (1990). Testosterone and personality among college students and military veterans. *Personality and Individual Differences, 11*, 1263-1269.

Douglas, V. I. (1984). Attentional and cognitive problems. In M. Rutter (Ed.), *Developmental Neuropsychiatry*, (pp. 280-329). New York: Churchill Livingstone.'

von Eye, A. (1990). *Introduction to Configural Frequency Analysis: The Search for Types and Antitypes in Cross-Classifications.* Cambridge: Cambridge University Press.

Eysenck, S. B. G., & Eysenck, H. J. (1975). *Manual of the Eysenck personality questionnaire.* London: Hodder & Stoughton.

Frankenhaeuser, M. (1983). The sympathetic-adrenal and pituitary-adrenal response to challenge: Comparison between the sexes. In T. M. Dembroski, T. H. Schmidt, & G. Blümchen (Eds.), *Biobehavioral Bases of Coronary Heart Disease*, (Vol. 2, pp. 91-105). Basel: Karger.

Gacono, C. B., & Meloy, J. R. (1994). *The Rorschach Assessment of Aggressive and Psychopathic Personalities.* Hillsdale, NJ: Erlbaum.

Gorenstein, E. E., & Newman, J. P. (1980). Disinhibitory psychopathology: A new perspective and a model for research. *Psychological Review, 87*, 301-315.

Gray, A., Jackson, D. N., & McKinlay, J. B. (1991). The relation between dominance, anger, and hormones in normally aging men: Results from the Massachusetts male aging study. *Psychosomatic Medicine, 53*, 375-385.

Hare, R. D. (1991). *The Hare Psychopathy Check List-Revised.* Toronto: Multi-Health Systems.

Hare, R. D., & Schalling, D. (1978). *Psychopathic Behavior. Approaches to Research.* Chichester: Wiley.

Hauser, P., Zametkin, A. J., Martinez, P., Vitiello, B., Matochik, J. A., Mixson, J., & Weintraub, B. D. (1993). Attention-deficit-hyperactivity disorder in people with generalized resistance to thyroid hormone. *The New England Journal of Medicine, 328*, 997-1001.

King, R. J., Jones, J., Scheuer, J. W., Curtis, D., & Zarcone, V. P. (1990). Plasma cortisol correlates of impulsivity and substance abuse. *Personality and Individual Differences, 11*, 287-291.

af Klinteberg, B. (1995). Biology, norms, and personality: A developmental perspective (Reports from the Department of Psychology No 804): Stockholm University.

af Klinteberg, B. (1996). Biology, norms, and personality: A developmental perspective. *Neuropsychobiology,* in press.

af Klinteberg, B., Andersson, T., Magnusson, D., & Stattin, H. (1993). Hyperactive behavior in childhood as related to subsequent alcohol problems and violent offending: A longitudinal study of male subjects. *Personality and Individual Differences, 15*, 381-388.

af Klinteberg, B., Hallman, J., Oreland, L., Wirsén, A., Levander, S. E., & Schalling, D. (1992). Exploring the connections between platelet monoamine oxidase activity and behavior II: Impulsive personality without neuropsychological signs of disinhibition in air force pilot recruits. *Neuropsychobiology, 26*, 136-145.

af Klinteberg, B., Humble, K., & Schalling, D. (1992). Personality and psychopathy of males with a history of early criminal behaviour. *European Journal of Personality, 6*, 245-266.

af Klinteberg, B., Levander, S., Oreland, L., Åsberg, M., & Schalling, D. (1987). Neuropsychological correlates of platelet monoamine oxidase (MAO) in female and male subjects. *Biological Psychology, 24*, 237-252.

af Klinteberg, B., & Magnusson, D. (1989). Aggressiveness and hyperactive behaviour as related to adrenaline excretion. *European Journal of Personality, 3*, 81-93.

af Klinteberg, B., & Magnusson, D. (1996). *Personality correlates of biochemical patterns at adult age and relationships with early behaviors.* Manuscript in preparation, Department of Psychology, Stockholm University.

af Klinteberg, B., Magnusson, D., & Schalling, D. (1989). Hyperactive behavior in childhood and adult impulsivity: A longitudinal study of male subjects. *Personality and Individual Differences, 10*, 43-50.

af Klinteberg, B., & Oreland, L. (1995). Hyperactive and aggressive behaviors in childhood as related to low platelet monoamine oxidase (MAO) activity at adult age: A longitudinal study of male subjects. *Personality and Individual Differences, 19*, 373-383.

af Klinteberg, B., Schalling, D., Edman, G., Oreland, L., & Åsberg, M. (1987). Personality correlates of platelet monoamine oxidase (MAO) activity in female and male subjects. *Neuropsychobiology, 18,* 89-96.

af Klinteberg, B., Schalling, D., & Magnusson, D. (1986). *Self-report assessment of personality traits. Data from the KSP Inventory on a representative sample of normal male and female subjects within a developmental project* (Reports from the project Individual Development and Adjustment 64): Department of Psychology, Stockholm University.

af Klinteberg, B., Schalling, D., & Magnusson, D. (1990). Childhood behaviour and adult personality in male and female subjects. *European Journal of Personality, 4,* 57-71.

von Knorring, A.-L., Hallman, J., von Knorring, L., & Oreland, L. (1991). Platelet monoamine oxidase activity in type I and type II alcoholism. *Alcohol and Alcoholism, 26,* 409-416.

von Knorring, L., & Oreland, L. (1996). *Platelet MAO activity in Type I/Type II alcoholics.* Manuscript. Department of Psychiatry, University of Uppsala.

von Knorring, L., Oreland, L., & von Knorring, A.-L. (1986). *Personality traits and psychopathology related to platelet MAO activity.* Paper presented at the Biological Psychiatry 1985, Philadelphia, Pennsylvania, USA.

von Knorring, L., Oreland, L., & von Knorring, A.-L. (1987). Personality traits and platelet monoamine oxidase activity in alcohol abusing teenage boys. *Acta Psychiatrica Scandinavica, 75,* 307-314.

von Knorring, L., von Knorring, A.-L., Smigan, L., Lindberg, U., & Edholm, M. (1987). Personality traits in subtypes of alcoholics. Journal of Studies on Alcohol, 48, 523-527.

Kruesi, M. J. P., Hibbs, E. D., Zahn, T. P., Keysor, C. S., Hamburger, S. D., Bartko, J. J., & Rapoport, J. L. (1992). A 2-year prospective follow-up study of children and adolescents with disruptive behavior disorders. *Archives of General Psychiatry, 49,* 429-435.

Levander, S., Mattson, Å., Schalling, D., & Dalteg, A. (1987). Psychoendocrine patterns within a group of male juvenile delinquents as related to early psychosocial stress, diagnostic classification, and follow-up data. In D. Magnusson & A. Öhman (Eds.), *Psychopathology: An Interactional Perspective,* (pp. 235-252). New York: Academic Press.

Lewis, C. E. (1991). Neurochemical mechanisms of chronic antisocial behavior (psychopathy): A literature review. *The Journal of Nervous and Mental Disease, 179,* 720-727.

Lidberg, L., Modin, I., Oreland, L., Tuck, J. R., & Gillner, A. (1985). Platelet monoamine oxidase activity and psychopathy. *Psychiatry Research, 16,* 339-343.

Lilienfeld, S. O. (1992). The association between antisocial personality and somatization disorders: A review and integration of theoretical models. *Clinical Psychology Review, 12,* 641-662.

Loeber, R. (1990). Development and risk factors of juvenile antisocial behavior and delinquency. *Clinical Psychology Review, 10,* 1-41.

Magnusson, D. (1988). Individual Development from an Interactional Perspective: A Longitudinal Study. In D. Magnusson (Ed.), *Paths Through Life,* (Vol. 1,). Hillsdale, NJ: Erlbaum.

Mason, J. W. (1975). Emotion as reflected in patterns of endocrine integration. In L. Levi (Ed.), *Emotions - Their Parameters and Measurement,* (pp. 143-181). New York: Raven Press.

McBurnett, K., Harris, S. M., Swanson, J. M., Pfiffner, L. J., Tamm, L., & Freeland, D. (1993). Neuropsychological and psychophysiological differentiation of inattention/overactivity and aggression/defiance symptom groups. *Journal of Clinical Child Psychology, 22,* 165-171.

McCord, J. (1993). Gender issues. In C. Culliver (Ed.), *Female Criminality: The State of the Art,* (pp. 105-118). New York: Garland Press.

McGee, R., Williams, S., & Silva, P. A. (1985). Behavioural and developmental characteristics of aggressive, hyperactive and aggressive-hyperactive boys. *Journal of the American Academy of Child Psychiatry, 23*, 270-279.

Moss, H. B., Guthrie, S., & Linnoila, M. (1986). Enhanced thyrotropin response to thyrotropin releasing hormone in boys at risk for development of alcoholism. *Archives of General Psychiatry, 43*, 1137-1142.

Murphy, D. L., Wright, C., Buchsbaum, M., Nichols, A., Costa, J. L., & Wyatt, R. J. (1976). Platelet and plasma amine oxidase activity in 680 normals: Sex and age differences and stability over time. *Biochemical Medicine, 16*, 254-265.

Olweus, D. (1986). Aggression and hormones: Behavioral relationship with testosterone and adrenaline. In D. Olweus, J. Block, & M. Radke-Yarrow (Eds.), *Development of Antisocial and Prosocial Behavior*, (pp. 51-72). New York: Academic Press.

Oreland, L. (1993). Monoamine oxidase in neuro-psychiatric disorders. In H. Yasuhara, S. H. Parvez, K. Oguchi, M. Sandler, & T. Nagatsu (Eds.), *Monoamine Oxidase: Basic and Clinical Aspects*, (pp. 219-247). Utrecht: VSP Press.

Oreland, L., & Hallman, J. (1995). The correlation between platelet MAO activity and personality - a short review of findings and discussion on possible mechanisms. In P. M. Yu, K. F. Tipton, & A. A. Boulton (Eds.), Progress in Brain Research: Vol. 106 *"Current neurochemical and pharmacological aspects of biogenic amines: their function, oxidative deamination and inhibition"*, (pp. 77-84). New York: Elsevier.

Robins, L. N. (1986). The consequences of conduct disorder in girls. In D. Olweus, J. Block, & M. Radke-Yarrow (Eds.), *Development of Antisocial and Prosocial Behavior* (pp. 385-409). New York: Academic Press.

Satterfield, J. H. (1987). Childhood diagnostic and neurophysiological predictors of teenage arrest rates: An eight-year prospective study. In S. A. Mednick, T. E. Moffitt, & S. A. Stack (Eds.), *The Causes of Crime*, (pp. 199-207). Cambridge: Cambridge University Press.

Schalling, D. (1993). Neurochemical correlates of personality, impulsivity and disinhibitory suicidality. In S. Hodgins (Ed.), *Mental Disorder and Crime*, (pp. 208-226). Newbury Park, Ca: Sage.

Schalling, D., Åsberg, M., Edman, G., & Oreland, L. (1987). Markers for vulnerability to psychopathology: Temperament traits associated with platelet MAO activity. *Acta Psychiatrica Scandinavica, 76*, 172-182.

Shapiro, D. (1965). *Neurotic Styles*. New York: Basic Books.

Shekim, W. O., Davis, L. G., Bylund, D. B., Brunngraber, E., Fikes, L., & Lanham, J. (1982). Platelet MAO in children with Attention Deficit Disorder and Hyperactivity: A pilot study. *American Journal of Psychiatry, 139*, 936-938.

Shekim, W. O., Hodges, K., Horwitz, E., Glaser, R. D., Davis, L., & Bylund, D. B. (1984). Psychoeducational and impulsivity correlates of platelet MAO in normal children. *Psychiatry Research, 11*, 99-106.

Stattin, H., & Magnusson, D. (1990). *Pubertal maturation in female development*. Hillsdale, NJ: Lawrence Erlbaum.

Taylor, E. (1988). Diagnosis of hyperactivity - A British perspective. In L. M. Bloomingdale & J. Sergeant (Eds.), *Attention Deficit Disorder: Criteria, Cognition, Intervention*, (pp. 141-159). Oxford: Pergamon Press.

Thorley, G. (1984). Review of follow-up and follow-back studies of childhood hyperactivity. *Psychological Bulletin, 96*, 116-132.

Tucker, D. M., & Williamsson, P. A. (1984). Asymmetric neural control systems in human self-regulation. *Psychological Review, 91*, 185-212.

Virkkunen, M., & Linnoila, M. (1993). Serotonin in personality disorders with habitual violence and impulsivity. In S. Hodgins (Ed.), *Mental Disorder and Crime*, (pp. 227-243). London: Sage publications.

Weiss, G., Hechtman, L., Milroy, T., & Perlman, T. (1985). Psychiatric status of hyperactives as adults: A controlled prospective 15 year follow-up of 63 hyperactive children. *Journal of the American Academy of Child Psychiatry, 24*, 211-220.

White, J. L., Moffitt, T. E., Caspi, A., Bartusch, D. J., Needles, D. J., & Stouthamer-Loeber, M. (1994). Measuring impulsivity and examining its relationship to delinquency. *Journal of Abnormal Psychology, 103*, 192-205.

Whybrow, P. C., & Prange, A. J. (1981). A hypothesis of thyroid-catecholamine receptor interaction. *Archives of General Psychiatry, 38*, 106-113.

Zahn, T. P., Kruesi, M. J. P., Leonard, H. L., & Rapaport, J. L. (1994). Autonomic activity and reaction time in relation to extraversion and behavioral impulsivity in children and adolescents. *Personality and Individual Differences, 16*, 751-758.

Zuckerman, M. (1991). *Psychobiology of Personality*. Cambridge: Cambridge University Press.

Author's note

The present research was financially supported by grants from the Swedish Council for Planning and Coordination of Research, the Swedish Council for Social Research, the Bank of Sweden Tercentenary Foundation, and the Swedish Medical Research Council. Special thanks are forwarded to Professor David Magnusson for constructive collaboration, to Professor Lars von Knorring for valuable comments on an earlier version of the manuscript, and to Assoc Professor Sigrid Gustafson for editing work.

CALLOUS-UNEMOTIONAL TRAITS AND CONDUCT PROBLEMS: APPLYING THE TWO-FACTOR MODEL OF PSYCHOPATHY TO CHILDREN

PAUL J. FRICK
Department of Psychology
University of Alabama
Tuscaloosa, USA.

INTRODUCTION

The concept of *psychopathy* has a long and prominent history in clinical psychology. Clinical reports spanning several decades describe the psychopathic personality as being characterized by pathological egocentricity, an absence of empathy, an absence of guilt, superficial charm, shallow emotions, an absence of anxiety, and the inability to form and sustain lasting and meaningful relationships (Cleckley, 1976; Hare, 1993; McCord & McCord, 1964). While these personality traits were often accompanied by severe antisocial and criminal behavior, such behavior was neither necessary or sufficient for most clinical definitions of psychopathy (Cleckley, 1976). Due to concerns over the level of inference required to assess psychopathic personality traits and thus the potential for unreliability (Robins, 1978), the third edition of the *Diagnostic and Statistical Manual of Mental Disorders* (DSM-III; American Psychiatric Association, 1980) and its later revisions (DSM-III-R; American Psychiatric Association, 1987; DSM-IV; American Psychiatric Association, 1994) broke with these early conceptualizations of psychopathy in their definitions of Antisocial Personalty Disorder (APD). In these definitions, a severe and chronic pattern of antisocial behavior was both the necessary and sufficient condition for a diagnosis of APD.

Hare (Hare, Hart, & Harpur, 1991), Lykken (Lykken, 1995), and others (Lilienfeld, 1994; Newman & Wallace, 1993) have argued that this behavioral definition of APD, while affording high reliability, may have dramatically altered the construct being measured. For example, Hare, Harpur and colleagues found that when sufficient items measuring both the chronic antisocial lifestyle of the APD criteria and the affective and interpersonal traits of psychopathy are included in a factor analysis, two separate dimensions emerge (Harpur, Hakstian, & Hare, 1988; Harpur, Hare, & Hakstian, 1989; Hare et al., 1990). Furthermore, these two dimensions appear to have divergent correlates. The APD symptoms are associated with adverse family background factors, low socioeconomic status, and low intelligence, whereas psychopathic traits are positively correlated with measures of narcissism and negatively correlated with measures of anxiety (Harpur et al., 1989). In addition, psychopathic traits predict several important antisocial outcomes, such as the number and variety of criminal offenses, level of violence and aggression, and risk for violent recidivism in released male inmates (see Hare et al., 1991).

D.J. Cooke et al. (eds.), Psychopathy: Theory, Research and Implications for Society, 161–187.

The purpose of this chapter is to summarize a line of research that has attempted to extend this focus on the two distinct dimensions of psychopathy to children. Most authors consider childhood conduct problems to be developmental precursors to adult psychopathy (e.g., Hinshaw, 1994). However, like the adult criteria for APD, most classification schemes for childhood conduct problems focus on the severity and chronicity of the antisocial behavior exhibited by the child and rarely focus on the interpersonal or affective features of psychopathy (Lahey, Loeber, Quay, Frick, & Grimm, 1992). Therefore, linking research on childhood conduct disorders to research on adult psychopathy crosses not only developmental boundaries but crosses key definitional boundaries as well. The line of research described in this chapter attempts to extend the definitional refinements of the two-factor model of psychopathy to children, so that research in children can begin to focus more closely on understanding the early development of psychopathic traits.

Before discussing this line of research, there have been legitimate concerns about applying the term *"psychopathy"* to children (see Quay, 1987). These concerns tend to focus on a) the negative connotations this term has for treatment success and overall long-term outcome and b) the implication of an intrinsic and biological basis to the dysfunction which ignores the substantial influence of a child's social context in the development of personality traits. The legitimate aspect of these concerns is that one should not simply assume that the negative prognosis found in research on adults with psychopathic features can be applied to children nor should one minimize the effects of a child's environmental context in the development of any personality trait, including those associated with psychopathy. Unfortunately, the common alternative to *explicitly* applying the concept of psychopathy to children is to *implicitly* consider all children with severe conduct problems as showing a *"childhood manifestation of psychopathy"* (e.g., Hinshaw, 1994; Richters & Cicchetti, 1993). This alternative is even more problematic. Based on the research reviewed in this chapter, many of the malignant, impairing, and unique dispositional features associated with the construct of psychopathy may only apply to a rather small subset of children with conduct disorders. Therefore, a large number of children with conduct disorders may be inappropriately considered as showing early signs of psychopathy. Hopefully, by being more precise in conceptualizing which children with conduct problems show early precursors to psychopathy, we may begin to address these critical questions of how changeable are these traits in children and how do dispositional factors interact with a child's social context in the developmental of these personality traits.

INITIAL CONSTRUCT DEVELOPMENT IN CHILDREN

Developing a Measurement Strategy

The first goal for extending the two-factor model of psychopathy to children was to answer two basic questions. First, could the interpersonal and affective features of psychopathy be measured reliably in children? Second, would they be separable from behavioral definitions of conduct problems in children? To address these issues, the Psychopathy Screening Device (PSD: Frick & Hare, in press) was developed to assess each aspect of psychopathy assessed by the Psychopathy Checklist-Revised (PCL-R; Hare, 1991). The PCL-R was used as the basis for developing the PSD because its content has proven broad enough to capture the two factors in adults (Harpur et al., 1989). With consultation from the author of the PCL-R (R.D. Hare, personal communication, November 1990), each of the 20 items on the PCL-R was made into an analogous question on the PSD that was worded to be relevant for children.

The assessment format of the PSD was designed to be different from the format of the PCL-R in several ways. First, for ease of administration the items were placed into a rating scale format in which each item was to be rated on a three-point scale as either 0 (*not at all true*), 1 (*sometimes true*), or 2 (*definitely true*). Second, two rating scale formats were developed, one to be completed by a child's parent and the other to be completed by a child's teacher. The explicit decision not to include a self-report format was based on research which has called into question the validity of children's self-report, especially that of young children, for the assessment of their emotional and behavioral functioning in general (Kamphaus & Frick, 1996), and for the assessment of their antisocial behavior specifically (Loeber, Green, Lahey, & Stouthamer-Loeber (1991). Furthermore, research suggests that parents and teachers are the optimal informants for reporting on childhood conduct problems (Loeber et al., 1991). Since a major initial focus of construct development was on the divergent validity of psychopathic traits from conduct problem behavior, it was important that the same assessment format be used to assess both dimensions of behavior.

Isolating the Two Dimensions in Child Samples

In the initial test of the PSD, Frick, O'Brien, Wootton, and McBurnett (1994) obtained parent and teacher PSD ratings on 92 clinic-referred children between the ages of 6 and 13. Children were consecutive referrals to two university-based outpatient child mental health clinics and the sample was predominantly male (84%) and white (82%), which reflected the referral base of the two clinics. A principal components analysis with an oblique (Promax) rotation was conducted on the PSD items using a combination of parent and teacher ratings for each item. A scree plot of the eigenvalues of each successive principal component extracted suggested that a two component solution seemed to be most appropriate. The first component (eigenvalue of 5.9) included items tapping poor impulse control, irresponsibility, and antisocial behavior. The second component (eigenvalue of 2.4) included items related to a callous and unemotional interpersonal style, very similar to the psychopathic traits isolated in adult samples. While these two dimensions were very similar in content to the dimensions which have emerged in adult samples (Harpur et al., 1989), one notable difference was that items related to narcissism (e.g., "Thinks he/she is more important than others") were more associated with the impulsive and antisocial behavior dimension in children, whereas in adults narcissistic traits tended to be more associated with callous and unemotional traits.

To test the divergent validity of these two dimensions, Frick et al. (1994) formed two scales based on this principal components analysis. One scale included those items (n=10) that were highly related to the first component (rotated loadings of > .40) but unrelated to the second component. This was labeled the Impulsive-Conduct Problems (I/CP) scale which had a coefficient alpha of .82. The second scale, the Callous Unemotional (CU) scale, consisted of those items (n=6) that were highly and uniquely related to the second component which had a coefficient alpha of .73. These two scales were significantly correlated (r=.50, p < .001) and the items which formed these scales are listed in Table 1.

TABLE 1. Items of the Psychopathy Screening Device which Form the Two Dimensions of Psychopathy in Children

Impulsive-Conduct Problems	*Callous-Unemotional Traits*
8. Brags about accomplishments	3. Concerned about schoolwork (I)
15. Becomes angry when corrected	12. Feels bad or guilty (I)
16. Thinks he/she is more important than others.	5. Emotions seem shallow
4. Acts without thinking	19. Does not show emotions
1. Blames others for mistakes	14. Acts charming in ways that seem
11. Teases other people	insincere
13. Engages in risky and dangerous behavior	18. Is concerned about the feelings of
2. Engages in illegal activities	others (I)
20. Keeps the same friends (I)	
9. Gets bored easily.	

Note. The dimensions were formed from a principal component analysis of combined parent and teacher ratings using an oblique (Promax) rotation described in Frick et al. (1994). Only items which had rotated factor loadings of .40 or greater on only one component are listed. (I) denotes items that were inversely scored prior to the principal components analysis.

The first test of the divergent validity of these two scales was in their association with traditional conduct problems measures. One measure was a combination of parent and teacher report of all symptoms included in the DSM-III-R criteria for ODD and CD based on a structured diagnostic interview (DISC-2.3; Shaffer, Fisher, Piacentini, Schwab-Stone, & Wicks, 1992). Two other measures of conduct problems included parent (CBCL-91, Achenbach, 1991) and teacher (CBRSC, Neeper, Lahey, & Frick, 1990) report of conduct problems from two standardized behavior rating scales. The I/CP scale of the PSD was highly correlated with these traditional conduct problems measures (.53 to .71) and it differentiated children with an ODD or CD diagnosis from other clinic-referred children (t(62)=5.6, p < .05). However, the CU scale was less strongly associated with traditional conduct problem measures (.30-.45) and this scale did not differentiate children with an ODD or CD diagnosis from other clinic-referred children (t(62)=1.4, p=ns).

From these initial analyses, it appeared that the I/CP scale was tapping a dimension of behavior that was similar to traditional conduct problem measures. To further support this contention, Frick et al. (1994) found that the I/CP scale and ODD/CD symptoms did not account for unique variance in the prediction of several important external criteria (e.g., sensation seeking, anxiety, intelligence, socio-economic status, family arrest history). Therefore, the I/CP scale of the PSD and ODD/CD symptoms seem to be measuring a similar construct. In contrast, the CU scale showed several areas of divergence from DSM-III-R conduct problem symptoms in the prediction of external criteria. The CU scale was negatively related to measures of anxiety and positively related to measures of sensation seeking behavior, whereas ODD/CD symptoms were positively associated with measures of anxiety and unrelated to measures of sensation seeking. There was also an interaction between ODD/CD symptoms and the CU scale for predicting intelligence test scores and a paternal criminal history. Specifically, children who were high on ODD/CD symptoms (met DSM-III-R criteria for a diagnosis of ODD or CD) but with low to moderate scores on the CU scale had significantly lower intelligence scores than a) children with an ODD/CD diagnosis and high scores on the CU scale and b) other clinic-referred children without conduct problems. In contrast, those children with a conduct problem diagnosis and high scores on the CU scale had a higher rate of paternal arrests (67%) compared to those children with only an ODD/CD diagnosis (21%).

In summary, Frick et al. (1992) found two correlated dimensions of behavior in clinic-referred children that were analogous in many respects to the two factors of psychopathy that have emerged in adult samples. One dimension included items tapping an impulsive, irresponsible, and antisocial behaviors that was highly related to DSM and other common definitions of childhood conduct problems. A second dimension included items tapping the callous and unemotional traits that have been hallmarks of clinical definitions of psychopathy and that were more divergent from traditional conduct problem definitions. One puzzling area of divergence between CU traits and ODD/CD symptoms was in the association of the two dimensions with a measure of sensation seeking behavior. In children, scores on the Sensation Seeking Scale for Children (SSSC; Russo et al., 1993) were more strongly associated with the CU scale than with the I/CP scale or ODD/CD symptoms. In adults, sensation seeking measures have typically been more strongly associated with the impulsive and antisocial dimension in the two-factor model (Harpur et al., 1989). This discrepancy could be explained by the fact that in the Frick et al. (1994) study, the association between sensation seeking and CU traits was largely attributable to the Thrill and Adventure Seeking scale of the SSSC. This aspect of sensation seeking tends to be less associated with poor impulse control and antisocial behavior than other aspects of sensation seeking, like boredom susceptibility and disinhibition (Levenson, 1990). Therefore, the difference in findings could be due to the focus on a different aspect of sensation seeking on the childhood version of the scale. In support of this possibility, the item on the PSD *"Gets bored easily"* susceptibility was associated with the other items on the I/CP scale (see Table 1).

Callous-Unemotional Traits and Subtypes of Children with Conduct Problems

In addition to isolating two correlated dimensions of behavior with distinct correlates, a major contribution of the two-factor model of psychopathy in adults has been its ability to identify individuals with an especially severe and chronic pattern of antisocial behavior (see Hare et al., 1990). The possibility that CU traits might also identify a severe group of children with conduct problems would be consistent with past subtyping attempts that have used interpersonal (e.g., undersocialized, aggressive) or affective (e.g., low anxiety) characteristics of the child with conduct problems to designate an especially severe and chronic pattern of behavior (Lahey et al., 1992). However, these past sub-typing approaches have captured only certain aspects of the relevant psychological dimensions included in adult conceptualizations of psychopathy.

To test the potential usefulness of CU traits in delineating a subgroup of children with conduct problems, Christian, Frick, Hill, Tyler, and Frazer (1995) studied 120 consecutive clinic-referrals between the ages 6 and 13 (mean = 8.68, sd=2.07). Children's scores on the I/CP and CU scales of the PSD and the number of ODD and CD symptoms endorsed as present by either parent and teacher were first standardized (z-scores) to equate for differences in variance on these measures. These standard scores were then subjected to the SAS clustering procedure FASTCLUS which places subjects into disjoint clusters based on the similarity of scores with others in that cluster. Using the procedures recommended by Bornstein (1988), four distinct clusters of children were isolated. In Table 2 several important characteristics of the four clusters are described.

TABLE 2. Results of a Cluster Analysis of the Two PSD Scales and DSM-III-R ODD and CD Symptoms.

	Clinic Control Cluster (n=39)	Callous-Unemotional Cluster (n=41)	Impulsive-Conduct Cluster (n=29)	Psychopathic Conduct Cluster (n=11)	F (3,116)
CU Scale of PSD	5.27 a	10.20 b	8.44 c	16.06 d	68.81 ***
(sd)	(2.27)	(2.34)	(2.33)	(1.94)	
I/CP Scale of PSD	7.89 a	13.92 b	19.94 c	22.35 c	80.68 ***
(sd)	(2.93)	(3.55)	(3.76)	(3.69)	
Number DSM-III-R					
Symptoms of ODD/CD	1.35 a	3.42 b	8.78 c	11.37 d	97.03 ***
(sd)	(1.64)	(2.12)	(2.51)	(2.89)	
Full Scale IQ	100.49 a	91.24 ab	88.52 b	100.00 a	7.31 ***
(sd)	(13.93)	(10.29)	(10.66)	(14.68)	
					X^2 (3, n=120)
ODD (%)	5% a	15% a	90% b	100% b	78.58 ***
CD (%)	0% a	0% a	45% b	55% b	45.71 ***
Either ODD or CD (%)	5% a	15% a	90% b	100% b	78.58 ***
Lifetime Police Contacts (%)	0% a (n=39)	5% a (n=39)	14% ab (n=29)	36% b (n=10)	6.13 *
Parent with APD (%)	8% a	10% a	14% ab	40% b	8.48 *

Note. These findings are a tabular summary of the results presented in Christian et al. (1995). All comparisons were conducted controlling for SES, Full Scale IQ, Age, and Gender using either an ANCOVA or a logistic regression procedure. The sample size differed for the analyses of parental APD due to the exclusion of 3 children for whom a biological parent was not available to provide a family history.

The first cluster (n=39) was a Clinic Control Cluster that had low scores on both PSD scales and also did not show many conduct problem symptoms. The second cluster (n=41), the Callous-Unemotional cluster, was somewhat higher on both PSD scales and also somewhat higher on number of conduct problem symptoms. However, their rate of conduct problems was still below the sample mean and very few of these children met DSM-III-R criteria for either an ODD (15%) or CD (0%) diagnosis. The final two clusters were of most interest. Both of theses clusters had high rates of conduct problem diagnoses. In the third cluster (n=29), labeled the Impulsive Conduct Cluster, 90% had an ODD diagnosis and 45% had a CD diagnosis. In the fourth cluster (n=11), the Psychopathic Conduct Cluster, all of the children had an ODD diagnosis and 55% had a CD diagnosis. Therefore, almost all of the children in the sample with a conduct problem diagnosis fell in the latter two clusters.

While both conduct problem clusters had high rates of DSM-III-R diagnoses, they had several distinguishing characteristics. First, the Psychopathic Conduct Cluster had much higher scores than all other clusters on the CU scale of PSD. Also, this cluster had a significantly higher rate of ODD and CD symptoms than any of the other clusters, including the Impulsive Conduct Cluster. This Psychopathic Conduct Cluster showed greater numbers of problems in three of the four specific domains of conduct problems studied. They showed more oppositional symptoms, more aggressive symptoms, and more covert-property destructive symptoms (see Frick et al., 1993 for the development of this method of dividing conduct problem symptoms). Therefore, this cluster of children with conduct problem diagnoses who were also high on the CU scale seemed to show a greater severity and variety of conduct problem behavior than other children with conduct problem diagnoses. This is an important finding given that the number and variety of conduct problems displayed is one of the most consistent predictors of the persistence of antisocial behavior (Loeber, 1982; 1991).

There were several other important differences between the two conduct problem clusters that are also described in Table 2. On both lifetime histories of police contacts and parental histories of APD, only the Psychopathic Conduct Cluster differed from the Clinic Control group. The difference between the two conduct problem groups approached significance for both variables (p< .07, p < .09), with the Psychopathic Conduct Cluster having more police contacts and a greater family history of APD than the Impulsive Conduct Cluster. Again, both early police contact (Loeber & Stouthamer-Loeber, 1987) and a family history of APD (Lahey et al., 1995) have been shown to predict stability in antisocial behavior. Interestingly, the Psychopathic Conduct Cluster had a significantly higher level of intelligence than the Impulsive Conduct Cluster. This finding seems to be discrepant from other indices of severity in that lower intelligence is often found to predict greater severity and persistence of conduct problems (Moffitt, 1993b). However, the differential association across clusters on both intelligence and parental APD could explain an intriguing and unexpected finding in the four-year longitudinal study conducted by Lahey et al. (1995). These authors reported an interaction between parental APD and intelligence for predicting the persistence of conduct disorders. Children with high intelligence showed less persistence *only in the absence of parental APD*. Those children with higher intelligence who also had a family history of APD, similar to our Psychopathic Conduct Cluster, actually showed the highest level of persistence in the study.

One prediction that was not supported by these data was that the Psychopathic Conduct Cluster would show an earlier age of onset to CD symptoms, based on past research showing that an earlier age of onset predicts persistence (Hinshaw, Lahey, & Hart, 1992; Moffitt, 1993a). However, this may have been a function of the age of the sample. The sample was largely a preadolescent sample (mean age 8.6) and therefore, most of the children with a conduct disorder would have fallen into the *"childhood-onset"* category of conduct disorder, which past research has found to be at high risk for persistence (Moffitt, 1993a). Within this early onset group, CU traits did not predict an *"extremely"* early age of onset. However, they did designate a group of children who showed many other characteristics associated with persistence. As a result, it may be that this subgroup of children with CU traits accounts for a significant proportion of the persistence associated with this early-onset pattern of conduct problem behavior.

Summary of Initial Construct Development in Children

Taken together, these initial studies with children provide preliminary support for extending the two-factor model of psychopathy to childhood. The basic features of the two-factor model in adults were supported in these clinic samples. Specifically, CU traits and an impulsive and antisocial pattern of behavior formed two distinct psychological dimensions with different correlates. Therefore, as was the case for adults, not all children with severe conduct problems show CU traits. The ones that do, however, seemed to show a potentially serious and chronic pattern of behavior, making these traits important for delineating unique subtypes of children with conduct disorders.

Given these promising findings, it is important to extend the theoretical framework for conceptualizing these two dimensions in both children and adults. Even in the adult literature where the two-factor model of psychopathy originated, there has been little conceptual clarity as to how the differential correlates to the two dimensions might be integrated into causal theories. It is also unclear how one should conceptualize the relationship between these two dimensions, since they are correlated. The major reason for this limited theoretical network is that the isolation of the two dimensions of psychopathy is fairly recent (Harpur et al., 1989). Also, much of the research that has used the PCL-R or its predecessor the PCL, one of the few assessment systems that adequately assesses both psychopathic traits and antisocial behavior, has used incarcerated male inmates (Hare et al., 1991). Therefore, there has been little research on psychopathic traits independent of antisocial behavior. Finally, even in this limited body research on male inmates, studies have rarely studied the differential correlates of the two dimensions in such a way that controls for the significant correlation between these two factors. Most studies using the PCL have used the total PCL score, which combines both dimensions, either to define psychopathic individuals (e.g., Hart, Forth, & Hare, 1990; Newman, Patterson, & Kosson, 1987) or to explain variation in external criteria (e.g., Hart, Kropp, & Hare, 1988). In the few studies that have studied the two dimensions separately, zero-order correlations between the two dimensions and external criteria are compared (e.g., Harpur et al., 1989). This methodology does not control for the correlation between the two dimensions themselves.

In the following sections I describe an emerging theoretical model which attempts to explain both the divergence and convergence of these two psychological constructs for explaining the development of conduct problems in children. In developing this model, I have tried to integrate three rich areas of research: research on psychopathy in adults, research on childhood conduct problems, and research on the temperamental styles of adults and children. One of the areas of great promise in extending the two-factor model to children is its potential for successfully pulling together these important lines of research. After an initial overview of the basic conceptual model, I provide a more in depth discussion of the basis for the key assumptions of the model and I provide some tests of the predictions which follow from this theoretical framework.

EXTENDING THE THEORETICAL FRAMEWORK OF THE TWO-FACTOR MODEL IN CHILDREN

An Overview of the Conceptual Model

In Figure 1, I outline a basic framework for conceptualizing the relationship between CU traits and conduct problems in children. A key assumption of this model is that conduct problems are an etiologically heterogeneous outcome that can result from a number of fairly distinct causal pathways, each involving different interactions of causal factors. In contrast, CU traits are a) viewed as a more etiologically homogeneous construct and b) delineate one of these causal pathways to conduct problems.

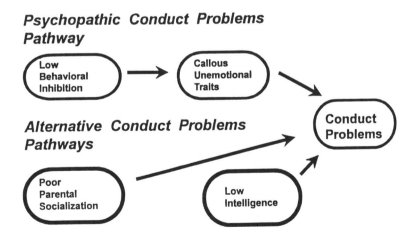

Figure 1. Basic conceptual framework for extending the two-factor model of psychopathy to children

CU traits are considered to develop partly as a function of a unique temperamental style, low behavioral inhibition, that makes a child more difficult to socialize. Once they develop, CU traits (e.g., an absence of empathy, a lack of guilt) make a child more likely to act against parental and societal norms and to violate the rights of others. However, there are other pathways involving other etiological factors that can also result in a child exhibiting conduct problems. From the cluster analysis described previously (see Table 2), it seems that only a minority of children with conduct disorders show high levels of CU traits, albeit a minority that may operate at quite a high cost to society. While this framework is admittedly simplistic, it does lead to several testable predictions that would not be explained well by existing theories of the development of conduct problems.

Behavioral Inhibition and CU Traits

One key assumption of the theoretical model outlined in Figure 1 is that CU traits are related to a unique temperamental style and, more specifically, to a style characterized by low behavioral inhibition. Many theorists have tried to account for the behavior of individuals with psychopathic traits through variations in a set of neurologically-based motivational systems which lead to stable temperamental styles (e.g., Cloninger, 1987; Gray, 1982; Lykken, 1995; Newman & Wallace, 1993). I will not attempt a complete integration of the many commonalities and differences on both the behavioral and neurological level in these theories. However, each of these theories focus on the presence of two distinct neurological systems that control appetitive and inhibitory drives.

The first neurological system controls appetitive drives and activates cues to reward and nonpunishment. This has been called the *"behavioral activation system"* by Gray (1982). A temperamental style characterized by overactivity of this appetitive system could lead to the tendency to overfocus on cues for potential rewards (Newman, Patterson, & Kosson, 1987), to the tendency to seek out stimulating activities (Cloninger, 1987; Zuckerman, 1979), and to difficulties delaying gratification and planning ahead (Hare et al., 1991; Newman & Wallace, 1993) that are all characteristic of antisocial adults. An analogous temperamental style has been identified in young children described as deficits in the *"effortful control of purposeful behavior"* which is characterized by developmentally inappropriate levels of poor planfullness, lack of foresight, inability to delay of gratification, and inability to resist temptation (e.g., Kochanska, 1993; Rothbart, 1989). Many children with extremes of this temperamental style may be diagnosed with Attention-deficit Hyperactivity Disorder (ADHD) (Barkley, 1994).

The second motivational system that is common across these theories is a separate neurological system that governs inhibitory drives. This system activates cues to punishment and non-reward and is labelled the *"behavioral inhibition system"* by Gray (1982). A temperamental style characterized by underactivity of this inhibitory system could lead to the lack of responsivity to cues to punishment (Newman & Wallace, 1993), to the lack of responsivity to cues to potential danger and harm (Cloninger, 1987), to the low fearfulness and low susceptibility to anxiety (Lykken, 1995), and to the abnormal processing of affective stimuli (Williamson, Harpur, &

Hare, 1991) that have been characteristic of people with psychopathic traits. Researchers on children's temperament have also documented variations in children's susceptibility to fearful arousal in response to novel or threatening situations that are a) present very early in life, b) associated with a distinct pattern of neurological functioning that would be consistent with the neurological underpinnings of the behavioral inhibition system, and c) relatively stable over the course of development (Kagan & Snidman, 1991; Kochanska, 1993; Rothbart, 1989).

While the presence of two distinct motivational systems has been well documented on an neuroanatomical level (Gray, 1982), it has been difficult to separate the activity of the two systems on a behavioral level, since they operate in an antagonistic fashion. As a result, it has been difficult to determine whether certain patterns of disinhibited behavior are a result of overactivity of the behavioral activation system, underactivity of behavioral inhibition system, or both (e.g., Oosterlaan & Sargeant, 1996). However, the two-factor model of psychopathy may provide a basis for studying the differential effects of these two motivational systems. Specifically, the impulsive and antisocial lifestyle dimension found in adults (Harpur et al., 1989) and the impulsive-conduct problems factor found in children (Frick et al., 1994) both focus on indicators of poor impulse control. Thus, it seems to be more related to overactivity of the behavioral activation system or to the temperamental dimension of poor effortful control of behavior. In samples of both adults and children, this dimension has been related to boredom susceptibility, failure to delay gratification, and poor planning abilities (Frick et al., 1994; Harpur et al., 1989) which have been defining features of this temperamental style (Kochanska, 1993). Since most traditional definitions of psychopathy and antisocial behavior in adults and most traditional definitions of conduct problems in children are highly correlated with the impulsive-antisocial dimension of psychopathy (Frick et al., 1994; Hare et al., 1991), they likely define a construct that is more related to overactivity of the behavioral activation system. This would be consistent with the finding that the vast majority of children with conduct disorders (90% in many clinic samples - Abikoff & Klein, 1992) are also diagnosed with ADHD.

CU traits, on the other hand, may focus on traits that are more specifically related to low levels of behavioral inhibition. This would be consistent with the work of Kochanska (1991; 1993; 1995) who contends that behavioral inhibition is critical in the development of the *"affective discomfort components of conscience"* (i.e., guilt, remorse, empathy) in young children. She found that children low in fearful inhibitions did not respond to the type of socialization practices (i.e., gentle non-power assertive discipline) that led to the development of conscience in more fearful children (Kochanska, 1991). She places this finding into a model in which a child must experience an optimal level of arousal in situations involving potential punishment, including social disapproval, in order to internalize parental norms for behavior. Either too little arousal (e.g., temperamentally low fearful inhibitions) or too much arousal (e.g., caused by harsh parental responses) can negatively affect internalization (Kochanska, 1993).

Influenced by this line of research, I propose that deficits in behavioral inhibition are directly related to the developmental of CU traits and only indirectly related to conduct problems (see Figure 1). This prediction of a mediational role of CU traits sets this model apart from other models that have attempted to link deficits in behavioral inhibition to the development of psychopathy and antisocial behavior in adults (Fowles, 1988; Lykken, 1995) or to the development of conduct problems in children (Milich, Hartung, Martin, & Haigler, 1994; Newman & Wallace, 1993; Quay, 1993). Considering CU traits as the more proximal consequence of this temperamental style would be consistent with several lines of research. First, Lahey et al. (1993) conducted a review of the neuropsychological correlates to conduct disorders in children and concluded that the neurochemical and autonomic irregularities that are thought to underlie deficits in the behavioral inhibition system are consistently associated with only a subgroup of children with conduct disorders; *"those described as undersocialized, aggressive, and psychopathic"* (p. 141). Second, studies that have tested children's responsiveness to punishment have found that an insensitivity to cues to punishment is only characteristic of a subset of children with conduct problems; namely, those who do not show high rates of emotional distress or anxiety accompanying their behavioral disturbance (Daugherty & Quay, 1991; O'Brien, Frick, & Lyman, 1994; Shapiro, Quay, Hogan, & Schwartz, 1988). One could argue that the subset of children with severe conduct problems who are less distressed by their behavior are most likely to show CU traits. Both of these lines of research provide only indirect evidence for a model in which CU traits designate a pathway to conduct problems that is related to deficits in behavioral inhibition. The most direct test of this assumption would be to test the prediction that a measure of low behavioral inhibition would be directly related CU traits but only indirectly related to conduct problems, whereas a measure of poor impulse control would be related to conduct problems irrespective of the presence of CU traits.

Behavioral Inhibition and Impulse Control: Differential Associations with CU Traits and Conduct Problems.

This prediction was tested in a sample of 131 consecutive referrals to an outpatient mental health clinic between the ages of 6 and 13. The measure of low behavioral inhibition was the Thrill and Adventure Seeking Scale (TAS) of the Sensation Seeking Scale for Children (SSSC; Russo et al., 1993). This scale measures a child's self-reported preference for engaging in novel and dangerous activities. As mentioned previously, this scale seems to be distinct from other aspects of sensation seeking behavior, like boredom susceptibility and behavioral disinhibition, which are more related to poor impulse control (Levenson, 1990). The measure of impulse control the number of Impulsivity-Hyperactivity (I-H) symptoms from the DSM-IV criteria for Attention-deficit Hyperactivity Disorder (ADHD; American Psychiatric Association, 1994) that were reported as being present by either the child's parent or teacher. In order to focus on the extremes of both dimensions, scores on the TAS and the number of I-H symptoms were dichotomized into those in the upper quartile of the sample and those in the lower three quartiles.

These data were first analyzed using a 2 X 2 logit model analysis in which elevations on the TAS scale and high rates of I-H symptoms were used to predict elevations on the CU scale of the PSD. From this analysis, a main effect for the TAS scale was found (X^2 (1, n=131)=4.18, p < .05) but there was no significant main effect for the I-H symptoms nor was there a significant interaction between the TAS scale and I-H symptoms. This effect remained significant when a logistic regression procedure was used to control for potentially confounding demographic variables (e.g., sex, ethnicity, age, socioeconomic status, and intelligence). More importantly, this main effect for the TAS scale also remained significant when controlling for the presence of a diagnosis of ODD or CD. Therefore, elevations on the TAS scale predicted the presence of CU traits independent of a diagnosis of ODD or CD.

A similar set of logit model analyses were conducted using the same predictors but using a diagnosis of ODD or CD as the criterion variable. Consistent with predictions, a very different pattern of results emerged. In the initial logit model analysis, there was a main effect for I-H symptoms in predicting an ODD/CD diagnosis (X^2 (1, n=131)= 7.38, p < .01) but there was no main effect for the TAS scale and no significant interaction. Again, this main effect remained significant after controlling for demographic variables and after controlling for elevations on the CU scale in logistic regression analyses. Taken together, these analyses indicate that TAS scale elevations, as a measure of low behavior inhibition, were associated with CU traits irrespective of the presence of conduct problems. However, low behavioral inhibition did not predict the presence of an ODD or CD diagnosis independent of CU traits, which would be consistent with the mediational role of CU traits outlined in Figure 1. In contrast, impulsivity predicted an ODD/CD diagnosis independent of CU traits but it did not predict CU traits independent of an ODD/CD diagnosis. Therefore, poor impulse control seems to be related to severe conduct problems in general and not to CU traits in the absence of such problems.

Sensitivity to Cues of Punishment and CU Traits.

In most theories of how low behavioral inhibition places a person at risk for developing CU traits, the critical mechanism is the lack of responsivity to cues of punishment (e.g., Kochanska, 1993; Lykken, 1995). In much of Gray's (1982) work, responsivity to cues of punishment and non-reward is a defining feature of the behavioral inhibition system. Therefore, another prediction that would follow from the model outlined in Figure 1 is that an insensitivity to cues of punishment, as a marker of low activity of behavioral inhibition system, should be directly related to CU traits and only indirectly related to conduct problems.

While not directly addressing the potential mediational role of CU traits, many authors have used a behavioral paradigm developed by Newman and colleagues (Newman, Patterson, & Kosson, 1987) and later extended to children by Quay and colleagues (Daugherty & Quay, 1991; Shapiro et al., 1988) to test antisocial individuals' reponsivity to punishment cues. In this paradigm, a person plays a game in which he or she can win points. The game is designed to provide the subject with a steadily decreasing ratio of rewarded (e.g., won points) to punished (lost points) trials, starting with a reward:punishment ratio of 9:1 in the first ten trials which gradually decreases in each successive ten trial block until the ratio is 1:9. As a result, a reward-oriented response set is established in the early trials which must be altered as the rate of punishment increases. In this task, a person can stop playing the game at any time. Low anxious adults with psychopathic traits (Newman et al., 1987) and children with conduct problems who were also low on anxiety played more trials on this task despite the increasing ratio of punished responses (Daugherty & Quay, 1991; O'Brien et al., 1994; Shapiro et al., 1988). However, for these results to fit with the model outlined in Figure 1, one must assume that isolating children with conduct problems who were also low on anxiety increased the likelihood that they exhibited CU traits.

To test this assumption directly, O'Brien and Frick (1996) employed this behavioral paradigm in a series of computer tasks administered to a sample of 92 consecutive clinic-referrals between the ages of 6 and 13 years, and 40 community volunteer children who were matched to the clinic group on age, gender, ethnicity, and socioeconomic status.

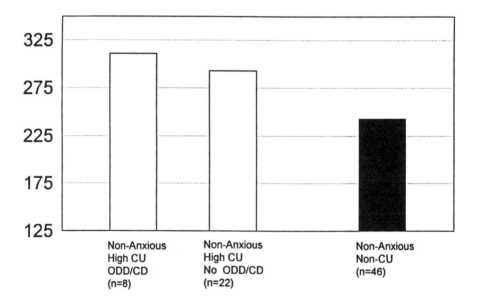

Figure 2. Number of trials played on Newman's Card Playing Task
Note. CU refers to elevations on the Callous-Unemotional scale of the PSD, ODD refers to Oppositional Defiant Disorder, and CD refers to Conduct Disorder. Data from O'Brian and Frick (1996).

As predicted, not all children with conduct problems showed the insensitivity to punishment. The non-anxious children with conduct disorders (n=9) played more trials than a) anxious children with conduct disorder (n=25), b) the clinic control group of non-anxious children with ADHD (n=18), and c) the normal control group (n=40) (F (3,88)=3.10, p < .05). It is interesting to note that the non-anxious ADHD group, who by definition exhibited high rates of impulsivity, did not play more trials than the normal control group. This suggests that performance on the task was not related to impulsivity. More importantly for the hypothesized mediating role of CU traits, almost all (89%) of the non-anxious children with conduct problems were high on CU traits. Furthermore, non-anxious children high on CU traits showed an insensitivity to punishment cues *irrespective of whether the child also had conduct problems*. This pattern is illustrated in Figure 2. Children high on CU traits both with (n=8) and without (n=22) an ODD/CD diagnosis played more trials than other non-anxious children (n=45) (F (2,72)=4.30, p < .01). Therefore, the inability to shift from a reward dominant response set in response to cues of punishment seemed to be more directly related to CU traits and only related to conduct problems in children with these traits.

Anxiety, CU Traits, and Conduct Problems.

If low levels of fearful inhibition is critical in the development of CU traits, it is hard to explain why many people with psychopathic traits show high scores on some measures of anxiety (see Lykken, 1995 for a review). In fact, many studies have used anxiety as a method of dividing individuals with psychopathic traits into those who do not show high levels of anxiety (*"primary psychopathy"*) and those who do show high levels of anxiety (*"secondary psychopathy"*) (see Newman & Wallace, 1993). Many theorists have proposed that there are two distinct forms of psychopathy (i.e., primary and secondary) that differ in their underlying motivational style (Lykken, 1995; Newman & Wallace, 1993). However, it is also possible that the apparent overlap between anxiety and psychopathy may be at least partly an artifact of two methodological issues.

First, as mentioned previously, most of the commonly used measures of psychopathy and antisocial behavior in adults, and conduct problems in children, tend to focus more on the person's impulsive and antisocial lifestyle rather than on CU traits (Frick et al., 1994; Hare et al., 1991). If one considers low anxiety as a marker of low behavioral inhibition (Gray, 1982; Newman & Wallace, 1993), and one considers this motivational tendency to be specifically related to CU traits and not to impulsive-antisocial behavior in general, one would expect that a) a negative correlation with anxiety would be specific to CU traits and b) the large number of people who show antisocial behavior without these traits may show elevated levels of anxiety. Second, some of the confusion may also lie in the imprecise definitions of anxiety; namely, the failure to distinguish between fearfulness and anxiety (Lilienfeld, 1994). Lilienfeld (1994) makes a distinction between fearfulness, which is defined as *"sensitivity to cues of impending danger"* (p. 31), and anxiety, which is defined as *"distress produced by the perception that danger and related consequences are inevitable"* (p. 31). As a result, a person with psychopathic traits could be low in fearfulness, a more specific marker of the behavioral inhibition system, but may score high on measures of trait anxiety or negative affectivity because of the significant and recurrent impairments (e.g., legal, occupational, and/or social difficulties) that often accompanies his or her behavior.

In an effort to clarify this issue, the differential association between a measure of anxiety, CU traits, and conduct problems was tested in the sample of 131 clinic-referred children described previously (Frick, Lilienfeld, & McBurnett, 1996). The measure of anxiety was the number of DSM-III-R symptoms of childhood anxiety disorders which was primarily composed of symptoms of Overanxious Disorder (e.g., worry about competence in numerous areas, worry about the future). This construct seems to capture the construct of negative affectivity. This measure of anxiety, based on the combined report of the child and his or her parent on a structured diagnostic interview, was uncorrelated with CU traits ($r=-.02$, $p=n.s$) but positively correlated with ODD and CD symptoms ($r=.37$, $p < .01$). However, when semi-partial correlations were calculated, an even greater degree of divergence was found. The negative correlation between anxiety and the CU scale increased to $-.28$ ($p<.01$) after controlling for the number of ODD/CD symptoms and the positive correlation between ODD/CD symptoms and anxiety climbed to $.51$ ($p<.001$) after controlling for CU traits. In statistical terms, the correlation between ODD/CD symptoms and CU traits *"suppressed"* the divergent associations with anxiety in the zero-order correlations.

In practical terms, this pattern of correlations suggests that as the number of conduct problems increased, children exhibited more emotional distress or anxiety. However, children *with similar levels of conduct problems* showed less distress when they were higher on CU traits. This suppressor effect is illustrated in Figures 3 and 4.

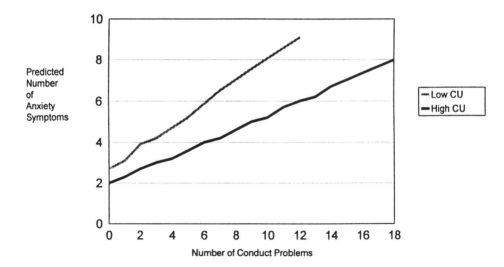

Figure 3. Predicted number of anxiety symptoms at each level of ODD/CD symptoms plotted separately for children above and below the median on CU traits

In Figure 3 the regression line for conduct problem symptoms predicting anxiety symptoms was plotted separately for children above the median on CU traits and for those below the median on CU traits. For both regression lines, there was a positive correlation between conduct problems and anxiety. However, in children low on CU traits, there was a greater slope to the regression line and these children consistently exhibited more anxiety at each level of conduct problem symptomology. In Figure 4 the regression line for CU traits predicting anxiety symptoms was plotted separately for children above the median and below the median on conduct problem symptoms. CU traits were inversely correlated with anxiety, especially for those children with high numbers of conduct problem symptoms. However, those children with high numbers of conduct problem symptoms were more anxious at each level of CU traits than children below the median of conduct problems.

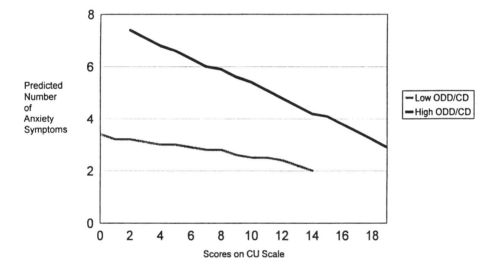

Figure 4. Predicted number of anxiety symptoms at each level of CU traits plotted separately for children above and below the median on number of ODD and CD symptoms

This pattern of associations has two important implications for the relationship between anxiety and the two-factors of psychopathy. First, it is consistent with the contention that many measures of anxiety assess the level of distress that a person experiences and this will increase with the severity of his or her behavioral disturbance, albeit to a somewhat lesser degree if he or she also shows CU traits. Second, this pattern of associations was quite different from the pattern of associations found for the TAS scale that was reported earlier from the same sample. The TAS scale, which seems to be a more specific measure of low behavioral inhibition, was positively correlated with CU traits but unrelated to conduct problems independent of CU traits. Therefore, consistent with the contention of Lilienfeld (1994), measures of negative affectivity and behavioral inhibition show a very different pattern of associations with CU traits and conduct problems.

Multiple Causal Pathways to Conduct Problems

To this point, the discussion has focused on the pathway to conduct problems in Figure 1 labeled the *"Psychopathic Pathway"* which is a) related to behavioral inhibition and b) mediated by the development of CU traits. However, this model also could have important implications for understanding causal factors that operate in the development of conduct problems for children without CU traits. The model outlined in Figure 1 has been described as a *"multiple pathway model"* to emphasize that the same causal factors may not operate in a similar manner for all children who develop conduct problems. This type of model is in contrast to many other theoretical models that, while considering multiple causal factors in the development of conduct problems, assume that causal factors operate in the same way for all children. These models, either explicitly or implicitly, assume that causal factors operate in an interchangeable and additive manner with increasing numbers of risk factors, irrespective of the type of risk factor, leading to an increasing probability that a child will develop conduct problems (e.g., Loeber, 1990). This type of model ignores a basic concept in the study of children's temperament that risk and protective factors may not operate in the same manner for all children but may vary depending on the child's temperament (Rothbart, 1989).

Parental Socialization Practices and Conduct Problems.

Integrating the role of parental socialization practices into this model can illustrate this issue. Any adequate explanation for the development of conduct problems must include the role of parental socialization practices (Frick, 1993; 1994). By their very nature, conduct problems represent a failure of the child to conform his or her behavior to the rules and expectations of society in general, or to some specific authority figure (e.g., parents or teachers). In many cultures, especially in most western cultures, the sole or primary responsibility for this socialization lies with the child's parents (Lykken, 1995). In addition to this intuitive link between ineffective parenting and conduct problems, breakdowns in parenting practices designed to socialize a child have been associated with the development of conduct problem behaviors in several hundred published studies (see Frick, 1994; Loeber & Stouthamer-Loeber, 1986 for reviews).

The processes through which dysfunctional parenting practices disrupt the socialization of the child has been the focus of many scholarly discussions in the child clinical (Patterson, 1986), developmental (Kochanska, 1993) and sociological (Wells & Rankin, 1988) literatures and therefore, will not be reviewed here. However, how these processes might interact with CU traits in the development of conduct problems is critical for the model outlined in Figure 1. In a traditional additive model, CU traits and dysfunctional parenting practices would be viewed as each placing a child at risk for developing conduct problems and together combine to be especially iatrogenic to the child. However, the multiple pathway model outlined in Figure 1, provides an alternative formulation. Dysfunctional parenting practices may play a major role in the development of conduct problems *primarily in children without CU traits*.

This prediction is consistent with Lykken's (1995) distinction between the *"sociopath"* and the *"primary psychopath"*. The primary psychopath, because of a *"hard-to-socialize temperament"*, is at high risk for developing antisocial behavior in most child-rearing environments. In contrast, the sociopath does not have this predisposing temperament. Instead, his or her antisocial behavior is a direct consequence of an inadequate child-rearing environment in which he or she is not socialized well by parents, other caretakers, or society. If one assumes that CU traits are a result of this hard-to-socialize temperament, which in the model outlined in Figure 1 is low behavioral inhibition, then one would predict that children with these traits would be at high risk for developing conduct problems in many child-rearing environments. Therefore, in children with CU traits, the quality of parenting practices would not be strongly associated with the development of conduct problems. In contrast, in children without these traits, who presumably are less likely to have this hard-to-socialize temperament, the quality of parenting should play a much greater role in the development of conduct problem behavior.

Wootton, Frick, Shelton, and Silverthorn (1995) tested this hypothesized interaction between parenting practices and CU traits in the prediction of conduct problems in a sample of 136 consecutive clinic referrals between the ages of 6 and 13 years, and 30 community children who were matched to the clinic group on age, gender, and ethnicity. The assessment of parenting was designed to tap the five dimensions of parental socialization practices that research has most consistently linked to the development of conduct problem behavior: lack of parental involvement with their child, failure to use positive control strategies (e.g, use of praise and other positive reinforcement) for discipline, poor parental monitoring and supervision of their child, parental inconsistency in discipline, and use of harsh physical discipline (Frick, 1994; Loeber & Stouthamer-Loeber, 1986). Each of these parenting constructs was assessed through two analogous assessment formats (Kuper, Wootton, & Frick, in press). A parental global report format had the child's parent or primary caretaker rate items on a five-point likert scale as to how frequently each parenting behavior *typically* occurs. A parental telephone interview format was also used in which a child's parent or primary caretaker completed four telephone interviews. Using this format, parents provided estimates on how frequently each parenting behavior had occurred within the *past three days*.

Wootton et al. (1995) found a significant interaction between a composite index of dysfunctional parenting practices and CU traits for predicting conduct problems. This interaction was found in separate multiple regression analyses using either the parenting composite based on the global report format or the parenting composite based on the telephone interview format. The form of this interaction is illustrated in Figure 5 using the results with the telephone interview format. In Figure 5 the regression line for the parenting composite predicting conduct problems after controlling for demographic variables is plotted separately for children high and low on CU traits. As would be predicted by Lykken's (1995) formulation, parenting was unrelated to conduct problems in children high on CU traits. The relatively flat regression line suggests that children high on CU traits showed high rates of conduct problems, irrespective of the quality of parenting they received (b=-.14, t=.68, p=ns). In contrast, increasing levels of problematic parenting predicted higher rates of conduct problems in children who were not elevated on CU traits (b=.47, t=2.51, p < .01).

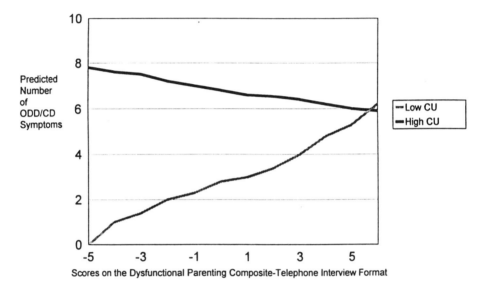

Figure 5. Predicted number of ODD/CD symptoms at each level of the Dysfunctional Parenting composite plotted separately for children elevated on CU traits (above 1 SD; n=48) and those not elevated on CU traits (n=107). Data are based on scatter plot in Figure 2 of Wootton et al. (1995)

These results are consistent with the predictions made from the multiple pathway model outlined in Figure 1. However, even if one rejects the theoretical context in which these results have been embedded, they have several practical implications. By ignoring the moderating influence of CU traits, past studies may have underestimated the association between problematic parenting and conduct problems for children without these traits and overestimated the association for children with CU traits. This could explain some of the inconsistencies in the literature regarding the strength of the association between parenting practices and conduct problem behavior (e.g., Frick et al., 1992; Laub & Sampson, 1986). Given these results, it is also possible that outcome studies may have underestimated the effects of treatments designed to enhance parental socialization strategies for many children with conduct problems by failing to account for the potential moderating role of CU traits on treatment effectiveness (Frick & O'Brien, 1994).

Intelligence and Conduct Problems.

It is important to emphasize that the multiple pathway model that is outlined in Figure 1 should not be considered a nature-vs-nurture conceptualization. In all pathways, there is almost assuredly an interaction between innate predispositions and environmental stressors, albeit different predispositions, different stressors, and different types of interactions in the various pathways. By focusing on parental socialization, this model has focused on a major environmental risk factor that may play an important role in the development of conduct problems in children without CU traits. However, even in children without CU traits, parental socialization practices may be more or less important depending on various child characteristics. For example, parental socialization practices may be very important for determining whether or not children with a temperamental style characterized by poor impulse control eventually develop conduct problems (Frick, 1994).

Another intrinsic risk factor that may place a child at risk for developing conduct problems independent of CU traits is intelligence. Two findings reported previously in this chapter support this contention. First, Frick et al. (1994) reported a significant interaction between CU traits and ODD/CD symptoms for predicting intelligence test scores. That is, children with an ODD or CD diagnosis without CU traits had lower intelligence scores than other clinic-referred children. They also had lower intelligence scores than children with ODD/CD who also were high on CU traits. In contrast, children with ODD/CD and CU traits did not differ from other clinic-referred children on their intelligence test scores. A similar pattern emerged in the cluster analysis of Christian et al. (1995). Children showing high rates of both conduct problems and CU traits had significantly higher intelligence test scores than children showing high rates of conduct problems without CU traits (see Table 2).

Moffitt (1993b) reviewed several decades of research that has linked lower intelligence to conduct problems, aggression, and delinquency. She also summarized numerous theories to explain how lower intelligence could lead to the development of conduct problems, such as impairing a child's ability to develop self-control, impairing a child's ability to delay gratification, impairing a child's ability to develop appropriate conflict resolution skills, impairing a child's ability to develop positive social relationships, or impairing a child's ability to succeed in school. While a definitive conclusion on which of these theories might best explain this relationship awaits further research, the data on the moderating role of CU traits suggest that, whatever the mechanism(s), it seems to operate primarily in the development of conduct problems in children without CU traits.

Summary and Implications for Future Research

Overall, the best summary of this line of research is the statement that an explicit extension of the two-factor model of psychopathy to children seems quite promising for advancing our understanding of antisocial youth. The theoretical model that I have outlined in Figure 1 to guide this extension to children should be viewed as a very simple heuristic. It was designed to emphasize two main points. First, by focusing on CU traits as at least partially separate from poor impulse control and conduct problem behavior, research may begin to focus on a unique causal pathway to conduct problems that is related to low behavioral inhibition. Second, this basic model was designed to emphasize the existence of multiple causal pathways to conduct problems, each involving a unique interaction of causal factors, with CU traits delineating one of these distinct causal pathways. Despite the promise of the two-factor model for enhancing our understanding of childhood conduct problems, it is also important to recognize that this model is still in its infancy. Much of the data presented in this chapter comes from one lab and used overlapping samples. Therefore, this conceptualization will and should undergo many revisions as more data accumulate.

However, the model does point the way to several important areas of research. First, it is critically important to more fully understand the link between low behavioral inhibition and the development of CU traits. For example, Kochanska (1995) has begun to focus on factors, such as secure parent-child attachment, that may enhance the development of the affective components of conscience in children who are temperamentally fearless. Alternatively, it is also quite possible that some children who are not low in behavioral inhibition develop CU traits, such as children from very abusive environments (see Kochanska, 1993). This issue again highlights that the model outlined in Figure 1 is not attempting to define purely *"biological"* or purely *"environmental"* pathways to conduct problems.

Second, it is important to study CU traits in the absence of poor impulse control and conduct problem behaviors. Most of the data presented in this chapter were obtained from clinic-referred children. In these samples it was rare for children high on CU traits not to also show high rates of impulsivity and conduct problems, although many children with conduct problems did not show CU traits. It is possible that CU traits rarely occur without impulsivity and conduct problems. However, it is also quite possible that this would only be found outside of a clinic setting. Studying CU traits in community samples and in isolation from impulsivity and conduct problems could provide some of the best tests of unique causal factors to this psychological dimension.

Third, it is important to explicitly test the predictive utility of CU traits. Christian et al. (1995) provided data to suggest that a subgroup of children with conduct problems who also exhibit CU traits show many of the characteristics that a) have predicted poor outcome in past longitudinal studies and b) make them more analogous to adults with psychopathy. However, both of these possibilities need to be tested directly in longitudinal research. An important question when testing the predictive validity of CU traits is determining whether or not CU traits *add* to the prediction of various outcomes, either independently or in combination with impulsivity, in comparison to proven predictors of persistence like the number, type, and severity of conduct problems (Loeber, 1982; 1991).

Fourth, the basic framework outlined in this chapter has only been used to test a limited number of causal factors involved in the development of conduct problems. Other potential causal mechanisms such as deficits in social cognition (Dodge & Coie, 1987) or the influence of a deviant peer group (Keenan, Loeber, Zhang, Stouthamer-

Loeber, & Van Kammen, 1995) need to also be tested in relation to CU traits. It is quite possible that, like parental socialization practices and intelligence, the study of *"alternative causal pathways"* will be enhanced by studying the interaction of various causal agents with CU traits for predicting the development of conduct problems.

Fifth, an important outcome of an improved understanding of the diverse causal pathways to conduct problems is an improved ability to match treatment to the specific attributes of the child with conduct problems. Successful treatment matching is admittedly a long way off given the need for more basic research on the divergent causal pathways. However, treatment outcome studies can begin to test the potential moderating role of CU traits in predicting the success of existing treatment techniques. For example, it would not be surprising if the absence of CU traits predicted a better outcome of family-based interventions for conduct problems, given the finding that dysfunction parenting was more strongly related to conduct problems in children without these traits.

All of these suggestions for future research highlight the promise of the two-factor model of psychopathy for advancing our understanding of the development of childhood conduct problems. The fulfillment of this promise is dependent on the adequate measurement and separation of these two dimensions for studying unique subgroups of children with conduct problems and for uncovering divergent associations with theoretically important external criteria. Undoubtedly, this early extension of the two-factor model to children has only scratched the surface of many important methodological and theoretical issues. However, the two-factor model is poised to make a significant contribution to the understanding of conduct problems by enhancing our ability to integrate a rich body of research on adult psychopathy, a rich body of research on childhood conduct problems, and a rich body of research on the temperamental styles of adults and children.

References

Abikoff, H., & Klein, R.G. (1992). Attention-deficit hyperactivity disorder and conduct disorder: Comorbidity and implications for treatment. *Journal of Consulting and Clinical Psychology, 60*, 881-892.

Achenbach, T.M. (1991). *The child behavior checklist-1991*. Vermont: University of Vermont.

American Psychiatric Association (1980). *Diagnostic and statistical manual of mental disorders, 3rd edition*. Washington, DC: Author.

American Psychiatric Association (1987). *Diagnostic and statistical manual of mental disorders* (3rd ed., rev.). Washington, DC: Author.

American Psychiatric Association (1994). *Diagnostic and statistical manual of mental disorders* (4th ed.). Washington, DC: Author.

Barkley, R.A. (1994). Impaired delayed responding: A unified theory of attention-deficit hyperactivity disorders. In D.K. Routh (Ed.), *Disruptive behavior disorders in childhood (pp. 11-58)*. New York: Plenum.

Bornstein, I.H. (1988). *Applied multivariate analysis*. New York: Springer-Verlag.

Christian, R., Frick, P.J., Hill, N., Tyler, L.A., & Frazer, D. (1995). *Psychopathy and conduct problems: II. Subtyping children with conduct problems based on their interpersonal and affective style*. Manuscript submitted for publication.

Cleckley, H. (1976). *The mask of sanity (5th edition)*. St. Louis, MO: Mosby.

Cloninger, C.R. (1987). A systematic method for clinical description and classification of personality variants. *Archives of General Psychiatry, 44*, 573-588.

Daugherty, T. K., & Quay, H. C. (1991). Response perseveration and delayed responding in childhood behavior disorders. *Journal of Child Psychology and Psychiatry, 32*, 453-461.

Dodge, K.A., & Coie, J.D. (1987). Social-information-processing factors in reactive and proactive aggression in children's peer groups. *Journal of Personality and Social Psychology, 53*, 1146-1158.

Fowles, D. C. (1988). Psychophysiology and psychopathology: A motivational approach. *Psychophysiology, 25*, 373-391.

Frick, P.J. (1993). Childhood conduct problems in family context. *School Psychology Review, 22*, 376-385.

Frick, P.J. (1994). Family dysfunction and the disruptive behavior disorders: A review of recent empirical findings. In T.H. Ollendick & R.J. Prinz (Eds.), *Advances in clinical child psychology, (Vol. 16, pp. 203-226)*. New York: Plenum.

Frick, P.J., & Hare, R.D. (in press). *The psychopathy screening device*. Toronto: Multi-Health Systems.

Frick, P.J., Lahey, B.B., Loeber, R., Stouthamer-Loeber, M., Christ, M.A.G., & Hanson, K. (1992). Familial risk factors to oppositional defiant disorder and conduct disorder: Parental psychopathology and maternal parenting. *Journal of Consulting and Clinical Psychology, 60*, 49-55. Frick, P.J., Lahey, B.B., Loeber, R., Tannenbaum, L., Van Horn, Y., Christ, M.A.G., Hart, E.A., & Hanson, K. (1993). Oppositional defiant disorder and conduct disorder: A meta-analytic review of factor analyses and cross-validation in a clinic sample. *Clinical Psychology Review, 13*, 319-340.

Frick, P.J., Lilienfeld, S.O., & McBurnett, K. (1996). *Anxiety, psychopathy, and antisocial behavior in three samples*. Manuscript in preparation.

Frick, P.J., & O'Brien, B.S. (1994). Conduct disorders. In R.T. Ammerman and M. Hersen (Eds.), *Handbook of child behavior therapy in the psychiatric setting* (pp. 199-216). New York: Wiley.

Frick, P.J., O'Brien, B.S., Wootton, J.M., & McBurnett, K. (1994). Psychopathy and conduct problems in children. *Journal of Abnormal Psychology, 103*, 700-707.

Gray, J. A. (1982). *The neuropsychology of anxiety: An enquiry into the functions of the septo-hippocampal system*. Oxford: Oxford University Press.

Hare, R.D. (1985). Comparison of procedures for the assessment of psychopathy. *Journal of Consulting and Clinical Psychology, 30*, 135-137.

Hare, R.D. (1991). *The Hare psychopathy checklist-revised*. Toronto: Multi-Health Systems.

Hare, R.D. (1993). *Without conscience: The disturbing world of the psychopaths among us*. New York: Pocket.

Hare, R.D., Harpur, T.J., Hakstian, A.R., Forth, A.E., Hart, S.D., & Newman, J.P. (1990). The revised Psychopathy Checklist: Reliability and factor structure. *Psychological Assessment, 2*, 338-341.

Hare, R.D., Hart, S.D., & Harpur, T.J. (1991). Psychopathy and the DSM-IV criteria for antisocial personality disorder. *Journal of Abnormal Psychology, 100*, 391-398.

Harpur, T.J., Hakstian, A.R., & Hare, R.D. (1988). Factor structure of the Psychopathy Checklist. *Journal of Consulting and Clinical Psychology, 56*, 741-747.

Harpur, T.J., Hare, R.D., & Hakstian, A.R. (1989). Two-factor conceptualization of psychopathy: Construct validity and assessment implications. *Psychological Assessment, 1*, 6-17.

Hart, S.D., Forth, A.E., & Hare, R.D. (1990). Performance of male psychopaths on selected neuropsychological tests. *Journal of Abnormal Psychology, 99*, 374-379.

Hart, S.D., Kropp, P.R., & Hare, R.D. (1988). Performance of male psychopaths following conditional release from prison. *Journal of Consulting and Clinical Psychology, 56*, 227-232.

Hinshaw, S.P. (1994). Conduct disorder in childhood: Conceptualization, diagnosis, comorbidity, and risk status for antisocial functioning in adulthood. In D.C. Fowles, P. Sutker, & S.H. Goodman, (Eds.), *Special Focus on Psychopathy and Antisocial Personality: A Developmental Perspective* (pp. 3-44). New York: Springer.

Hinshaw, S.P., Lahey, B.B., & Hart, E.L. (1993). Issues of taxonomy and comorbidity in the development of conduct disorder. *Development and Psychopathology, 5*, 31-49.

Kagan, J., & Snidman, N. (1991). Temperamental factors in human development. *American Psychologist, 46*, 856-862.

Kamphaus, R.W., & Frick, P.J. (1996). *Clinical assessment of child and adolescent personality and behavior.* Boston: Allyn & Bacon.

Keenan, K., Loeber, R., Zhang, Q., Stouthamer-Loeber, M., & Van Kammen, W.B. (1995). The influence of deviant peers on the development of boys' disruptive and delinquent behavior: A temporal analysis. *Development and Psychopathology, 7*, 715-726.

Kochanska, G. (1991). Socialization and temperament in the development of guilt and conscience. *Child Development, 62*, 1379-1392.

Kochanska, G. (1993). Toward a synthesis of parental socialization and child temperament in early development of conscience. *Child Development, 64*, 325-347.

Kochanska, G. (1995). Children's temperament, mothers' discipline, and security of attachment: Multiple pathways to emerging internalization. *Child Development, 66*, 597-615.

Lahey, B.B., Hart, E.L., Pliszka, S., Applegate, B., & McBurnett, K. (1993). Neurophysiological correlates of conduct disorder: A rationale and a review of research. *Journal of Clinical Child Psychology, 22*, 141-153.

Lahey, B.B., Loeber, R., Hart, E.L., Frick, P.J., Applegate, B., Zhang, Q., Green, S.M., & Russo, M.F. (1995). Four-year longitudinal study of conduct disorder in boys: Patterns and predictors of persistence. *Journal of Abnormal Psychology, 104*, 83-93.

Lahey, B.B., Loeber, R., Quay, H.C., Frick, P.J., & Grimm, J. (1992). Oppositional defiant and conduct disorders: Issues to be resolved for DSM-IV. *Journal of the American Academy of Child and Adolescent Psychiatry, 31*, 539-546.

Laub J.H., & Sampson, R.J. (1988). Unraveling families and delinquency: A reanalysis of the Gluecks' data. *Criminology, 26*, 355-380.

Levenson, M.R. (1990). Risk taking and personality. *Journal of Personality and Social Psychology, 58*, 1073-1080.

Lilienfeld, S.O. (1994). Conceptual problems in the assessment of psychopathy. *Clinical Psychology Review, 14*, 17-38.

Loeber, R. (1982). The stability of antisocial and delinquent child behavior: A review. *Child Development, 53*, 1431-1446.

Loeber, R. (1990). Development and risk factors of juvenile antisocial behavior and delinquency. *Clinical Psychology Review, 10*, 1-41.

Loeber, R. (1991). Antisocial behavior: More enduring than changeable? *Journal of the American Academy of Child and Adolescent Psychiatry, 30*, 393-397.

Loeber, R., Green, S. M., Lahey, B. B., & Stouthamer-Loeber, M. (1991). Differences and similarities between children, mothers, and teachers as informants on disruptive child behavior. *Journal of Abnormal Child Psychology, 19*, 75-95.

Loeber, R., & Stouthamer-Loeber M. (1986). Family factors as correlates and predictors of juvenile conduct problems and delinquency. In M. Tonry & N. Morris (Eds.), *Crime and justice* (Vol. 17, pp. 29-149). Chicago: University of Chicago Press.

Loeber, R., & Stouthamer-Loeber, M. (1987). Prediction. In H.C. Quay (Ed.), *Handbook of juvenile delinquency* (pp. 325-382). New York: Wiley.

Lykken, D.T. (1995). *The antisocial personalities.* Hillsdale, NJ: Erlbaum.

McCord, W. & McCord, J. (1964). *The psychopath: An essay on the criminal mind.* Princeton, NJ: Van Nostrand.

Milich, R., Hartung, C.M., Martin, C.A., & Haigler, E.D. (1994). Behavioral disinhibition and underlying processes in adolescents with disruptive behavior disorders. In D.K. Routh. (Ed.), *Disruptive behavior disorders in childhood (pp. 109-138).* New York: Plenum.

Moffitt, T.E. (1993a). Adolescence-limited and life course persistent antisocial behavior: A developmental typology. *Psychological Review, 100,* 674-701.

Moffitt, T.E. (1993b). The neuropsychology of conduct disorder. *Development and Psychopathology, 5,* 135-152.

Neeper, R., Lahey, B.B., & Frick, P.J. (1990). *The comprehensive behavior rating scale for children.* San Antonio, TX: The Psychological Corporation.

Newman, J. P., Patterson, C. M., & Kosson, D. S. (1987). Response perseveration in psychopaths. *Journal of Abnormal Psychology, 96,* 145-148.

Newman, J.P., & Wallace, J.F. (1993). Diverse pathways to deficient self-regulation: Implications for disinhibitory psychopathology in children. *Clinical Psychology Review, 13,* 699-720.

O'Brien, B.S., & Frick, P.J. (1996). Reward dominance: Associations with anxiety, conduct problems, and psychopathy in children. *Journal of Abnormal Child Psychology, 24,* 223-240.

O'Brien, B.S., Frick, P.J., & Lyman, R.D. (1994). Reward dominance among children with disruptive behavior disorders. *Journal of Psychopathology and Behavioral Assessment, 16,* 131-145.

Oosterlaan, J. & Sargeant, J.A. (1996). Inhibition in ADHD, aggressive, and anxious children: A biologically based model of child psychopathology. *Journal of Abnormal Child Psychology, 24,* 19-38.

Patterson, G.R. (1986). Performance models for antisocial boys. *American Psychologist, 41,* 432-444.

Quay, H.C. (1987). Patterns of delinquent behavior. In H.C. Quay (Ed.), *Handbook of juvenile delinquency* (pp. 118-138). New York: Wiley.

Quay, H.C. (1993). The psychobiology of undersocialized aggressive conduct disorder. *Development and Psychopathology, 5,* 165-180.

Richters, J.E., & Cicchetti, D. (1993). Mark Twain meets DSM-III-R: Conduct disorder, development, and the concept of harmful dysfunction. *Development and Psychopathology, 5,* 5-30.

Robins, L. N. (1978). Etiological implications in childhood histories relating to antisocial personality. In R. D. Hare & D. Schalling (Eds.), *Psychopathic behavior: Approaches to research* (pp. 255-272). New York: Wiley.

Rothbart, M.K. (1989). Temperament in childhood: A framework. In G.A. Kohnstamm, J.A. Bates, & M.K. Rothbart (Eds.), *Temperament in childhood (pp.59-73).* New York: Wiley.

Russo, M. F., Stokes, G. S., Lahey, B. B., Christ, M. A. G., McBurnett, K., Loeber, R., Stouthamer-Loeber, M., & Green, S. M. (1993). A sensation-seeking scale for children: A further refinement and psychometric development. *Journal of Psychopathology and Behavioral Assessment, 15,* 69-86

Shaffer, D., Fisher, P., Piacentini, J.C., Schwab-Stone, M., & Wicks, J. (1992). *National Institute of Mental Health Diagnostic Interview Schedule for Children, Version 2.3.* New York: Columbia University.

Shapiro, S. K., Quay, H. C., Hogan, A. E., & Schwartz, K. P. (1988). Response perseveration and delayed responding in undersocialized aggressive conduct disorder. *Journal of Abnormal Psychology, 97,* 371-373.

Shelton, K.K., Frick, P.J., & Wootton, J.M. (in press). The assessment of parenting practices in families of elementary school-aged children. *Journal of Clinical Child Psychology*.

Wells, L.E., & Rankin, J.H. (1988). Direct parental controls and delinquency. *Criminology, 26,* 263-285.

Williamson, S., Harpur, T.J., & Hare, R.D. (1991). Abnormal processing of affective words by psychopaths. *Psychophysiology, 28,* 260-273.

Wootton, J.M., Frick, P.J., Shelton, K.K., Silverthorn, P. (1995). *Problematic parenting and childhood conduct problems: The moderating role of child temperament.* Manuscript submitted for publication.

Zuckerman, M. (1979). *Sensation-seeking: Beyond the optimal level of arousal.* Hillsdale, NJ: Erlbaum.

COMORBIDITIES AND BIOLOGICAL CORRELATES OF CONDUCT DISORDER

KEITH MCBURNETT and LINDA PFIFFNER
University of California,
Irvine, USA.

ESTIMATING DEVELOPMENTAL RISK FOR PSYCHOPATHY USING SUBTYPES, COMORBIDITIES, AND BIOLOGICAL CORRELATES OF CONDUCT DISORDER

Chronic antisocial syndromes in adulthood are preceded by antisocial behavior in childhood and adolescence (Robins, 1966, 1978). The near-universality of this sequence is codified in the DSM-IV (American Psychiatric Association, 1994) definition of Antisocial Personality Disorder (APD), in the diagnostic criterion requiring that Conduct Disorder (CD) originated before the age of 15 years. Unlike the diagnostic category of APD, psychopathy is measured dimensionally, and it has no essential diagnostic requirements even when dimension score cutpoints are applied to make a categorical distinction. Documentation of youthful onset can only raise the dimensional score by affecting the two (of a total of 20) items from the Hare Psychopathy Checklist-Revised PCL-R (Hare, 1991) that refer to antisocial behavior during the developmental period—early behavior problems and juvenile delinquency. Yet, developmental origin is just as axiomatic for psychopathy as for APD (Hare, 1970).

More research in recent years has been devoted to CD than to emergent psychopathy. Because of this, a large portion of what might be inferred about early psychopathy must at present be based on studies of CD. We know that individuals who never exhibit the kind of behavior that would justify the CD diagnosis during the developmental period (up to age 18) will almost certainly not become psychopaths. However, what we would most like to know is not which children will not become psychopaths, but which will. Given that adult psychopathy and APD are stunningly untouched by any known therapy or medication, scarce preventive resources would best be directed in large, sustained, and undiluted doses toward youths known to be in the early stages of psychopathy (or APD). CD can be diagnosed with good reliability (Lahey et al., 1994). If the prevalence of CD were not so high, CD would be an excellent identifier of risk for psychopathy. The problem is that increased antisocial behavior is so common among adolescents that it might be considered a normal stage of development. Even the very serious diagnosis of CD, using strict DSM criteria, is estimated to apply to between 6% to 16% of males and 2% to 9% of females under the age of 18 (American Psychiatric Association, 1994). If prevalence of APD is estimated at 3% of adult males and 1% of adult females (American Psychiatric Association, 1994), and the prevalence of psychopathy is thought to be lower than for APD, then it becomes clear that most children with CD will not become psychopaths.

189

D.J. Cooke et al. (eds.), Psychopathy: Theory, Research and Implications for Society, 189–203.
© *1998 Kluwer Academic Publishers. Printed in the Netherlands.*

The goal of much research with CD is to find ways of better predicting antisocial risk. This discussion will outline three nonexclusive strategies for increasing the resolution of the diagnostic lens of CD and its power to focus on psychopathic risk. The first strategy is to examine the effects of co-existing diagnoses, or *comorbidity*. The second is to divide CD into *subtypes* that have some validity for risk prediction. The third is to consider the CD diagnosis to be a measure of behavioral disturbance analogous to the Factor II of the PCL-R, one that is limited in its predictive utility without the concurrent use of a measure of the interpersonal and psychopathic personality characteristics associated with Factor I.

COMORBIDITY

Despite its status as an APD criterion, CD is not the only childhood diagnosis that presages psychopathy. In the DSM-IV, CD is one of three disorders classified under Attention and Disruptive Behavior Disorders, each posing some risk for chronic antisocial behavior. For example, Attention-deficit Hyperactivity Disorder (ADHD) is estimated to lead to APD in 25% of cases (Barkley, 1990) on the basis of existing outcome studies.[1] Thus, on a purely statistical basis, ADHD may provide as good or better predictive validity as does CD.[2] The third disorder in this group is Oppositional Defiant Disorder (ODD). ODD and CD have a hierarchical relationship in that CD subsumes ODD. When CD is diagnosed, the diagnosis of ODD is not given, even if warranted. CD is considered to be a severe form or advanced progression of ODD.

The symptoms of these disorders follow different developmental courses. ADHD is a chronic condition whose pathophysiology is believed to involve the frontal lobes and their modulation of diencephalic and limbic systems involved in motor control and emotion. ADHD always begins in early childhood (generally by age seven, often at much younger ages), and is often life-long, at least in residual form. Its symptoms of inattention/disorganization, which are clearly linked to academic problems, tend to be life-long but can appear less prominent once an individual discontinues school. On the other hand, the hyperactivity/impulsivity symptoms of ADHD reliably diminish somewhat over the course of childhood (perhaps benefiting from the frontal maturation and mylenization that continues into the third decade of life), particularly those symptoms involving gross motor hyperactivity. CD can begin at any age. Some symptoms of CD can and sometimes do occur in toddlers, but many CD symptoms can only be achieved (with rare exceptions) in adolescence. In its most common and benign form, CD begins and ends over a brief period of adolescence. Less commonly, it begins in early childhood and is preceded or accompanied by ODD, but in this form it appears more likely to persist into adulthood.

For the purposes of considering what implications comorbidity in childhood has for the development of psychopathy, we will be concerned with four combinations:

---

[1] By contemporary diagnostic standards, the outcome studies of ADHD that have been reported to date are inadequate for estimating the relative risk that childhood ADHD poses for adult psychopathy, because these studies either failed to fully account for the comorbidity of CD and CD's precursor, ODD, in the subject selection process.
[2] The predictive power that ADHD has for adult antisocial behavior is thought to derive largely from the high rates of comorbidity of the other child behavior disorders (CD and ODD).

ADHD without CD, CD without ADHD, ADHD plus CD, and the benign state of having neither ADHD nor CD. The information that comes with knowing the diagnostic status of a case is not limited to the disorders that are present, but also builds from knowing which disorders have been ruled out. (For example, because ADHD and CD in combination are known to pose an extremely high risk, a child with ADHD who has been evaluated and found to *not* have CD or ODD can be said to have a relatively benign prognosis in many respects and to probably not fall among the estimated 25% of youths with ADHD who will develop APD.) We do not treat ODD separately here because it has received less research, and because for the most part, it can be assumed to carry similar but milder implications as CD.

Let us first simply inspect the similarity of content between psychopathy features and child disorder symptoms. The characteristics of adult psychopathy appear to be better represented by the combination of ADHD and CD than by CD alone (see Table 1).

Turning to empirical studies, without going into detail we can summarize the evidence as follows. ADHD is more dangerous when accompanied by CD than when it occurs alone. Compared to ADHD in the absence of CD, the comorbid condition is marked by greater social impairment, greater likelihood of persistence, poorer adult adjustment, and higher rate of adult antisocial behavior (August, Stewart & Holmes, 1983; Hart et al., in press; Loney, Kramer & Milich, 1981; Taylor, Sandberg, Thorley & Giles, 1991). Looking at the mirror image, CD is more dangerous when accompanied by ADHD than when it occurs alone. Compared to CD in the absence of ADHD, the comorbid condition is marked by younger age of onset, greater social impairment, greater likelihood of persistence, more physical aggression, and greater antisocial versatility (Farrington, Loeber & Van Kammen, 1990; Loeber, 1988; Magnusson & Bergman, 1990; Moffitt, 1990; Offord, Sullivan, & Abrams, 1979; Schachar, Rutter & Smith, 1981; Walker, Lahey, Hynd & Frame, 1987). Again, it would appear that the greatest risk for psychopathy would occur in youngsters with comorbid ADHD and CD.

A third approach would be to examine whether biologically based characteristics of psychopathy are best represented by a single disorder or by the comorbid condition. Here we will argue that arousal deficits are associated with CD, executive neuropsychological impairment is associated with ADHD, and both of these are associated with antisocial behavior. First, though, the discussion must briefly digress to the issue of whether psychopaths have abnormal frontal lobe development. When psychopathic prisoners are compared to nonpsychopathic prisoners on neuropsychological tests thought to measure frontal abilities or executive functions, the groups often are found to be equivalent (e.g., Hare, 1984).

However, if frontal abnormalities are prevalent among the larger population of individuals prone to criminal behavior and antisocial conduct (and high ratings on Factor 2 of the PCL-R), and not *specifically* associated with the kind of personality features tapped by Factor I items that are the major divergence between psychopathic and nonpsychopathic prisoners, then frontal abnormalities would not be found in this kind of design because they would be represented in both experimental groups.

TABLE 1. Correspondence of Psychopathy Features with Attention and Disruptive Behavior
　　　　Disorder Symptoms

Psychopathy features (PCL-R Items)	ODD/CD Symptoms	ADHD Symptoms
Factor I items		
Glibness/superficial charm		Tangentially represented by "Often talks excessively"
Grandiose sense of self-worth		
Pathological lying	Often lies to obtain goods or favors or to avoid obligations (i.e., "cons" others) (CD)	
Conning/manipulative	Often lies to obtain goods or favors or to avoid obligations (i.e., "cons" others) (CD)	
Lack of remorse or guilt		
Shallow affect		
Callous/lack of empathy		
Failure to accept responsibility for own actions	Often blames others for his mistakes or misbehavior (ODD)	
Factor II items		
Need for stimulation/proneness to boredom	No equivalent symptom, but can be inferred from the context of some CD symptoms	Often avoids, dislikes, or is reluctant to engage in tasks that require sustained mental effort; often "on the go" or acts as if "driven by a motor;" often has difficulty awaiting turn
Parasitic lifestyle		
Poor behavior controls	Often loses temper; actively defies or refuses to comply with adult requests or rules; often touchy or easily annoyed by others; often angry and resentful (ODD). Often bullies, threatens or intimidates others; often initiates physical fights; has used a weapon; has been physically cruel to people (CD).	
Early behavioral problems	All symptoms of CD	
Lack of realistic long-term goals		
Impulsivity	No equivalent symptom, but can be inferred from the context of some CD symptoms	Often blurts out answers, often has difficulty awaiting turn, often interrupts or intrudes on others
Irresponsibility		Tangentially represented by "Often does not follow through on instructions and fails to finish"
Juvenile delinquency	Illegal CD symptoms	
Revocation of conditional release		
Remaining items		
Promiscuous sexual behavior	Has forced someone into sexual activity (CD)	
Many short-term marital relationships		
Criminal versatility	Multiple CD symptoms	

Secondly (and less appreciated in the literature), the clinical neuropsychological tests that have been developed with brain-injured populations have ceiling effects that make them insensitive to subtle differences in adult executive abilities. Elementary-school-age children with ADHD often perform poorly on these neuropsychological tests compared to age peers, but interestingly, such performance deficits tend *not* to be found in older children and adolescents with ADHD much past the age range of 10-12 years at which normal children master these tasks and match the performance of adults (McBurnett et al., 1993). As children with ADHD—whose executive test performance lags that of their age peers by 1-3 years—mature beyond the normal mastery age by at least a similar interval, they may also master the tests while still harboring executive abilities that are mildly impaired, relative to their chronological peers without ADHD. This subtle impairment may continue into adulthood, unmeasureable by standard clinical tests but functionally manifesting as difficulty *or inconsistency* in setting goals, following plans, generating and following organizational strategies, inhibiting distractions and temptations, monitoring multiple responsibilities, and adhering to time constraints and schedules, *particularly* in functional domains without strong inherent motivation for the individual.

For the sake of argument, let us refrain from assuming that psychopaths have impaired or inconsistent executive functions, and acknowledge only that any psychopaths who *do* have such problems will be even more likely to live an erratic, disorganized, present-focused, and impulsive lifestyle. A biological correlate of psychopathy that is observed with greater consistency is physiological underarousal. In several paradigms measuring electrodermal activity (EDA), psychopaths tend to be less active and responsive than nonpsychopaths (reviewed by Hare, 1978). Which child condition(s) might have the most complete representation of these biological abnormalities associated with psychopathy and chronic antisocial behavior? In one study of 57 normal and clinic-referred children, parent and teacher ratings were used to divide children into groups based on whether they showed behaviors predominantly characteristic of ADHD, behaviors predominantly characteristic of ODD/CD, behaviors characteristic of both ADHD and ODD/CD, or none such behavior (McBurnett et al., 1993). Children were tested on an executive function task (the Wisconsin Card Sorting Test, WCST) while their EDA was measured. ANOVAs found that ODD/CD behavior was associated with lower electrodermal responding, and ADHD behavior was associated with poorer WCST performance. There were no interaction effects. This suggests that ADHD and CD have unique neuropsychological and psychophysiological features, and that an additive (comorbid) model is necessary to account for the co-occurrence of those features. Moreover, the findings suggest that whatever etiological risks for psychopathy are posed or signaled by low executive and electrodermal functioning, those risks are elevated in children with symptoms of both ADHD and CD in the age range used in this study (5-12 years). In a large study of male adolescents in New Zealand, those with symptoms of both ADHD and CD performed more poorly on the WCST and on other tests of executive function than youths with either CD alone or ADHD alone, and the poorer executive performance was associated with early onset of delinquency (Moffit & Henry, 1989; Moffit & Silva, 1988). This study makes a strong case that at least one form of neuropsychological risk for antisocial behavior is concentrated in the comorbid condition of ADHD and CD, although the risk is not specifically established for psychopathy.

SUBTYPING

The heterogeneity problem in CD has a long history, and several strategies have been proposed for dividing CD into more homogenous subtypes. As reviewed by Quay (1986), multivariate analyses of childhood problem behavior items across the last fifty years have replicated with a remarkable degree of consistency a factor fitting the rubric of Undersocialized Aggressive CD, characterized by aggressive, disruptive, noncompliant, hyperactive, and restless behavior; often associated with psychopathic features such as poor attachment and lack of remorse for wrongdoing; and observed in children of all ages including very young children. The other CD pattern that has been replicated across several studies (but not as consistently as the Undersocialized pattern) fits the label of Socialized CD, characterized by more covert antisocial and rule-breaking behavior and by capacity for social bonding and remorse for wrongdoing, and more typical of older children and adolescents. These patterns have inspired researchers to propose methods of classifying CD cases into more homogeneous subtypes. Within studies, subtyping approaches have often received empirical validation, but their acceptance has been limited by lack of diagnostic reliability and methodological standardization across clinicians and studies.

Subtyping in DSM

The DSM-III (American Psychiatric Association, 1980) presented a method of categorizing CD using what amounted to a two-by-two factorial design in which the factors were socialization and aggression (whether these were present or absent in a given case of CD). Thus, there were four subtypes: Undersocialized Aggressive, Undersocialized Nonaggressive (for which few cases were found), Socialized Aggressive, and Socialized Nonaggressive. DSM-III-R (American Psychiatric Association, 1987) retained the subtypes for which there was the most empirical support. These were Solitary Aggressive Type and Group Type (which corresponded roughly to Socialized Nonaggressive Type, but expanded to include youths whose conduct problems occurred mainly as a group activity with peers, regardless of the degree of aggressiveness). Thus the *de facto* categories in DSM-III-R were psychopathic and delinquent CD, not dissimilar to the empirically derived patterns just described, and the chief distinguishing characteristic was socialization. Despite a considerable amount of biological and other research supporting the validity of the socialization dimension, no reliable means of operationalizing the distinction was ever agreed upon by researchers. The current DSM-IV (American Psychiatric Association, 1994) uses age of onset of CD (by age 10, or later) to distinguish a Childhood-Onset Type from an Adolescent-Onset Type. This scheme certainly has an advantage of reliable classification. It also gains validity from studies showing that early onset CD tends to be accompanied by ADHD, to show a strong bias toward male gender, and to follow a long-term developmental course marked by greater severity and versatility of antisocial behavior with advancing age (Hinshaw, 1994; Moffitt, 1990, 1993). Adolescent-Onset CD does not have such a strong association with ADHD, and it is distributed more evenly across genders. These youths are more likely to exhibit covert forms of antisocial behavior rather than aggression, and they are more likely to desist spontaneously at some time during the teen years. By inference, children with Childhood-Onset CD appear to have the greater risk of developing psychopathy. By no means, however, is it clear that all or even most children with early CD become psychopaths, even though most will face great difficulty adjusting to society.

Studies of CD have used not only these subtyping systems, but several others, including anxious v. nonanxious (subtyping by comorbid anxiety) and psychopathic v. neurotic. Quite obviously, these different methods are not independent, and several seem to map onto each other to some degree. CD groups variously described in different studies as undersocialized, aggressive, nonanxious, and psychopathic, tend to bear certain descriptive and empirical resemblances to each other and to adult psychopaths. On the milder side of the fence, there are similarities among groups described as socialized, nonaggressive, anxious, and neurotic. Three published reviews of the biological correlates of CD (Lahey, Hart, Pliszka, Applegate & McBurnett, 1993; Lahey, McBurnett, Loeber & Hart, 1995; McBurnett & Lahey, 1994) reached a similar set of tentative conclusions. Biologically, two subtypes of CD can be differentiated, distinguished by low vs. high psychobiological tone.[3] CD groups defined as undersocialized, psychopathic, aggressive, or nonanxious tend to have low arousal and/or reactivity of the sympathetic branch of the autonomic nervous system and of the hypothalamic-pituitary-adrenal axis (HPA, the system that provides multi-level feedback regulation of cortisol). Summing across the results of several studies, the ordinal ranking of the means of some biological variables suggests that socialized/neurotic/anxious/nonaggressive CD groups exhibit the highest arousal or reactivity, normal controls or non-CD clinic controls occupy an intermediate position, and undersocialized/psychopathic/nonanxious/aggressive groups have the lowest arousal or reactivity. In spite of large individual differences in arousal and reactivity, group mean differences are sometimes large enough to be statistically significant when the comparison groups are non-CD controls, but the largest group differences often occur in comparisons between the two CD subtypes. An important corollary is that any biological study of CD that fails to differentiate subtypes runs the risk of averaging extremely low and extremely high values together and finding no differences from controls. This can lead to the mistaken generalization that youths with CD have an average level of arousal that does not differ from that of non-CD youths.

---

[3] A crucial gap in our understanding of the psychobiology of CD exists regarding the temporal stability and developmental staging of variations in autonomic and HPA tone. In particular, it is not known whether CD youths who exhibit higher arousal do so over the entire developmental period and into adulthood, or only during a circumscribed epoch.

Cortisol and CD subtypes

For this paper we focused on cortisol as an indicater of arousal and as a validator of CD subgrouping distinctions. We computed effect sizes for several studies of CD and cortisol, and we conducted new analyses of the data from a previous study of CD and salivary cortisol (McBurnett et al., 1991). Together, these studies demonstrate the utility of several designs that are more likely to concentrate psychopaths or pre-psychopaths into a single experimental group: (a) grouping by childhood history of DSM-III CD subtype, (b) grouping by adult status of violent APD, (c) grouping by comorbid anxiety, and (d) grouping by DSM-IV CD subtype.

No subtyping

Three cortisol studies have been reported that did not subtype CD, and none of these found the CD diagnosis to have any statistically significant effect on cortisol. Kruesi, Schmidt, Donnelly, Euthymia et al. (1989) compared a highly aggressive group of 19 children with mixed disruptive behavior disorders (most of whom had CD) to 19 normal controls, mean age 10.5 years. The groups did not differ on 24-hour urinary free cortisol (UFC), and the size of the diagnostic effect on cortisol was negligible (Cohen's d = .06 in favor of the clinical group). Scerbo & Kolko (1994) compared 19 children with CD to 11 clinic-referred children without CD, mean age 11.18 years. Mean salivary cortisol concentration in the CD group was lower than in the non-CD group (d = -.17), but this small difference was not statistically significant. Targum, Clarkson, Magac-Harris, Marshall & Skwerer (1990) compared 11 adolescents with CD to 11 adolescents with major depression, mean age 15.4 years. Some differences in cortisol output occurred between the groups that would be classified as moderately-sized effects, but these were not statistically significant (there was *greater* 24-hour UFC excretion by the CD group, d = .64, and *lower* 8 am serum cortisol in the CD group, d = -.63). Regardless, the use of a clinical comparison group that itself may be associated with HPA disruption makes any findings uninterpretable.

GROUPING BY DSM-III SUBTYPE HISTORY AND BY ADULT VIOLENT APD STATUS

Virkkunen (1985) reported an important study of adult male offenders. Among 73 habitually violent male offenders, those who had the DSM-III subtype of Undersocialized Aggressive CD in childhood (n = 31) excreted only about half the amount of free cortisol in 24-hour urine as those who did not meet criteria for the subtype, a large and statistically significant effect (d = 1.23). Analyses using concurrent adult diagnoses found that the mean 24-hour UFC from a group of 34 male offenders diagnosed as having APD with habitually violent tendencies was about half that found in five other experimental groups. The violent APD group effect on cortisol was large and statistically significant compared to APD offenders without habitually violent tendencies (n = 20, d = 1.73), to offenders with intermittent explosive disorder (n = 39, d = 1.85), to other violent offenders (n = 17, d = 1.67), to recidivous arsonists (n = 10, d = 2.84), and to psychiatric male personnel (n = 15, d = 2.33). Both the concurrent and retrospective analyses suggest that it is those individuals characterized by both poor socialization *and* aggression who show the biological abnormality reflected in low cortisol levels. Not coincidentally, the subtypes of CD (Undersocialized Aggressive) and of APD (with habitual violence, a clinical determination not formalized in DSM APD) are the DSM-III niches most likely to apply to psychopaths.

Grouping by comorbid DSM-III-R anxiety disorder

McBurnett et al. (1991) compared 7 children with DSM-III-R CD but no DSM-III-R anxiety disorder to 11 children diagnosed with CD and a comorbid anxiety disorder, mean age 9.4 years. A 2 x 2 ANOVA (CD v. no CD, anxiety disorder v. no anxiety disorder) found a statistically significant effect for the interaction of CD and anxiety, but no main effect for CD (thus supporting the validity of subtyping). When the two CD subgroups were compared to each other, the concentration of cortisol in saliva was significantly lower in the CD subgroup that was free from anxiety. The effect of this subtyping was large (d = 1.3). (Mean salivary cortisol concentrations in children without CD, whether or not these children had an anxiety disorder, fell in the range between the two CD subtypes.) Moreover, the children with CD but not anxiety had more contacts with police, more suspensions from school, and more nominations by their classmates for being *"meanest"* and for *"fights most"* than children with both CD and an anxiety disorder (Walker et al., 1991).[4] This behavioral evidence identifies the non-anxious CD group as the one at highest risk for developing psychopathy.

These data came from one small sample of clinic-referred children with CD, but within that limitation they provide strong support for using comorbid anxiety as a subtype criterion. In the adult literature, not coincidentally, subtyping by anxiety has sometimes been found to sharpen the relationship between psychopathy and psychobiological effects (Arnett, Howland, Smith & Newman, 1993; Smith, Arnett & Newman, 1992; Newman, Kosson & Patterson, 1992). Subtyping by anxiety is attractive from a theoretical view. There is a long history of characterizing psychopaths as being abnormally low in anxiety and differentiating primary from secondary psychopaths on that basis (Blackburn, 1975; Cleckley, 1982; Lykken, 1957). To the extent that CD symptoms reflect unbridled instrumental behavior, and anxiety symptoms reflect sensitivity to threat and punishment and behavioral restraint, subtyping CD by anxiety fits Gray's (1982, 1987) two-factor theories of neural control systems (the Behavioral Activation System and the Behavioral Inhibition System) and of personality (Impulsivity and Anxiety) (see also (Fowles, 1980, 1983; McBurnett, 1992; Quay, 1988). But subtyping by anxiety is beset by several problems. First, being less visible to adult informants (parents and teachers), anxiety is not as straightforward to measure in children as is disruptive behavior. Second, anxiety is not a unitary construct, and there is evidence that anxiety's relationship to psychopathy differs according to whether anxiety is a trait rather than a state (Levenson, Keihl & Fitzpatrick, 1995; Spielberger, Kling & O'Hagan, 1978) or whether anxiety is of the somatic rather than psychic variety (Schalling, 1978), or whether anxiety measures are

---

[4] Other analyses highlight an association between low cortisol and aggression. Across all subjects (n = 67), cortisol was significantly and inversely related to peer nominations for *"meanest"* (-.39), nominations for *"fights most"* (-.40), and number of aggressive CD symptoms reported by parents (-.41), but insignificantly to number of nonaggressive symptoms (-.08; Lahey & Loeber, 1991; McBurnett et al., 1990).

tapping behavioral inhibition or subjective distress (Frick, this volume). This complexity may relate to why, when Gray's theory predicts orthogonality between impulsive CD and anxiety, CD and anxiety symptoms are sometimes found to be positively correlated. Methods of measuring anxiety and behavioral inhibition must be reliable and unconfounded by the negative mood states that often arise from the consequences of CD behavior and the circumstances in which these children and families often find themselves, in order to be empirically and theoretically adequate for testing risk for psychopathy.

Grouping by DSM-IV subtype

Using the same data from the McBurnett et al. (1990) study, and cortisol obtained from some of these same children two years later, we analyzed the effects of subtyping CD by DSM-IV subtype. The methods for diagnosis, collection of salivary cortisol, and radioimmunoassay are detailed in the original report. Briefly, diagnoses were based on multi-informant structured interviews, rating scales, and history, and kappa statistics for cross-diagnostician agreement were high. Cortisol concentration was determined from a single sample of saliva collected during the second year clinic visit. The time of day varied across the midmorning to early afternoon hours. The diurnal rhythm of cortisol release has been widely described, but across the hours that cortisol was collected in this study, children's cortisol maintains a relatively steady plateau (Puig-Antich et al., 1989). Consistent with that data, we found no significant relationship between salivary cortisol concentration and time of collection. We conducted our data analyses with and without time of collection as a covariate, and the results were similar. In order to validly use parametric statistics, we normalized the cortisol concentration values, which were positively skewed and leptokurtic in raw form, using Blom's (Blom, 1958) procedure. Based on the discussion up to this point, it was reasonable to hypothesize that children with Childhood-Onset CD would have the lowest salivary cortisol concentration.

Children who received a CD diagnosis during any one of five annual evaluations conducted over a six-year interval (no evaluations were conducted in the fifth year), and who had at least one symptom of CD before the age of 10 (satisfying the criterion for Childhood-Onset Type) formed one group; those who were asymptomatic for CD through their 10th birthday but who later developed CD formed a second group; and children who did not meet criteria for CD at any of the assessments formed a third group. Of the 27 children who received a CD diagnosis at least once, only four were not reported to have exhibited at least one CD criterion before age 10. Because of this limitation on cell size, the results for the Adolescent-Onset group should be regarded cautiously until they are replicated with a larger sample.

The mean salivary cortisol concentration in milligrams per deciliter was 0.77 for the Adolescent-Onset group (n = 4), 0.17 for the clinic control group (n = 36), and -0.50 for the Childhood-Onset group (n = 23). The group effect was statistically significant in a one-way ANCOVA, $F (3, 61) = 4.60$, $p < .01$, with age as a covariate (it was also significant without the covariate). Planned comparisons among the age-adjusted means found the Childhood-Onset group to have significantly lower salivary cortisol concentration than both the Adolescent-Onset group ($t = 2.21$, $p = .03$) and the clinic control group (t = 2.69, p = .009). The effect size for the subtyping comparison (Childhood-Onset vs. Adolescent Onset) was large (d = 1.2).

At the fourth annual assessment, saliva samples were collected from 42 subjects, 40 of whom had given saliva in the second year and two of whom provided saliva for the first time. On the assumption that salivary cortisol concentration is related to trait arousal, and that the mean of repeated samples yields a more precise estimate of the trait, we used all available cortisol data as an estimate of HPA arousal in a second round of analyses. Thus, for the 40 subjects who gave saliva in both years, we used the mean of the two values, and we used the one available value for the 27 subjects who gave saliva in only one year. The relationship between group membership and cortisol concentration in these analyses was similar but more precise than in the previous analyses. The normalized mean concentration was 0.91 in the Adolescent-Onset group (n = 4), 0.21 in the clinic control group (n=38), and -0.67 in the Childhood-Onset (n=25) group. The group effect was significant in the ANCOVA, F (3, 63) = 10.74, p < .0001. Planned comparisons of the age-adjusted means found the Childhood-Onset group to have significantly lower cortisol than the Adolescent-Onset group (t = 3.22, p = .002) and the clinic control group (t = 4.2, p < .0001). The effect size for the subtyping comparison (Childhood-Onset vs. Adolescent Onset) was large (d = 1.73).

MEASUREMENT OF PSYCHOPATHIC CHILD PERSONALITY

The third and last approach to identifying those youths who are most at risk for adult psychopathy is to use a measure of psychopathic personality in addition to the CD diagnosis. Hare (1991) and others have criticized the DSM-III-R diagnostic criteria for APD as being overly focused on the easily identifiable unstable, antisocial behavior of the psychopath and short-shrifting the callous, manipulative, and narcissistic personality features. In an effort to maximize diagnostic reliability, the critique goes, the APD criteria predominantly assesses those features of psychopathy tapped by Factor II items from the PCL-R.

An analogous situation exists regarding the DSM criteria for CD. All of the CD behavioral criteria represent major violations of the basic rights of others or of age-appropriate societal norms. Even when ADHD and ODD symptoms are included, the DSM-IV disruptive behavior items correspond poorly to the Factor I items (see Table 1). The ADHD item of *"often talks excessively"* is only distantly related in content to psychopathic glibness and superficial charm. The PCL-R items of pathological lying and conning/manipulative are jointly represented by a single CD item that does not include the readiness to lie without apparent motivation that is part of the former item. Based on this lopsided correspondence to the PCL-R factors, we would predict that young people who meet diagnostic criteria for CD have an elevated risk for being diagnosed with APD and receiving high ratings on Factor II of the PCL-R in adulthood, particularly if they also meet diagnostic criteria for ADHD. But because these diagnoses are unselective for the Factor I traits, the population of youths who meet diagnostic criteria for CD (with or without ADHD) will include some who possess Factor I traits— future adult psychopaths—and some who do not—future adults with APD, perhaps, but not future psychopaths.

The adaptation of the PCL-R for children (Frick, this volume; Frick, O'Brien, Wooten & McBurnett, 1994) is a promising recent development for increasing the specificity of risk prediction for psychopathy. Because this approach is covered at length in the paper by Frick in this volume, it need not be discussed here.

SUMMARY

To summarize: The commonly occurring comorbid condition of ADHD and CD is more topographically similar to psychopathy than either disorder alone. Compared to each disorder alone, the comorbid condition has special risks that are consistent with the development of psychopathy: higher aggression, greater persistence, broader antisocial versatility, greater social impairment, and higher eventual rate of adult antisocial behavior. The dampened EDA that is characteristic of adult psychopathy appears to be a correlate only of CD/ODD symptoms. Subtle dysfunction in executive functions is a correlate of ADHD symptoms. Such dysfunction does not appear to be a distinguishing feature that is specific to adult psychopathy, but the kinds of functional impairment that it may engender are consistent with the kinds of difficulties frequently exhibited by psychopaths. Both sets of biological risks are to be found in comorbid ADHD and CD.

There is some validity to the generalization that subtypes of CD that are defined as aggressive, psychopathic, unsocialized, or nonanxious tend to bear some resemblance to each other and to adult psychopathy by virtue of showing underarousal or underactivity in biological systems (the sympathetic ANS and the HPA axis). This is particularly evident when they are contrasted with their corresponding opposite subtype. New analyses conducted for this paper demonstrated that children with DSM-IV Childhood-Onset CD have lower levels of daytime salivary cortisol than other clinic-referred children without CD. The Childhood-Onset Type was also tentatively shown to have lower cortisol levels than children with Adolescent-Onset Type (who appear on the basis of this small sample of Adolescent-Onset Type to have relatively high cortisol levels). The effect sizes (Cohen's d) found with cortisol by constituting CD subgroups were 1.23 for childhood history of DSM-III Undersocialized Aggressive CD in adult prisoners, 1.3 for comorbidity of anxiety disorder in children with DSM-III-R CD, and 1.2 and 1.73 for DSM-IV subtypes in two sets of salivary cortisol analyses.

Although the DSM-IV subtyping method has the advantage of high reliability, it cannot be expected to apply only to youths who are psychopathic or pre-psychopathic, chiefly because this method does not provide any means of discriminating individuals who have the psychopathic personality features associated with Factor I of the PCL-R. The use of comorbid ADHD as a subtyping criterion has the empirically validated advantages of concentrating behavioral and biological risks for psychopathy, and it has better content validity for emergent psychopathy than does CD or ADHD alone. Content validity for psychopathy can be maximized by adding a measure of psychopathic personality, such as the PSD, to the diagnostic procedure. This approach is also beginning to accumulate construct validity in empirical studies (Frick, this volume; Frick et al., 1994).

References

American Psychiatric Association. (1980). *Diagnostic and Statistical Manual of Mental Disorders, Third Edition*. Washington, DC: APA.

American Psychiatric Association. (1987). *Diagnostic and Statistical Manual of Mental Disorders, Third Edition-Revised*. Washington, DC: APA.

American Psychiatric Association. (1994). *Diagnostic and Statistical Manual for Mental Disorders, Fourth Edition*. Washington, D.C.: APA.

Arnett, P. A., Howland, E. W., Smith, S. S., & Newman, J. D. (1993). Autonomic responsivity during passive avoidance in incarcerated psychopaths. *Personality and Individual Differences, 14*(1), 173-184.

August, G. J., Stewart, M. A., & Holmes, C. S. (1983). A four- year follow-up of hyperactive boys with and without conduct disorder. *British Journal of Psychiatry, 143*, 192-198.

Barkley, R. A. (1990). *Attention deficit hyperactivity disorder: A handbook for diagnosis and treatment*. New York: Guilford Press.

Blackburn, R. (1975). An empirical classification of psychopathic personality. *British Journal of Psychiatry, 127*, 456-460.

Blom, G. (1958). *Statistical estimates and transformed beta variables*. New York: Wiley.

Cleckley, H. (1982). *The mask of sanity*. (revised ed.). St. Louis: C.V. Mosby.

Farrington, D. P., Loeber, R., & Van Kammen, W. B. (1990). Long term criminal outcomes of hyperactivity-impulsivity-attention deficit and conduct problems in childhood. In L. N. Robins & M. R. Rutter (Eds.), *Straight and devious pathways to adulthood* (pp. 62-81). New York: Cambridge University Press.

Fowles, D. C. (1980). The three arousal model: Implications of Gray's two -factor learning theory for HR , electrodermal activity, and psychopathy. *Psychophysiology, 17*, 87-104.

Fowles, D. C. (1983). Motivational effects on HR and electrodermal activity: Implications for research in personality and psychopathology. *Journal of Research in Personality, 17*, 48-71.

Frick, P. J., O'Brien, B. S., Wooten, J. M., & McBurnett, K. (1994). Psychopathy and conduct problems in children. *Journal of Abnormal Child Psychology, 103*, 700-707.

Gray, J. A. (1982). *The neuropsychology of anxiety: An inquiry into the functions of the septo-hippocampal system*. Oxford: Oxford University Press.

Gray, J. A. (1987). *The psychology of fear and stress*. (2 ed.). Cambridge: Cambridge University Press.

Hare, R. D. (1970). *Psychopathy: Theory and research*. New York: Wiley.

Hare, R. D. (1978). Electrodermal and cardiovascular correlates of psychopathy. In R. D. Hare & D. Schalling (Eds.), *Psychopathic behaviour: Approaches to research* . Chichester: John Wiley & Sons.

Hare, R. D. (1984). Performance of psychopaths on cognitive tasks related to frontal lobe function. *Journal of Abnormal Psychology, 93*, 133-140.

Hare, R. D. (1991). *The Hare Psychopathy Checklist—Revised*. Toronto: Multi-Health Systems.

Hart, E. L., Lahey, B. B., Loeber, R., Applegate, B., Greeen, S. M., & Frick, P. J. (in press). Developmental change in attention-deficit hyperactivity disorder in boys: A four-year longitudinal study. *Journal of Abnormal Child Psychology*.

Hinshaw, S. P. (1994). Conduct disorder in childhood: Conceptualization, diagnosis, comorbidity, and risk status for antisocial functioning in adulthood. In D. C. Fowles, P. Sutker, & S. H. Goodman (Eds.), *Progress in experimental personality and psychopathology research* . New York: Springer.

Kruesi, M. J., Schmidt, M. E., Donnelly, M., Euthymia, D., & others. (1989). Urinary free cortisol output and disruptive behavior in children. *Journal of the American Academy of Child & Adolescent Psychiatry, 28*(3), 441-443.

Lahey, B. B., Applegate, B., Barkley, R. A., Garfinkel, B., McBurnett, K., Kerdyk, L., Greenhill, L., Hynd, G. W., Frick, P. J., Newcorn, J., Biederman, J., Ollendick, T., Hart, E. L., Perez, D., Waldman, I., & Shaffer, D. (1994). DSM-IV Field Trials for Oppositional Defiant Disorder and Conduct Disorder in children and adolescents. *American Journal of Psychiatry, 151*(8), 1163-1171.

Lahey, B. B., Hart, E. L., Pliszka, S., Applegate, B., & McBurnett, K. (1993). Neurophysiological correlates of conduct disorder: A rationale and a review of research. *Journal of Clinical Child Psychology, 22*(2), 141-153.

Lahey, B. B., McBurnett, K., Loeber, R., & Hart, E. L. (1995). Psychobiology. In G. P. Sholevar (Ed.), *Conduct disorders in children and adolescents* (pp. 27-44). Washington, DC: American Psychiatric Press.

Levenson, M. R., Keihl, K. A., & Fitzpatrick, C. M. (1995). Assessing psychopathic attributes in a noninstitutionalized population. *Journal of Personality & Social Psychology, 68*(1), 151-158.

Loeber, R. (1988). Behavioral precursors and accelerators of delinquency. In W. Buikhuisen & S. A. Mednick (Eds.), *Explaining criminal behavior* (pp. 51-67). Leiden: Brill.

Loney, J., Kramer, J., & Milich, R. S. (1981). The hyperactive child grows up: Predictors of symptoms, delinquency, and achievement at follow-up. In K. D. Gadow & J. Loney (Eds.), *Psychosocial aspects of drug treatment for hyperactivity* (pp. 381-415). Boulder, CO: Westview Press.

Lykken, D. T. (1957). A study of anxiety in the sociopathic personality. *Journal of Abnormal and Social Psychology, 55*, 6-10.

Magnusson, D., & Bergman, L. R. (1990). A pattern approach to the study of pathways from childhood to adulthood. In I. Robins & M. Rutter (Eds.), *Straight and devious pathways from childhood to adulthood* (pp. 101-115). Cambridge: Cambridge University Press.

McBurnett, K. (1992). Psychobiological theories of personality and their application to child psychopathology. In B. B. Lahey & A. Kazdin (Eds.), *Advances in Child Clinical Psychology* (Vol. 14, pp. 107-164). New York: Plenum Press.

McBurnett, K., Harris, S. M., Swanson, J. M., Pfiffner, L. J., Freeland, D., & Tamm, L. (1993). Neuropsychological and psychophysiological differentiation of inattention/overactivity and aggression/defiance symptom groups. *Journal of Clinical Child Psychology, 22*, 165-171.

McBurnett, K., & Lahey, B. (1994). Psychophysiological and neuroendocrine correlates of conduct disorder and antisocial behavior in children and adolescents. In D. C. Fowles, P. Sutker, & S. Goodman (Eds.), *Progress in experimental personality & psychopathology research* (pp. 199-232). New York: Springer Publishing Company.

McBurnett, K., Lahey, B. B., Frick, P. F., Risch, S. C., Loeber, R., Hart, E. L., Christ, M. A. G., & Hanson, K. S. (1991). Anxiety, inhibition, and conduct disorder in children: II. Relation to salivary cortisol. *Journal of the American Academy of Child and Adolescent Psychiatry, 30*, 192-196.

Moffit, T. E., & Henry, B. (1989). Neuropsychological assessment of executive functions in self-reported delinquents. *Development and Psychopathology, 1*, 105-118.

Moffit, T. E., & Silva, P. A. (1988). Self-reported delinquency, neuropsychological deficit, and history of attention deficit disorder. *Journal of Abnormal Child Psychology, 16*, 553-569.

Moffitt, T. E. (1990). Juvenile delinquency and attention deficit disorder: Boys' developmental trajectories from age 3-15. *Child Development, 61*, 893-910.

Moffitt, T. E. (1993). Adolescence-limited and life-course-persistent antisocial behavior: A developmental taxonomy. *Psychological Review, 100*, 674-701.

Newman, J., Kosson, D. S., & Patterson, C. M. (1992). Delay of gratification in psychopathic and nonpsychopathic offenders. *Journal of Abnormal Psychology, 101*(4), 630-636.

Offord, D. R., Sullivan, K., N, A., & Abrams, N. (1979). Delinquency and hyperactivity. *Journal of Nervous and Mental Disease, 167*, 734-741.

Puig-Antich, J., Dahl, R., Ryan, N., Novacenko, H., Goetz, D., Goetz, R., Twomey, J., & Klepper, T. (1989). Cortisol secretion in prepubertal children with major depressive disorder. *Archives of General Psychiatry, 46*, 801-809.

Quay, H. C. (1986). Classification. In H. C. Quay & J. S. Werry (Eds.), *Psychopathological disorders of childhood* (3 ed., pp. 1-34). New York: John Wiley & Sons.

Quay, H. C. (1988). The behavioral reward and inhibition system in childhood behavior disorders. In L. M. Bloomingdale (Ed.), *Attention deficit disorder: New research in attention, treatment and psychopharmacology* (Vol. 3, pp. 176-186). Oxford: Pergamon Press.

Robins, L. N. (1966). *Deviant children grown up.* Baltimore: Williams & Wilkins.

Robins, L. N. (1978). Aetiological implications in studies of childhood histories relating to antisocial personality. In R. D. Hare & D. Schalling (Eds.), *Psychopathic behaviour: Approaches to research* . Chichester: John Wiley & Sons.

Scerbo, A. S., & Kolko, D. J. (1994). Salivary testosterone and cortisol in disruptive children: Relationship tp aggressive, hyperactive and internalizing behaviors. *Journal of the American Academy of Child & Adolescent Psychiatry, 3*(8), 1174-1184.

Schachar, R., Rutter, M., & Smith, A. (1981). The characteristics of situationally and pervasively hyperactive children: Implications for syndrome definition. *Journal of Child Psychology and Psychiatry, 22*, 375-392.

Schalling, D. (1978). Psychopathy-related personality variables and the psychophysiology of socialization. In R. D. Hare & D. Schalling (Eds.), *Psychopathic behaviour: Approaches to research* . Chichester: John Wiley & Sons.

Smith, S., Arnett, P., & Newman, J. P. (1992). Neuropsychological differentiation of psychopathic and non-psychopathic criminal offenders. *Personality and Individual Differences, 13*, 1233-1243.

Spielberger, C. D., Kling, J. K., & O'Hagan, S. E. J. (1978). Dimensions of psychopathic personality: Antisocial behaviour and anxiety. In R. D. Hare & D. Schalling (Eds.), *Psychopathic behaviour: Approaches to research* . Chichester: John Wiley & Sons.

Targum, S. D., Clarkson, L. L., Magac-Harris, K., Marshall, L. E., & Skwerer, R. G. (1990). Measurement of cortisol and lymphocyte subpopulations in depressed and conduct-disordered adolescents. *Journal of Affective Disorders, 18*(91-96).

Taylor, E., Sandberg, S., Thorley, G., & Giles, S. (1991). *The epidemiology of childhood hyperactivity.* London: Institute of Psychiatry.

Virkkunen, M. (1985). Urinary free cortisol secretion in habitually violent offenders. *Acta Psychiatrica Scandinavica, 72*(1), 40-44.

Walker, J. L., Lahey, B. B., Hynd, G. W., & Frame, C. L. (1987). Comparison of specific patterns of antisocial behavior in children with conduct disorder or with or without coexisting hyperactivity. *Journal of Consulting and Clinical Psychology, 55*, 910-913.

Walker, J. L., Lahey, B. B., Russo, M., Frick, P. J., Christ, M. A. G., McBurnett, K., Loeber, R., Stouthamer-Loeber, M., & Green, S. (1991). Anxiety, inhibition, and conduct disorder in children: I. Relations to social impairment and sensation seeking. *Journal of the American Academy of Child and Adolescent Psychiatry, 30*, 187-191.

Hare, R. D. (1984). Performance of psychopaths on cognitive tasks related to frontal lobe function. *Journal of Abnormal Psychology, 93*, 133-140.

PSYCHOPATHY IN ADOLESCENCE: ASSESSMENT, VIOLENCE, AND DEVELOPMENTAL PRECURSORS

ADELLE E. FORTH and HEATHER C. BURKE
Department of Psychology
Carleton University
Ottawa, Canada.

INTRODUCTION

Psychopathy is a serious personality disorder that first manifests itself early in life and persists throughout most of the lifespan. Most clinicians and researchers agree that psychopathy is associated with a constellation of affective, interpersonal, and behavioral characteristics, central to which are a profound lack of remorse or guilt and a callous disregard for the feelings, rights, and welfare of others (Cleckley, 1976; Hare, 1991; Tennent, Tennent, Prins, & Bedford, 1990). Individuals with this disorder are typically described as impulsive, selfish, deceitful, sensation-seeking, and irresponsible. Given these characteristics it is not surprising that psychopaths commit a disproportionate amount of serious repetitive crime and violence and frequently come into contact with the criminal justice system. Despite a substantial body of work dealing with psychopathy in adults, surprisingly little work has focused on the precursors of this disorder. Understanding the antecedents of psychopathy may lead not only to a better understanding of its etiology but also its treatment and perhaps, ultimately, its prevention.

The goal of the present chapter is to consider several lines of research that have dealt with identifying aspects of psychopathy in adolescents. This chapter is organized into three major sections. The first section contains a discussion of issues involved in the assessment of psychopathy in adolescents and describes an adaptation of the Hare Revised Psychopathy Checklist (PCL-R; Hare, 1991) for this age group. In the second section, research on the association between psychopathy and criminal conduct in the adolescent offender, with a particular emphasis on violence, is reviewed. Finally the third section deals with research on the family background factors associated with the psychopathic adolescent offender.

Assessment of Psychopathy in Adolescence

Although the concept of psychopathy has undergone a long and somewhat confusing evolution, there is consensus among clinicians and researchers that the central features of this disorder must include both personality and behavioral characteristics (Davies & Feldman, 1981; Gray & Hutchinson, 1964; Lay, 1995; Tennent et al., 1990). Despite this agreement, one of the largest obstacles to research in this area has been the use of a variety of different assessment procedures and terms (Lilienfeld, 1994) including:

D.J. Cooke et al. (eds.), Psychopathy: Theory, Research and Implications for Society, 205–229.

psychopath, sociopath, dyssocial personality disorder, and antisocial personality disorder. Although these terms all share an emphasis on socially-deviant behavior, only the concept of psychopathy reflects both the affective and interpersonal characteristics that have traditionally been considered central to this disorder. In contrast, the concepts of sociopathy and antisocial personality disorder, although popular, rely almost exclusively on easily measured behavioral criteria, particularly delinquent and criminal behaviors, and disregard critical personality characteristics. Such practices make it difficult to distinguish between, for example, the violent offender and the psychopathic violent offender. The PCL-R measures both the behavioral and personality characteristics associated with psychopathy (Cleckley, 1976; McCord & McCord, 1964). It consists of 20 items that are scored on a 3-point scale on the basis of a semi-structured interview and collateral information. Total scores range from 0 to 40, with 0 indicating a complete lack of psychopathic characteristics whereas 40 indicates an individual with virtually all the characteristics of the prototypical psychopath. A cutoff score of 30 has proven useful for the diagnosis of psychopathy.

Factor analytic studies of the PCL-R have revealed a two factor structure. Both these factors are considered essential to the diagnosis of psychopathy (Hare et al., 1990). Factor 1 reflects interpersonal and affective characteristics of psychopathy, such as egocentricity, callousness, and manipulativeness. This factor strongly correlates with self-report measures of machiavellianism, narcissism, empathy, and anxiety. Factor 2 reflects behavioral characteristics of psychopathy, such as impulsivity, chronic instability, an irresponsible lifestyle, and antisocial behavior. The PCL-R been used extensively in research with adult forensic populations and there exists considerable evidence attesting to its reliability and validity (Hare, 1991; 1996; Hare et al., 1990; Harpur, Hakstian, & Hare, 1988; Kosson, Smith, & Newman, 1990; Wong, 1984).

When applying an assessment procedure that has been developed for one population to a different population, it is important to show that the same construct is being measured. Although the *Diagnostic and Statistical Manual of Mental Disorders* (DSM-IV, American Psychiatric Association [APA], 1994) does not permit a diagnosis of antisocial personality disorder unless the individual is at least 18 years of age, most clinicians and researchers agree that the personality traits and behaviors that define psychopathy are first manifested early in life. Unfortunately, there is currently little empirical research in this area. To date, there have been three published studies using a modified PCL-R with adolescents. Forth, Hart, and Hare (1990) used a modified 18-item version of the PCL-R to assess psychopathy in 75 male young offenders in a maximum-security Canadian institution. The modifications included deleting items reflecting a parasitic lifestyle (item 9) and many short term marital relationships (item 17). In addition, the scoring of items relating to criminal history was also modified. The findings from this study will be discussed in more detail below.

The two other studies that used the PCL-R with adolescents examined the association between psychopathic characteristics and moral development in delinquent and nondelinquent youth. Trevothan and Walker (1989) used the same modified 18-item PCL-R as Forth et al. (1990) to assess 29 male young offenders from the same population that Forth et al. studied. In addition, they also tested 15 nondelinquent adolescent controls. They found that psychopathic young offenders did not differ from other offenders or controls on measures of moral reasoning involving hypothetical dilemmas. However, when real-life moral dilemmas were discussed, they were more likely to express egotistic concerns in their decision-making than were the nonpsychopathic offenders or controls. Chandler and Moran (1990) used a similar (17-item) modification of the PCL-R to assess 60 male juvenile delinquents and 20 nondelinquent controls in the United States who were matched for age, race, education, and socioeconomic level. They found no association between psychopathy and measures of moral reasoning. However, juveniles receiving high psychopathy ratings obtained lower scores on the California Personality Inventory (CPI; Gough, 1957) measure of socialization, and higher scores on the personal autonomy scale, compared to other juveniles.

As a result of experience using the modified version of the PCL-R and feedback from other researchers, further modifications were made in order to facilitate scoring with adolescents. This modified version of the PCL-R was named the Psychopathy Checklist: Youth Version (PCL:YV; Forth, Kosson, & Hare, 1994). Item descriptions have been modified to take into account the restricted life experience of adolescents and scoring has been altered to have increased emphasis on relations with peers, family, and school adjustment. For example, in scoring item 2 (grandiose sense of self-worth), more emphasis was placed on short-term goals and less focus on long-term occupational goals. More emphasis was placed on small-scale conning behaviors and manipulative attempts to gain prestige among peers for item 5 (conning/manipulation). In assessing adults, item 9 (parasitic lifestyle) is determined primarily on the basis of occupational history. Since adolescents tend to have restricted work experience an increased emphasis was placed on being parasitic towards peers, girlfriends, and parents. All casual sexual activities were included in scoring item 11 (promiscuous sexual behavior). More emphasis was placed on whether goals were consistent with school performance for scoring item 13 (lack of realistic long-term goals). Additional sources of evidence were included for item 15 (irresponsibility), including failure to fulfill treatment/institutional obligations. Item 17 (many short-term marital relationships) was scored 0 if sexual relationships were stable and long-term (4 months or longer); 1 if the individual had significant stability problems within sexual relationships, and 2 if the individual had three or more short-term relationships or if long-term relationships were extremely unstable. This item was omitted if the individual had never established a sexual relationship. For item 18 (juvenile delinquency), any violent offences were scored a 2, nonviolent offences a 1, and no offences prior to age 18 as a 0. For item 20 (criminal versatility), four or more types of offences were scored 2, three types of offences 1, and less than two types of offences 0. For the purposes of this chapter, research using both the earlier 18-item PCL-R modification and the 1994 PCL:YV will be reviewed.

Prevalence of Psychopathic Characteristics

Data from a number of studies are summarized in Table 1. These studies represent data collected from male samples from three settings: incarcerated youth, youth in open custody or on probation, and community youth. The studies were as follows: (1) Subjects in the Forth et al. (1990) study consisted of 75 young offenders incarcerated in a maximum security institution in British Columbia. Their ages ranged from 13 to 20 ($M = 16.3$, $SD = 1.1$); 75% were Caucasian; (2) Subjects in the Forth (1995a) were 106 young offenders incarcerated in two secure custody facilities in Ontario. Their ages ranged from 15 to 19 ($M = 17.5$, $SD = .8$); 80% were Caucasian. A community sample of 50 adolescents were also assessed in this study.

TABLE 1. Mean and Standard Deviation (in parenthesis) for
PCL:YV Total and Factor Scores and Baserates Across Studies

Setting and Study	Total	Factor 1	Factor 2	Baserate
Incarcerated Settings				
Forth et al. (1990)	26.28 (7.57)	8.94 (3.95)	13.71 (3.06)	35
Forth (1995a)	26.52 (6.04)	10.73 (3.09)	13.04 (3.06)	32
Laroche (1996)	22.95 (6.52)	7.56 (3.11)	12.09 (3.13)	18
Probation Settings				
Bailey (1994)	23.62 (6.53)	8.38 (2.88)	12.09 (2.98)	15
Kosson (1996)	21.41 (7.76)	8.56 (3.67)	9.92 (3.41)	9
Community Settings				
Toupin et al. (1995)	16.95 (8.56)	6.42 (4.17)	8.85 (3.81)	7
Forth (1995a)	3.98 (3.74)	.74 (1.04)	2.89 (2.66)	0

Note. Baserate is percent of subjects with a PCL:YV total score of 30 or greater. The Forth et al. (1990) used the 18-item modification of the PCL-R. Scores for this sample are pro-rated out of 40.

Their ages ranged from 13 to 19 ($M = 17.2$, $SD = 1.6$). This sample included youth from community centers, youth employment centers, and advertisements in local newspapers; (3) Offenders in the Laroche (1996) study consisted of 106 young offenders in a secure detention facility in Quebec. Their ages ranged from 14 to 17 ($M = 16.1$, $SD = 1.1$); 43% were Caucasian. All were recently convicted of a violent offense; (4) Subjects in the Bailey (1994) study consisted of 26 young offenders residing in two open custody facilities in Ontario. Their ages ranged from 16 to 18; 85% were Caucasian; (5) The sample in the Kosson (1996) study were 67 adolescents on probation in North Carolina. Their ages ranged from 12 to 16 ($M = 14.5$; $SD = 1.1$); 33% were Caucasian; (6) Subjects in the Toupin, Mercier, Déry, Côté, and Hodgins (1995) study were 52 youth undergoing treatment at a facility in Quebec. Their ages ranged from 13 to 17 ($M=15.2$, $SD = 1.2$); 100% were Caucasian. All had a diagnosis of conduct disorder according to DSM-III-R criteria (APA, 1987). Descriptive statistics for the PCL:YV total, Factor 1, and Factor 2 scores are provided in Table 1 across the three settings. A preliminary investigation of the factor structure of the PCL:YV was conducted by Forth (1995a). A two-factor solution was computed using principal-components analysis with an oblique rotation of the factors. The observed factor structure of the PCL:YV corresponds closely to the factor structure of the PCL-R found with adult offenders described by Hare et al. (1990). As can be seen, there is substantial variability in the mean PCL:YV total and factor scores across the settings. As expected, the mean score was highest among the secure custody young offenders. This is not surprising considering that only the most violent or recidivistic youth are sent to secure custody. In contrast, the mean score for the community youth was lowest, particularly in the Forth (1995a) study. Most of these youth had no significant problems at school or in the community. Research with adult noncriminal samples has shown a similar low score on measures of psychopathy (Forth, Brown, Hart, & Hare, 1996). The relatively high score seen in the Toupin et al. (1995) study is not surprising since all the youth were diagnosed with conduct disorder.

Although for some research and clinical applications, a categorical diagnosis of psychopathy is desirable, specific cutoffs for use with the PCL:YV have not yet been established. For comparison purposes with data reported on adult offenders, the baserate of psychopathy using a cutoff of 30 or greater is presented in the Table 1 across the studies.

The noncriminal adolescent samples provide information on whether some general characteristics of adolescence may be associated with psychopathy. For example, one might expect the mean score for items such as sensation-seeking, impulsivity, and irresponsibility to be higher in samples of male adolescents than in adults. In the community samples, the following items had the highest means: item 3 (need for stimulation), item 10 (poor behavioral controls), item 12 (early behavioral problems) and item 14 (impulsivity). With respect to demographic characteristics, there was no association between age and PCL:YV total or factor scores. The average correlation between age and PCL:YV total scores was .08.

Reliability of PCL:YV

Measures of internal consistency (Cronbach alpha), item homogeneity (mean inter-item correlation), and interrater reliability (Pearson correlation) of the PCL:YV total scores are presented in Table 2. The alpha and mean inter-item correlations for PCL:YV total scores suggest that in adolescent samples the PCL:YV has adequate internal consistency and is a relatively homogeneous scale. The interrater correlations were very high across all the studies. Although not presented in the Table, interrater correlations were slightly lower for Factor 1 scores as compared to Factor 2 scores. There were no substantial differences in the interrater correlations, alpha, or mean inter-item correlations across the three settings. Measures of internal consistency (Cronbach alpha), item homogeneity (mean inter-item correlation), and interrater reliability (Pearson correlation) of the PCL:YV total scores are presented in Table 2. The alpha and mean inter-item correlations for PCL:YV total scores suggest that in adolescent samples the PCL:YV has adequate internal consistency and is a relatively homogeneous scale. The interrater correlations were very high across all the studies. Although not presented in the Table, interrater correlations were slightly lower for Factor 1 scores as compared to Factor 2 scores. There were no substantial differences in the interrater correlations, alpha, or mean inter-item correlations across the three settings.

TABLE 2. Reliabilities of PCL:YV Total Scores Across Studies

Setting and Study	Alpha	Interitem r	Interrater r
Incarcerated Settings			
Forth et al. (1990)	.90	.33	.90
Forth (1995a)	.75	.13	.92
Laroche (1996)	.83	.19	.98
Probation Settings			
Bailey (1994)	.84	.20	.96
Kosson (1996)	.85	.24	.91
Community Settings			
Toupin et al. (1995)	.88	.29	--
Forth (1995a)	.77	.17	.93

Note. The *N*s for the interrater correlations were as follows: Forth et al. (1990) 75; Forth (1995a), 45; Laroche (1996), 38; Bailey (1994), 10; Kosson (1996), 18; Forth (1995a) community youths, 25.

The alpha and mean inter-item correlations for PCL:YV total scores suggest that in adolescent samples the PCL:YV has adequate internal consistency and is a relatively homogeneous scale. The interrater correlations were very high across all the studies. Although not presented in the Table, interrater correlations were slightly lower for Factor 1 scores as compared to Factor 2 scores. There were no substantial differences in the interrater correlations, alpha, or mean inter-item correlations across the three settings.

Association Between Psychopathy and Conduct Problems

Many studies have demonstrated that children with antisocial problems are at a higher risk for antisocial problems during adulthood (Huesmann, Eron, Lefkowitz, & Walder, 1984; Robins, 1966; West & Farrington, 1973). The importance of early antisocial behavior is made explicit in the DSM-IV which includes as one of its criteria for APD conduct problems prior to age 15. However, at least half of children and adolescents with severe conduct problems do not become antisocial adults (White, Moffitt, Earls, Robins, & Silva, 1990).

The DSM-IV diagnostic criteria for conduct disorder (CD) requires 3 of 15 symptoms be present over the course of the last year (c.f., DSM-III-R which requires 3 of 13 criteria be present over 6 months). The criteria are currently separated into four main categories: serious violations of rules (3 symptoms), deceitfulness or theft (3 symptoms), destruction of property (2 symptoms), and aggressive conduct (7 symptoms). In contrast to previous versions of conduct disorder, there is now no attempt to differentiate socialized and unsocialized or aggressive and nonaggressive types. Instead, the subtype classification is based on age of symptom onset, with the childhood-onset type having one symptom prior to age 10 and the adolescent-onset type with no symptoms present prior to age 10.

A moderate relation has been reported between symptoms of antisocial personality disorder and PCL-R total scores in adults (Hare, 1991; Harpur et al., 1988). Several studies have examined a comparable association between the PCL:YV and symptoms of CD. In Forth et al. (1990) the correlation between DSM-III-R CD symptoms and the 18-item modification of the PCL-R scores was $r = .64$. Table 3 presents the correlation between PCL:YV scores and the total CD symptoms, the number of aggressive CD symptoms, drug use, and alcohol use from the Forth (1995a) study. Among both young offenders and community adolescents, PCL:YV total scores were significantly correlated with the total number of CD symptoms and with the number of aggressive CD symptoms.

TABLE 3. Correlations Between PCL:YV Total and Factor Scores and Conduct Disorder Symptoms and Measures of Substance Use (Forth, 1995a)

Measure	Total	Factor 1	Factor 2
Number of CD symptoms			
Young offenders	.52***	.31**	.54***
Community youth	.75***	.66***	.71***
Number of aggressive CD symptoms			
Young offenders	.47***	.32**	.31**
Community youth	.38**	.42**	.38**
MAST			
Young offenders	.23**	.06	.32**
Community youth	.48***	.33**	.52***
DAST			
Young offenders	.27**	.10	.34**
Community youth	.56***	.41**	.52***

Note. CD = DSM-IV conduct disorder ; MAST = Michigan Alcohol Screening Test; DAST = Drug Abuse Screening Test. * $p < .05$, ** $p < .01$, *** $p < .001$ (one-tailed)

In the young offender sample, Factor 2 (social deviant factor) was more strongly correlated with the number of CD symptoms present than with Factor 1 (interpersonal/affective factor). Toupin et al. (1995) reported a similar pattern of correlations in their sample of conduct disordered youth.

In the Forth (1995a) study, nearly all the adolescent offenders met the DSM-IV diagnosis of CD (97%). Moreover, although the mean PCL:YV score was very low for the community youth, 20% of these youth met the criteria for CD. These results point to the over inclusive nature of CD. An asymmetric relationship has consistently been reported between antisocial personality disorder as measured by the DSM criteria and psychopathy as measured by the PCL-R (Hare, 1996). A similar asymmetric relation has also emerged when comparing the DSM CD and PCL:YV psychopathy. All the psychopathic young offenders in the Forth (1995a) study met the DSM-IV criteria for CD; however, only 30% of the CD young offenders met the criteria for psychopathy as measured by the PCL:YV (using a cutoff of 30 or greater).

Examination of the CD criteria reveal that the symptoms are primarily focused on antisocial behaviors. Thus youth diagnosed with CD all engage in socially deviant behavior; however, the majority of CD youth do not possess the interpersonal and affective traits associated with prototypical psychopathy. The above findings suggest that CD and adolescent psychopathy, as with antisocial personality disorder and adult psychopathy, are constructs that cannot be used interchangeably.

Lynam (1996) has suggested that children who demonstrate symptoms of conduct problems and a combination of hyperactivity, impulsivity, and attention deficits are at greatest risk for engaging in persistent antisocial behavior. He also speculates that this combination of symptoms manifested during childhood may identify those children who later manifest the symptoms of psychopathy in adulthood. To date, only one study has investigated the association between psychopathy and hyperactivity. McBride and Hare (1996) examined the prevalence of attention deficit disorder (APA, 1980) in a sample of 189 adolescent offenders attending a sex offender treatment program. The assessment of psychopathy was based on the PCL:YV completed on the basis of institutional file information. Correlational analysis revealed that psychopathy was significantly related to the presence or absence of attention deficit disorder ($r = .38$).

Psychopathy has also been associated with substance use in adult offenders (Hart, Forth, & Hare, 1991; Hart & Hare, 1989; Hemphill, Hart, & Hare, 1994; Smith & Newman, 1990). As can be seen in Table 3, a positive association, similar to that observed in adult offenders, was found with the PCL:YV total and Factor 2 scores and measures of alcohol and drug use. In the community youth, Factor 1 and substance use were also significantly related.

Past researchers have found only low to moderate correlations between self-report measures of psychopathy and the PCL-R in adult offenders (see Harpur et al., 1988; Hart et al., 1991). Psychological tests such as the Minnesota Multiphasic Personality Inventory (Hathaway & McKinley, 1940), the Millon Clinical Multiaxial Inventory (Millon, 1987), and CPI have all been found to correlate more strongly with the social deviant facet of psychopathy than with the interpersonal and affective facet. Sullivan (1996) examined the association between the Minnesota Multiphasic Personality Inventory-Adolescent Version (MMPI-A; Butcher et al., 1992) and the PCL:YV in a sample of 95 male young offenders. Significant correlations were found between PCL:YV total scores and the Psychopathic Deviate scale ($r = .23$), Conduct Problems content scale ($r = .29$), Alcohol/Drug Acknowledgment scale ($r = .34$), and the Anger content scale ($r = .34$). Consistent with research with adult offenders, these scales were more highly correlated with Factor 2 than with Factor 1 of the PCL:YV. Moreover, the presence or absence of psychopathy as assessed using the PCL:YV could not be accurately predicted by the MMPI-A as indicated by measures of diagnostic efficiency. Given these problems, the MMPI-A should not be used to assess psychopathy in adolescent populations.

Association with Criminal Behavior

Recent research has pointed to the importance of the construct of psychopathy in the criminal justice system (see Hare, 1996). While the presence of psychopathic traits in adult offenders has indisputable effects on judicial outcomes, possessing psychopathic characteristics also has a significant impact on judicial decisions for juvenile forensic populations. For example, the presence of psychopathy has been considered one factor in the decision to transfer a youth charged with a serious offense to adult court (see Zinger & Forth, 1996). Although most adolescents who engage in criminal conduct desist as they enter adulthood, some adolescents become chronic offenders.

Moffit (1993) has proposed a developmental taxonomy that differentiates between antisocial adolescence-limited versus life-course-persistent behavior patterns. She suggests that a relatively small group of adolescents are highly antisocial individuals who will remain extremely antisocial even later in life and across a variety of situations (see also Farrington, Ohlin, & Wilson, 1986; Wolfgang, Figlio, & Sellin, 1972). In contrast, many adolescents are temporarily involved with antisocial behavior, usually as a result of situational factors. The psychopathic young offender in theory fits into her life course-persistent antisocial group, persisting in criminal activity well into adulthood. By contrast, the nonpsychopathic young offender is most likely to fit into the adolescence-limited antisocial group, and unlike the persistent group, will likely desist from criminal activity after adolescence.

The characteristics that define psychopathy are compatible with a criminal lifestyle and a lack of concern for societal norms. A strong relation between psychopathy, criminal behaviors, and violence has consistently been found in adult offender populations (see Hare, Forth, & Strachan, 1992 and Hart & Hare, in press for review). For example, research in adult populations has found that psychopaths start committing crime at an earlier age, are more likely to fail on conditional release, commit a larger number of crimes, are more versatile in their offending, and are more likely to engage in institutional violence than are other offenders (Hare & McPherson, 1984; Serin, 1991, 1996; Serin, Peters, & Barbaree, 1990; Wong, 1984).

To examine this issue, research investigating the relationship between PCL:YV total and factor scores and a number of measures of criminal conduct is reviewed: a) age of onset, b) frequency of nonviolent and violent criminal behaviors, and c) versatility of nonviolent and violent criminal behaviors. Forth et al. (1990) reported a correlation of $r = -.25$ between psychopathy and the age of first arrest. The association between a variety of measures of criminal behavior and psychopathy is presented in Table 4 (Forth, 1995a). To avoid overlap between items on the PCL:YV that were directly associated with antisocial behaviors, item 18 (juvenile delinquency), item 19 (revocation of conditional release), and item 20 (criminal versatility) were excluded from each participant's PCL:YV total and Factor 2 scores. Analyses reveal significant negative correlations between age of onset for both nonviolent and violent antisocial behaviors and the PCL:YV in both young offenders and community youth. The average age of onset for nonviolent criminal behaviors in the low psychopathy group (PCL:YV scores ≤ 22) was 11.9 years, as compared to 9.3 years for the high psychopathy group (PCL:YV scores ≥ 30), almost 3 years earlier. A similar age-related difference was found with age of onset for violent criminal behaviors, with the less psychopathic group starting at age 14.5, over two years later than the more psychopathic group with an onset at age 12.1. In summary, youth with psychopathic characteristics tend to start their criminal careers at a younger age.

TABLE 4. Correlations between PCL:YV total and factor scores and measures of self-report antisocial behaviors (Forth, 1995a)

Measure	Total	Factor 1	Factor 2
Number of Nonviolent Offences			
Young offenders	.31**	.16	.37***
Community youth	.75***	.60***	.73***
Number of Violent Offences			
Young offenders	.25**	.24*	.23*
Community youth	.40**	.35**	.38**
Age of Onset for Nonviolent Offences			
Young offenders	-.33***	-.14	-.41***
Community youth	-.40***	-.30*	-.45**
Age of Onset for Violent Offences			
Young offenders	-.26**	-.14	-.29**
Community youth	-.01	-.17	-.21
Versatility of Nonviolent Offences			
Young offenders	.35***	.15	.46***
Community youth	.69***	.58***	.68***
Versatility of Violent Offences			
Young offenders	.28**	.22*	.32**
Community youth	.54***	.40**	.53***

Note. PCL:YV items 18, 19, and 20 deleted from scales; community sample $n = 41$ for age of onset for nonviolent offending; $n = 17$ for age of onset for violent offending. * $p < .05$, ** $p < .01$, *** $p < .001$ (one-tailed).

There is also evidence that psychopathic youth engage in a greater number of nonviolent and violent delinquent behaviors than nonpsychopathic youth. Toupin et al. (1995) in their study of 52 conduct disordered youth reported a correlation of $r = .46$ between PCL:YV total score and the number of delinquent acts and $r = .30$ with the number of aggressive behaviors.

As can be seen in Table 4, PCL:YV scores were significantly related to all measures of delinquent behaviors. It was also found that young offenders in the high psychopathic group were convicted of significantly more offences, on average, than had those in the low psychopathic group (*M*s = 8.1 and 12.5, respectively).

PCL:YV total scores were also correlated with the number of different types of nonviolent and violent antisocial behaviors committed (i.e., versatility). With respect to different types of aggressive behavior, young offenders scoring high on the PCL:YV were more likely to have threatened others with a weapon, be sexually assaultive, commit robbery and arson. Moreover, in the high psychopathy group, almost two-thirds (64%) of young offenders had engaged in 10 or more violent behaviors, compared to about one-third (37%) of the young offenders in the low psychopathy group (Forth, 1995a). Clearly, psychopathy is associated with the most serious offences in this sample.

Although aggressive behavior within dating relationships rarely come to the attention of the criminal justice system, the use of self-report questionnaires provides some information on the prevalence of this form of violence. The association between psychopathy and dating violence was measured in the Forth (1995a) study. Psychopathy was not significantly related to the total number of physically aggressive acts (as measured by a modified Conflict Tactics Scale, Straus, 1979) within dating relationships in this sample. However, psychopathic youth admitted engaging in more coercive and controlling behaviors with their girlfriends than the nonpsychopathic youth. Significant correlations were obtained between the PCL:YV total scores and several measures from the Psychological Maltreatment of Woman Inventory (PMWI; Tolman, 1989), including the total score (r = .20), the dominance-isolation subscale (r = .18), and the verbal-emotional abuse subscale (r = .19). None of the PMWI scales were significantly related to Factor 2 scores, but, all were significantly correlated with Factor 1 scores (rs = .28, .28, and .24, respectively). Psychopathic young offenders were more likely to control their partner's autonomy by limiting her social network, restricting her activities, and demanding obedience from her. This is not surprising given that psychopaths are often described as dominant, grandiose, and callous (Cleckley, 1976).

The extent to which psychopathic youth harm their victims has only recently been investigated. Gretton, McBride, Lewis, O'Shaughnessy, and Hare (1994) found that adolescent sex offenders diagnosed as psychopathic by the PCL:YV threatened their victims more and used more severe violence during the commission of their acts than did nonpsychopathic sex offenders.

Research with adult violent offenders suggests that the antisocial behavior of psychopaths is motivated by different factors than those that motivate nonpsychopaths. Recent studies have found that the violence of adult psychopaths seems to be motivated primarily for instrumental (e.g., material gain, revenge) rather than for reactive (e.g., strong emotional arousal) reasons (Cornell et al., 1996; Dempster, Lyon, Sullivan, & Hart, 1996; Serin, 1991; Williamson, Hare, & Wong, 1987). One study has examined the motive for offending in psychopathic adolescent offenders. Dempster and Hart (1996) used the Crime Classification Manual (Douglas, Burgess, Burgess, & Ressler, 1992) to classify the motive for offending in 43 male young offenders charged with murder or attempted murder. A modified PCL-R was coded retrospectively based on institutional files. Young offenders whose offences were classified as Sexual Homicide and Criminal Enterprise were more instrumental and goal-directed than the Personal Cause or Group Case subjects. Compared to the other categories Sexual Homicide participants scored significantly higher on psychopathy.

Over the past decade there has been considerable research examining the predictive validity of the PCL-R in male offender and forensic psychiatric patients (see Hart & Hare, in press). Two studies have examined the association between psychopathy and recidivism in male young offenders. Forth et al. (1990) found that 71 of 75 offenders were released from secure custody during a 16 to 24 month follow-up period; 79% of them committed a new offense. Modified PCL-R total scores were correlated (r = .26) with the number of post-release violent offenses. Gretton et al. (1994) reported preliminary data from a sample of 112 male adolescent sex offenders assessed using the PCL:YV. The mean PCL:YV score based on a retrospective file review was 21.4 (SD = 7.2) with 25% being classified as psychopathic (PCL:YV score ≥ 27). The latter group caused significantly more problems during treatment. This sample has since been increased to 189 subjects who have been followed up on average for 34 months (Heather Gretton, April 6, 1996, personal communication). Offenders in the high psychopathy group recidivated more rapidly than the other offenders, on average within 16.2 months versus 26.7 months for offenders in the low psychopathy group. The rate of nonviolent recidivism was twice as high for the high psychopathy group (66% in the high psychopathy group versus 27% in the low psychopathy group), while the rate of violent recidivism was almost triple for the high psychopathy group (31% versus 12%, respectively). In contrast, the rates for sexual recidivism were comparable for the high and low psychopathy groups (10% versus 16%, respectively).

Age-Related Change In Criminal Behavior

Hare and his colleagues (Hare et al., 1992; Hare, McPherson, & Forth, 1988) have studied age-related changes in criminality in both psychopathic and nonpsychopathic adult offenders. The results from these studies have found that psychopathic offenders committed more offenses than other offenders until about age 40. At this age, the conviction rate for nonviolent, but not for violent, convictions for psychopaths drops to the same level as that of other offenders. The psychopath's capacity to engage in violence across the lifespan is supported by a study by Harris, Rice, and Cormier (1991). In a sample of 166 male adult forensic patients released from a forensic psychiatric hospital, the probability of violent failure was examined for 5 year periods from between age 25 and age 40. Psychopaths were significantly more likely to recidivate violently across all the age periods compared to nonpsychopaths.

Given these age-related effects in adult psychopathy, Forth (1995b) examined the age-related changes in criminal behavior in the sample of young offenders from the Forth et al. (1990) study. The participants were assessed using the modified 18-item version of the PCL-R as young offenders and followed up into early adulthood. The offenders were divided into a high psychopathy group (n = 23; score of ≥ 30) and a low psychopathy group (n = 40; score ≤ 24). Official criminal records were used to code the mean number of nonviolent and violent offenses and mean time spent incarcerated:

these were broken into three 2.5-year periods from age 13 to age 20.5. To compensate for individual differences in the amount of time spent incarcerated, the offense data were converted to the number of offenses committed per 6 months free. The majority of young offenders in this sample persisted into an adult criminal career (86%). This high rate of persistence was not unexpected given the lengthy history of antisocial behavior displayed by the sample.

Figures 1 and 2 present the rates of nonviolent and violent offenses for offenders in both groups across the age periods.

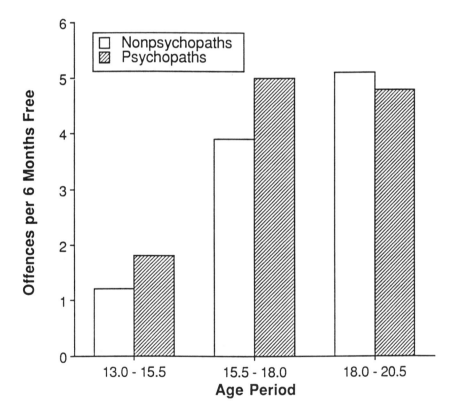

Figure 1. Mean Number of Nonviolent Offenses per 6 Month Free by Psychopaths and Nonpsychopaths From Age 13 to 20.5.

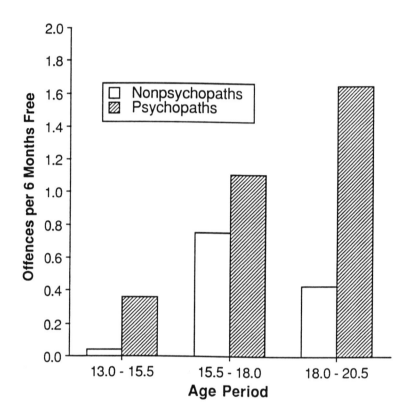

Figure 2. Mean Number of Violent Offenses per 6 Months Free by Psychopaths and Nonpsychopaths From Age 13 to 20.5.

Not surprisingly, all offenders engaged in the highest rate of offending during the later age periods. Although the psychopathic offenders committed more nonviolent offending during the first two age periods, this effect was not statistically significant. The group differences were significant for violent offenses, however, as psychopathic offenders engaged in more violent offenses during the first and last age periods. The percentage of those in both groups who committed at least one violent offense was also analyzed. The offenders in the high psychopathy group were more likely to have committed a violent offense (52%, 64%, and 48% of the individuals committed a violent offense in each of the three age periods) as compared to those in the low psychopathy group (12%, 54%, and 33%, respectively). These preliminary results confirm that the propensity for violence in psychopathic youth remains relatively persistent. However, further research following these offenders as they age is needed to confirm this persistence into adulthood.

Developmental Correlates of Adolescent Psychopathy

Despite quite widespread agreement about what constitutes the construct of psychopathy and the psychopath's characteristic pattern of offending, the etiology of the psychopathic personality remains largely unknown (Hare, 1996). It seems probable that, like other psychological disorders, there are several groups of factors which impact on its onset and presentation, including environmental and biological factors.

Recently there has been a resurgence of interest in the environmental precursors to psychopathy. Family background represents one of the most important environmental agents. Understanding how familial factors impact on the development of a psychopathic personality could facilitate a greater understanding of the developmental pathways of psychopathy and assist in identification of risk factors associated with this disorder. This knowledge is essential if treatment and prevention strategies are going to be developed to offset or mitigate the expression of psychopathic traits in youth.

Considerable research has demonstrated a link between dysfunction in the family and delinquency and the perpetration of violence (Garbarino & Plantz, 1986; Lewis, Shanok, Pincus, & Glaser, 1979; Loeber & Stouthamer-Loeber, 1986; Widom, 1989). However, relatively little research has examined whether psychopaths have dysfunctional family backgrounds. The research that has been done, though, has shown no decisive link between family history and the presence of psychopathy in adults (Cleckley, 1976; Hare, 1970).

Investigating this relationship in adolescents may yield a stronger association than in adults since adolescent may have better recall of their familial experiences. Moreover, there is often more detailed corroborative information about family circumstances within the institutional files of adolescent offenders than for adult offenders. Until recently, no retrospective research with adolescent psychopaths has been completed. The empirical studies investigating the relationship between adolescent psychopathy and family background will be reviewed. Due to the dearth of research, studies which examine the family background of adult psychopaths and children who exhibit psychopathic traits will also be considered.

McCord and McCord (1964) conducted an extensive review of the literature on antecedents to psychopathy. The authors concluded that there may be three causal patterns associated with psychopathy. Parental rejection was deemed a major contributor in each of these etiological pathways. They identified the paths as: (1) severe rejection; (2) mild rejection with neurological damage; and (3) mild rejection with a psychopathic parent, erratic discipline and a lack of parental supervision.

Hare (1970) in his review of the research concluded that parental substance abuse and having an antisocial or psychopathic parent, accompanied by inconsistent discipline, were related to psychopathy. Hare outlines how delayed or inconsistently administered discipline may contribute to the development of psychopathy in some individuals. He also points out that many individuals from homes with inconsistent discipline do not develop a psychopathic personality, and suggests that there may be an interaction between genetic vulnerability or predisposition and environmental factors.

If we assume that psychopaths do not acquire conditioned fear responses readily (perhaps for congenital reasons), then it would follow that the timing of punishment for these individuals would be even more crucial than it would be for other persons. That is, for punishment to have any effect at all in producing resistance to temptation in psychopaths, it would have to occur reliably at some optimal point in the response sequence. The combination of poor fear conditionability and inefficient punishment techniques could therefore be important determinants of psychopathy. (Hare, 1970, p. 106)

Hare (1970) also speculated that parental separation was related to psychopathy. This was subsequently corroborated by Wong (1984). Wong examined a random sample of 315 male adult offenders using the Psychopathy Checklist (PCL; Hare, 1980). In an extreme groups analysis, psychopaths were more likely to be raised by an individual other than their biological parents and tended to leave home earlier than nonpsychopaths. There was, however, no evidence that psychopaths were more likely to have been physically abused.

Adults. Three studies have used retrospective self-report in adult offenders to investigate the link between family background and psychopathy, with mixed results. Hare, McPherson, and Forth (1984) retrospectively investigated the family background and criminal records of 315 male adult offenders. Psychopathy was assessed using the PCL using a diagnostic cutoff for psychopaths as 32. Hare et al. found that no family background variables were related to psychopathy. A poor family background was, however, associated with the emergence of early criminality (i.e., formal contact with the criminal justice system) in nonpsychopaths but not in psychopaths.

A study of 107 adult male offenders (DeVita, Hare, & Forth, 1990) examined the association between family background, psychopathy (using the PCL-R), and criminal behavior. The family background variables coded from institutional files included: lack of supervision, physical punishment, verbal abuse, parental rejection, parental criminality, parental alcoholism, marital discord, broken homes, and parental mental illness. They found that a lack of parental supervision and paternal rejection were related to psychopathy, confirming the observations of McCord and McCord (1964).

Generally, a poor family background was associated with increased offending (i.e., total number of official charges or convictions prior to age 20) and earlier age of onset of criminality in nonpsychopaths, but had no impact on the criminality of psychopaths. For example, nonpsychopaths from a poor family background were first arrested, on average, at age 15, compared to age 22 for those from less dysfunctional backgrounds. In contrast, family environment had no influence on psychopaths. Psychopaths from a poor family background were first arrested about age 12, whereas those from less troubled families were first arrested at age 13. Although not statistically significant, an interesting interaction between family background and psychopathy was found with respect to violent offences. Specifically, psychopaths from poor backgrounds were more likely (73%) to commit a violent offence than psychopaths from less troubled backgrounds (39%). In contrast, nonpsychopaths from poor or fair backgrounds committed few violent offences (33% from poor and 20% from fair family backgrounds).

Marshall and Cooke (1996) examined family background and psychopathy of 105 convicted adult male offenders within the Scottish prison system. Offenders were interviewed and assessed using the Childhood Experiences of Care and Abuse (Bifulco, Brown, & Harris, 1994) and the PCL-R. A large number of family background measures were coded including parental rejection, parental neglect/indifference, parental supervision/control, discord/tension in the home, physical abuse, and sexual abuse. Prior to examining the correlation of childhood factors to psychopathy scores, item 12 *"early behavioral problems"* and item 18 *"juvenile delinquency"* were removed.

Using regression analysis, seventy percent of PCL-R total scores were predicted by a combination of poor discipline, poor school experience, and parental rejection. These researchers investigated whether differential family background variables predicted PCL-R Factor 1 and Factor 2 scores. Only 6% of the variance in Factor 2 scores could be accounted for by school experience after Factor 1 was entered into the equation. Over a third (35%) of Factor 1 scores could be predicted by inconsistent discipline, child antipathy (child rejection of parent), physical abuse, and social factors after Factor 2 was entered into the equation. The largest contributor to Factor 1 scores was inconsistent discipline, by itself accounting for 26% of the variance in the scores. This finding corresponds to the conclusions of Hare (1970).

The above research on the association between family background and psychopathy has obtained inconclusive results, with the study by Marshall and Cooke (1995) reporting an association and the study by DeVita et al. (1990) finding no evidence that family dysfunction was related to psychopathy. Due to the lack of corroborative information in the institutional files relating to family background, most of the information to assess these factors were based on self-reports by the offender of their family history. The reliability and validity of retrospective recall has been widely questioned (see Widom & Shepard, 1996 for recent discussion). Moreover, in light of the association between psychopathy and deceitfulness, the issue of intentional distortion of information is of a particular concern (Hare, Forth, & Hart, 1989).

Children. The association between psychopathic characteristics and parenting practices has also been studied in children. A recent study by Wooton, Frick, Shelton, and Silverthorn (in press) investigated the interaction between parenting practices, the callous/unemotional factor from the Psychopathy Screening Device (PSD; see Frick, O'Brien, Wootton, & McBurnett, 1994 for a description of this scale) and conduct problems in a sample of 6 to 13 year-old clinic-referred ($n = 136$) and volunteer children ($n = 30$). Ineffective parenting, as defined as a lack of supervision, a lack of involvement, and inconsistent or harsh discipline, was associated with conduct problems only in children who scored low on the callous/unemotional factor of the PSD. In children who scored high on the callous/unemotional factor of the PSD, the number of conduct problems was not related to the quality of parenting they experienced. Wooten et al. suggest that antisocial behaviors in children lacking in empathy and guilt is associated with an etiological pathway different from those children who do exhibit these traits.

Adolescents. Three studies have examined the association between family background and psychopathy in adolescent offenders. In a study by McBride and Hare

(1996), participants were 189 adolescent male (ages 12-18) who attended an adolescent sex offender treatment program between 1985 and 1993. Family background and PCL:YV assessments were completed based on institutional file information. Family background variables included: number of years at home with both parents, history of physical and sexual abuse, history of Attention Deficit Disorder (ADD), maternal and paternal adversity (defined as a combination of parental criminality, violence, drug abuse, and alcoholism). Correlational analyses revealed that psychopathy was significantly related to maternal adversity ($r = .22$), paternal adversity, ($r = .21$), physical abuse ($r = .33$), and sexual abuse ($r = .16$), and presence or absence of ADD ($r = .38$). Using a stepwise regression analysis to predict PCL:YV scores, a combination of parental adversity, physical abuse, and ADD accounted for 22% of the variance.

Laroche and Toupin (1996) also examined the association between parental characteristics and parent-child relationships and psychopathy in a sample of 60 adolescent male offenders. Parental characteristics included the mother's psychopathology (i.e., affective, psychotic, anxiety, substance abuse) and father's antisocial or psychopathic personality. The parent-child relationship included an evaluation of supervision, physical and nonphysical punishment, communication, attachment, rules and family activities as well as a measurement of affection, rejection, and control. Twenty-five of the offenders were classified as psychopathic and 35 nonpsychopathic using the PCL:YV. Twenty-one mothers and nine fathers of nonpsychopathic offenders and 15 mothers and seven fathers of psychopathic offenders participated in the study. Nonpsychopathic offenders were more likely to be adequately supervised by their parents, which was consistent with some previous findings (DeVita et al., 1992). Nonpsychopaths also participated in more familial activities than the psychopathic offenders. No differences were detected between the two groups on any of the other parent-child relationship or on any of the parental characteristics.

Burke and Forth (1996) investigated the relationship between psychopathy, family background, and violence in 106 male young offenders from two secure correctional institutions and 50 community male adolescents. Subjects were assessed for psychopathy using the PCL:YV on the basis of interview and file information. Family dysfunction was also measured using interview and institutional file information. The following family history variables were assessed: physical abuse, sexual abuse, marital discord, antisocial parents, parental alcoholism, inconsistent discipline, inadequate parental supervision, neglect, early parental separation, and psychological maltreatment. A global family background score was calculated by summing all the standardized family background variables. Since self-report measures were utilized, self-deception and impression management were assessed using the Balanced Inventory of Desirable Responding (BIDR Version 6-40 A; Paulhus, 1991). The samples did not differ significantly in self-deception or impression management scores.

Global family background was significantly correlated with PCL:YV scores (excluding items 12 [early behavior problems] and 18 [juvenile delinquency]) for the whole sample ($r = .53$). For Factor 1, the association with family background was $r = .44$, while for Factor 2 (excluding items 12 and 18) it was $r = .55$. Family background was only associated with Factor 2 for young offenders ($r = .24$) and not with PCL-:YV total or Factor 1 scores. For community youth, global family dysfunction was related to PCL:YV total scores ($r = .56$), Factor 1 ($r = .41$), and Factor 2 ($r = .46$) scores. To summarize, Factor 2 rather than Factor 1 is more strongly related to overall family dysfunction, particularly for young offenders as compared to the community youth.

For the young offenders, no family background variables predicted PCL-YV total, Factor 1 or Factor 2 scores. By contrast, in the community adolescents, all the family background variables together accounted for almost half the variance in psychopathy ($R^2 = .49$, $p < .01$). Forty-three percent of this variance in PCL-YV total scores could be attributed to antisocial parents, inconsistent discipline, and parental alcoholism ($p < .0001$). For Factor 2, just over half of the variance (51%) could be accounted for by all the variables ($p < .001$). Again, a large proportion of the variance (40%, $p < .0001$) was attributed to the same variables: antisocial parents, inconsistent discipline, and parental alcoholism. In contrast, for Factor 1, 27% of the variance was explained by antisocial parents, psychological abuse, neglect, parental alcoholism, parental separation, and sexual abuse ($p < .05$). Of this variance in Factor 1, 22% of the 27% was attributable to antisocial parents, parental alcoholism, and sexual abuse ($p < .001$). Therefore, the strongest predictors of psychopathy in community youth appears to be antisocial parents, inconsistent discipline, and parental alcoholism, while for young offenders, no family background variables seem to be related to psychopathy.

From the literature reviewed, it seems clear that several family background variables are linked to psychopathy: parental rejection, parental antisocial personality, parental substance abuse, inconsistent discipline, lack of supervision, parental separation, physical abuse, and sexual abuse. However, for many of these variables (parental separation, parental rejection, physical abuse, and sexual abuse) the relationship to psychopathy is not consistently found across different samples - with perhaps one third or fewer of the investigations of these variables showing a significant relationship with psychopathy. The following factors seem to have a stronger link: having an antisocial or psychopathic parent, parental alcoholism, inconsistent discipline and a lack of supervision. At least half of the studies examining these variables demonstrated a significant association with psychopathy.

It seems likely that no one variable or combination of family background variables is responsible for the development of psychopathy. Perhaps there are multiple developmental pathways to psychopathy some of which involve family background and others in which psychopathy emerges irrespective of family background. For example, the developmental precursors for Factor 1 and Factor 2 traits may differ. Factor 2, the social deviance aspect of psychopathy that is similar to the antisocial personality disorder found in most offenders, may be linked more strongly to family background or other environmental factors. In contrast, Factor 1, the interpersonal and affective facet which is necessary for a diagnosis of psychopathy but not for antisocial personality disorder, may be independent of family history. If so, the causal origins of Factor 1 traits are more likely to be tied to biological factors. Recent research on the genetics of personality have consistently reported heritability coefficients ranging from .4 to .6 for most personality traits and little influence of family environmental factors (DiLalla, Carey, Gottesman, & Bouchard, 1996; Tellegen et al., 1988). Other researchers have also speculated about the differential contribution for the development of the two facets of psychopathy. For example, Wootton et al. (in press) suggests that factors such as a lack of normal fear response may mediate the development of such traits of callousness and unemotionality.

The cross-sectional design used in all the studies allow only correlational conclusions to be drawn, therefore, causality cannot be determined. Consequently, even though some family background variables appear to be related to psychopathy, we cannot be certain whether the family dysfunction preceded the psychopathic personality traits, whether the psychopathic personality indeed caused or contributed to the dysfunction, or if other factors not studied resulted in this personality disorder. Only in a prospective longitudinal design in which participants are followed from conception to early adulthood, can the family background and psychopathic traits be monitored so that etiological pathways may be established.

SUMMARY AND CONCLUSIONS

The current chapter provides evidence that the concept of psychopathy can be extended from adults to adolescents. The overall pattern of associations between the PCL:YV and a variety of external criteria was theoretically consistent with the construct of psychopathy. The association between psychopathy and violent behaviors seen across the studies is particularly noteworthy. Similar psychopathy-violence associations have been found in adult offenders, suggesting that violence is an integral part of the behavioral repertoire of individuals who are psychopathic. Finally, in some studies psychopathic characteristics were found to be predicted by various family background variables.

Though promising, the findings reviewed in this chapter are most appropriately seen as simply the beginning of the theoretical and empirical research in the area. Additional work needs to be done to clarify a number of the issues explored here. First, assessment research on more representative and larger community samples would enable a broader range of generalizations to be made about the correlates of psychopathy. Second, an important avenue for future research would be to determine the extent to which psychopathic youth manifest the same physiological, cognitive, and affective deficits that discriminate between adult psychopaths and nonpsychopaths (see chapters by Hare et al. and Newman). Third, preliminary research points towards a different etiological pathway for the development of the distinct facets of psychopathy. This provides a potential bases for understanding the development of this disorder and offers impetus for future research. Finally and most importantly, while adult psychopathic offenders may indeed be resistant to the effects of treatment (Hemphill, 1992; Ogloff, Wong, & Greenwood, 1990; Rice, Harris, & Cormier, 1992), psychopathic young offenders may be more malleable and may benefit more from treatment. Given the implications that psychopathy has for society in general and the criminal justice system in particular, future research initiatives are needed to address issues surrounding the development of effective intervention and management strategies for psychopathic youth. The only way to resolve these issues is to obtain further empirical evidence via additional research.

References

American Psychiatric Association. (1980). *Diagnostic and statistical manual of mental disorders* (3rd ed.). Washington, DC: American Psychiatric Association.

American Psychiatric Association. (1987). *Diagnostic and statistical manual of mental disorders* (3rd ed. rev.). Washington, DC: American Psychiatric Association.

American Psychiatric Association. (1994). *Diagnostic and statistical manual of mental disorders* (4th ed.). Washington, DC: American Psychiatric Association.

Bailey, D. (1994). *Assessment of psychopathy in young offenders.* Unpublished Honours thesis, Carleton University, Ottawa, Ontario, Canada.

Bifulco, A., Brown, G.W., & Harris, T. (1994). Childhood experiences of care and abuse (CECA): A retrospective interview measure. *Journal of Child Psychology and Psychiatry, 35,* 1419-1435.

Burke, H.C., & Forth, A.E. (1996). *Psychopathy and familial experiences as antecedents to violence: A cross-sectional study of young offenders and nonoffending youth.* Unpublished manuscript, Carleton University, Ottawa, Ontario, Ontario.

Butcher, J.N., Williams, C.L., Graham, J.R., Tellegen, A., Ben-Porath, Y., & Kaemmer, B. (1992). *MMPI-A (Minnesota Multiphasic Personality Inventory- Adolescent Manual for adminstration, scoring, and interpretation.* Minneapolis: University of Minnesota Press.

Chandler, M., & Moran, T. (1990). Psychopathy and moral development: A comparative study of delinquent and nondelinquent youth. *Development and Psychopathology, 2,* 227-246.

Cleckley, H. (1976). *The mask of sanity.* (5th ed.). St. Louis, MO: Mosby.

Cornell, D.G., Warren, J., Hawk, G., Stafford, E., Oram, G., & Pine, G. (1996). Psychopathy in instrumental and reactive violent offenders. *Journal of Consulting and Clinical Psychology, 64,* 783-790.

Davies, W., & Feldman, P. (1981). The diagnosis of psychopathy by forensic specialists. *British Journal of Psychiatry, 138,* 329-331.

Dempster, R.J., & Hart, S.D. (1996, March). *Utility of the FBI's Crime Classification Manual: Coverage, reliability, and validity for adolescent murderers.* Paper presented at the Biennial Meeting of the American Psychology-Law Society (APA Div. 41), Hilton Head, South Carolina.

Dempster, R.J., Lyon, D.R., Sullivan, L.E., & Hart, S.D. (1996, August). *Psychopathy and instrumental aggression in violent offenders.* Paper presented at the Annual Meeting of the American Psychological Association, Toronto, Ontario.

DiLalla, D.L., Carey, G., Gottesman, I.I., & Bouchard, T. J., Jr. (1996). Heritability of MMPI personality indicators of psychopathology in twins reared apart. *Journal of Abnormal Psychology, 105,* 491-499.

DeVita, E., Forth A.E., & Hare, R.D. (1990). Family background of male criminal psychopaths.[Abstract]. *Canadian Psychology, 31,* 346.

Douglas, J.E., Burgess, A.W., Burgess, A.G., & Ressler, R.K. (1992). *The crime classification Manual: A standard system of investigating and classifying violent crimes.* New York: Lexington.

Farrington, D.P., Ohlin, L.E., & Wilson, J.Q. (1986). *Understanding and controlling crime: Toward a new research strategy.* New York: Springer-Verlag.

Forth, A.E. (1995a). *Psychopathy and young offenders: Prevalence, family background, and violence.* Program Branch Users Report. Ottawa, Ontario, Canada: Minister of the Solicitor General of Canada.

Forth, A.E. (1995b, November). *Psychopathy in adolescent offenders: Assessment, family background, and violence.* Lecture presented at the NATO ASI on Psychopathy: Theory, research, and implications for society, Alvor, Portugal

Forth, A.E., Brown, S.L., Hart, S.D., & Hare, R.D. (1996). The assessment of psychopathy in male and female noncriminals: Reliability and validity. *Personality and Individual Differences, 20,* 531-543.

Forth, A.E., Hart, S.D., & Hare, R.D. (1990). Assessment of psychopathy in male young offenders. *Psychological Assessment: A Journal of Consulting and Clinical Psychology, 2,* 342-344.

Forth, A.E., Kosson, D.S., & Hare, R.D. (1994). *The Psychopathy Checklist: Youth Version.* Unpublished test manual, Carleton University, Ottawa, Ontario.

Frick, P., O'Brien, B., Wootton, J., & McBurnett, K. (1994). Psychopathy and conduct problems in children. *Journal of Abnormal Psychology, 103,* 700-707.

Garbarino, J., & Plantz, M.C. (1986). Child abuse and juvenile delinquency: What are the links? In J. Garbarino, C.J. Schellenbach & J.M. Sebes (Eds.), *Troubled youth, troubled families* (pp. 27 - 39). New York: Aldine deGryter.

Gough, H. (1957). *Manual for the California Psychological Inventory.* Palo Alto: Consulting Psychologists Press.

Gray, K.C., & Hutchinson, H.C. (1964). The psychopathic personality: A survey of Canadian psychiatrists' opinions. *Canadian Psychiatric Association Journal, 9,* 452-461.

Gretton, H., McBride, M., Lewis, K., O'Shaughnessy, R., & Hare, R.D. (1994, March). *Patterns of violence and victimization in adolescent sexual psychopaths.* Paper presented at the Biennial Meeting of the American Psychology-Law Society (Div. 41 of the American Psychological Association), Santa Fe, New Mexico.

Hare, R.D. (1970). *Psychopathy: Theory and research.* New York: John Wiley & Sons, Inc.

Hare, R.D. (1980). A research scale for the assessment of psychopathy in criminal populations. *Personality and Individual Differences, 1,* 111-119.

Hare, R.D. (1991). *The Hare Psychopathy Checklist - Revised.* Toronto Ontario: Multi-Health Systems.

Hare, R.D. (1996). Psychopathy: A clinical construct whose time has come. *Criminal Justice and Behavior, 23,* 25-54.

Hare, R.D., Forth, A.E., & Strachan, K. (1992). Psychopathy and crime across the lifespan. In R. DeV. Peters, R. J. McMahon, & V. L. Quinsey (Eds.), *Aggression and violence throughout the life span* (pp. 285-300). Newbury Park, CA: Sage.

Hare, R.D., Harpur, T.J., Hakstian, A.R., Forth, A.E., Hart, S.D., & Newman, J.P. (1990). The Revised Psychopathy Checklist: Reliability and factor structure. *Psychological Assessment: A Journal of Consulting and Clinical Psychology, 2,* 338-341.

Hare, R.D., Forth, A.E., & Hart, S.D. (1989). The psychopath as prototype for pathological lying and deception. In J.C. Yuille (Ed.), *Credibility assessment* (pp. 24-49). Dordrecht, The Netherlands: Kluwer.

Hare R.D., & McPherson L.M. (1984). Violent and aggressive behavior by criminal psychopaths. *International Journal of Law and Psychiatry, 7,* 35-40.

Hare R.D., McPherson, L.M., & Forth A.E. (1984). *Early criminal behavior as a function of family background.* Unpublished manuscript, University of British Columbia, Vancouver, B.C.

Hare, R.D., McPherson, L.E., & Forth, A.E. (1988). Male psychopaths and their criminal careers. *Journal of Consulting and Clinical Psychology, 56,* 710-714.

Harpur, T.J., Hakstian, R., & Hare, R.D. (1988). Factor structure of the Psychopathy Checklist. *Journal of Consulting and Clinical Psychology, 56,* 741-747.

Harris, G.T., Rice, M.E., & Cormier, C.A. (1991). Psychopathy and violent recidivism. *Law and Human Behavior, 15,* 625-637.

Hart, S.D., Forth, A.E., & Hare, R.D. (1991). The MCMI-II as a measure of psychopathy. *Journal of Personality Disorders, 5,* 318-327.

Hart, S.D., & Hare, R.D. (1989). Discriminant validity of the Psychopathy Checklist in a forensic psychiatric population. *Psychological Assessment: A Journal of Consulting and Clinical Psychology, 1,* 211-218.

Hart, S.D., & Hare, R.D. (in press). Psychopathy: Assessment and association with criminal conduct. In D. M. Stoff, J. Brieling, & J. Maser (Eds.), *Handbook of antisocial behavior.* New York: Wiley.

Hathaway, S.R., & McKinley, J.C. (1940). A multiphasic personality schedule (Minnesota): I. Construction of the schedule. *Journal of Psychology, 10,* 249-254.

Hemphill, J. (1992). *Psychopathy and recidivism following release from a therapeutic community treatment program.* Unpublished Master's thesis. University of Saskatchewan, Saskatoon, Saskatchewan, Canada.

Hemphill, J., Hart, S.D., & Hare, R.D. (1994). Psychopathy and substance use. *Journal of Personality Disorders, 8,* 169-180.

Huesmann, L.R., Eron, L.D., Lefkowitz, M.M., & Walder, L.O. (1984). Stability of aggression over time and generations. *Developmental Psychology, 20,* 1120-1134.

Kosson, D.S., Smith, S.S., & Newman, J.P. (1990). Evaluation of the construct validity of psychopathy in Black and White male inmates: Three preliminary studies. *Journal of Abnormal Psychology, 99,* 250-259.

Kosson, D.S. (1996). [PCL:YV scores from a probation sample]. Unpublished raw data. Finch University of Health Sciences, Chicago, Illinois.

Laroche, I. (1996). Les composantes psychologiques et comportementales parentales associées à la psychopathie du contrevenant juvénile. Unpublished doctoral thesis. University of Montreal, Montreal, Quebec.

Laroche, I., & Toupin, J. (1996, August). *Psychopathic delinquents: A family contribution?* Paper presented at the XXVI International Congress of Psychology, Montreal, Quebec.

Lay, P. (1995). *The Psychopathy Checklist Revised (PCL-R) User Survey.* Unpublished Honours thesis, Carleton University, Ottawa, Ontario.

Lewis, D.O., Shanok, S.S., Pincus, J.H., & Glaser, G.H. (1979). Violent delinquents. Psychiatric, neurological, psychological, and abuse factors. *Journal of the American Academy of Child Psychiatry, 18,* 307-319.

Lilienfeld, S.O. (1994). Conceptual problems in the assessment of psychopathy. *Clinical Psychology Review, 14,* 17-38.

Loeber, R., & Stouthamer-Loeber, M. (1986). Family factors as correlates and predictors of juvenile conduct problems and delinquency. In M. Tonry & N. Morris (Ed.), *Crime and Justice* (Vol. 7, pp. 219-339). Chicago: University of Chicago Press.

Lynam, D.R. (1996). Early identification of chronic offenders: Who is the fledging psychopath? *Psychological Bulletin, 120,* 209-234.

Marshall, L., & Cooke, D. (1995, November). *The role of childhood experiences in the etiology of psychopathy.* Paper presented at NATO Advanced Studies Institute on Psychopathy, Alvor, Portugal.

McBride, M E& Hare, R.D. (1996). *Precursors of psychopathy and recidivism.* Unpublished manuscript, University of British Columbia, Vancouver, B.C.

McCord, W., & McCord, J. (1964). *The psychopath: An essay on the criminal mind.* Princeton, NJ: Van Nostrand.

Millon, T. (1987). *Manual for the Millon Multiaxial Inventory-II* (2nd ed.). Minneapolis: National Computer Systems.

Moffit, T.E. (1993). Adolescence-limited and life-course-persistent antisocial behavior: A developmental typology. *Psychological Review, 106,* 674-701.

Ogloff, J., Wong, S., & Greenwood, A. (1990). Treating criminal psychopaths in a therapeutic community program. *Behavioral Sciences and the Law, 8,* 81-90.

Paulhus, D.L. (1991). *Balanced Inventory of Socially Desirable Responding.* Unpublished test, University of British Columbia, British Columbia, Canada

Rice, M.E., Harris, G.T., & Cormier, C.A. (1992). An evaluation of a maximum security therapeutic community for psychopaths and other mentally disordered offenders. *Law and Human Behavior, 16,* 399-412.

Robins, L.N. (1966). *Deviant children grown up: A sociological and psychiatric study of sociopathic personality.* Baltimore, MD:Williams & Wilkins.

Serin, R.C. (1991). Psychopathy and violence in criminals. *Journal of Interpersonal Violence, 6,* 423-431.

Serin, R.C. (1996). Violent recidivism in criminal psychopaths. *Law and Human Behavior, 20,* 207-217.

Serin, R.C., Peters, R.D., & Barbaree, H.E. (1990). Predictors of psychopathy and release outcome in a criminal population. *Psychological Assessment: A Journal of Consulting and Clinical Psychology, 2,* 419-422.

Smith, S.S., & Newman, J.P. (1990). Alcohol and drug abuse/dependence disorders in psychopathic and nonpsychopathic criminal offenders. *Journal of Abnormal Psychology, 99,* 430-439.

Straus, M. (1979). Measuring family conflict and violence: The Conflict Tactics Scale. *Journal of Marriage and the Family, 41,* 75-88.

Sullivan, L.E. (1996). *Assessment of psychopathy using the MMPI-A: Validity in male adolescent forensic patients.* Unpublished Master's thesis, Simon Fraser University, Burnaby, British Columbia.

Tellegen, A., Lykken, D.T., Bouchard, T.J., Wilcox, K.J. Segal, N.J. & Rich, S. (1988). Personality similarity in twins reared apart and together. *Journal of Personality and Social Psychology, 54,* 1031-1039.

Tennent, G., Tennent, D., Prins, H., & Bedford, A. (1990). Psychopathic disorder: A useful clinical concept? *Medicine, Science, and the Law, 30,* 38-44.

Tolman, R.M. (1989). The development of a measure of psychological maltreatment of women by their partners. *Violence and Victims, 4,* 159-177.

Toupin, J., Mercier, H., Déry, M., Côté, G., & Hodgins, S. (1995, November). *Validity of the PCL-R for adolescents.* Paper presented at the NATO ASI on Psychopathy: Theory, research, and implications for society, Alvor, Portugal

Trevethan, S.D., & Walker, L.J. (1989). Hypothetical versus real-life moral reasoning among psychopathic and delinquent youth. *Development and Psychopathology, 1,* 91-103.

West, D.J., & Farrington, D.P. (1973). *Who becomes delinquent.* London: Heineman Educational Books.

White, J.L., Moffit, T.E., Earls, F., Robins, L., & Silva, P.A. (1990). How early can we tell?: Predictors of childhood conduct disorder and adolescent delinquency. *Criminology, 28,* 507-533.

Widom, C.S. (1989). Does violence beget violence: A critical examination of the literature. *Psychological Bulletin, 106,* 3-28.

Widom, C.S., & Shepard, R.L. (1996). Accuracy of adult recollections of childhood victimization: Part 1. Childhood physical abuse. *Psychological Assessment, 8,* 412-421.

Williamson, S.E., Hare, R.D., & Wong, S. (1987). Violence: Criminal psychopaths and their victims. *Canadian Journal of Behavioral Science, 19,* 454-462.

Wolfgang, M.E., Figlio, R.M., & Sellin, T. (1972). *Delinquency in the birth cohort.* Chicago: University of Chicago Press.

Wong, S. (1984). *Criminal and institutional behaviors of psychopaths*. Program Branch Users Report. Ottawa, Ontario, Canada: Minister of the Solicitor General of Canada.

Wootton, J.M., Frick, P.J., Shelton, K.K., & Silverthorn, P. (in press). Ineffective parenting and childhood conduct problems: The moderating role of callous-unemotional traits. *Journal of Consulting and Clinical Psychology*.

Zinger, I., & Forth, A.E. (1996). *Psychopathy and Canadian criminal proceedings: A review of case law and psychological research*. Unpublished manuscript, Carleton University, Ottawa, Ontario.

Authors' notes

Preparation of this chapter and some of the research presented herein were supported by grants to the first author from the Ministry of Solicitor General of Canada and by the Faculty of Social Sciences, Research Grants, Carleton University. The opinions expressed are those of the authors and do not necessarily represent the opinions or policies of the Ministry of Solicitor General.

We wish to thank Shelley Parlow and John Logan for their comments on the chapter. We are also grateful to Dr. David Kosson, Dr. Jean Toupin and Irene Laroche for making their data available to us.

Correspondence should be addressed to A. Forth, Department of Psychology, Carleton University, Ottawa, Ontario, Canada K1S 5B6 (e-mail: forth@ccs.carleton.ca).

MAJOR MENTAL DISORDER AND CRIME: AN ETIOLOGICAL HYPOTHESIS

SHEILAGH HODGINS
Université de Montréal
Montréal, Canada.

GILLES CÔTÉ
Université du Québec à Trois-Rivières
Trois-Rivières, Canada.

JEAN TOUPIN
Université de Sherbrooke
Sherbrooke, Canada.

INTRODUCTION

Evidence has been accumulating since the 1960's indicating that greater proportions of persons who suffer from major mental disorders than non-disordered persons commit crimes, commit crimes of violence, and behave aggressively towards others. Three types of investigations have addressed the relation between the major mental disorders and crime: follow-up studies of psychiatric patients discharged to the community; studies of the prevalence of the major mental disorders among convicted offenders; and investigations of unselected birth cohorts comparing the prevalence of criminality among persons with major disorders and with no disorders. A fourth type of investigation has examined aggressive behavior.

Studies of psychiatric patients discharged to the community

In the 1960's and 1970's many follow-up studies were conducted in the U.S. in which the criminal activity of persons who had been discharged from psychiatric wards was compared to that of persons living in the communities surrounding the hospitals (Durbin, Pasewark, & Albers, 1977; Giovanni & Gurel, 1967; Rappeport & Lassen, 1965; 1966; Sosowsky, 1974; 1978; 1980; Steadman, Cocozza & Melick, 1978; Zitrin, Hardesty, Burdock, & Drossman, 1976). All of these investigations documented higher rates of criminality among the former patients than among the non-disordered population in the community where the patients lived. However, because of the methodology of these investigations, the conclusions which can be drawn about the association between major mental disorders and crime are limited. For example, the diagnoses of the discharged patients are often not reported, and it is likely that the samples are not comparable with respect to the proportions of subjects with various diagnoses. Subject attrition was relatively high. In many instances, criminal records were available for only one state (for a further discussion, see Hodgins, 1993).

Three recent investigations have overcome these problems. Lindqvist and Allebeck (1990) followed all inpatients in Stockholm county with a diagnosis of schizophrenia who were born between 1920 and 1959 and discharged in 1971. Patients were re-diagnosed by an independent clinician, using DSM-III criteria, and 85% (644) met the criteria for schizophrenia. These 644 patients were then followed for 14 years.

D.J. Cooke et al. (eds.), Psychopathy: Theory, Research and Implications for Society, 231–256.
© *1998 Kluwer Academic Publishers. Printed in the Netherlands.*

The relative risk of a criminal offense among these schizophrenics as compared to the general Swedish population was 1.2 for the men and 2.2 for the women. However, the schizophrenics *"committed four times as many violent offenses as the general population"* (pp. 346-347). This finding is important considering the fact that subjects who had committed a homicide were excluded from this sample because they were hospitalized outside of Stockholm county. [1]

In a carefully designed investigation, Link and his co-workers (Link et al., 1992) examined the criminality of psychiatric patients compared to subjects who lived in the same neighborhood of New York but who had never received any mental health treatment. Four groups were followed: (1) patients who received psychiatric treatment for the first time in the year preceding the study; (2) patients who were in treatment during the previous year and once before; (3) former patients who received no treatment in the previous year; and (4) a community sample with no history of psychiatric treatment. Among the patients, 34% had received a diagnosis of major depression, 19% schizophrenia, 10% another psychotic disorder and 37% another mental disorder. While 6.7% of the community cohorts had been arrested and 6.0% of the first contact patients, 12.1% of the repeat treatment patients and 11.7% of the former patients had been arrested. The arrests of the patients were more likely to have been for felonies and for violent behavior than the arrests of the subjects in the community sample.

A follow-up study conducted in Finland examined all 281 males released from a forensic hospital. Seventy percent had a history of at least one violent offense. During the first year in the community after discharge, the patients were 300 times more likely than the males in the general population to commit a homicide. During the follow-up period that averaged 7.8 years, the increased risk of committing a homicide for the discharged male patients was 53 times that for the general Finnish male population (Tiihonen, Hakola, Eronen, Vartiainen, & Ryynänen, in press). While the odds ratios reflect the greatly increased risk of violent crime among patients with a history of violence, it is important to note that the numbers of homicide offenders are low (97 before, 7 during follow-up).

Studies of the mental health of offenders

Looking at the same problem from the opposite point of view are the studies of mental disorder among convicted offenders. Recent studies of representative samples of U.S. prison inmates (Collins & Schlenger, 1983; Daniel, Robins, Reid, & Wilfley, 1988; Hyde & Seiter, 1987; Neighbors, Williams, Gunnings, Lipscomb, Broman, & Lepkowski, 1987; Robins & Regier, 1991) and Canadian penitentiary inmates (Hodgins & Côté, 1990; Motiuk & Poporino, 1991) have revealed higher prevalence rates of mental disorders, and particularly of the major disorders within these facilities than in

---

[1] The difficulties in tracking discharged patients with major mental disorders and accurately documenting their criminal records is described by Belfrage (1994). As he notes, it is essential to construct a non-biased sample of patients or at least to accurately describe the sample, for example noting if certain categories of violent patients have been excluded, and to take account of the loss of subjects due to the high death rates in this population.

the general population. [2] In our study of Canadian penitentiary inmates, we were able to confirm that in the large majority of cases the major mental disorder was present before the incarceration. These five investigations all employed the same diagnostic criteria, and standardized, reliable and valid diagnostic instruments. These same instruments have been used to examine the prevalence of mental disorders in the general population. Consequently, comparisons between the prevalence of disorders among inmates and in the general population, controlling for gender and age, can be made with some confidence.

In addition to these studies showing that major mental disorders are more prevalent among incarcerated offenders in North America than in the general population, four investigations suggest that the prevalence of the major disorders is even higher among homicide offenders. These four studies differ from most investigations of homicide offenders which include only compilations of the psychiatric and psychological assessments conducted at the request of the court. These latter samples are biased and represent only a small proportion of homicide offenders. In contrast are three studies from Scandinavian where the diagnoses of all persons accused of homicide are established by several mental health professionals after intensive inpatient evaluations and consultations with family members, colleagues from work, and others who knew the accused well. These diagnoses are thought to represent the diagnoses present at the time of the offense. A study of all homicide offenders in Copenhagen over a 25 year period revealed that 20% of the men and 44% of the women were diagnosed psychotic (Gottlieb, Gabrielsen & Kramp, 1987). A similar investigation was conducted in Northern Sweden between 1970 and 1981 (Lindqvist, 1986). Thirty-four of the 64 (53%) individuals who were convicted of committing a homicide, were found to suffer from a major mental disorder. Eronen, Tiihonen and Hakola (1996) have studied all the 1423 homicide offenders in Finland over a 12 year period. Schizophrenia with no secondary diagnosis of an alcohol use disorder was found to have increased the risk of homicide 6.4 times among men and 5.3 times among women. Schizophrenia with a secondary diagnoses of alcohol increased the risk of homicide by 16.6 times in men and 84.6 times in women. The fourth study examined a representative sample of incarcerated homicide offenders and found that 35% met DSM-III criteria for a major mental disorder (lifetime) (Côté & Hodgins, 1992).

Studies of the prevalence of criminality in unselected birth cohorts

In 1975, Ortmann (1981) examined the criminality of all persons born in Copenhagen in 1953. Although the subjects were only 23 years of age, he found that more of those who had been admitted to a psychiatric ward with a diagnosis of a major mental disorder, as compared to subjects who had never been admitted, had been registered for a criminal offense.

An investigation of an unselected birth cohort composed of all 15,117 persons born in Stockholm in 1953 and still living there in 1963 showed that subjects who develop major mental disorders are at significantly increased risk for criminality as

---

[2] Among incarcerated offenders in England (Gunn, Maden, & Swinton, 1991) and Scotland (Cooke, 1994), there are few cases of major mental disorders.

compared to non-disordered persons. Among the male subjects, 31.7% of those with no mental disorder and no retardation as compared to 50.0% of those who developed major disorders were registered for a criminal offense by the age of 30. Among the female subjects, 5.8% of the non-disordered women as compared to 19.0% of those who developed major mental disorders were registered for a criminal offense by age 30. Both the men and the women who developed major disorders were found to be at even greater risk for violent crimes, than for non-violent crime. The offenders with major mental disorders committed, on average, as many or more offenses than the non-disordered offenders. They committed all types of crimes (Hodgins, 1992). The relation between socioeconomic status and criminality within the different groups was examined. Among both the men and women with no disorder and no handicap, there are highly statistically significant relations between socioeconomic status of the family of origin and criminality of the subject. Also, among the subjects with no disorder or handicap, significantly more of the offenders, as compared to the non-offenders, were raised in families who received social welfare payments. However, among the males with major mental disorders there was no relation between socioeconomic status and criminality. Among the women with major mental disorders, there was a significant relationship but in the opposite direction of that which might be expected. A higher socio-economic status of the family of origin was associated with criminality among these women. These findings have now been replicated with a Danish birth cohort composed of 324,401 subjects followed to age 43 (Hodgins, Mednick, Brennan, Schulsinger & Engberg, in press). An examination of a Finnish birth cohort composed of 11,017 males and females followed to age 28 again found that a greater proportion of those who developed major mental disorders, as compared to non-disordered subjects, had been convicted of at least one criminal offense (Tiihonen, Isohanni, Koiranen, Moring, Rantakallo, submitted).

Conclusion

Three types of investigations have compared the prevalence of criminality and violence among persons suffering from major mental disorders and those with no disorders: follow-up studies of patients with major mental disorders discharged from psychiatric wards to the community; investigations of the mental health of representative samples of convicted offenders; and four studies of unselected birth cohorts. All three types of investigations indicate that persons suffering from one or other of these three mental disorders are more likely than non-disordered persons to commit crimes and to perpetrate acts of violence.

AGGRESSIVE BEHAVIOR AMONG PERSONS WITH MAJOR MENTAL DISORDERS

Link et al. (1992) noted that the subjects with major mental disorders were not being arrested for trivial behaviors. They suggested that the higher rates of violent crime resulted from the fact that more of the patients than the non-disordered community controls behaved aggressively, hurt a victim seriously, and more often used weapons. These findings are consistent with an older study (Steadman & Felson, 1984), also carried out in New York city, in which more ex-patients reported behaving violently and reported incidents involving weapons than did subjects in a matched community sample. In this investigation it was found that police were less likely to arrest a former patient than a subject with no history of mental disorder for an offense involving a firearm.

A recent U.S. publication (Swanson, Holzer, Granju, & Jono, 1990) compared reports of aggressive behavior among subjects in the ECA study with and without mental disorders. The ECA was designed to document the prevalence of mental disorder in a representative sample of the U.S. population (Robins, et al., 1984). Lay interviewers conducted interviews with the identified subjects in their homes using the Diagnostic Interview Schedule (Robins, Helzer, Croughan, & Ratcliff, 1981). Among the subjects diagnosed as having a major mental disorders about 13% of the men and 10% of the women reported interpersonal aggressive behavior during the year preceding the interview. However, only 2.7% of the non-disordered men and 1.1% of the women reported behaving aggressively during the same period (Swanson et al., 1990). The rates of aggressive behavior reported by the non-disordered subjects in the ECA study are low in comparison to what has been found in other U.S. investigations (see for example, Straus, Gelles & Steinmetz, 1980). For example, investigations of conjugal violence employ interview protocols which have been carefully designed specifically to elicit information about aggressive behavior towards spouses and children. In the U.S., such investigations generally find that between 30% and 40% of adult men and women report physically aggressive behavior towards another person during the preceding months (O'Leary, Barling, Arias, & Rosenbaum, 1989; Elliot, Huizinga, & Morse, 1986). These self-reports are corroborated by victim reports. The differences in rates of aggressive behavior obtained in the ECA study and the family violence studies may be due to small differences in the questions asked. Alternatively, the differences could be due to a refusal on the part of a certain proportion of non-disordered subjects to report past aggressive behavior. Another difficulty inherent in these investigations is the comparability of self-reports of subjects with major mental disorders, antisocial personality disorder, and no disorder. While many subjects fear that they may get into trouble if they report aggressive behavior, it is not clear if persons with different disorders and those with no disorder bias their reports in similar ways.

A recent investigation followed-up patients who had been consecutively admitted to psychiatric wards in three different U.S. cities. All patients were included in the study except those with a primary diagnosis of mental retardation. [3] Information on aggressive behaviors was collected both from the subjects themselves and from collaterals who had contact with the subjects. It was found that during the two months . prior to admission, 34.8% of the women and 39.0% of the men reported at least one violent incident. During the two months after discharge, 32.8% of the women and 22.4% of the men reported behaving violently at least once (Steadman, et al., 1993). However, the rate of violence increased by 25.6% when the information from the

---

[3] This is an applied study of the predictors of violence, and not an epidemiological study of aggressive behavior among persons with major mental disorders. As the authors themselves have repeatedly pointed out, this is a biased sample of persons with mental disorders as those who behave aggressively are more likely to be admitted to a psychiatric ward than are non-aggressive persons with the same disorders.

collaterals was combined with the self-report data from the patients (Steadman et al., 1994).

Conclusion

There is evidence to suggest that the prevalence of aggressive behavior is higher among persons suffering from major mental disorders than among non-disordered community controls. However, for the moment the validity of these reports remain an issue. As previously noted, self report data from severely disordered and non-disordered persons may not be comparable.[4] On the other hand, the validity of information from collaterals has only recently been examined. They may think, for example, that by reporting aggressive behavior, their disordered relative or friend will receive better or more mental health services even if, as was done in the investigation of Steadman and colleagues, they are told that this not the case.

WHY ARE PERSONS WHO SUFFER FROM MAJOR MENTAL DISORDERS AT HIGH RISK TO COMMIT CRIMES?

A number of explanations have been advanced in attempts to explain the criminality and violence of persons suffering from major mental disorders. One hypothesis proposes that the police discriminate against persons with mental disorders. One study (Teplin, 1984) found that police in the U.S. were more likely to arrest a suspect with a major mental disorder than one with no disorder. However, other evidence (Link et al., 1992; Steadman & Felson, 1984) suggests that persons with major mental disorders are less likely to be arrested for trivial offenses and even for offenses involving weapons than are persons with no disorders. Further, in many countries police have discretionary powers allowing them to divert suspects of all but the most serious offenses to the health system rather than charging them with a criminal offense. Such diversion affords positive discrimination to persons with major disorders. If this hypothesis of police or judicial discrimination explained the results of the follow-up studies of patients discharged from psychiatric wards, of the diagnostic studies of incarcerated offenders, and the birth cohort studies, it would imply that the police and judicial systems in all the different countries where these investigations were conducted had the same bias or prejudice against the mentally disordered. This is highly unlikely.

Another hypothesis proposes that alcohol and/or drugs when used by persons with major mental disorders lead to crime and violence. The role of alcohol and drugs in determining the illegal behaviors of persons with major mental disorders is complex and difficult to clarify (Hodgins, 1994a). Persons with major mental disorders are more likely than non-disordered persons to develop substance use disorders (Drake et al., 1990; Mueser et al., 1990; Regier et al., 1990). However, the rates of substance use disorders among persons with major mental disorders vary by sample, by regions, by time period, by disorder, and by gender. Among persons with major disorders, those who have secondary diagnoses of alcohol or drug use disorders are at higher risk than those with the same major disorder but no history of substance abuse, to commit crimes

---

[4] Controlling for Social Desirability as Link et al. have done may not adequately address the problem.

and/or to behave violently. However, those with only the major disorder (and no secondary substance abuse) are still at higher risk than non-disordered persons to commit crimes and/or behave violently (Hodgins, 1994a; Eronen, Tiihonen, Hakola, 1996; Swanson, 1993). It is not known whether it is a history of abuse or intoxication at the time of the illegal act or both that are important in increasing the likelihood of illegal behavior (Beaudoin, Hodgins, & Lavoie, 1993).

Another hypothesis proposes that certain symptoms are associated with violence among persons with major mental disorders. Link and Stueve (1994) have shown that threat/control overide symptoms[5] are associated with aggressive behaviors while other types of psychotic symptoms are not. Another group of researchers (Swanson, Borum, Swartz, & Monahan, submitted), using the data from the Epidemiological Catchment Area project, have also found that symptoms of threat/control overide increased the risk of assaultive behavior. This association between threat/control overide symptoms is limited to self reports. A British group studying persecutory delusions has found no relation when assessments of symptoms and behaviors are made by clinicians based on information provided by patients, family members and hospital staff (Wessely, Buchanan, Reed, Cutting, Everitt, Garety, & Taylor, 1993). These findings underline the difficulty of examining the relationship between paranoid-type symptomatology and illegal behavior. While this hypothesis may well explain some of the violent behavior of persons with major mental disorders, it is unlikely to explain all of the illegal behavior. Both data collected prospectively (the Swedish cohort study) and retrospectively (our penitentiary study, the ECA data) document illegal or antisocial behavior on the part of some persons with major mental disorders long before the onset of psychotic symptoms. Further, if patients can report delusions as determinants of aggressive behavior, then in the Canadian system they would not be held responsible for their behavior. Yet, data show that many more offenders with major mental disorders are incarcerated (Hodgins & Côté, 1990), than are excused from criminal responsibility (Hodgins & Webster, 1992). Consequently, while threat/control overide and/or paranoid-type symptoms may play a role in determining some of the aggressive behavior of some individuals who suffer from major mental disorders, they do not explain the observed relation between the major disorders and crime.

TWO TYPES OF OFFENDERS WITH MAJOR MENTAL DISORDERS:

Early and late-starters

We have proposed a more parsimonious hypothesis to explain the relation between the major mental disorders and criminality. Recent findings suggest that there are two types of persons who develop major mental disorders and who commit crimes. The *"early starters"* display a stable pattern of antisocial behavior from a young age and through adulthood. As noted by Robins and McEvoy (1990) antisocial children are exposed to alcohol and drugs earlier than other children, and many become substance abusers and

---

[5] Link and Stueve (1994) have defined threat/control overide symptoms as positive responses to the following questions: (1) how often have you felt that your mind was dominated by forces beyond your control? (2) how often have you felt that thoughts were put into your head that were not your own? (3) How often have you felt that there were people who wished to do you harm?

criminals. The *"late-starters"* begin offending in adulthood as the symptoms of the major mental disorder emerge. Both paranoid-type symptoms and intoxication may play a role in the illegal behaviors of the *"late-starters"*.

Evidence from the Swedish cohort study

The Swedish cohort (Hodgins, 1992; 1993; 1995) initially provided evidence for the existence of the two types of offenders among the subjects who developed major mental disorders. Among the males with no mental disorder or intellectual handicap, a decreasing proportion, varying from 10.8% before age 15 to 6.4% after age 21, were first convicted of a criminal offense. However, among the males who developed a major mental disorder 15.9% were first convicted before age 15, 15.9% between the ages of 15 and 18, 6.1% between the ages of 19 and 21 years, and 12.2% after the age of 21. Among the non-disordered non-handicapped females, between one and two percent committed their first offense at the four age periods. Among the women who developed major mental disorders, 5.1% were first convicted before the age of 15, 2.5% between the ages of 15 and 18 years, 5.1% between the ages of 19 and 21 years, and 6.3% after 21 years. These data which had been collected prospectively from official records, demonstrated that among subjects who would eventually develop major mental disorders and commit crimes there were two groups: those who began offending in early adolescence and those who began offending in adulthood. In addition, we noted that early abuse of alcohol and/or drugs was associated with criminality. Among the male offenders with a major mental disorder, 37% had been identified by the social agency for abuse as children or young adolescents as opposed to 7% of the men with a major disorder who did not have a criminal record. Among the women, the comparable figures were 27% and 5%.

Evidence from a study of incarcerated male offenders

We then looked for these two types, early and late-starters, among offenders with major mental disorders. We (Hodgins & Côté, 1990) examined a representative sample of 495 male penitentiary inmates in Québec. Each subject was diagnosed using the Diagnostic Interview Schedule (Robins et al., 1981). One-hundred and nine of these men met criteria for having had at least one episode of a major mental disorder during their life (MMD). Two of the subjects with a major mental disorder and three other subjects did not complete the part of the diagnostic interview which assesses antisocial personality disorder (APD). The prevalence of APD was found to be similar among inmates with major mental disorders and those with no major disorder. Of the 349 non-disordered inmates, 59.6% received a diagnosis of APD as compared to 66.0% of the inmates with a major mental disorder ($X^2(1, N = 456) = 1.57, p = $ n.s.).

Complete criminal records for all subjects were obtained from the Correctional Services of Canada. Among the offenders with major mental disorders, those with APD differed from those without APD as to age of onset and severity of their criminal careers. Proportionately, more of the MMD inmates with APD, as compared to the MMD inmates without APD, had a juvenile record (87.3% versus 27.8% $X^2(1, N = 107) = 38.48, p < .01$), and, on average, they were younger when first sentenced to a penitentiary ($M = 24.7$ years ($SD = 5.9$) versus $M = 30.4$ years ($SD = 9.6$); $t(49.04) = $

-3.31, $p < .01$). In order to control for age, the number of convictions was divided by the number of years between the subject's 18th birthday and the date the criminal records were extracted. Among the offenders with major mental disorders, those with APD, compared to those without APD, had accumulated more convictions ($M = 2.28$ versus $M = 0.71$; $t(101.57) = 3.29$, $p < .001$), and more convictions for non-violent crimes ($M = 1.71$ versus $M = 0.26$; $t(76.92) = 3.59$, $p < .001$). However, the MMD men with and without APD had been convicted, on average, of similar numbers of violent offenses ($M = 0.57$, versus $M = 0.44$, $t(54.53) = 0.51$, $p = $ n.s.).

While the men with major mental disorders and APD began their criminal careers earlier and were convicted of more offenses than those with major disorders but no APD, the proportions of offenders in each of these groups who committed different types of offenses were very similar. The only statistically significant difference is for robbery and theft once the level of significance was adjusted to account for multiple comparisons. However, these differences must be interpreted cautiously as the numbers of subjects who committed certain types of offenses, for example arson, are low. Thus, among the men with major mental disorders similar proportions of those with and without APD committed various types of offenses, but those with APD committed more offenses than those without. This is not surprising given that those with APD necessarily reported antisocial behavior before age 15, more of them had juvenile records, and that they were first convicted in adult court, on average, at a younger age than those without APD.

Now consider comparisons between the offenders with a major mental disorder and APD and the non-disordered offenders with APD. No differences were found between these two groups as to the mean number of convictions, mean number of convictions for violent crimes, and mean number of convictions for non-violent offenses. Not only were these two groups of offenders with APD similar as to numbers of convictions, no differences were found in the proportions of subjects in each group who were convicted of different types of offenses. Thus the offenders with a major mental disorder and APD had criminal histories very similar to offenders with APD but no major disorder. This is illustrated in Figure 1. In this figure the criminality of the four groups of male offenders, non-disordered with and without APD, and major mental disorder, with and without APD, is presented. Not only are the patterns of convictions of the offenders with APD similar whether or not a major mental disorder is present, the severity of early antisocial behavior is also similar. The diagnosis of APD requires three symptoms of antisocial behavior before the age of 15. Twelve questions about different types of antisocial behavior including truancy, expulsion from school, lying, stealing and fighting, were put to the subjects. Each item the subject endorsed was given a score of 1. The offenders with major mental disorders and APD obtained scores similar to those of the non-disordered offenders with APD, ($M = 7.14$ ($SD = 2.46$) versus $M = 6.55$ ($SD = 2.49$), $t(277) = 1,74$, $p = $ ns). These scores are indicative of a stable pattern of antisocial behavior in childhood and/or early adolescence (Hodgins & Côté, 1993a & b).

Conclusion

These findings led us to hypothesize that among offenders with major mental disorders there are two distinct types, the early starter or antisocial type and the late-starter. We proposed that the early-starters are characterized by a stable pattern of antisocial behavior in childhood and adolescence, long before the symptoms of the major mental disorder developed. The late-starters, in contrast, show no evidence of antisocial behavior before the onset of the symptoms of the major mental disorder.

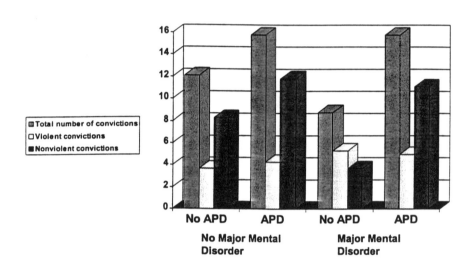

Figure 1. Number of convictions by mental disorder: Male penitentiary inmates

WHAT ARE THE DIFFERENCES BETWEEN THE EARLY AND LATE-STARTERS?

Evidence from a study of men suffering from schizophrenia

We examined a sample of 74 male schizophrenics recruited at the time of discharge from one forensic hospital and two psychiatric hospitals. Their diagnoses were all confirmed using the Schedule for Schizophrenia and Affective Disorders (SADS) (Endicott & Spitzer, 1978) and the Research Diagnostic Criteria (Endicott & Spitzer, 1979; Spitzer, Endicott & Robins, 1978) (for a detailed description of this sample see Hodgins, Toupin, Fiset, & Moisan, 1995). Twenty of these men received a diagnosis of APD, and 54 did not. The 20 who received the diagnosis of APD endorsed, on average, 5.5 of 11 items descriptive of antisocial behavior before the age of 15, while the 54 others endorsed, on average, 2.9 items ($t(55) = 4.36$, $p = .000$). These two groups of subjects did not differ as to age, socio-economic status, years of education, or the percent who had never been gainfully employed. No differences could be detected in the presentation of schizophrenic symptoms using either the SADS' items or the Positive and Negative Symptom Scale (Kay, Fiszbein, & Opler, 1987). Scores for social handicaps and life skills were equivalent for the two groups. However, the schizophrenic men who reported early antisocial behavior had slightly higher scores for interpersonal social skills than did those who reported little or no early antisocial behavior. Those who reported early antisocial behavior were significantly more likely to have a secondary diagnosis of an alcohol use disorder (45.0% versus 20.4%, X^2(1, N = 74) = 4,49, p = .03), and of a drug use disorder (70.0% versus 38.9%, X^2(1, N = 74) = 5.67, p = .02). Further, more of those who had reported antisocial behavior before the age of 15 than those who reported little or no antisocial behavior before age 15, had a juvenile record (47.4% versus 18.0%, X^2(1, N = 56) = 4.98, p = .03), and they had been first convicted in adult court at a younger age than those who reported little or no antisocial behavior (20.9 years versus 25.7 years, t(38.85) = -2.73, p =.009). As well, they had accumulated more convictions (7.6 versus 1.7, t(20.87) = 3.20, p = .004), more convictions for non-violent offenses (7.4 versus 1.5, t(20.70) = 3.25, p =.004), but similar numbers of convictions for violent offenses (0.2 versus 0.2).

Conclusion

Again, these findings confirmed the existence of early and late-starters among persons with major mental disorders who committed crimes. Further, this study showed that at least among schizophrenics who were functioning at their optimal level in the weeks preceding discharge from hospital, no differences in the presentation of the schizophrenic symptoms were evident for the early and late-starters. The differences were restricted to age of onset of antisocial behavior, type and intensity of criminal activities.

Evidence from a study of men with schizophrenia: Neuropsychological test performance study

A sub-group of 30 of the schizophrenic men from this study were compared to 30 non-disordered men on a test of neurological soft signs [6] and a battery of neurospychological tests[7]. The men with schizophrenia compared to the non-disordered men showed significantly more soft signs (Braun, Hodgins, Lapierre, Toupin, Léveillée, & Constantineau, in press), and more impairment on every neuropsychological test (Hallé, Fiset, Hodgins, Toupin, & Braun, 1996).

However, among the 30 schizophrenic men, performance on these tests differed depending on their history of early antisocial behavior. Those with APD (n = 8) showed fewer neurological soft signs and less impairment on neuropsychological tests than did those with no history of childhood antisocial behavior (n = 23). Given the small number of subjects, these findings remain tentative. However, they concur with results from another study with only a small number of subjects (Rasmussen, Levander, & Sletvold, 1995) in suggesting that men who are both antisocial from a young age and schizophrenic evidence less brain damage than men with schizophrenia and no childhood or adolescent history of antisocial behavior (but significantly more than non-disordered men). There is a good deal of evidence indicating that among men with schizophrenia, more severe brain abnormalities are associated with social withdrawal

---

[6] NKI Neurological Scale of Soft Signs (Brizer, Convit, & Krakowski, 1987; Convit, Jaeger, & Lin, 1988; Krakowski, Convit, Jaeger, Lin, & Volavka, 1989).

[7] Controlled Oral Word Association, Rey Complex Figure Test, Wisconsin Card Sorting Test, Go-no-go, Trail Making Test, Picture Arrangement, Picture Arrangement Inertia, Porteus Mazes.

and fewer social contacts while less severe abnormalities are associated with a higher level of social functioning and more social contacts (Andreasen et al., 1992). However, this higher level of social functioning is associated with antisocial behavior, including both substance abuse (Hallé et al., 1996; Laroche, Hodgins, & Toupin, 1995) and aggressive behavior (Léveillée, 1994; Rasmussen et al., 1995).

Evidence from a study of male offenders with schizophrenia: Psychosocial functioning

Another group of researchers (Schanda, Födes, Topitz, & Knecht, 1992) have also compared early and late-starting schizophrenic offenders. Early-starters as compared to late-starters scored higher on measures of sociability/withdrawal and social-sexual functioning in adolescence, performed more poorly at school, and scored higher on measures of sociability/withdrawal, peer relationships, and social-sexual adjustment in adulthood.

WHO ARE THE EARLY-STARTERS?

Several longitudinal prospective investigations conducted in Denmark (Høgh & Wolfe, 1983), England (Farrington, 1983), Finland (Pulkkinen, 1988), New Zealand (Moffitt, 1990), Norway (Olweus, 1993), Poland (Zabczynska, 1977), Sweden (Janson, 1982; Stattin & Magnusson, 1991), and the U.S. (Blumstein, Farrington, & Moitra, 1985; Cline, 1980; Patterson & Yoerger, 1993; Robins & Ratcliff, 1979) of unbiased cohorts have identified a small group of boys who are characterized by stable antisocial behavior from a young age through adulthood (for a review, see Hodgins, 1994b). These males commit most of the crime (see for example, Stattin & Magnusson, 1991). Despite the fact that these investigations have been conducted in countries with very different cultures, criminal justice, social and health systems, the findings have been similar. Our next step was to determine if the early-starting offenders who develop major mental disorders are similar to these other antisocial children.

Evidence from the Swedish cohort

We examined this question using the Swedish cohort. A review of the longitudinal investigations identified several factors which characterized antisocial children who became adult recidivistic offenders. These factors were extracted from the available record data: pregnancy complications, birth complications, birth weight, social class of the family of origin, school performance (in grades 6 and 9), school conduct as evaluated by the teacher (in grades 6 and 9), intelligence measured at age 13, conduct problems noted in the community by age 12, conduct problems noted in the community from ages 13 to 18, family problems brought to the attention of the social agency, individual problems (other than conduct problems) brought to the attention of the social agency. (For a detailed description of the methodology see Kratzer & Hodgins, in press).Figures 2 and 3 present the percentage of subjects who have a criminal record by age 30 as a function of the total score on these indices of childhood problems. As can be observed and as would be expected from previous research, among the non-disordered males and females, there is a linear relation between the number and severity of childhood problems and the percentage of subjects who have a criminal record as adults.

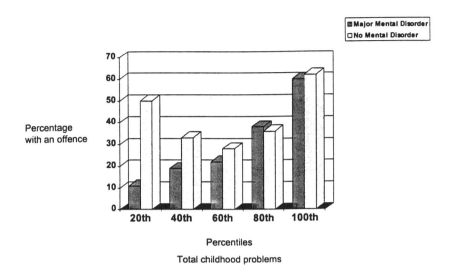

Figure 2. Crimes and childhood problems: Male subjects

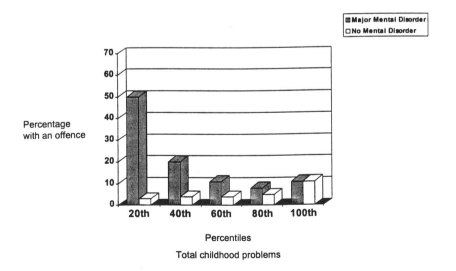

Figure 3. Crimes and childhood problems: Female subjects

Further, there are many fewer females than males who display these childhood problems. This confirms findings from many other investigations (see for example, Hodgins, 1994b). However, among the subjects who eventually developed major mental disorders, the relation is bimodal suggesting the existence of two sub-groups. The first group (noted on the right of figures) includes subjects with many childhood problems. Among this group, as among the non-disordered offenders, the more problems, the greater the likelihood that the subject will have a criminal record as an adult. A second group is evident on the left of the figures. This groups includes subjects who, according to the variables measured, showed no or very few difficulties in childhood, but as adults they developed a major mental disorder and committed crimes. Among the women, the sub-group with no childhood problems includes more subjects than does the early antisocial group.

We hypothesized that among those who developed major mental disorders and offended, the subjects with many childhood problems would in fact be early-starters while those with few or no problems in childhood would be late-starters. In order to test this hypothesis, the percentile scores on the indices of childhood problems were split at the median. None of the male subjects with scores of childhood problems which fell below the median (the subjects depicted on the left of figure 2) were convicted of an offense before the age of 18 years, and all but one was first convicted after the age of 21. This contrasts strongly with the male subjects who had scores of childhood problems above the median. Among these subjects 68.5% were convicted of an offense before the age of 18. The male offenders with high scores, as compared to the offenders with low scores, came from families of lower social class, obtained lower scores on an individual intelligence test, obtained lower marks in school, demonstrated behavior problems at school and in the community, had more individual problems (other than conduct), and came from families with more problems. These findings need to be replicated with a larger cohort. Despite the fact that the cohort was composed of over 15,000 subjects, not many developed a major mental disorder, committed a crime, and had complete data necessary for all of the childhood indices. From these findings, we conclude that the early-starters are similar to other antisocial children.

Are these findings consistent with knowledge about the development of the major mental disorders?

This finding that among children who will develop major mental disorders there exists a sub-group who are antisocial as children is consistent with what is known about the development of these disorders. In a review of the studies which compare the development of children of schizophrenic mothers to that of children of non-disordered mothers, it was noted that a sub-group of the children of schizophrenic mothers were characterized by aggressive behavior (Asarnow, 1988). In the only one of these studies of high risk children in which the subjects have passed through the age of risk for schizophrenia, two distinct developmental pathways to the disorder have been identified. The subjects who developed schizophrenia with predominately positive symptoms were described in early adolescence as overactive, irritable, distractible, and aggressive (Cannon, Mednick, & Parnas, 1990). It is interesting to note in light of our previous findings that these subjects evidenced less severe brain abnormalities than did the others who also developed schizophrenia.

Aggressive or antisocial behavior is not only evident among a sub-group of children who will develop schizophrenia, but also among children with affective symptoms. In children and adolescents suffering from depression, rates of conduct disorder are very high. In a review of the literature on this issue, Angold and Costello (1993) concluded that among children with depression rates of co-morbid conduct disorder/oppositional defiant disorder ranged from 21% to 83%, comorbidity with anxiety disorder ranged from 30% to 75%, and comorbidity with attention deficit disorder ranged from 0% to 57.1%. A recent retrospective study of childhood mental health records showed that one-third of a sample of bipolar patients had been seen as children, most for externalizing disorders (Manzano & Salvador, 1993). A prospective study has now shown similar results (Carlson & Weintraub, 1993).

Are the early-starters psychopaths?

Côté and Lesage (1995) have recently completed a study that allowed us to answer this question. The subjects were all males, recruited in a penitentiary or a psychiatric hospital, who met criteria for a major mental disorder in the month preceding their incarceration or hospitalization. The sample of subjects from the hospital was constructed to match the penitentiary sample as to type of disorder (psychotic [schizophrenia, other psychoses, or delusional disorder], or major affective disorder) and age (18-24 years, 25-34 years, 35-44 years, 45 years and older). Subjects recruited in the penitentiary had been incarcerated longer (median, 4 months) than the other subjects had been hospitalized (median, 1 month).

Eighty-eight of these men had been convicted of at least one offense. We divided them into two groups, early and late-starters. The early starters were defined as those who reported having engaged in at least three types of antisocial behavior before the age of 15, and the late-starters as those who reported two or fewer antisocial behaviors before age 15. By this criterion, 37.5% of the subjects were classified as early-starters and the others as late-starters. As we had previously done, we accorded one point to each item describing antisocial behavior before the age of 15. The mean score for the early-starters was 4.0 (SD = 1.4), and for the late-starters 0.9 (SD = 0.8) (t(44.79) = -11.81, p = .000)[8].

Not surprisingly, the early-starters had a lower level of education than the late-starters (M = 8.6 (SD = 2.4) versus M = 10.5, (SD = 2.7); t(85) = 3.39, p = .001), and more of them had never been employed (39.4% versus 14.5%; X^2(1, N = 88) = 7.01, p = .008).

As we had previously found, more of the early-starters than the late-starters (39.4% versus 12.7%) had a juvenile record (X^2(N = 88) = 8.35, p = .004), and their age at first conviction in adult court was younger than that for the late-starters (M = 20.3 (SD = 4.6) versus M = 25.1 (SD = 10.1); t(81.45) = 3.03, p = .003). Despite the fact that the early-starters began their criminal careers at a younger age than did the late-starters,

---

[8] By definition none of the late-starters met criteria for APD. All but four of the early-starters were diagnosed APD.

the early-starters and late-starters had been convicted, on average, of similar numbers of offenses (M = 26.0 (SD = 19.2) versus M = 18.9 (SD = 33.9); t(86) = -1.09, p = ns), and similar numbers of non-violent offenses (M = 20.5 (SD = 18.4) versus M = 15.4 (SD = 32.7), t(86) = -.82, p = ns). Unlike our previous findings, in this study, the early-starters had committed, on average, more violent offenses than the late-starters (M = 5.5 (SD = 3.7) versus M = 3.6 (SD = 4.7); t(86) = -2.04, p = .05). While all but one of the early-starters had been convicted of a violent offense, 29% of the late-starters had not committed a violent offense. The proportion of subjects in the two groups who were convicted for different types of offenses differed only for assaults; 81.1% of the early-starters, as compared to 29.1% of the late-starters, had been convicted for assault ($X^2(N$ =88) = 28.15, p = .000).

      This study differs from all other investigations in this area of research by the quality of the diagnoses. Unlike our penitentiary study in which we used the DIS, and the Swedish cohort study which uses file diagnoses, this investigation included lengthy (five to six hours if necessary) interviews by experienced clinicians using the Structured Clinical Interview for DSM-III-R (SCID) (Spitzer, Williams, Gibbon, & First, 1992; Williams et al., 1992). (The kappas measuring inter-diagnostician agreement varied from 0.78 to 1.00 for the major disorders.) This costly investment in hiring experienced diagnosticians and using a standardized clinical interview protocol led to results never before obtained. While the percentages of early and late-starters who had a major affective disorder (63.6% versus 54.5%), and a psychotic disorder (36.4% versus 45.5%) did not differ ($X^2(N$ = 88) = .70, p = ns), the percentages with different types of psychoses did differ. Among the early-starters with a psychotic disorder, 25.0% suffered from schizophrenia and 50.0% from delusional disorder while among the late-starters, 48.0% suffered from schizophrenia and 20.0% from delusional disorder. The difficulty of identifying delusional disorder cannot be over-estimated. This disorder is characterized by systematic delusions, beliefs that could possibly be true except that they are based on a false premise. The delusions are not bizarre, and consequently, it is often difficult to ascertain whether or not they are true. Subjects with this disorder maintain a relatively high level of psychosocial functioning, and only seldom experience hallucinations. For example, one offender in this study had convinced both the penitentiary staff and the news media that he was being persecuted by the Royal Canadian Mounted Police force because he was a political refugee. Only after several hours was the interviewer able to understand that none of the story was true. The systematic delusion is the only remarkable symptom of delusional disorder. In the case of recently incarcerated offenders, the paranoia is no doubt increased by their latest experiences with the police and the courts, and their new surroundings. Consequently, persuading these subjects who were convinced that they were being persecuted to provide sufficient information to a stranger who was trying to discover if their story was true or not, took considerable patience, clinical skill, and tenacity.

      Not only did the early and late-starters differ as to the principal diagnosis, but also with respect to secondary diagnoses. As we had previously found, more of the early-starters than the late-starters had a history of substance abuse. While 66.7% of the early-starters met criteria for alcohol abuse and/or dependence, this was the case for only 45.5% of the late-starters ($X^2(1$, N = 88) = 3.73, p = .05). For drug abuse and/or dependence the difference between the two groups was even greater; 81.8% of the early starters as compared to 52.7% of the late-starters ($X^2(1, N = 88) = 7.54, p = .006$). In fact, all but one of the early-starters (97.0%) as compared to two-thirds of the late-starters met criteria for alcohol and/or drug abuse and/or dependence ($X^2(1, N = 88) = 9.85, p = .002$).

Finally, these same subjects were rated on the revised version of the Psychopathy Checklist (Hare, 1991). Raters were trained to use the French version of the PCL-R (Côté & Hodgins, in press). Both file data and interview data were used to make the ratings. The kappa measuring inter-rater reliability for the total score was 1.0 (0-19, 20-40), and the correlations were r = .91 for factor I, and r = .92 for factor II. None of the late-starters and only two of the early-starters scored above 30 on the PCL-R indicating that they met criteria for a diagnosis of psychopathy. As would be expected, the early-starters scored higher than the late-starters (total score $M = 18.9$ ($SD = 7.2$) versus $M = 11.1$ ($SD = 6.1$), $t(86) = -5.42, p = .000$; score factor 1 $M = 5.5$ ($SD = 3.1$) versus $M = 3.7$ ($SD = 2.6$), $t(86) = -2.89, p = .005$; score factor 2 M 10.2 ($SD = 3.8$) versus $M = 5.3$ ($SD = 3.5$), $t(86) = -6.05, p = .000$).

Conclusion

This study of male offenders with major mental disorders again confirms the existence of the early and late-starters, the differences in their patterns of criminality, and provides the first evidence that these two groups may differ as to type of psychotic symptomatology. This finding corresponds to results from two other types of investigations. One, the studies of the development of schizophrenia have identified a sub-group of males characterized by aggressive behavior in childhood, predominately positive (paranoid) symptomatology, and less severe brain abnormalities than other schizophrenics. Two, this finding is consistent with results from investigations which have demonstrated an association between threat/control overide symptoms and/or paranoid symptoms and violent behavior (Link & Stueve, 1994; Swanson, 1993). As can be seen, much more is understood about the criminality and violence associated with schizophrenia spectrum disorders than that associated with the major affective disorders.

Evidence from a study of violent adolescent boys

In order to again verify our findings we looked at the same phenomenon from the opposite point of view. A sample of 85 adolescents convicted of a violent offense was examined using the SCID and the PCL-R adolescent form (for details of the procedure see Toupin, Déry, Pauzé, Fortin, & Mercier, 1995). Of these 85 boys, 29% obtained scores on the PCL-R of 30 or above, 29% obtained scores between 20 and 29, and 42% less than 20. None received a diagnosis of a major mental disorder. There were not even any differences on numbers or severity of symptoms of psychosis, depression or mania. These results could be due to the age of the subjects or alternatively, they could be interpreted as suggesting that there is no overlap between psychopathy and major mental disorders.

CONCLUSIONS

The studies described above have lead us to hypothesize that among subjects who will develop major mental disorders in adulthood and commit offenses there are two distinct types who follow different developmental pathways. The first is the early-starter, the child who displays a stable pattern of antisocial behavior which is identifiable at a young age and which persists across the lifespan. This type of child shows conduct problems at home and at school, poor academic performance, and most likely has an IQ score slightly below the normal. He/she may well come from a family characterized by multiple problems. Our work to date suggests that the behavior and academic performance of the early-starters may be indistinguishable from other children who present antisocial behavior. The second type of offender with a major mental disorder presents no behavior or academic problems as a child, either at home or at school. He/she, it appears, passes through childhood and early adolescence without any difficulties that would attract attention or warrant intervention. However, by late adolescence or early adulthood, a major mental disorder develops and offending begins.

We further hypothesize that alcohol and drug use, and threat/control overide and paranoid symptomatology are associated with the illegal behaviors of these two groups of subjects but in different ways. Antisocial children are exposed earlier than other children to alcohol and drugs (Robins & McEvoy, 1990), and throughout adolescence and adulthood abuse often becomes a part of their antisocial lifestyle. The late-starters, we hypothesize, may be more likely to use alcohol and drugs in attempts to reduce symptoms. Intoxication may, however, increase symptoms and lead to illegal behavior. While it is reasonable, given the available evidence, to hypothesize that intoxication and threat/control overide and/or paranoid symptoms play a role in the criminal behavior of the late-starters, this may not be true for the early-starters. Our recent finding of a large number of subjects with delusional disorders among the early-starters is perplexing. Have the paranoid-type symptoms been present as long as the antisocial behavior? Do the symptoms simply increase the severity and frequency of the criminal behaviors or are these symptoms associated exclusively with aggressive or violent behavior and not with non-violent offending?

We have presumed throughout our work that the DSM-III and DSM-III-R diagnoses of APD identify early-starters. The prevalence of APD is much higher among persons with major mental disorders than in the general population in which it has been estimated to affect 4.5% of men and 0.8% of women (Robins, Tipp, & Przybeck, 1991). We have previously demonstrated that the prevalence of APD among both men and women with schizophrenia is at least five times higher than among non-disordered persons (Hodgins, Toupin, & Côté, in press). Looking at this same phenomenon from the opposite point of view, the ECA data showed that among men with APD the prevalence of schizophrenia was seven times that in the general population, and among women with APD it was almost 12 times more prevalent (Robins, Tipp, & Przybeck, 1990). Thus schizophrenia and what was labeled APD (DSM-III) are co-occurring much more frequently than would be expected by chance. The epidemiological findings on the co-occurence of depression and conduct disorder in children, and the findings on criminality among persons with major affective disorders are suggestive of a disproportionate number of antisocial persons among those suffering from major affective disorders.

As noted, our findings to date suggest that in childhood, the early-starters present like other antisocial children. As a group, antisocial children are characterized by persistent antisocial behavior, poor school performance, lower than normal IQ scores, and deficits in neuropsychological testing (Moffitt, 1990; Toupin et al., 1995). Most of the males go on to become repetitive offenders in adulthood, and most of the males and the females show serious antisocial behavior in adulthood (Farrington, 1983; Hodgins, 1994b; Janson, 1982; Moffitt, 1990; Robins & Ratcliff, 1979; Stattin & Magnusson, 1991), and significant psychosocial maladaptation (Quinton, Pickles, Maughan, & Rutter, 1993). As we have previously argued (Hodgins, 1994b), however, antisocial children are a heterogeneous group. This fact has been recently discussed by Rutter (1996) and further supported by examination of the Virginia Twin Registry adolescent sample (Silberg et al., 1996). Among antisocial children, there is a sub-group who have attention deficit disorder in addition to their conduct problems (Farrington, Loeber, & Van Kammen, 1990), a sub-group who are mentally retarded (Hodgins, 1994b; Kratzer & Hodgins, in press), another sub-group with very distinctive neuroendocrinological functioning which appears to be related to a hereditary form of early onset alcoholism (Virkkunen et al., 1994a & b), another sub-group who develop major mental disorders in adulthood, and others who appear to develop into adults with APD and substance abuse problems. Regardless of the additional problems, for example, mental retardation or major mental disorder, the early antisocial behavior is highly predictive of adult criminality and socially maladaptive behavior (Hodgins, 1994b; Kratzer, Hodgins, in press).

While all available data suggest that psychopaths must be among this group of antisocial children, no prospective study has isolated such a sub-group among antisocial children. What is perplexing is the finding that these antisocial children, as a group, demonstrate deficits on neuropsychological tests and lower than average IQ scores (Moffitt, 1990; 1993), while adult males who obtain scores of 30 or higher on the PCL-R do not show either deficits on standard neuropsychological tests nor lower than average IQ scores (Hart, Forth, & Hare, 1990; Lapierre, Braun, & Hodgins, 1995). It could be simply that in studies of antisocial children, the analyses of the neuropsychological and IQ test results have not been conducted and presented in a way that allows homogeneous sub-groups of subjects to emerge. Results are always presented as group means, the antisocial children's test results compared to the non-antisocial children's test results. Reanalysis of existing data could easily test this hypothesis. Alternatively, it could be that men who are rated as psychopaths showed these deficits as children, but outgrew them[9]. Only a prospective, longitudinal study could test this hypothesis.

---

[9] Such a change in cognitive functioning from childhood to adulthood could be due to maturation or to the fact that different cortical structures may be associated with the same function in childhood and adulthood. Weinberger (1987) has reviewed the primate literature noting that some cognitive functions are associated with different cortical structures before and after puberty. If the childhood structure is abnormal or damaged,

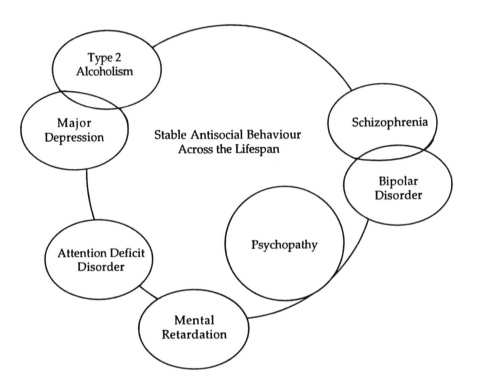

Figure 4. A schema of the overlap between stable and antisocial behavior and other mental disorders.

Figure 4 presents our synthesis of current findings. There is considerable evidence, as noted previously, from several different cultures, that a small proportion of boys and an even smaller proportion of girls display a stable pattern of antisocial behavior from a young age through adulthood. This group, however, is heterogeneous and includes several distinctive sub-groups. We speculate that those who become psychopaths (PCL-R score of 30 or higher) are among these children. This hypotheses, like the others which we have advanced, awaits empirical testing.

---

only the behavior in childhood not in adulthood is affected. (The opposite has also been shown to be true.)

References

Andreasen, N. C. et al., (1992). Hypofrontality in neuroleptic-naive patients and inpatients with chronic schizophrenia. *Archives of General Psychiatry, 49*, 943-958.

Angold, A., & Costello, E. J. (1993). Depressive comorbidity in children and adolescents: Empirical, theoretical, and methodological issues. *American Journal of Psychiatry, 150*, 1779-1791.

Asarnow, J. R. (1988). Children at risk for schizophrenia. Converging lines of evidence. Schizophrenia Bulletin, 14, 613-631.

Beaudoin, M. N., Hodgins, S., & Lavoie, F. (1993). Homicide, schizophrenia, and substance abuse or dependency. *Canadian Journal of Psychiatry, 38*, 541-546.

Belfrage, H. (1994). Criminality and mortality among a cohort of former mental patients in Sweden. *Nordik Journal of Psychiatry, 48*, 343-347.

Blumstein, A., Farrington, D. P., & Moitra, S. (1985). Delinquency careers: Innocents, desisters, and persisters. In M. Tonry and N. Morris (Eds.), *Crime and Justice: An Annual Review of Research, vol. 6.* Chicago: University of Chicago Press.

Braun, C., M. J., Hodgins, S., Lapierre, D., Toupin, J., Léveillée, S., & Constantineau, C. (in press). Neurological soft signs in schizophrenia. *Archives of Clinical Neuropsychology.*

Brizer, D. A., Convit, A., Krakowski, M., & Volavka, J. (1987). A rating scale for reporting violence on psychiatric wards. *Hospital and Community Psychiatry, 38*, 769-770.

Cannon, T. D., Mednick, S., & Parnas, J. (1990). Antecedents of predominantly negative and predominantly positive symptom schizophrenia in a high risk population. *Archives of General Psychiatry, 47*, 622-632.

Carlson, G. A., & Weintraub, S. (1993). Childhood behavior problems and bipolar disorder - relationship or coincidence? *Journal of Affective Disorders, 28*, 143-153.

Cline, H. F. (1980). Criminal behavior over the life span. In O.G. Brim, Jr. and J. Kagan (Eds.), *Constancy and Change in Human Development* (pp. 641-674). Cambridge, MA: Harvard University Press.

Collins, J. J., & Schlenger, W. E. (1983). *The Prevalence of Psychiatric Disorder Among Admissions to Prison.* Paper presented at the 35th Annual Meeting of the American Society of Criminology, Denver.

Convit, A., Jaeger, J., & Lin, S. (1988). Prediction of violence in psychiatric inpatients. In. T.E. Moffitt and S.A. Mednick (Eds.), *Biological Contributions to Crime Causation* (pp. 223-245). The Netherlands: Martinus Nijhoff.

Cooke, D. J. (1994). *Psychological disturbance in the Scottish prison system: Prevalence, precipitants and policy.* The Scottish Office: Edinburgh.

Côté, G., & Hodgins, S. (in press). *L'Échelle de psychopathie de Hare.* Toronto: Multi-Health Systems.

Côté, G., & Hodgins, S. (1992). The prevalence of major mental disorders among homicide offenders. *International Journal of Law and Psychiatry, 15*, 89-99.

Côté, G., & Lesage, A. (1995). *Diagnostics complémentaires et adaptation sociale chez des détenus schizophrènes ou dépressifs.* Report commissionned by the FRSQ/CQRS.

Daniel, A. E., Robins, A. J., Reid, J. C., & Wilfley, D. E. (1988). Lifetime and six-month prevalence of psychiatric disorders among sentenced female offenders. *Bulletin of the American Academy Psychiatry and Law, 16*, 333-342.

Drake, R. E., Osher, F. C., Noordsy, D. L., Hurlbut, S. C., Teague, G. B., & Beaudett, M. S. (1990). Diagnosis of alcohol use disorders in schizophrenia. *Schizophrenia Bulletin, 16*, 51-67.

Durbin, J. R., Pasewark, R. A., & Albers, D. (1977). Criminality and mental illness: A study of current arrest rates in a rural state. *American Journal of Psychiatry, 134*, 80-83.

Elliot, D. S., Huizinga, D., & Morse, B. J. (1986). Self-reported violent offending: Descriptive analysis of juvenile violent offenders and their offending careers. *Journal of Interpersonal Violence, 4*, 472-514.

Endicott, J., & Spitzer, R. L. (1979). Use of the RDC and SADS in the study of affective disorders. *American Journal of Psychiatry, 136*, 52-56.

Endicott, J., & Spitzer, R. L. (1978). A diagnostic interview: The schedule for affective disorders and schizophrenia. *Archives of General Psychiatry, 35*, 837-844.

Eronen, M., Tiihonen, J., & Hakola, P. (1996). Schizophrenia and homicidal behavior. *Schizophrenia Bulletin, 22.*

Farrington, D. P. (1983). Offending from 10 to 25 years of age. In K.T. Van Dusen and S.A. Mednick (Eds.), *Prospective Studies of Crime and Delinquency* (pp. 17-37). The Hague: Kluwer-Nijhoff.

Farrington, D. P., Loeber, R., & Van Kammen, W. B. (1990). Long-term criminal outcomes of hyperactivity-impulsivity-attention deficit and conduct problems in childhood. In. L.N. Robin and M. Rutter (Eds.), *Straight and Devious Pathways from Childhood to Adulthood* (pp. 62-81). Cambridge: Cambridge University Press.

Giovanni, J. M., & Gurel, L. (1967). Socially disruptive behaviour of ex-mental patients. *Archives of General Psychiatry, 17*, 146-153.

Gottlieb, P., Gabrielsen, G., & Kramp, P. (1987). Psychotic homicides in Copenhagen from 1959 to 1983. *Acta Psychiatrica Scandinavica, 76*, 285-292.

Gunn, J., Maden, T., & Swinton, M. (1991). *Mentally Disordered Prisoners*. London: Home Office.

Hallé, P., Fiset, S., Hodgins, S., Toupin, J., & Braun, C. (submitted). *Neuropsychological test performance of male schizophrenics with and without co-morbid drug use disorders.*

Hare, R. D. (1991). The Hare Psychopathy Checklist Revised. Toronto: Multi-Health Systems, Inc.

Hart, S., Hare, R. D., & Forth, A. (1990). Performance of criminal psychopaths on selected neuropsychological tests. *Journal of Abnormal Psychology, 99*, 374-379.

Hodgins, S. (1995). Major mental disorder and crime: An overview. *Psychology, Crime and Law, 2*, 5-17.

Hodgins, S. (1994a). Letter to the Editor. *Archives of General Psychiatry, 51*, 71-72.

Hodgins, S. (1994b). Status at age 30 of children with conduct problems. *Studies of Crime and Crime Prevention, 3*, 41-62.

Hodgins, S. (1993). The criminality of mentally disordered persons. In S. Hodgins (Ed.), *Mental Disorder and Crime* (pp. 1-21). Newbury Park, California: Sage.

Hodgins, S. (1992). Mental disorder, intellectual deficiency and crime: Evidence from a birth cohort. *Archives of General Psychiatry, 49*, 476-483.

Hodgins, S., & Côté, G. (1993a). The criminality of mentally disordered offenders. *Criminal Justice and Behavior, 28*, 115-129.

Hodgins, S., & Côté, G. (1993b). Major mental disorder and APD: A criminal combination. *Bulletin of the American Academy of Psychiatry and the Law, 21*, 155-160.

Hodgins, S., & Côté, G. (1990). The prevalence of mental disorders among penitentiary inmates. *Canada's Mental Health, 38*, 1-5.

Hodgins, S., Mednick, S. A., Brennan, P. A., Schulsinger, F., & Engberg, M. (in press). Mental disorder and crime: Evidence from a birth cohort. *Archives General of Psychiatry.*

Hodgins, S., Toupin, J., & Côté, G. (in press). Schizophrenia and antisocial personality disorder: A criminal combination. In L.B. Schlesinger (Ed.), *Explorations in Criminal Psychopathology: Clinical Syndromes with Forensic Implication.*

Hodgins, S, Toupin, J., Fiset, S., & Moisan, D. (1995). *Une comparaison des soins externes offerts aux patients souffrant de troubles mentaux graves pendant 24 mois suite à leur sortie d'un centre hospitalier*. Report commissioned by the Conseil Québécois de la Recherche Sociale.

Hodgins, S., & Webster, C. D. (1992). *The Canadian data base: Patients held on Lieutenant-Governors' Warrants*. Ottawa: Department of Justice of Canada.

Høgh, E., & Wolf, P. (1983). Violent crime in a birth cohort: Copenhagen 1953-1977. In K. Teilmann Van Dusen and S. A. Mednick (Eds.), *Prospective Studies of Crime and Delinquency* (pp. 249-267). Boston: Kluwer-Nijhoff.

Hyde, P. S., & Seiter, R. P. (1987). *The Prevalence of Mental Illness Among Inmates in the Ohio Prison System*. The Department of Mental Health and the Ohio Departments of Rehabilitation and Correction. Interdeparmental Planning and Oversight Commitee for Psychiatric Services to Corrections.

Janson, C.-G., (1982). *Delinquency Among Metropolitan Boys* (Research Report No. 17). Stockholm, University of Stockholm, Department of Sociology.

Kay, S. R., Fiszbein, A., & Opler, L. A. (1987). The positive and negative syndrom scale (PANSS) for schizophrenia. *Schizophrenia Bulletin, 13*, 261-276.

Krakowski, M. I., Convit, A., Jaeger, J., Lin, S., & Volavka, J. (1989). Neurological impairment in violent schizophrenic inpatients. *American Journal of Psychiatry, 146*, 849-853.

Kratzer, L., & Hodgins, S. (in press). Adult outcomes of childhood conduct problems. *Journal of Abnormal Child Psychology*.

Lapierre, D., Braun, C. M., & Hodgins, S. (1995). Ventral frontal deficits in psychopathy: Neuropsychological test findings. *Neuropsychologia, 33*, 139-151.

Laroche, I., Hodgins, S., & Toupin, J. (1995). Liens entre les symptômes et le fonctionnement social chez des personnes souffrant de schizophrénie ou de trouble affectif majeur. *Canadian Journal of Psychiatry, 40*, 27-34.

Léveillée, S. (1994). *Évaluation multidimensionnelle du support social des schizophrènes*, Doctorat thesis. Université de Montréal.

Lindqvist, P. (1986). Criminal homicide in Northern Sweden 1970-In 1981: Alcohol intoxication, alcohol abuse and mental disease. *International Journal of Law and Psychiatry, 8*, 19-37.

Lindqvist, P., & Allebeck, P. (1990). Schizophrenia and assaultive behaviour: the role of alcohol and drug abuse. *Acta Psychiatrica Scandinavica, 82*, 191-195.

Link, B. G., Andrews, H., & Cullen, F. T. (1992). The violent and illegal behaviour of mental patients reconsidererd. *American Sociological Review, 57*, 275-292.

Link, B. G., & Stueve, A. (1994). Psychotic symptomes and the violent/illegal behavior of mental patients compared to community control. In. J. Monahan and H. Steadman (Eds.), *Violence and Mental Disorder. Developments in Risk Assessment.* (pp. 137-159). Chicago: University of Chicago Press.

Manzano, J., & Salvador, A. (1993). Antecedents of severe affective (mood) disorders. Patients examined as children or adolescents and as adults. *Acta Paedopsychiatrica, 56*, 11-18.

Moffitt, T. E. (1993). Adolescence-limited and life-course-persistent antisocial behavior: A developmental taxonomy. *Psychological Review, 100*, 674-701.

Moffitt, T.E. (1990). The neuropsychology of delinquency: A critical review of theory and research. In N. Morris and M. Tonry (Eds.), *Crime and Justice* (Vol. 12, pp. 99-169). Chicago, IL: University of Chicago Press.

Motiuk, L., & Poporino, F. (1991). *The Prevalence, Nature and Severity of Mental Health Problems Among Federal Male Inmates in Canadian Penitentiaries*. Correctional Services of Canada Research Report, no. 24.

Mueser, K. T., Yarnold, P. R., Levinson, D. F., Singh, H., Bellack, A. S., Kee, K., Morrison, R. L., & Yadalam, K. G. (1990). Prevalence of sbustance abuse in schizophrenia. *Schizophrenia Bulletin, 16*, 31-56.

Neighbors, H. W., Williams, D. H., Gunnings, T. S., Lipscomb, W. D., Broman, C., & Lepkowski, J. (1987). *The Prevalence of Mental Disorder in Michigan Prisons.* Final report submitted to the Michigan Department of Corrections, MI.

O'Leary, K. D., Barling, J., Arias, I., & Rosenbaum, A. (1989). Prevalence and stability of physical aggression between spouses: A longitudinal analysis. *Journal of Consulting and Clinical Psychology, 57*, 263-268.

Olweus, D. (1993). Bully/victim problems among schoolchildren: Long-term consequences and an effective intervention program. In S. Hodgins (Ed.), *Mental Disorder and Crime* (pp. 317-349). Newbury Park, CA: Sage.

Ortmann, J. (1981). Psykisk ofvigelse og kriminel adfaerd en under sogelse af 11533 maend fodt i 1953 i det metropolitane omrade kobenhaun. Forksningsrapport, 17.

Patterson, G. R., & Yoerger, K. (1993). Developmental models for delinquent behavior. In S. Hodgins (Ed.). *Mental Disorder and Crime* (pp. 140-172). Newbury Park, California: Sage.

Pulkkinen, L. (1988). Delinquent development: Theoretical and empirical considerations. In M. Rutter (Ed.), *Studies of Psychosocial Risk. The Power of Longitudinal Data* (pp. 184-199). Cambridge: Cambridge University Press.

Quinton, D., Pickles, A. R., Maughan, B., & Rutter, M. (1993). Partners, peers and pathways: Assortative pairing and continuities in conduct disorder. *Developmental Psychopathology, 5*, 763-783.

Rappeport, J. R., & Lassen, G. (1966). The dangerousness of female patients. A comparison of the arrest rate of discharged psychiatric patients and the general population. *American Journal of Psychiatry, 123*, 413-419.

Rappeport, J.R., & Lassen, G., (1965). Dangerousness arrest rate comparisons of discharged patients and the general population. *American Journal of Psychiatry, 121*, 776-783.

Rasmussen, K., Levander, S., & Sletvold, H. (1995). Aggressive and non-aggressive schizophrenics: Symptom profile and neuropsychological differences. *Psychology, Crime, and Law, 15*, 119-129.

Regier, D. A., Farmer, M. E., Rae, D. S., Locke, B. Z., Keith, S. J., Judd, L. L., & Goodwin, F. K. (1990). Comorbidity of mental disorders with alcohol and other drug abuse. *Journal of the American Medical Association, 264*, 2511-2518.

Robins, L. N., Helzer, J. E., Croughan, J., & Ratcliff, K. S. (1981). National Institute of Mental Health Diagnostic Interview Schedule: It's history, characteristics, and validity. *Archives of General Psychiatry, 38*, 381-389.

Robins, L. N., Helzer, J. E., Weissman, M. M., Orvaschel, H., Gruenberg, E., Burke, J. D., & Regier, D. A. Jr. (1984). Lifetime prevalence of specific psychiatric disorders in three sites. *Archives of General Psychiatry, 41*, 949-958.

Robins, L. N., & McEvoy, L. (1990). Conduct problems as predictors of substance abuse. In Robins, L.N. & Rutter, M. (Eds.), *Straight and Deviant Pathways from Childhood to Adulthood* (pp. 182-204). Cambridge: Cambridge University Press.

Robins, L. N., & Ratcliff, K. S. (1979). Risk Factors in the continuation of childhood antisocial behavior into adulthood. *International Journal of Mental Health, 7*, 96-116.

Robins, L. N., & Regier, D. A. (1991). *Psychiatric Disorders in America: The Epidemiologic Catchment Area Study.* New York: The Free Press.

Robins, L. N., Tipp. J., & Przybevk, T. (1991). Antisocial personality. In L.N. Robins and D.A. Regier (Eds.). *Psychiatric disorders in America* (pp. 258-290). New York: The Free Press.

Robins, L. N., Tipp, J., & Przybeck, T. (1990). Antisocial personality. In L. N. Robins and D. A. Regier (Eds.), *Psychiatric Disorder in America* (pp. 258-290). New York: MacMillan/Free Press.

Rutter, M. (1996). Concepts of antisocial behaviour, of cause, and of genetic influences. In. G.R. Bock and J.A. Goode (Eds.), *Genetics of Criminal and Antisocial Behaviour* (pp. 1-15). New York: Johns Wiley & Sons.

Schanda, H., Födes, P., Topitz, A., & Knecht, G. (1992). Premorbid adjustment of schizophrenic criminal offenders. *Acta Psychiatrica Scandinava, 86,* 121-126.

Silberg, J., Meyer, J., Pickles, A., Simonoff, E., Eaves, L., Hewitt, J., Maes, H., & Rutter, M. (1996). Heterogeneity among juvenile antisocial behaviours: Findings from the Virginia twin study of adolescent behavioural development. In. G.R. Bock and J.A. Goode (Eds.), *Genetics of Criminal and Antisocial Behaviour* (pp. 76-92). New York: Johns Wiley & Sons.

Sosowsky, L. (1980). Explaining the increased arrest rate among mental patients: A cautionary note. *American Journal of Psychiatry, 137,* 1602-1605.

Sosowsky, L. (1978). Crime and violence among mental patients reconsidered in view of the new legal relationship between the state and the mentally ill. *American Journal of Psychiatry, 135,* 33-42.

Sosowsky, L. (1974). *Violence and the Mentally Ill, in Putting State Mental Hospitals Out of Business - The Community Approach to Treating Mental Illness in San Mateo County* (pp. 17-33). Berkeley, California: University of California Graduate School of Public Policy.

Spitzer, R. L., Endicott, J., & Robins, E. (1978). Research diagnostic criteria: Rationale and reliability. *Archives of General Psychiatry, 35,* 773-782.

Spitzer, R. L., Williams, J. B. W., Gibbon, M., & First, M. B. (1992). The structured clinical interview for DSM-III-R (SCID) I: History, rationale and description. *Archives of General Psychiatry, 49,* 624-629.

Stattin, H., & Magnusson, D. (1991). Stability and change in criminal behaviour up to age 30. The *British Journal of Criminology, 31,* 327-345.

Steadman, H. J., Cocozza, J. J., & Melick, M. E. (1978). Explaining the increased arrest rate among mental patients: The changing clientele of state hospitals. *American Journal of Psychiatry, 135,* 816-820.

Steadman, H. J., & Felson, R. B. (1984). Self-reports of violence. Ex-mental patients, ex-offenders, and the general population. *Criminology, 22,* 321-342.

Steadman, H. J., Monahan, J., Appelbaum, P. S., Grisso, T. Mulvey, E. P., Roth, L. H., Robbins, P. C., & Classen, D. (1994). Designing a new generation of risk assessment research. In J. Monahan and H.J. Steadman (Eds.), *Violence and Mental Disorder: Developments in Risk Assessment* (pp. 297-318). Chicago: The University of Chicago Press.

Steadman, H. J., Monahan, J., Robbins, P. A., Applebaum, P., Grisso, T., Klassen, D., Mulvey, E., & Roth, L. (1993). From dangerousness to risk assessment: Implications for Appropriate research stategies. In S. Hodgins, (Ed.), *Mental Disorder and Crime* (pp. 39-62). Newbury Park, Ca.: Sage.

Straus, M.A., Gelles, R.J., & Steinmetz, S.K. (1980). *Behind Closed Doors: Violence in the American Family.* New York: Doubleday/Anchor.

Swanson, J. W. (1993). Alcohol abuse, mental disorder, and violent behavior. *Alcohol Health & Research World, 17,* 123-132.

Swanson, J., Borum, R., Swartz, M., & Monahan, J. (submitted). *Psychotic Symptoms and disorders and the risk of violent behavior in the community.*

Swanson, J., Holzer, C., Ganju, V., & Jono, R. (1990). Violence and psychiatric disorder in the community: Evidence from the epidemiological catchment area surveys. *Hospital and Community Psychiatry, 41,* 761-770.

Teplin, L. (1984). Criminalizing mental disorder: The comparative arrest rate of the mentally ill. *American Psychologist, 39,* 794-803.

Tiihonen, J., Isohanni, M., Koiranen, M., Moring, J., & Rantakallio, P. (submitted). *Specific mental disorders and criminality. A 25-year prospective study of an unselected birth cohort.*

Tiihonen, J., Hakola, P., Eronen, M., Vartiainen, H., & Ryynänen, O.-P. (in press). Risk of homicidal behavior among discharged forensic psychiatric patients. *Forensic Science International.*

Toupin, J., Déry, M., Pauzé, R., Fortin, L., & Mercier, H. (1995). *Social and Psychological Correlates of Conduct Disorder in Children.* Poster presented at the 42nd annual meeting of The American Academy of Child and Adolescent Psychiatry, New Orleans.

Virkkunen, M., Rawlings, R., Tokola, R., Poland, R. E., Guidotti, A., Nemeroff, C., Bissette, G., Kalogeras, K., Karonen, S.-L., & Linnoila, M. (1994a). CSF biochemistries, glucose metabolism, and diurnal activity rhythms in alcoholic, violent offenders, fire setters, and healthy volunteers. *Archives of General Psychiatry, 51,* 20-27.

Virkkunen, M., Kallio, E., Rawlings, R., Tokola, R., Poland, R. E., Guidotti, A., Nemeroff, C., Bissette, G., Kalogeras, K., Karonen, S.-L., & Linnoila, M. (1994b). Personality profiles and state aggressiveness in finnish alcoholic, violent offenders, fire setters, and health volunteers. *Archives of General Psychiatry, 51,* 28-33.

Weinberger, D. R. (1987). Implications of normal brain development for the pathogenesis of schizophrenia. *Archives of General Psychiatry, 44,* 660-669.

Wessely, S., Buchanan, A., Reed, A., Cutting, J., Everitt, B., Garety, P., & Taylor, P. J. (1993). Acting on delusions. I. Prevalence. *British Journal of Psychiatry, 163,* 69-76.

Williams, J. B. W., Gibbon, M., First, M. B., Spitzer, R. L., Davies, M., Borus, J., Howes, M. J., Kane, JH., Pope, H. G., Jr., Rounsaville, B., & Wittchen, H. U. (1992). The structured clinical interview for DSM-III-R (SCID). II. Multisite test-retest reliability. *Archives of General Psychiatry, 49,* 630-636.

Zabczynska, E. (1977). A longitudinal study of development of juvenile delinquency. *Polish Psychological Bulletin, 8,* 239-245.

Zitrin, A., Hardesty, A. S., Burdock, E. T., & Drossman, A. K. (1976). Crime and violence among mental patients. *American Journal of Psychiatry, 133,* 142-149.

Authors' notes

This chapter was prepared with a grant to the authors from the Fonds pour la Formation de Chercheurs et l'Aide à la Recherche. Financial support for each of the studies reported herein, acknowledged in other publications, came from the Social Sciences and Humanities Research Council of Canada, the Conseil Québécois de la Recherche Sociale, the Fonds de Recherche en Santé du Québec, and Correctional Services of Canada.

We would like to thank John Monahan for his helpful comments on an earlier version of the manuscript.

Correspondence concerning this article should be addressed to Dr. S. Hodgins, Department of Psychology, Université de Montréal, C.P. 6128, succ. Centre-ville, Montréal (Québec) H3C 3J7.

COMORBIDITY OF PSYCHOPATHY WITH MAJOR MENTAL DISORDERS

NORBERT NEDOPIL, MATTHIAS HOLLWEG, JULIA HARTMANN
and ROBERT JASER
Abteilung für Forensische Psychiatrie,
Psychiatrische Klinik der Universität München,
Germany.

INTRODUCTION

A considerable number of patients with major mental disorders seen by the forensic psychiatrist, or being treated in forensic hospitals, have a comorbidity with other disorders. This comorbidity has a significant influence on clinical outcome, criminal relapse, on detention rate and length of detention (Lindquist & Allebeck. 1989; Soyka et al., 1994). In addition, comorbidity has an influence on the assessment of criminal responsibility: In a recent study, patients suffering from schizophrenia and antisocial personality disorder (APD) were more often held to be responsible or to have diminished responsibility while patients who received the diagnosis of schizophrenia alone were considered to be irresponsible for their criminal acts (Nedopil, 1996b). The group of patients suffering from that comorbidity was, however, relatively small. Only 5 out of the 41 schizophrenics assessed as a consequence of violent crimes had a comorbid antisocial personality disorder.

Schizophrenia has been associated with a higher risk of violence. The percentage of aggressive individuals among schizophrenic patients, especially of those suffering from paranoid schizophrenia, has been shown to be several times higher than that in the general population in several studies (Böker & Häfner, 1973; Häfner & Böker, 1982; Monahan, 1991; Monahan & Steadman, 1994; Côté & Hodgins, 1992, Hodgins, 1995). Psychopathy is also associated with a high risk of criminality, and especially, of violent criminality (Hare, 1984; Hare, 1993; Hart et al., 1994). Schizophrenia and antisocial personality disorder are the two most frequent diagnoses found in aggressive individuals seen by the forensic psychiatrist. They differ, however, not only in psychopathology but also in many other clinical features: e.g., course, relapse rates and treatability. A comorbidity of the two disorders can not only affect the assessment of responsibility but may also affect outcome of treatment and risk of relapse. The outcome of treatment for schizophrenic patients, and the future course of their diseases, are quite variable. While 10-20% will recover from the disease even without treatment and 30-60% will profit from treatment, 20-40% will continue to be disturbed regardless of treatment (Caroner et al., 1991; Kaplan et al., 1994). Especially in forensic settings, the patients who will not improve with neuroleptic treatment cause a major problem, because they can hardly be integrated into other treatment programs; they continue to be dangerous and thereby are poor prospects for release.

D.J. Cooke et al. (eds.), Psychopathy: Theory, Research and Implications for Society, 257–268.
© 1998 *Kluwer Academic Publishers. Printed in the Netherlands.*

Psychopathy is regarded as being an almost untreatable disturbance of personality; psychopaths lack insight into their own disorder (Hare, 1993; Dolan & Coid, 1993). It could be hypothesized that psychopathic character traits interfere, not only with the compliance of schizophrenic patients, but also with treatment outcome.

Considering this empirical knowledge it seemed worthwhile to examine the following hypotheses:

1. Does a comorbidity of psychopathy with major mental disorders lead to an increased relapse into criminality than the major mental disorder itself, or — for that matter — than psychopathy itself?

2. Does such a comorbidity have an influence on the clinical and court judgment of responsibility?

3. Does comorbidity have an influence on treatment programs, on compliance and on the results of treatment?

Psychopathy — personality traits or disorder?

When looking more closely at the concept of psychopathy and comparing the original idea of Cleckley (1976) to the current concept (Hare, 1993), one becomes aware that psychopathy today is not seen as a disorder in a clinical sense, but rather as a personality structure of not yet known roots; this contrasts with Cleckley's (1976) conception, he considered psychopaths to be mentally ill individuals who were disguised behind a *"mask of sanity"*.

If today's concept is true, then any concept, or even any hypothesis of comorbidity, would be a contradiction in itself. If psychopathy is not a disorder, it cannot be co-ocurrent — in the sense of comorbidity — *with another* disorder. Although it is not regarded as a disorder, it is seen as an entity in categorical terms, and substantial research is being carried concerning the morphological, functional and biochemical dysfunction in psychopathic individuals (see other chapters in this book). Intrator (1993) found a difference of regional cerebral blood flow between psychopaths on one side and controls and substance abusers on the other. Psychopaths had a relative greater rCBF in some parts of the occipital region and an activation of rCBF on the frontal subcortical regions during emotional stimulation, while rCBF did not change in controls during the same tasks. Some authors claim low 5-hydroxy indolacetic acid (5-HIAA) levels in the cerebrospinal fluid of APD patients (Virkunnen et al., 1994, a&b). These findings are, however, not very conclusive, since low 5-HIAA and low serotonergic turnover is observed in many clinical conditions, like anxiety disorder, obsessive compulsive disorder, some form of major depression, aggression and violent suicide, to name just a few (Linnoila et al., 1983; Van Praag, 1994; Lester, 1995).

Today's concept of psychopathy is greatly influenced by the development of the Psychopathy Checklist Revised (PCL-R; Hare 1990). The PCL-R has been proven to be one of the most powerful instruments for predicting future offending, psychopathy, as diagnosed by a score over 30 on the PCL-R, being the condition most closely related to criminal recidivism.

So the Psychopathy Checklist Revised is a very valid and very useful tool to identify persons in risk for relapse into criminality and for causing social and personal harm and — if I understand it correctly — it has been conceptualized for that purpose

(Hare, 1993). The items of the Checklist — and the underlying concept of psychopathy — however, cover, such a large number of different personality traits that they can hardly be conceived as an entity. I fear that the idea of psychopathy as a special character entity may lead to the same problems clinical research had, and still has, with the concept of schizophrenia. More than ten years ago, Karl Leonhard, one of the most renowned researchers in that field, argued that one of the few things people in schizophrenia research agreed upon, was, that schizophrenia is not a disease entity, but a cluster of similar psychopathological syndromes of different etiologies and genetics. So research to find a common biological, psychodynamic or genetic cause would always remain inconclusive.

To substantiate this view on psychopathy some current and historical concepts of personality disorders should be examined. If we compare the items of the PCL to the criteria in different diagnostic instruments, we find that psychopathy always borrows from several disorders classified separately in those classifications or typologies: In DSM-IV (1994) it has not only a substantial overlap with the Antisocial Personality Disorder but also with the Narcissistic and to a lesser degree with the Histrionic Personality Disorder.

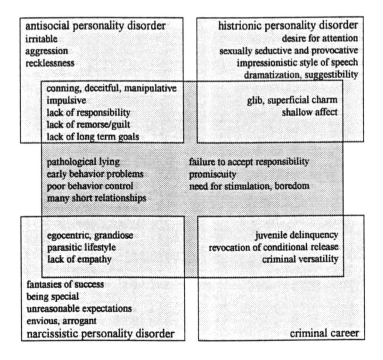

Figure 1. Psychopathy and DSM-IV

It also has three items concerning criminal career, which are not found in any of the other classifications, and there are always a few items that are not included in any of the other nosological systems. In ICD-10 (1991) Narcissistic Personality Disorder does not exist, the greatest overlap is with the Histrionic Personality Disorder, but psychopathy borrows also from the Dissocial and to some extend from the Impulsive type. Overlaps with the Hysterical type of personality can also be demonstrated with the historical typologies of Kurt Schneider (1923) and Karl Leonhard (1976).

In Schneiders typology the major overlap exists with the Gemütsarmer Psychopath, which is translated into English as *"affectionless psychopath"*.

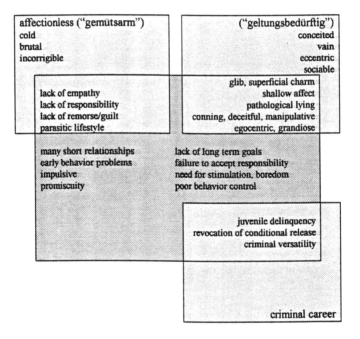

Figure 2. Psychopathy and Schneider's typology

The *"Gemütsarmer Psychopath"* would be quite different from what we see when we describe psychopaths according to the PCL-R. They lack the histrionic traits that enable psychopaths — as defined by Hare — to persuade other people, to fool even professionals and to find victims so easily.

Psychopathy in that sense covers a whole spectrum of personality traits and is not — contrary to the typologies of authors such as Schneider, Leonhard or Cloninger (1993) — seen as an extreme ideal type of personality traits or as the extreme position in a multidimensional view or a multifactorial concept of human personality. It does not strive to set limits to other personality disorders, and it is not part of a classification system or of a typology that tries to include all personality disorders.

Reformulating the hypothesis

What do these introductory remarks have to do with comorbidity or, perhaps more accurately, with co-ocurrence? If one looks at the items of the PCL-R and at the personality traits that lay behind them more closely, there is an astonishing mixture of features that contrast quite clearly with most of the symptoms of the major disorders. That notion becomes most evident when the scrupulous guilt feelings of depressive patients are opposed to the characteristics of psychopaths. Criteria like lack of remorse or guilt and shallow affect do not seem to be compatible with the diagnosis of a major depression. Manic patients rarely have criminal careers (Nedopil, 1996). Less than one per cent of the 2500 offenders assessed for criminal courts in the department of forensic psychiatry at the University of Munich received the diagnosis of a manic episode. If one looks at schizophrenia, the disorder most prone to be associated with criminality or aggressive crimes, there is some overlap of symptoms with psychopathy but the majority of symptoms — especially the basic symptoms and the negative symptoms — contradicts the essential features of psychopathy.

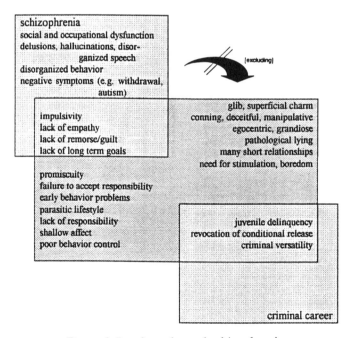

Figure 3. Psychopathy and schizophrenia

Difficulties arise also with organic disorders or with substance dependency syndromes. If these disorders reach a degree of clinical relevance they interfere with most of the activities that make psychopaths dangerous for their environment.

If this theoretical analysis was true, the following hypothesis seem to be justified:

1) The combination of personality traits that portrait psychopathy are incompatible with major mental disorders or,

2)   If psychopaths become seriously mentally ill, their risk of relapse into continuous criminal behavior is reduced.

Analysis of psychiatric assessments for criminal courts

This hypothesis could be proven if only a very small number of patients would manifest a co-occurrence of psychopathy and major mental disorder, whereas a substantial number of psychopathic individuals would also receive the diagnosis of a personality disorder.

There are some difficulties to really prove this hypothesis empirically from our own data at present because the PCL-R was translated into German only two years ago and has only been used in a preliminary experimental version for one and a half years. Therefore, the number of individuals assessed with the PCL-R is relatively small. Nonetheless, we have been using a very extensive 512-item documentation system for more than ten years (Nedopil & Graßl, 1987). Data obtained from this documentation have been included in a second part of this paper.

The hypothesis was tested on two samples: Sample 1 consisted of 131 individuals who were assessed with an experimental translation of the PCL-R, 50 of them for the prediction of future of offending, 81 for criminal responsibility.

TABLE 1. co-occurrence of psychopathy and personality disorders in patients with major mental disorders

Diagnosis	n	PCL-R score > 25	Dyssocial PD	Histrionic PD
Schizophrenia	16	2	4	1
Dementia	16	2	4	2
Dependence	23	3	2	3
Minimal brain dysfunction[1])	13	5	7	3
Personality disorder	42	14		
No diagnosis	37	4		

The mean score of all patients on the PCL-R was 18.1 ($\pm$ 6.4). We set the cutoff point at 25, as is done by a number of European authors (Kullgren, 1995; See Cooke, this volume), and which corresponds to a score of one standard deviation above the mean in our population. With this cutoff point only two schizophrenics and two patients with organic brain syndrome could be considered as psychopaths. Five patients with minimal brain dysfunction (see footnote 1 for an explanation), 14 individuals with personality disorders and 4 individuals without any clinical diagnoses had a score over

---

[1] The term *"minimal brain dysfunction"* appears somewhat outdated, but had an important meaning in categorizing disorders for German courts. It was similar in concept to attention deficit, hyperactivity disorder combined with some sort of history of birth complications and/or soft neurological signs. The diagnosis was given during the childhood of these individuals and was only included into the forensic assessment if the individual had a record of seeing a pediatrician, child psychiatrist or child psychologist who had established the diagnosis.

25. There was a substantial larger number of co-occurrences of schizophrenia with personality disorders when using the diagnosis of personality disorder according to clinical diagnostic systems like ICD-10 or DSM-IV, than when using the PCL-R criteria for psychopathy. Four schizophrenics were also diagnosed as Dissocial and one as Histrionic Personality Disorder according to ICD-10.

The distribution of scores among schizophrenics resembled quite clearly the distribution of those without diagnosis, whereas those with organic brain dysfunctions were more evenly distributed in all score categories (fig. 1). The diagnosis of Dissocial Personality Disorder and of Histrionic Personality disorder deserves some further attention. Four individuals had a co-occurrence of Dissocial personality and schizophrenia, another 4 one of Dissocial personality and dementia, and 2 of the Dissocial personalities were also dependent. Four individuals received the diagnosis of being both Dissocial and histrionic. Of the histrionic personality disorders one was also diagnosed as schizophrenic, 3 as dependent, two had minimal brain dysfunction and two were slightly demented.

At first glance the hypothesis, that psychopathy is rarely associated with major mental disorder has gained some empirical support. In order to find out whether the hypotheses could be tested on a larger sample we used 554 individuals assessed for crimes of violence, the assessments being documented on a comprehensive documentation system. Considering the population we examined the data are neither representative of criminals, psychopaths, patients with APD or mentally ill criminals, but they constitute a sample large enough, to find some preliminary indication of the value of the hypothesis, that criminality, psychopathy and major mental disorder is a rather rare combination. The diagnoses of these individuals are shown on table 5.

TABLE 2. Diagnoses of individuals assessed for criminal responsibility

Diagnosis	
Psychosis	45
Dementia	56
Dependence	95
Minimal brain dysfunction	19
Personality disorder	171
Dyssocial personality disorder	42
Histrionic personality disorder	57
No diagnosis	207
All diagnoses for 554 patients	593

Note. Only 39 probands received more than one diagnosis. The concept of comorbidity was not applied in German psychiatry until 1993. The assessments date back as far as 1982, therefore, most individuals received only one diagnosis

Although the PCL-R was not used in that sample the documentation used, the documentation Forensic Psychiatric Documentation System, the FPDS, contains most of the items of the Psychopathy Checklist Revised. The FPDS has an elaborate description of 512 items and good inter-rater reliability (Nedopil & Graßl, 1988; Kröber et al., 1995). Twelve of the 20 items of the PCL-R can also be found in the FPDS with identical wordings, five other items were very similar (Table 6) and were also rated with this documentation.

TABLE 3. Comparison of items from the FPDS and the PCL-R

FPDS	PCL-R
Identical Items	
1) Manipulative	conning/deceitful/manipulative
2) Lying	pathological lying
3) Impulsivity	impulsivity
4) Justifying, excusing, trifling	failure to accept responsibility
5) Lack of affect	shallow affect
6) Lack of empathy	lack of empathy
7) Egocentric	egocentric/ grandiose
8) Without long-term planning	lack of long term goals
9) Behavior problems during childhood)	early behavior problems (stealing, running away, skipping school)
10) Delinquency before the age of 18	juvenile delinquency
11) Criminal versatility	criminal versatility
12) Promiscuity	promiscuity
Similar Items	
13) Many social intrigues	glib
14) Demonstrative, eccentric	grandiose
15) unreliable	deceitful
16) without inner relations to legal norms	lack of responsibility
17) lack of self reproach	lack of remorse/guilt
Additional Items	
18) desire for admiration	
19) demanding attention	
Items of the PCL-R that are not in the FPDS	
	revocation of conditional release
	many short relationships
	need for stimulation/boredom
	parasitic lifestyle
	poor behavior control

Two items closely related to the concept of psychopathy were also included in our evaluation. The PCL-R was constructed to detect psychopaths whereas the FPDS, a large comprehensive rating scale is not focused on one particular disorder. So the method of rating and the data obtained with these instruments may be quite different and have to be interpreted with great caution. On the other hand the evaluation of these 19 items could give some indication whether the hypothesis, I set forth, should be further investigated. The items were evaluated alternatively as present or not present. Using 19 items the highest possible score would amount to 19.

In order to identify those individuals who might be close to psychopathy we defined that they should have a higher score than one standard deviation above the mean of the total group. The mean was 2.3, the standard deviation 2.4, so all individuals with 5 or more points were tentatively considered as psychopaths. Although 5 might seem to be a rather low score, it gains some face value, when comparing some individuals who were also rated with the PCL-R. Also the percentage of psychopaths defined by this FPDS-psychopathy score and the percentage of psychopaths in the group assessed with the PCL-R are quite similar. In the latter group 16 out of 81, that is 20 percent were identified as psychopaths. In the larger sample 86, that is 16 %, had a score of 5 or higher. The mean scores assessed with the FPDS-psychopathy in the different diagnostic categories lead to a similar rank orders as those assessed with the PCL-R (Fig. 2).

In the former group schizophrenics had the lowest average score with only three of them scoring higher than 5. Patients with organic brain syndrome had a lower average value than individuals without diagnosis. Personality disorders had the highest average value followed by patients with minimal brain dysfunction and individuals with alcohol or drug dependence.

With this procedure the following distribution of psychopathic individuals can be found in the different diagnostic groups (table 7):

TABLE 4. Major mental disorders and Psychopathy according to FPDS scores

Diagnosis	n (total)	FPDS-psychopathy score > 5	% of diagnosis
Schizophrenia	45	3	7%
Dementia	56	8	14%
Dependence	95	28	27%
Minimal brain dysfunction	19	7	37%
Personality disorders	171	41	25%
No diagnosis	207	27	8%

The relative distributions of psychopathic individuals in the different diagnostic categories are the same in this sample as in the sample where the PCL-R was used (Fig 2).

DISCUSSION

Our data suggest that there is a significant co-occurrence of psychopathy with substance dependence and other personality disorders but a much lower co-occurrence with dementia and an even lower one with schizophrenia.

The number of individuals suffering from more than one disorder becomes considerably higher, when one uses clinical classifications like DSM-IV or ICD-10. This is especially true for the major mental disorders. It does not seem to be reasonable to talk about a co-occurrence of psychopathy with several personality disorders, since there is a significant overlap of symptoms and of diagnostic concepts between psychopathy and Dissocial, Histrionic or Narcissistic personality disorder. Comorbidity in the population assessed or treated by forensic psychiatrists is rather frequent, if one uses clinical classifications but is rather infrequent for the major disorders when using the concept of psychopathy.

These findings should be discussed carefully, since they are only preliminary, but they receive both theoretical and empirical evidence, e.g. activation patterns as measured by PET scan are quite different in schizophrenics than in psychopaths (Intrator, 1993), and it can hardly be understood, how these patterns could interact. In a recent study on relapse rates of 685 released forensic patients Rice et al., (1995) also found a smaller than expected number of schizophrenics who had a PCL-R score of more than 25. So their data seem to confirm the initial hypothesis of this paper. Only thirteen of the 161 schizophrenics were also psychopaths according to that definition. Moreover the authors found, that schizophrenics relapsed less frequently than other patients into violent crimes. Psychopathy accounted more for the relapse than schizophrenia.

Even if our findings and hypotheses were confirmed in other studies, it would not reduce the usefulness of the PCL-R in forensic practice. Warren (1971) stressed that typologies are only useful for the purpose they have been developed for and should not be applied universally. The concept of psychopathy, the identification of psychopathic individuals and the quantification of their abnormality are useful guidelines in dealing with the clientele of the forensic psychiatrist or psychologist, when questions of management and prediction are to be solved. This appears to be true regardless of the presence or absence of a major mental disorder. But the question whether this concept describes a clinical entity or a combination of malignant character traits remains unresolved for me. Only if the first assumption was correct, we should continue to reflect a concept of comorbidity of psychopathy with major mental disorders.

References

American Psychiatric Association (1994). *Diagnostic and Statistical Manual of Mental Disorders, 4th edn.* (DSM-IV). Washington, D.C.;: APA,.

Böker, W., & Häfner, H. (1973). *Gewalttaten Geistesgestörter.* Berlin, Heidelberg, New York,: Springer,.

Carone, B. J., Harrow, M., & Westermayer, J. F. (1991). Posthospital course and outcome of schizophrenia. *Archives of General Psychiatry, 48,* 247-251.

Cleckley, H. (1976). *The mask of sanity:* An attempt to clarify some issues about the so called psychopathic personality (5th ed, 1st ed 1941). St. Louis: Mosby.

Cloninger, C. R., Svrakic, D. M., & Przybeck, T. R. (1993). A psychobiological model of temperament and character. *Archives of General Psychiatry, 50*, 975-990.

Côté, G., & Hodgins, S. (1992). The prevalence of major mental disorders among homicide offenders. *International Journal of Law and Psychiatry, 15*, 89-99.

Dilling, H., Mombour, W., & Schmidt, M. H. (1991). *Internationale Klassifikation psychischer Störungen ICD-10*. Bern, Göttingen, Toronto: Huber.

Dolan, B., & Coid, J. (1993). *Psychopathic and Antisocial Personality Disorder, Treatment and Research Issues*. London: Gaskell.

Häfner, H., & Böker, W. (1982). *Crimes of violence by mentally abnormal offenders*. The psychiatric epidemiological study in the Federal German Republic. Cambridge: Cambridge University Press.

Hare, R. D. (1990). *The Hare Psychopathy Checklist - Revised*. Niagara Falls, Toronto: Multi-Health Systems.

Hare, R. D. (1993). *Without conscience*. New York, London, Toronto: Pocket Books.

Hare, R. D. (1984). Violent and aggressive behavior by criminal psychopaths. *International Journal of Law and Psychiatry, 7*, 35-50.

Hart, S. D., Hare, R. D., & Forth, A. E. (1994). Psychopathy as a risk marker for violence: Development and validation of a screening version of the Revised Psychopathy Checklist. In J. Monahan & H. J. Steadman (Eds.), *Violence and Mental Disorder* (pp. 81.98). Chicago: University of Chicago Press.

Hodgins, S. (1995). *Major mental disorder and crime: An overview*. Psychology, Crime and Law, 2, 5-17.

Intrator, J. (1993). *Cerebral activation of lexical decision in psychopaths using single photon emission tomography* Dept. Psychiatry, Bronx VA Medical Center, New York, NY, Oct. 14, 1993, Regional Conference of the IALMH Munich, Germany.

Kaplan, H. J., Sadock, B. J., & Grebb, J. A. (1994). *Synopsis of Psychiatry. (7th ed.)*. Baltimore, Hong Kong, London, Sidney: Williams & Wilkins,.

Kröber, H. L., Faller, U., & Wolf, J. (1994). *Nutzen und Grenzen standardisierter Schuldfähigkeitsbegutachtung. Eine Überprüfung des forensisch-psychiatrischen Dokumentation-ssystems*. Monatsschrift für Kriminologie und Strafrechtsreform, 77, 339-352.

Kullgren, G. (1995). *Personality disorders among 1255 male criminal offenders undergoing forensic psychiatric investigation*. International Congress of the IALMH, Tromsö, Norway, June 26, 1995.

Leonhard, K. (1976). *Akzentuierte Persönlichkeiten*. Stuttgart, New York, 2.Aufl.: Gustav Fischer,.

Leonhard, K. (1980). *Aufteilung der endogenen Psychosen*. Leipzig,: Akademie Verlag, 5.Aufl.

Lester, D. (1995). The concentration of neurotransmitter metabolites in the cerebrospinal fluid of suicidal individuals: a meta-analysis. *Pharmacopsychiatry, 28*, 45-50.

Lindquist, P., & Allebeck, A. (1989). Schizophrenia and assaultive behaviour: the role of alcohol and drug abuse. *Acta Psychiatr.Scand., 82*, 191-195.

Linnoila, M., Virkunnen, M., Scheinin, M., Nuutila, A., Rimon, R., & Goodwin, F. (1983). Low cerebrospinal fluid 5-hydroxyindoleacetic acid concentration differentia. *Life Sciences, 33*, 2609-2614.

Monahan, J., & Steadman, H. J. (1994). *Violence and Mental Disorder*. Chicago: University of Chicago Press.

Nedopil, N. (1996a). *Forensische Psychiatrie*. Stuttgart, New York: Thieme.

Nedopil, N. (1996b). Violence of psychotic patients - how much responsibility can be attributed? *International Journal of Law and Psychiatry, 17*, in press.

Nedopil, N., & Graßl, P. (1988). Das Forensisch-Psychiatrische Dokumentationssystem (FPDS). *Forensia, 9,* 139-147.

Nedopil, N., Graßl, P., & Mende, W. (1987). Le forensic psychiatric documentation systeme (FPDS),developpement et première application. *Acta Psychiatica Belgica, 87,* 93-112.

Praag, H. v. (1994). 5-HT-related anxiety- and/or aggression-driven depression. *Int. J. Clin. Psychopharmacology, Suppl.1,* 5-6.

Rice, M. E., & Harris, G. T. (1995). Psychopathy, Schizophrenia, Alcohol Abuse and Violent Recidivism. *International Journal of Law and Psychiatry, 18(3),* 333-342.

Schneider, K. (1923). *Die psychopathischen Persönlichkeiten.* Leipzig,: Thieme, (9. Aufl., 1950, Deuticke, Wien).

Soyka, M. (1994). Substance abuse and dependency as a risk factor for delinquency and violent behavior in schizophrenic patients - how strong is the evidence? *Journal of Clinical Forensic Medicine, 1,* 3-7.

Virkunnen, M., Kallio, E., Rawlings, R., Tokula, R., Poland, F. E., Guidotti, A., Nemeroff, C., Bisette, G., Kalegeras, K., Karonen, S.-L., & Linnoila, M. (1994a). Personality profiles and state aggressiveness in Finnish alcoholic, violent offenders, fire setters and healthy volunteers. *Archives of General Psychiatry, 51,* 28-33.

Virkunnen, M., Rawlings, R., Tokula, R., Poland, R. E., Guidotti, A., Nemeroff, C., Bisette, G., Kalegeras, K., Karonen, S.-L., & Linnoila, M. (1994b). CSF Biochemistries, glucose metabolism, and diurnal activity rhythms in alcoholic, violent offenders, fire setters and healthy volunteers. *Archives of General Psychiatry, 51,* 20-27.

Warren, M. Q. (1971). Classification of offenders as an aid to efficient management and effective control. *J. Criminal Law, Criminology and Police Science, 62,* 239-258.

PSYCHOPATHY AND PERSONALITY DISORDER: IMPLICATIONS OF INTERPERSONAL THEORY

RONALD BLACKBURN
Department of Clinical Psychology
University of Liverpool
United Kingdom.

INTRODUCTION

The concept of a personality type distinguished by a callous disregard for the feelings of others, egocentricity, and impulsive social rule-breaking has been elaborated by clinicians and behavioral scientists for over fifty years (e.g., Cleckley, 1976; Gough, 1948; McCord & McCord, 1964). Yet despite a surge of theory-driven research during the 1960s and 1970s, progress in understanding psychopathy has been slow. Not only have most of the earlier theories proved to be limited in illuminating the concept, the field has also been hampered by lack of agreement as to which attributes are the most prototypical indicators of psychopathy (Hare & Cox, 1978; Hare, Hart & Harpur, 1991).

The operationalization of the construct through the development of the Psychopathy Checklist (PCL: Hare, 1980) and the Psychopathy Checklist-Revised (PCL-R: Hare, 1991; Hare, Harpur, Hakstian, Forth, Hart & Newman, 1990) therefore promises to bring some order to a field known more for conceptual confusion. Accumulating data on the behavioral and personality correlates of the checklist suggest that it now provides a focus for refining the construct and for amplifying knowledge of causal psychological processes (Hare, in press). Relationships with criminal recidivism and violence also demonstrate its predictive utility (Hare, McPherson & Forth, 1988; Harris, Rice & Cormier, 1991; Kosson, Smith & Newman, 1990; Serin, 1996). Although PCL-R items define two oblique factors, and Factor 1 (callous and remorseless style of relating to others) comes closer to the core attributes of the concept than Factor 2 (socially deviant lifestyle), the correlates of the full scale and factor subscales support the validity of the PCL-R as a homogeneous measure of a unidimensional construct (Harpur, Hare & Hakstian, 1989).

As a concept of abnormal personality, however, psychopathy cannot be considered in isolation from the wider domain of individual differences, and there are several outstanding issues about its relation to other disorders of personality and to personality structure more generally. In this chapter, I argue that psychopathy is most appropriately construed as a dimension of personality disorder and that this dimension is represented primarily within the space of an established system for describing personality, the interpersonal circle. I will summarize some research on the classification of abnormal personality in mentally disordered offenders and its relation

269

D.J. Cooke et al. (eds.), Psychopathy: Theory, Research and Implications for Society, 269–301.
© *1998 Kluwer Academic Publishers. Printed in the Netherlands.*

to the PCL, and present some work on the interpersonal model of personality and its implications for understanding psychopathy. Although I do not propose a novel theory of psychopathy, I believe that the interpersonal model offers a coherent framework for the development of such a theory.

PSYCHOPATHY AND PERSONALITY DISORDER

The psychiatric classification of personality disorders follows a Kraepelinian model in identifying several discrete categories at a single level of analysis, antisocial personality disorder (APD) being the current synonym for psychopathy (American Psychiatric Association, 1994). The criteria for the DSM-III, DSM-III-R, and DSM-IV versions of APD have been criticized for the relative absence of personality traits considered central to psychopathy (Blackburn, 1988; Hare et al., 1991; Millon, 1981). Nevertheless, Cleckley (1976) considered the DSM-II version to be *"a recognizable entity in a fairly large group of different and distinct disorders"* (p.134). Hare and Hart (1993) similarly describe psychopathy as *"a specific form of personality disorder... similar in many respects to the category antisocial personality disorder"* (p. 104). However, the assumption of a *"distinct entity"* raises questions about the degree of specificity of the concept, and whether it may alternatively be represented as a dimension rather than a categorical entity.

The question of specificity is to some extent a semantic one that goes to the heart of the confusion that has characterized the history of the concept. The literal meaning of *"psychopathic"* is simply *"psychologically damaged"*, and in German psychiatry, where the term originates, psychopathic personality was a generic term denoting a heterogeneous group of abnormal personalities defined by personality deviation, not antisocial behavior (Schneider, 1923/1950). Paradoxically, Schneider's psychopathic personalities became the wider class of personality disorders in current European and American psychiatric classifications. Narrower use of the terms psychopathic, sociopathic, or antisocial personality to refer to a specific kind of socially deviant individual reflects the persisting influence in Anglo-American psychiatry of the nineteenth century notion of *"moral insanity"*. This entails the inference of psychological abnormality from socially unacceptable behaviors (Millon, 1981; Pichot, 1978). Antisocial acts, however, have multiple determinants and belong in a different conceptual domain from that of personality dispositions. They are not in themselves a logical basis for inferring personality deviation (Blackburn, 1988).

North American concepts of psychopathic personality, such as that of Cleckley, are hybrids in the Schneiderian and moral insanity traditions insofar as personality traits define a specific antisocial type. The recent APD category of the DSM, on the other hand, lies more within the moral insanity tradition, emphasizing as it does socially deviant behaviors. The effect of the relative absence of psychopathic personality traits among the criteria for APD is apparent from its relation to the PCL and PCL-R. Although categorical diagnoses of APD correlate in the region of 0.5 with total PCL scores, correlations are stronger with Factor 2 than with Factor 1 (Hare, 1991; Hare et al., 1991), and only a minority of those diagnosed as APD are identified as psychopaths on the recommended PCL-R cut-off score of 30 or more (Hart & Hare, 1989; Hart, Forth & Hare, 1991).

However, etymological niceties notwithstanding, restricting the term psychopath to those exhibiting the personality traits identified as central by Cleckley and others does not guarantee its distinctiveness from other personality disorders. The relation of the PCL to personality disorders other than APD has so far received only limited attention in research, but traits associated with psychopathy can be detected among the criteria for several DSM-III and DSM-IV personality disorders, notably histrionic (superficial charm, insincerity, egocentricity), narcissistic (grandiosity, lack of empathy, exploitativeness), borderline (impulsivity, anger, suicidal gestures) and paranoid (mistrust). Cleckley's distinct entity therefore seems broader than a single category of personality disorder.

The PCL might therefore be expected to correlate with other personality disorders apart from APD, and the available evidence bears this out. In a forensic psychiatric sample, Hart and Hare (1989) found that the PCL correlated significantly with categorical diagnoses of APD and histrionic disorder (of three categories examined) and with prototypicality ratings of antisocial, histrionic, narcissistic and avoidant disorders, the latter correlation being negative. Five of nine disorders examined correlated with Factor 1, while Factor 2 correlated only with APD. Hart et al. (1991) found that the PCL-R correlated with six of the 13 personality disorder scales of the MCMI-II (narcissistic, antisocial, sadistic, passive-aggressive, borderline, paranoid). Whereas eight disorders were correlated with Factor 2, only one correlated with Factor 1, in this case sadistic disorder. Correlations of the screening version of the PCL (PCL:SV) with both interview-derived and MCMI-II measures of DSM-III-R are also reported by Hart, Hare & Forth (1994). The PCL:SV correlated with six of the 13 interview measures and seven of the 13 MCMI-II scales. Although Hart and Hare (1989) argued that the magnitude of the correlations was sufficiently low to support the discriminant validity of the PCL, the data overall challenge the assumption that psychopathy is one distinct category among several categories of personality disorder. On the contrary, they seem consistent with the view that psychopathy is a superordinate dimension of personality deviation pervading many of the currently recognized disorders (Blackburn, 1993a).

These findings are not surprising given high rates of comorbidity among personality disorders in general (Clark, Watson & Reynolds, 1995; Clarkin & Kendall, 1992; Tyrer, 1988a). As Clarkin and Kendall (1992) note, recurring patterns of comorbidity are likely to reflect the organization of underlying dimensions, and arguments favoring a dimensional approach to the classification of personality disorders have been advanced increasingly in recent years (Blackburn, 1988; Tyrer, 1988a; Widiger, 1991). It has also been proposed that the dimensions most relevant to personality disorders are the Big Five factors of extraversion, agreeableness, neuroticism, conscientiousness, and openness to experience (Widiger & Frances, 1994; Wiggins & Pincus, 1994). The relation of these to psychopathy is considered later in the chapter.

It has to be noted that although the PCL is a dimensional measure, the appropriateness of construing psychopathy in terms of a dimension rather than a category is contentious. Harris, Rice and Quinsey (1994) applied taxometric methods to the PCL-R and found evidence for a taxon, apparently supporting the notion of a discrete entity. However, this conclusion is tentative because the discriminating items came primarily from PCL-R Factor 2. Hare believes that the dimensional or categorical nature of the underlying construct remains an open question (Hare, in press; Hare & Hart, 1993).

Although proponents of dimensional analysis argue that dimensional description is consonant with the assumption that personality dysfunctions differ quantitatively rather than qualitatively from normality, the distinction between dimensions and categories is less absolute than commonly supposed. A category may represent a combination of attributes that are continuously distributed throughout the population at large, and in the case of psychopathy, it is manifestly not the case that egocentricity, callousness, impulsivity, and so forth, are the exclusive property of those processed by the criminal justice or mental health systems. The notion of a category of psychopathic personality need not, then, imply any sharp discontinuity in the distribution of deviant personality traits. Nevertheless, naturally occurring types (or taxa) of personality disorder are likely to reflect the interaction of several dimensions.

PERSONALITY DISORDER IN MENTALLY DISORDERED OFFENDERS

My research has centered on the contribution of personality deviation to antisocial behavior and particularly on the utility of the North American concept of psychopathic personality in this context. This research has been undertaken with adult male mentally disordered offenders (MDOs) detained in maximum security psychiatric hospitals in England (the special hospitals) because of presumed dangerousness. The 1983 Mental Health Act for England and Wales differentiates categories of mental disorder. Two thirds of patients fall in the legal category of *mental illness* (MI), which covers the most serious mental disorders, and about a quarter in the category of *psychopathic disorder* (PD). The latter is defined in the Act as "*a persistent disorder or disability of mind, whether or not including significant impairment of intelligence, which results in abnormally aggressive or seriously irresponsible conduct on the part of the person concerned*".

It will be apparent that this legal definition makes little contact with the current North American concept of psychopathy, and in practice, those in the PD category are clinically heterogeneous. Coid (1992) found that less than a quarter met PCL criteria of psychopathy, and only 38% met DSM-III criteria for APD. Most of these patients are not, then, psychopathic in the current sense, but they are often described indiscriminately as "*psychopaths*". To add to the confusion, this label is still commonly used interchangeably with "*personality disorder*" in Britain. However, personality dysfunction is not confined to PD patients, and many in the MI category also have comorbid personality disorders. Tyrer (1988b), for example, found that 56% of MI patients met criteria of personality disorder on the Personality Assessment Schedule. Blackburn, Crellin, Morgan & Tulloch (1990) also identified 65% of MI patients as personality disordered on the MCMI-1. The MI and PD patients differed only on the antisocial and passive-aggressive disorder scales. The two medicolegal categories are also not differentiated by the PCL (Howard, 1990; O'Kane, Fawcett & Blackburn, 1996). These findings are consistent with the argument that personality disorders and mental illness belong in different universes of discourse and hence frequently coexist

(Foulds, 1971). Some of our studies of personality deviation have therefore included both PD and MI patients.

Much of our research has operationalized psychopathic traits by means of self-report scales. Self-report measures of personality have played a significant role in establishing the relevance of individual differences to criminal behavior (Andrews & Wormith, 1989), but Hare and his colleagues have long questioned the usefulness of such scales in psychopathy research (Hare, 1991, in press; Hare & Hart, 1993; Hart et al., 1991). They argue that because untruthfulness is among the traits of psychopathy, psychopaths are likely to falsify personality questionnaires. Self-report scales often used to define psychopathy correlate only modestly with clinical ratings of psychopathy (Hare, 1985), and the relationship is due largely to correlations with Factor 2 of the PCL rather than Factor 1 (Hare, 1991; Harpur et al., 1989; Hart et al., 1991). However, there are several reasons for doubting that this can be attributed simply to untruthfulness. First, self-report measures of personality are less concerned with verifiable facts than with beliefs about the sort of person one is. Hogan and Nicholson (1988) argue that responses to items on personality questionnaires are not, in fact, *"self-reports"* but are rather *"...self-presentations formally identical to responses to questions in an employment interview"* (p.625). Given that the demands of personality questionnaires and interviews are similar, there seems no reason why psychopaths should present themselves differently in response to one rather than the other. Second, low correlations between self- and observer ratings are not unique to psychopathy research, and this is a perennial issue in personality assessment (Becker, 1960). Gifford (1994) demonstrates some of the reasons, and notes both methodological and philosophical objections to the assumption that observer ratings are necessarily more valid or *"true"* than self-ratings.

Although attributes such as lack of empathy are not easily measured by self-report, trait measures whose content is more closely related to the concept of psychopathy, such as machiavellianism and narcissism, have somewhat stronger associations with Factor 1 of the PCL-R (Hare, 1991). Hare (1991) also reports a correlation between a self-report scale of psychopathy (SRP-II) and total PCL-R of .54 (N = 100), correlations with Factors 1 and 2 being .50 and .44, respectively. Considering the typical validity coefficients of self-report scales, these coefficients must be considered impressive. They suggest that it is not the self-report method *per se* which is problematic in the assessment of psychopathy so much as the relevance of some of the measures used. The scales employed in my own studies may suffer from the same limitations, but our results suggest that they permit valid generalizations about personality deviation.

An empirical classification of personality types among mentally disordered offenders

A basic assumption underlying my research is that theoretical clinical categories, such as the concept of psychopathic personality, are hypotheses about naturally occurring patterns of attributes, and that the methods of numerical taxonomy provide a means of validating such constructs (Blashfield, 1980; Lorr, 1983). A primary aim has therefore been to reduce the heterogeneity of the mentally disordered offender population by means of cluster analysis applied to personality test data. It may be noted that this approach seeks to identify a homogeneous class of psychopathic *individuals*, i.e. a taxon, by reference to multidimensional data.

My initial studies tested Megargee's hypothesis that violent offenders can be divided into overcontrolled and undercontrolled types (Megargee, 1966). Undercontrolled offenders, according to Megargee, have weak inhibitions against aggression, and hence respond aggressively with some regularity. They are also likely to be identified as psychopaths. Overcontrolled offenders, in contrast, have strong inhibitions, and aggress only when anger arousal is sufficiently intense to overcome inhibitions. They are therefore expected to attack others rarely, but with extreme intensity when they do, and should be found more commonly among those who have been extremely assaultive or homicidal. Supporting the hypothesis, I found that extreme assaultives among MDOs were significantly more controlled, inhibited, and defensive on the MMPI than moderate assaultives (Blackburn, 1968). They were also less likely to have a prior criminal record or to be diagnosed clinically as psychopaths. I later tested the theory further through cluster analysis of MMPI profiles of homicidal patients (Blackburn, 1971). This, however, produced two undercontrolled and two overcontrolled types. One undercontrolled type was defined by the well known *"49"* profile associated in clinical lore with psychopathic personality (i.e., combined elevations on the Psychopathic Deviate and Hypomania scales), the other by a highly deviant profile which includes abnormal scores on most other clinical scales. Of the overcontrolled groups, one was defined by a defensive *"hypernormal"* pattern, the other mainly by marked social introversion.

TABLE 1. Rotated factor loadings of SHAPS scales in patient and normal samples

SHAPS Scale	Patients (N = 499)		Normals (N = 238)	
	I	II	I	II
Lie	-.74	-.05	-.55	-.03
Anxiety	.68	.65	.54	.76
Extraversion	.35	-.84	.48	-.76
Hostility	.76	.28	.72	.44
Shyness	.27	.86	-.01	.89
Depression	.58	.72	.42	.78
Tension	.66	.56	.53	.63
Psychopathic Deviate	.61	.39	.62	.29
Impulsivity	.92	-.06	.92	-.05
Aggression	.86	.14	.86	.11
% variance	45	29	38	32

Note. SHAPS=Special Hospitals Assessment of Personality and Socialisation

Subsequent research has relied on a shorter questionnaire, the SHAPS (Special Hospitals Assessment of Personality and Socialisation: Blackburn, 1979a; 1987) which focuses more specifically on psychopathy-related traits such as impulsivity and hostile interpersonal attitudes, but which also contains measures of two of the Big Five dimensions, neuroticism and extraversion. The 213 items are drawn mainly from the MMPI but some are from the Buss-Durkee Hostility Inventory and a factor scale developed by Peterson, Quay and Cameron (1959) described as Psychopathy. Two factors underlie the 10 SHAPS scales (Blackburn, 1979a; 1986), the first being defined by impulsivity, aggression, hostility, and negatively by the Lie scale, and labeled *impulsive aggression* or *psychopathy* (Table 1). The second factor is defined by introversion, social anxiety, and proneness to dysphoric mood, and is labeled *Withdrawal versus Sociability*. These factors are consistent across several samples of MDOs, but also hold up in a normal sample of male volunteers (Table 1). The factors represent 45° rotations in the two-dimensional space of neuroticism and extraversion (Kassebaum, Couch & Slater, 1959). They therefore seem equivalent to Gray's impulsivity and anxiety dimensions (Gray, 1987), which are held to be manifestations of the Behavioral Activation System (BAS) and Behavioral Inhibition System (BIS), respectively. Given the contribution of hostility and aggression to the first factor, the SHAPS dimensions may be higher order factors incorporating agreeableness-disagreeableness as well as neuroticism and extraversion, but the relationship of the SHAPS to a measure of the Big Five remains to be tested.

These two factors are virtually identical to the two largest factors in the MCMI-1 personality disorder scales (Blackburn, 1996). The aggression dimension corresponds to an MCMI-1 factor described by Retzlaff and Gibertini (1987) as *labile-restrained* (passive-aggressive, paranoid, borderline, antisocial, avoidant versus compulsive), the withdrawal dimension corresponding to an *aloof-social* factor (schizoid, schizotypal, avoidant versus histrionic and narcissistic). Two scales, B (Belligerence) and W (Withdrawal), were developed to measure these factors (Blackburn, 1987), but the studies summarized below are based mainly on factor scores.

The earlier fourfold typology is consistently reproduced by cluster analyses of the SHAPS factors. The four patterns were distinguished among patients in the legal category of psychopathic disorder (Blackburn, 1975), demonstrating homogeneous subgroups within this category, but they also constitute the main patterns of personality deviation among MDOs as a whole (Blackburn, 1986). I have described the four classes as: (1) *Primary Psychopaths* (P; impulsive, aggressive, hostile, extraverted, self-confident, low to average anxiety); (2) *Secondary Psychopaths* (S; hostile, impulsive, aggressive, socially anxious, withdrawn, moody, low in self esteem): (3) *Controlled* (C; defensive, controlled, sociable, nonanxious); (4) *Inhibited* (I; shy, withdrawn, controlled, moderately anxious, low self esteem). The four groups represent combinations of extremes on the two SHAPS factor dimensions. P and S score towards the impulsive-aggressive extreme of the first factor, but are distinguished by the withdrawal-sociability dimension, P being socially uninhibited, S withdrawn and anxious. The C and I groups score at a low level on the aggression factor, but are also differentiated by withdrawal-sociability.

The classification has been replicated in research in the English prison system on *"normal"* murderers (McGurk, 1978), violent offenders (Henderson, 1982), and also unselected prisoners (McGurk and McGurk, 1979). The typology is therefore robust and represents the main personality types identifiable through self-report measures in prison and forensic psychiatric populations. These patterns are also recovered from cluster analysis of MCMI-1 personality disorder scales (Blackburn, 1996). The same types seem likely to emerge among antisocial populations from any comprehensive set of self-report measures of personality deviation because of the common influence of the two Big Five dimensions of neuroticism and extraversion. However, the sources of differentiation do not lie directly in these factors, but rather in their interaction in the aggression and withdrawal dimensions.

Differences on a number of variables have been found between the two *"psychopathic"* groups and C and I, but also between P and S. Although the groups are represented throughout the MDO population, P and S are more predominant in the legal category of psychopathic disorder than among the mentally ill (Blackburn, 1986, 1996). In one study (Blackburn, 1975), P and S were also found to have earlier criminal careers, although P had more convictions for violent crimes. Recent unpublished work tends to confirm these findings. P and S also score higher on the aggressive or antisocial personality disorder scale of the MCMI-1 (Blackburn, 1996). However, where P are also narcissistic and histrionic, S are passive-aggressive, avoidant, schizoid, dependent, and paranoid. The I group is also schizoid, avoidant, schizotypal, and passive aggressive, but differs from S in having low scores on the antisocial scale. Controlled patients score highest on the compulsive disorder scale, but show the least signs of personality disorder more generally.

Secondary psychopaths, who are characterized by the most deviant MMPI and SHAPS profiles, are also typically most deviant in other respects. The EEG abnormalities claimed in the older clinical literature to be common among psychopaths are most likely to be found in this group (Blackburn, 1979b; Howard, 1984), and they are also the least autonomically aroused (Blackburn, 1979b). In a delinquent sample, Gillham (1978) also found that S reported the least vivid emotional imagery. Primary psychopaths differ from S in having higher levels of cortical and autonomic arousal (Blackburn, 1979b), and score highest on Zuckerman's Sensation Seeking Scale (Blackburn, 1978). While the controlled group shows little distinctive that would not be anticipated from their denial of strong emotional reactions or socially improper behavior, the inhibited group was found by Henderson (1982) to include prisoners who were the least socially skilled.

P and S also describe themselves as more dominant in both threatening and affiliative settings, but differences between the psychopathic and nonpsychopathic groups are more apparent in threatening situations (Willner & Blackburn, 1988). On the other hand, S describe the most intense anger in response to verbal or physical threat (Blackburn & Lee-Evans, 1985). A study in an American prison also found that secondary psychopaths who are low in intelligence tend to be more violent than other inmates within the prison setting (Heilbrun and Heilbrun, 1985).

These findings overall support the validity of this empirically derived classification in discriminating classes of personality deviation among offenders. The first group has been described as *primary* psychopaths because it is distinguished by a pattern of traits that closely approximate the characteristics held to define the psychopath by the McCords and Cleckley. In particular, their hostile alienation from others, impulsivity, aggression, and a relative absence of anxiety or social inhibition are consistent with this concept. Findings that this group is distinguished by narcissism, sensation seeking, interpersonal dominance, and violent criminality strengthens this interpretation. The *secondary* psychopaths share some of these traits, but differ in showing extreme social anxiety and traits of schizoid, avoidant and passive-aggressive personality disorders. The differences between the two groups are in accord with the distinction made by Lykken (1957), who proposed that Cleckley psychopaths could be divided according to high and low trait anxiety, and this distinction was followed by several investigators until recently. It has, however, fallen into disfavor because it implies that there are two kinds of *"psychopath"*. This objection has some force in the context of the North American use of the term, although it has to be noted that in introducing the primary-secondary psychopath distinction, Karpman (1948) was following Schneider's broader use of the term psychopath. Nevertheless, although the label *"secondary psychopath"* may be misleading, the group it refers to is very real, and whatever the appropriate term, this is a clinically distinct and deviant group which seems to be prevalent among offenders.

The Psychopathy Checklist in mentally disordered offenders

The classification described above is *"objective"* insofar as it divides the population of MDOs into homogeneous groups on the basis of naturally occurring similarities of group members in their patterns of self-report. It has already been noted that the classification generalizes to other self-report measures, but its utility would clearly be strengthened if those identified as psychopaths were shown to correspond to psychopaths identified by the PCL. Some data are available to examine this question, but characteristics of PCL-defined psychopaths in this population will first be described.

There have been a few studies of the PCL in the special hospitals (e.g., Howard, 1990; O'Kane et al., 1996), but the most extensive was carried out by Coid as part of a survey of violent offenders and patients beginning in the mid 1980s. An initial report has been published (Coid, 1992) but the material reported here is derived from ongoing analyses of the data (Coid & Blackburn, in preparation). The sample consists of 86 male PD patients. Coid derived scores on the original 22-item PCL from interview and case records, but these have been reduced to the 20 items of the PCL-R. The mean PCL-R score is 21.60 ($SD = 9.08$), and 18 patients (21%) have a total score of 30 or more. No interrater reliability data were collected in this study, but the alpha coefficient is .91, and the factor structure is similar to that reported by others. Principal components analysis yielded three factors according to the scree test, accounting for 57% of the variance, and the first two rotated factors correspond to the social deviance and callous, remorseless factors identified by Hare et al. (1990). The present analyses, however, use the item scoring for the two factors derived by Hare et al. (1990). Alpha coefficients for Factor 1 (callous, etc.) and Factor 2 (social deviance) scores are .82 and .88, respectively, and the correlation between them is .63, slightly higher than that usually reported. There is a significant negative correlation between age and PCL-R total score ($r(84) = -.30$, $p < .001$) and scores on Factor 2 ($r(84) = -.37$, $p < .001$), and age was therefore entered as a covariate in most of the following analyses. PCL-R total scores were dichotomized at the recommended cutoff of 30 to form psychopathic ($n = 18$) and nonpsychopathic ($n = 68$) groups.

TABLE 2. Age at first conviction and mean convictions
of PCL-R groups

Criminal convictions	Psychopaths (n = 18)	Nonpsychopaths (n = 68)	F(1,83)
Age at first	13.61	18.29	7.72*
Total	16.56	6.32	27.86**
Violence	2.50	1.99	<1.0
Sex	1.44	0.88	1.49
Burglary	9.28	2.13	26.50**
Arson	0.22	0.28	<1.0
Property damage	0.56	0.49	<1.0
Fraud	1.61	0.10	21.90**
Robbery	0.72	0.28	3.53
Drug/Alcohol	0.17	0.10	<1.0

Note. PCL-R=Psychopathy Checklist-Revised.
** = p < .0001; * = p < .01

Also obtained in this study were criminal record information, DSM-III personality disorder diagnoses derived from a semi-structured interview (SCID-II), and lifetime DSM-III Axis I diagnoses made from research diagnostic criteria. Psychopaths in this population are broadly comparable to those in North American penal populations (e.g., Kosson et al., 1990) in being significantly more criminally inclined than nonpsychopaths (Table 2). Psychopaths have a higher mean number of convictions, and began their criminal careers at an earlier age than nonpsychopaths. Their greater number of convictions is due particularly to a high rate of burglary offences, but they also have more convictions for fraud and marginally more for robbery. However, psychopaths are not differentiated by violent or sexual offences.

Lifetime comorbidity data reveal that several psychopaths have a history of some form of Axis-I disorder. For example, 39% have a history of alcohol abuse, a third have experienced dysthymic disorder, and a fifth have a history of schizophrenic and depressive symptoms. However, the only significant differences lie in the higher prevalence of drug abuse in psychopaths (28%) compared to nonpsychopaths (7%: $X2(1) = 5.58$, $p < .05$), and in a more frequent history of somatization disorder in psychopaths (22% vs 3%: $X2(1) = 8.15, p < .01$).

Comparisons on categorical diagnoses of personality disorder (Table 3) indicate that most psychopaths, but less than a quarter of nonpsychopaths meet criteria for APD ($X2(1) = 30.27$, $p < .0001$), consistent with North American findings (Hare, 1991). Psychopaths are also more likely to meet criteria for paranoid ($X2(1) = 5.52, p < .05$), narcissistic $(X2(1) = 4.17, p < .05)$ and passive-aggressive $(X2(1) = 4.86, p < .05)$ disorders. Although many nonpsychopaths also exhibit borderline and narcissistic disorders, psychopaths meet criteria for more categories of disorder overall (means = 3.61 and 2.50: $t(84) = 2.87, p < .01$).

TABLE 3. Percentages of PCL-R groups in DSM-III personality disorder categories and correlations of PCL-R with personality disorder dimensional scores

Category	Psychopaths (n = 18)	Nonpsychopaths (n = 68)	Correlations PCL-R Total	Factor 1	Factor 2
Paranoid	50	22	.38***	.37*** .	34***
Schizoid	0	16	-.09	-.10	-.11
Schizotypal	6	22	-.13	-.16	-.12
Histrionic	22	10	.10	.19	.06
Narcissistic	66	40	.32**	.38***	.25*
Antisocial	94	24	.83***	.57***	.87***
Borderline	67	53	.36***	.17	.46***
Avoidant	6	9	-.15	-.31**	-.03
Dependent	11	22	-.32**	-.41***-.23*	
Compulsive	6	16	-.20	-.20	-.14
Passive-Aggressive	33	12	.31**	.25*	.35**

Note. PCL-R=Psychopathy Checklist-Revised.
*** = p < .001; ** = p < .01; * = p < .05 (N = 83).

However, correlations with dimensional scores (i.e. sums of all criteria within each category) indicate an association of the PCL-R with seven of the 11 disorders (Table 3). PCL-R total score correlates positively with paranoid, narcissistic, antisocial, borderline and passive-aggressive disorders, and negatively with dependent disorder. This is broadly consistent with previous reports (Hart & Hare, 1989; Hart et al., 1994), as is the positive correlation of Factor 1 with paranoid, narcissistic, antisocial, and passive-aggressive disorders, and the negative correlation with avoidant and dependent disorders. However, where Hart and Hare (1989) found that Factor 2 correlated significantly only with APD, in the present sample this factor also correlates positively with paranoid, narcissistic, borderline, and passive-aggressive disorders, and negatively with dependent disorder. The differences may reflect the lower base rate of psychopathy in the Hart and Hare sample, or the relatively greater correlation between PCL-R Factors 1 and 2 in the present sample. Nevertheless, the finding that both Factors 1 and 2 are associated with more than half of the DSM-III personality disorders is again consistent with the notion that psychopathy is a broad dimension of personality disorder.

The SHAPS classification and the PCL-R

What then of the relation of the PCL to the SHAPS typology described earlier? Two previous studies provide some evidence on this. First, an association has been found between the SHAPS impulsive aggression factor and the PCL. Kuriychuk (1990) found a correlation of .48 ($n = 60$: $p < .001$) between PCL total and the B (Belligerence) factor scale in a mixed sample of inmates and prison staff. Among inmates, however, the association was stronger with PCL Factor 2 ($r(38) = .36$, $p < .05$) than with Factor 1 ($r(38) = .30$, n.s.). O'Kane et al. (1996) similarly found that B correlated with total PCL-R score ($r(37) = .34$, $p < .05$) and PCL-R Factor 2 ($r(37) = .36$, $p < .05$), but not with PCL-R Factor 1 ($r(37) = .19$, n.s.).

Kuriychuk also compared SHAPS types derived from B and W scores with PCL classification of psychopaths. Although there was an overlap between SHAPS classification as a primary psychopath and identification as a psychopath by the PCL, secondary psychopaths were predominantly nonpsychopaths according to PCL criteria. In the O'Kane et al. sample, only one patient attained a PCL-R score of 30, precluding any direct comparison of classifications. When SHAPS factor scores were used to classify patients using an algorithm derived from an earlier study, there were no significant differences between the means of the four SHAPS groups on the PCL-R.

MMPI data were collected in Coid's study, but these were taken from psychology department files and in many cases had been obtained some years prior to the study. Because of organizational changes, we are currently unable to locate many of these records for further analysis. Nevertheless, we attempted to test the relationship of the SHAPS typology to PCL-R classification by estimating SHAPS factors from the eight SHAPS scales contained in the MMPI (this excludes the hostility and aggression scales), and by deriving the four types from factor scores through a nonhierarchical clustering procedure (k-means). The SHAPS types were then compared on the PCL-R and on personality disorder and criminality variables. The main interest is in whether primary psychopaths correspond to PCL-R psychopaths but also of concern is whether or not SHAPS secondary psychopaths are *"psychopathic"*. The data were therefore examined by means of planned orthogonal comparisons of P with the other three groups (S, C and I) and of S with C and I. The remaining orthogonal comparison is between the C and I groups.

There are several significant correlations between SHAPS measures and the PCL-R, although the relationships are of modest magnitude. PCL-R total score correlates with Impulsivity ($r(76) = .23$, $p < .05$), Extraversion ($r(76) = .26$, $p < .05$), and with the SHAPS Withdrawal factor ($r(76) = -.27$, $p < .05$). PCL-R Factor 1 also correlates with Extraversion ($r(76) = .26$, $p < .05$) and the Withdrawal factor ($r(76) = -.32$, $p < .01$), and with Shyness ($r(76) = -.23$, $p < .05$) and Anxiety ($r(76) = -.23$, $p < .05$). PCL-R Factor 2 correlates with Psychopathic Deviate ($r(76) = .23$, $p < .05$) and with Impulsivity ($r(76) = .24$, $p < .05$). The negative correlation of PCL-R Factor 1 with Anxiety (neuroticism) and the correlation of PCL-R Factor 2 with the *Pd* scale and Impulsivity are consistent with other reports (Hare, 1991). The correlation of PCL-R total and Factor 1 with Extraversion and Withdrawal is less consistent, but may reflect the negative correlation of Factor 1 with Anxiety and Shyness (*i.e.,* neurotic introversion). This could be interpreted as indirect support for the hypothesis that psychopathy is related to a weak Behavioral Inhibition System (Fowles, 1988). However, an association between PCL-R total and the SHAPS aggression factor in this sample is limited to the small correlation with Impulsivity.

TABLE 4. Means of SHAPS groups on PCL-R

| PCL-R | Groups | | | | Orthogonal comparisons | | |
| | P | S | C | I | P vs S,C,I | S vs C,I | C vs I |
	(n = 20)	(n = 21)	(n = 26)	(n = 13)	F(1,75)	F(1,75)	F(1,75)
Total	25.70	20.38	20.81	17.00	10.01**	<1.0	4.06*
Factor 1	11.40	8.67	10.08	7.85	8.24**	<1.0	5.04*
Factor 2	10.35	8.48	7.46	6.46	6.91**	1.41	1.96

Note. SHAPS=Special Hospitals Assessment of Personality and Socialisation; PCL-R = Psychopathy Checklist-Revised. P=Primary Psychopath; S=Secondary Psychopath; C=Controlled; I=Inhibited. ** = $p < .01$; * = $p < .05$

A significant relationship of the SHAPS typology to the PCL-R is nonetheless apparent from Table 4. Primary psychopaths attain the highest scores on PCL-R total and on both Factors 1 and 2, and the comparison with the other three groups yields significant effects for all three scores. The comparison of S with C and I did not yield a significant effect, but C has higher scores than I on PCL-R total and Factor 1. A significant association of the SHAPS and PCL-R classifications is also clear from Table 5, which indicates that 45% of primary psychopaths are also classified as psychopaths by the PCL-R, compared with 14% of secondary psychopaths, 12% of controlled patients, and none of the inhibited group. Primary psychopaths, then, are significantly more likely to meet the PCL-R criterion of psychopathy, but secondary psychopaths cannot be regarded as psychopathic in these terms, consistent with the findings of Kuriychuk (1990).

TABLE 5. Cross-tabulation of SHAPS and PCL-R classifications

PCL-R	Primary Psychopaths (n = 20)	Secondary Psychopaths (n = 21)	Controlled (n = 26)	Inhibited (n = 13)
Psychopaths	9	3	3	0
Nonpsychopaths	11	18	23	13

Note. SHAPS=Special Hospitals Assessment of Personality and Socialisation; PCL-R=Psychopathy Checklist-Revised. $X^2(3) = 13.21$: $p < .005$

When the data of Table 5 are reduced to a 2 X 2 table by combining S, C and I to form a single nonpsychopathic group, the overall agreement between the SHAPS and

PCL-R in classifying patients as psychopaths or nonpsychopaths is 79%, but kappa is a modest .38. In terms of predicting PCL-R classification from SHAPS classification, indices of diagnostic efficiency are: sensitivity .60, specificity .83, positive predictive value .45, and negative predictive value .90. Classifying patients as psychopaths on the basis of a SHAPS primary psychopath pattern is therefore likely to identify *nonpsychopaths* relatively effectively (specificity, negative predictive value), but many patients identified as primary psychopaths by the SHAPS will not be identified as psychopaths by the PCL-R (positive predictive value). The SHAPS *"misses"* differ from the *"hits"* in being older (mean ages 41.5 and 29.9, respectively) and relative latecomers to crime, but their level of convictions for sexual and violent offences is similar to that of SHAPS primary psychopaths with higher PCL-R scores. Despite not meeting PCL-R criteria of psychopathy, this group is deviant in several respects, but small numbers preclude reliable conclusions.

TABLE 6. Percentages of SHAPS groups in DSM-III
personality disorder categories

Category	Primary Psychopaths (n = 20)	Secondary Psychopaths (n = 21)	Controlled (n = 26)	Inhibited (n = 13)
Paranoid	30	38	27	0
Schizoid	0	29	4	31
Schizotypal	5	29	23	15
Histrionic	20	14	15	0
Narcissistic	65	29	50	31
Antisocial	55	38	31	15
Borderline	50	67	54	46
Avoidant	10	19	0	0
Dependent	30	29	15	8
Compulsive	15	19	12	15
Passive-Aggressive	15	24	12	15
Total categories	3.00	3.38	2.42	1.85

Note. SHAPS=Special Hospitals Assessment of Personality and
Socialisation.

Similarities of primary psychopaths to PCL-R psychopaths are also seen in comparisons of SHAPS groups on personality disorders and criminal history. Categorical personality disorder diagnoses of the four SHAPS groups are shown in Table 6. Although no single category is unique to any particular group, narcissistic, antisocial, borderline and paranoid disorders are the most frequent categories diagnosed among primary psychopaths, while borderline, antisocial, and paranoid disorders are the most frequent among secondary psychopaths. Secondary psychopaths also meet criteria for more categories of disorder than members of other groups. Comparisons of the number of criteria within each category (dimensional scores) indicate that relative to the other three groups, primary psychopaths exhibit more criteria for antisocial personality disorder ($p < .05$), and fewer traits of schizoid ($p < .001$) and schizotypal ($p < .01$) personality. They are also marginally more narcissistic and histrionic ($p < .10$). Secondary psychopaths are more avoidant ($p<.01$), paranoid ($p < .05$), and dependent ($p < .05$) than C and I, while C are more narcissistic ($p < .05$) and less schizoid ($p < .05$) than I. Although there are some differences between these results and previous findings using the MCMI-1 (Blackburn, 1996), these findings overall strengthen the evidence that the SHAPS types reflect distinguishable patterns of personality disorder.

SHAPS primary psychopaths also resemble PCL-R psychopaths in displaying higher levels of criminality. In particular, they have a higher mean number of convictions (10.20) than S, C and I (means = 5.95, 8.62, and 4.62, respectively: $F(1,76) = 4.98$, $p < .05$), and were on average first convicted at an earlier age ($p < .05$). However, although P also have the highest means for burglary and robbery, the differences are not significant. The remaining three groups do not differ in type of conviction, except that the controlled group has the highest mean number of convictions for fraud, while S and I have no convictions in this category. That the controlled group contains most of the fraudsters seems consistent with their low impulsivity and anxiety and with their relatively high score on PCL-R Factor 1 (Table 4).

Although the SHAPS primary psychopath group overlaps significantly with PCL-R psychopaths, the two classifications clearly produce differences in terms of personality disorder and criminality. It might be argued that this reflects limitations of the SHAPS in identifying psychopathic traits. However, the differences between the two classifications may be more readily interpreted in terms of the dimensions of personality deviation they are tapping. To examine this further, we factor analyzed the dimensionalized personality disorder measures. The scree test suggested three factors accounting for 53% of the variance. The rotated factors can be described broadly as impulsivity or *acting out* (antisocial, borderline, paranoid, narcissistic, passive-aggressive), emotional reactivity or *sensitivity* (avoidant, dependent, compulsive), and *withdrawal* versus spontaneity (schizotypal, schizoid versus histrionic).

There are clear differences in the pattern of associations of the PCL-R and SHAPS with personality disorder dimensions (Table 7). PCL-R total and both PCL-R factors correlate highly with the acting-out dimension. PCL-R total and Factor 1 are also negatively correlated with the sensitivity dimension, but the PCL-R is unrelated to the withdrawal dimension. In contrast, the SHAPS is related to all three personality disorder dimensions, but more particularly to sensitivity (Shyness, Depression, Tension, Anxiety, and the Aggression factor) and withdrawal (Shyness, Introversion, and the Withdrawal factor) and only modestly to the acting-out dimension (Psychopathic Deviate and Impulsivity). Individuals identified as psychopaths by the PCL-R and as primary psychopaths by the SHAPS will therefore occupy overlapping but not identical locations within the space of the three personality disorder dimensions. Although relatively small, the correlations of the SHAPS scales suggest an identification of the personality disorder dimensions with some of the Big Five personality factors.

TABLE 7. Correlations of PCL-R and SHAPS with personality disorder factors

Scale	Acting-out	Sensitivity	Withdrawal
PCL-R			
Total	.71***	-.32**	-.03
Factor 1	.60***	-.42**	-.07
Factor 2	.70***	-.19	-.03
SHAPS			
Lie	-.01	-.25*	-.04
Anxiety	-.02	.38**	.13
Extraversion	.11	-.11	-.34**
Shyness	-.04	.26*	.26*
Depression	.02	.26*	.18
Tension	.06	.42***	-.02
Psychopathic Deviate	.27*	.06	.01
Impulsivity	.24*	.19	.08
Factor 1 (Aggression)	.18	.30**	-.05
Factor 2 (Withdrawal)	-.13	.20	.32**

Note. PCL-R=Psychopathy Checklist-Revised; SHAPS=Special Hospitals Assessment of Personality and Socialisation.
*** = $p < .001$; ** = $p < .01$; * = $p < .05$ (N = 78).

The personality disorder factors do not align clearly with the SHAPS aggression and withdrawal factors, but the Anxiety and Extraversion scales have relatively strong correlations with the sensitivity and withdrawal dimensions, respectively. It is therefore likely that the latter dimensions of personality disorder are significantly related to neuroticism and introversion-extraversion. The acting out dimension seems most likely to represent the agreeableness-disagreeableness factor. In these terms, then, psychopathy as measured by the PCL-R is related primarily to disagreeableness and a low level of neuroticism. The SHAPS is primarily measuring neuroticism and extraversion and taps agreeableness only moderately.

This identification of the personality disorder dimensions is necessarily tentative. The equation of the first dimension with agreeableness rests in part on its small correlation with the Psychopathic Deviate scale, and although a relation of the second and third dimensions to neuroticism and extraversion seems more apparent, the MMPI records from which the relevant measures are derived were generally completed some time before the personality disorder interviews. It is conceivable that this has attenuated observed relationships, but further analysis with SHAPS data obtained concurrently will be necessary to clarify this. The association of the personality disorder dimensions with these three of the Big Five factors, however, agrees broadly with recent proposals (Widiger & Frances, 1994). Trull (1992), for example, found that these three factors had the strongest relation to personality disorder measures.

The apparent negative relation of the PCL-R, and particularly Factor 1, to neuroticism or anxiety also agrees with several findings (Hare, 1991), and the proposal that the PCL-R is closely related to agreeableness is consistent with the antagonistic, hostile, and callous attributes that define the disagreeableness pole of this factor. Although evidence on the relation of the PCL-R to current measures of the Big Five is limited, Harpur, Hart and Hare (1994) report a correlation of -.47 ($p<.05$) with the agreeableness factor of the NEO-PI in a sample of 28 inmates. This was the only correlation with the Big Five reaching a significant level. Agreeableness also most clearly distinguished psychopathic from nonpsychopathic inmates. Harpur et al. (1994) additionally carried out a regression analysis of the PCL-R and the Big Five in a student sample, and found that the role of agreeableness in predicting PCL scores was moderated by the neuroticism and conscientiousness dimensions, low scores on the latter dimensions increasing the predictability of the PCL-R from the Big Five.

Harpur et al. (1994) were primarily concerned with the predictability of the PCL-R from the Big Five. The focus here, however, is on the role of psychopathy in a dimensional model of personality deviation. Although it is apparent that the relation of the PCL-R to the Big Five is complex, it seems plausible to construe the PCL-R as a dimension of personality deviation within the space of the Big Five that is most closely related to agreeableness. Because agreeableness is an interpersonal dimension *par excellence*, this suggests an understanding of psychopathy in terms of interpersonal theory.

A COGNITIVE-INTERPERSONAL MODEL OF PSYCHOPATHY AND PERSONALITY DISORDER

The Interpersonal Circle

Although the empirical typology of personality deviation derived from the SHAPS reflects interactions of some of the Big Five personality dimensions, the SHAPS was developed essentially as a pragmatic instrument not tied to a particular theory of personality. In recent years, I have been interested in the potential of interpersonal theory for understanding personality disorders in general and psychopathy in particular.

The theory originated in the 1950s with Sullivan (1953) and Leary (1957) and has been developed more recently by Carson (1970) and Wiggins (Wiggins, 1982; Wiggins & Pincus, 1994; Wiggins & Trapnell, 1996). Sullivan integrated psycho-analysis with social psychology, and argued that the focus of psychopathology should be on what people are doing in their social interactions and relationships rather than on socially decontextualized individual behavior. He saw most psychiatric problems as the outcome of early distortions in relationships which are perpetuated into adult life.

Leary (1957) extended these ideas to an interpersonal theory of personality that has had a lasting impact in psychology (Wiggins, 1982). The basis is a descriptive scheme taking the form of the interpersonal circle. Intercorrelations of interpersonal behaviors typically produce a circular array, or circumplex, around a two-dimensional space. The two dimensions defining the space are first, the degree of power or control in an interaction (dominance versus submission), and second, the kind of affiliation (hostile versus friendly or nurturant). These dimensions represent the themes most commonly negotiated in social encounters, and the varying blends of these in interpersonal exchanges account for the circular ordering. The circumplex is illustrated by relationships between observer ratings of patient behavior found in a recent study (Figure 1). It will be noted that behaviors are similar to, and positively correlated with those adjacent around the circle, and negatively related to those opposite.

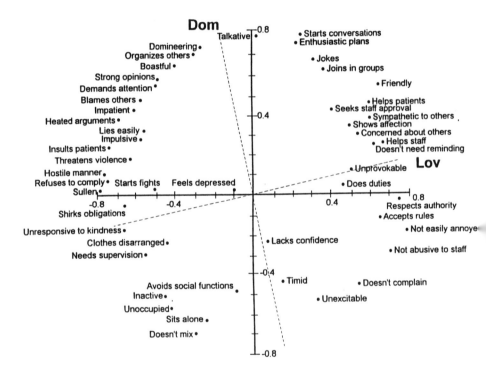

Figure 1. Plot of loadings of items (paraphrased) of the Chart of Interpersonal Reactions in Closed Living Environments (CIRCLE) on the first two principal components. Dotted lines are preliminary estimates of the optimal rotations of the Dominant-submissive (Dom) and Hostile-nurturant (Lov) axes (N = 210).

Note. From "Rating scales for measuring the interpersonal circle in forensic psychiatric patients," by R. Blackburn and S. J. Renwick, 1996, *Psychological Assessment, 8,* 76-84. Copyright 1996 by the American Psychological Association, Inc.

Some investigators work with the four quadrants of hostile-dominant, friendly-submissive, and so on, while others differentiate 32 points around the circle. Our own work follows Wiggins (Wiggins, 1982; Wiggins, Phillips, & Trapnell, 1989) in focusing on octants identified as dominant, coercive, hostile, etc. in Figure 2. However, the terminology differs from that of Wiggins. The octant labeled *coercive*, for example, is described by Wiggins as *arrogant-calculating* (and by Leary as *competitive-narcissistic*). Coercive is preferred here because the use of threats or punishments to gain compliance (Tedeschi, 1983) seems central to many of the behaviors making up this octant in our own work (Figure 1).

This descriptive system now has a firmly established empirical basis (Wiggins, 1982). The units of analysis may be dyadic interactions at the microanalytic level, but the system also applies to personality traits, or *interpersonal styles*. Adaptive responses to differing situational demands call for a repertoire of interpersonal skills represented at all parts of the circle. However, as a result of developmental experiences, people tend to acquire a distinctive style emphasizing a particular area of the circle. The more consistent or extreme a style, the narrower is the range of interactions on which the person relies. This follows from the circumplex structure in which segments of the circle are positively associated with adjacent segments, and negatively associated with opposite segments. A person with an extreme dominant style, for example, is someone whose interactions are marked by a high frequency of dominant exchanges. Such a person will also show coercive and sociable characteristics quite often, but submissive, withdrawn or compliant behavior infrequently. The individual's behavior will hence be rigid and inflexible.

The notion of inflexible interpersonal styles is consistent with the current concept of personality disorders as inflexible traits, and because these disorders are defined prominently by interpersonal dysfunction, several workers from Leary onwards have suggested that the interpersonal circle provides a basis for describing and classifying them (e.g., Blackburn, 1988; Kiesler, 1986; Widiger & Frances, 1985; Wiggins, 1982; Wiggins and Pincus, 1989). Classes of personality disorder would hence be represented as prototypical styles at different points around the circle. However, recent work suggests that personality disorders are more comprehensively described by the Big Five personality dimensions (Soldz, Budman, Demby, & Merry, 1993; Widiger & Frances, 1994; Wiggins & Pincus, 1994). Only two of these, extraversion and agreeableness, are represented within the interpersonal circle, corresponding approximately to axes falling between the coercive and hostile octants of Figure 2 (disagreeableness) and between the dominant and sociable octants (extraversion). Nevertheless, the evidence indicates that interpersonal dysfunction is central to histrionic, narcissistic, dependent, avoidant, schizoid, and antisocial personality disorders (Wiggins & Pincus, 1994).

Dominance and nurturance as rotational variants of extraversion and agreeableness may also have *"conceptual priority"* in the five-factor model of personality (Wiggins & Trapnell, 1996). Wiggins (1991) proposes that these interpersonal dimensions are concrete representations of the metaconcepts of *agency* (dominance) and *communion* (nurturance) that pervade the humanities and social sciences and have counterparts in many theories of personality. Agency (versus passivity) refers to a condition of being a differentiated individual and is manifest in strivings for mastery and power that enhance that differentiation. Communion (versus dissociation) is a condition of being part of a larger social or spiritual entity and is manifest in strivings for intimacy and solidarity with that larger entity. Wiggins argues that the other three of the Big Five are dimensions that either facilitate or interfere with agentic or communal strivings.

Interpersonal styles thus express fundamental motivational concerns. Wiggins notes that agency and communion are prominently represented in the social exchange theory of Foa and Foa (1974) by the resources of *status* (esteem, regard) and *love* (acceptance, liking), and proposes that variations in style around the interpersonal circle can be conceptualized in terms of the extent to which these resources are granted or denied to the self and others. A coercive style (Figure 2)), for example, entails the granting of both status and love to the self, but the denial or witholding of both to others. A dominant style differs in that love is granted to others, while a hostile style grants status but not love to self while denying both to others. This conceptualization provides a framework for understanding the dysfunctional traits that define personality disorders in terms of what is communicated in interpersonal transactions.

Psychopathy and the interpersonal circle

Psychopathy is identified particularly by interpersonal characteristics such as callous indifference to the effects of behavior on others, lack of affectional bonds, and manipulation or exploitation. Such characteristics are readily located as combinations of hostility and dominance in the interpersonal circle. It is therefore proposed here that psychopathy as a *dimension* corresponds broadly to the coercive-compliant axis of the circle. This is consistent with the evidence that psychopathy as measured by the PCL-R is closely related to agreeableness. It also broadly follows Leary (1957), although he located psychopathy more towards hostility (the aggressive-sadistic octant in his terms). However, because the location of an *individual* in the circle is defined by two orthogonal dimensions, those who are highly coercive will display varying interpersonal styles around the hostile-dominant quadrant, depending on their degree of withdrawal-gregariousness.

Only a few studies have so far examined this interpersonal conception of psychopathy, but the results are relatively consistent. A demonstration of the relationship between psychopathy and the interpersonal circle was reported by Blackburn & Maybury (1985). We obtained nurse ratings of Cleckley's criteria of psychopathy together with observer ratings of aggression and sociability, and several self-report personality measures, and extracted the first two principal components, which is a common means of identifying a circumplex. The relationship between these measures clearly corresponded to the interpersonal circle, with Cleckley's criteria falling around the hostile octant. However, cluster analysis of the observer ratings indicated two groups scoring high on the Cleckley measure of psychopathy. One psychopathic group was aggressive (coercive) and relatively gregarious. Most also belonged in the SHAPS primary psychopath group. The other psychopathic group was withdrawn and less aggressive, but did not correspond clearly to a specific SHAPS group.

Subsequent support for a relationship of psychopathy to the circle was provided by Harpur et al. (1989), who reported correlations of PCL scores with both self-ratings and observer ratings on Wiggins' Interpersonal Adjective scales (IAS), the most widely used measure of the circle. Psychopathy clearly projected onto the hostile-dominant quadrant. Factor 1 correlated with self-ratings of hostility (.26) and dominance (.35), hence falling within the coercive octant. Factor 2 was more closely related to hostility, while total PCL fell between the hostile and coercive axes. Correlations of the PCL with observer ratings of interpersonal style were somewhat stronger and consistently within the coercive octant, correlations of PCL total with hostility and dominance being .46 and .45, respectively.

Hart and Hare (1994) also recently reported correlations of the PCL-SV with interview-based ratings of Wiggins' IAS in a small sample of prisoners. They found that the PCL aligned closely with the coercive-compliant axis. However, it also correlated negatively with the conscientiousness factor of the Big Five.

Interpersonal style, personality disorder, and antisocial behavior

In recent work, we have expanded our earlier findings by developing a nurse rating scale to measure the interpersonal circle (Blackburn & Renwick, 1996). This instrument is described as CIRCLE (Chart of Interpersonal Reactions in Closed Living Environments), and the 49 items are relatively specific behaviors rated in terms of frequency. These map onto a two-dimensional space as required by the circumplex model (Figure 1). It will be noted that behaviors in the upper left (hostile-dominant) quadrant of Figure 1 are readily associated with psychopathy, notably *"shirks obligations"*, *"lies easily"*, *"impulsive"*, *"blames others"*, and *"demands attention"*. Items are grouped into eight scales to mark the octants around the circle, and the relationship between them meets the geometric requirements of a circumplex (Blackburn & Renwick, 1996).

Several investigations have examined the relation of personality disorder categories to self ratings of interpersonal style (e.g., DeJong, Brink, Jansen & Schippers, 1989; Morey, 1985; Soldz et al., 1993; Wiggins & Pincus, 1989). These studies support the general proposition that personality disorders have significant stylistic interpersonal components, and this has been replicated using CIRCLE ratings rather than self-reports (Blackburn, in press). Figure 2 shows the relationship of the MCMI-1 scales of personality disorder to CIRCLE dimensions. Although the MCMI-1 measures do not coincide precisely with the equivalent DSM-III disorders, of interest here is the location of *"acting out"* disorders, which were suggested earlier to be related to agreeableness. These disorders clearly project onto the hostile-dominant quadrant, the antisocial or aggressive category falling within the coercive octant. The relatively strong association of histrionic and narcissistic disorders with dominance appears to reflect the correlation of these MCMI-1 scales with extraversion (Blackburn, 1996). The lack of any distinct projection of the borderline disorder scale on the circle is consistent with evidence that this scale is related strongly to neuroticism, a dimension theoretically orthogonal to the dimensions of the circle (Wiggins & Pincus, 1994). The SHAPS groups described earlier are also differentiated by their interpersonal styles as assessed by CIRCLE (Blackburn, 1993b). Primary psychopaths attain the highest scores on the coercive scale, but their modal style is predominantly dominant-gregarious.

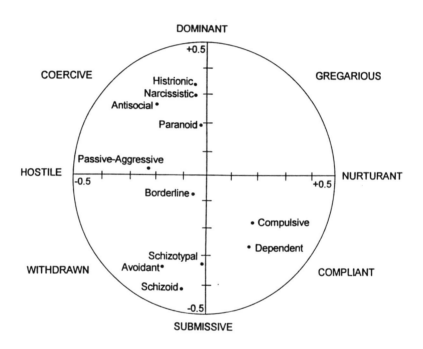

Figure 2. Correlations of personality disorder scales of the Millon Clinical Multiaxial Inventory (MCMI - 1) with the coordinates of the Chart of Interpersonal Reactions in Closed Living Environments (CIRCLE) (N = 104).

This pattern coincides with their self-reported extraversion and narcissism. Secondary psychopaths are also coercive, but differ from primary psychopaths in being more submissive and withdrawn. However, they have the least distinctive interpersonal style, perhaps reflecting the extreme neuroticism defining this group. The interpersonal characteristics of the controlled and inhibited groups are also broadly consistent with their self-report patterns. Controlled patients are rated on average as nurturant, compliant and gregarious, while inhibited patients are withdrawn, submissive and compliant.

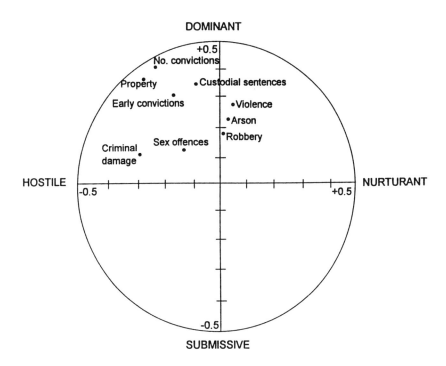

Figure 3. Correlations of criminal history variables with the coordinates of the Chart of Interpersonal Reactions in Closed Living Environments (CIRCLE) (N = 59).

The association of psychopathy and acting-out disorders with hostile-dominant interpersonal styles suggests that criminal behavior may also be related to the circle. We therefore recently examined the relation of CIRCLE to criminal history. Among patients in the legal category of psychopathic disorder, there are several relatively strong correlations between interpersonal style and criminality (Figure 3). A coercive interpersonal style is clearly associated with more persistent criminality as reflected in total number of convictions, convictions for property offences (burglary, theft, robbery), and a history of convictions at an early age. These are the variables we found to be most strongly related to the PCL-R in this population (Table 2). However, violence falls within the dominant-friendly quadrant, suggesting correlates with extraversion as much as with disagreeableness, and it will be recalled that the more extreme scores on the PCL-R in this population did not distinguish the most violent offenders.

These correlations are interesting because CIRCLE ratings were obtained on average six years after the patient's most recent criminal conviction. It is possible that they reflect an *effect* of differential treatment of the more criminally inclined within the secure hospital system and the development of coercive-dominant styles as coping strategies by such individuals. However, an absence of any relationship of interpersonal style with duration of detention argues against this (Blackburn & Renwick, 1996). It is therefore likely that these findings represent a causal relation between interpersonal style and criminality and indicate the relative consistency of interpersonal style over time.

The only data we have at present on the relation of the PCL-R to CIRCLE comes from a sample of 40 male mentally disordered offenders, half of them mentally ill and half in the psychopathic disorder category, who were assessed with the PCL-R by means of interview and case record review (O'Kane et al., 1996). The mean PCL-R score is 15.50 (SD = 5.69), which is substantially lower than that of the sample described earlier, and only one patient scores at the cutoff score of 30. This is not due to any difference between the mentally ill and psychopathic disorder patients, nor to low rater reliability, the correlation between two raters being .91. Alpha coefficients for PCL-R total and for Factors 1 and 2 are .73, .74, and .65, respectively, and the correlation between Factors 1 and 2 is .35 (p<.05). Whether the low mean score reflects sampling bias, recent changes in the population, or a threshold effect in rating psychopathic traits is unknown.

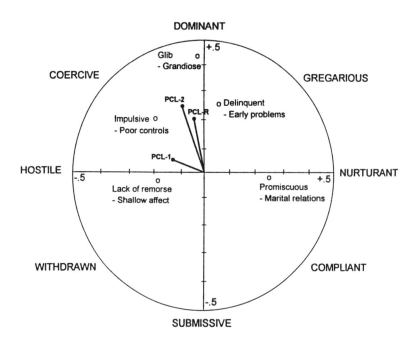

Figure 4. Correlations of the Psychopathy Checklist-Revised (PCL-R), factors 1 (PCL-1) and 2 (PCL-2), and PCL-R item clusters (0) with the coordinates of the Chart of Interpersonal Reactions in Closed Living Environments (CIRCLE) (N = 40).

The projection of the PCL-R measures on the circle is again as predicted in the hostile-dominant quadrant, but the relationships are generally weak (Figure 4). However, when PCL-R items were clustered by means of elementary linkage analysis, they fell into five distinguishable groups, and scores on these clusters are differentially related to the circle (Figure 4). Glibness and grandiosity are closely related to dominance, but lack of remorse, shallow affect and callousness are more closely related to hostility. The latter is consistent with our earlier findings (Blackburn & Maybury, 1985), as is the relation of impulsivity and poor behavior controls to the coercive octant. The results are also consistent with the suggestion that psychopaths are not homogeneous in interpersonal style and that high scorers on the PCL-R may vary in their location around the hostile-dominant quadrant. However, in view of the size of the current sample and range restriction in PCL-R scores, firm generalizations are not warranted.

The evidence reviewed above lends some support to the proposal that psychopathy is primarily an interpersonal dimension associated with the hostile-dominant quadrant of the interpersonal circle and with the personality dimension of agreeableness. Because the interpersonal circle assesses only two of the Big Five dimensions of personality, discrimination within socially deviant populations needs to take account of *intra*personal factors. For example, data presented earlier appears to support an association of psychopathy with low levels of anxiety or neuroticism. Nevertheless, interpersonal theory has implications for the explanation of psychopathy and for possible intervention strategies.

Interpersonal style, cognition, and personality disorder

Perhaps because of the influence of psychodynamic thinking and positivism, most theories of psychopathy have been bottom-up rather than top-down. For example, explanations have commonly emphasized affective deficits and associated psychophysiological or neuropsychological processes (Blackburn, 1993a). However, the cognitive revolution has demonstrated that affect needs to be seen in terms of top-down processes because cognitions are emergent properties with the causal power to determine emotional and social responses (Sperry, 1993). Although a biological basis to personality dimensions is generally acknowledged, an understanding of disorders of personality may more readily be found in dysfunctional cognitions.

Beck and Freeman (1990) have developed the best known cognitive theory of personality disorder. They propose that each personality disorder represents a generalized behavior strategy dictated by cognitive schemata that are organized around a general theme of the nature of self and others. The core beliefs of antisocial personalities, for example, relate to looking out for oneself and an entitlement to break rules. This, however, seems to be little more than a translation of DSM-III criteria. A more process oriented model which is underpinned by research in social cognition comes from interpersonal theorists.

In Wiggins' analysis of the motivational significance of the interpersonal circle (Wiggins & Trapnell, 1996), a coercive style represents the granting of status and love to the self and denial of these to others. Concerns about power and status in social hierarchies (agency) in the context of rejection or avoidance of intimacy (communion) would therefore be expected to be central to psychopathy, although variations might be anticipated depending on how close the individual falls to dominance or hostility. More dominant psychopaths (who seem close to SHAPS primary psychopaths), for example, might be expected to form intimate ties, i.e., grant love to others, while still being egocentric and concerned about status in interactions. As suggested by Figure 4, superficial charm and grandiosity may in particular characterize this subgroup. Psychopaths characterized by a more hostile style, on the other hand, may be more callous and concerned with avoiding intimacy. This concept of psychopathic personality is exemplified in Leary's identification of psychopaths as aggressive-sadistic (Leary, 1957). As he puts it, *"The essence of the psychopathic state is active aggression. These patients avoid anxiety and maintain security by avoiding dependent or tender feelings and by integrating critical, punitive relations with others."* (p. 347). Millon (1981) offers a similar account of the aggressive or antisocial personality, proposing that the aggression of such individuals is a pre-emptive counterattack in the face of anticipations that others will exploit, dominate and brutalize them. These conceptions imply that much of the behavior of psychopaths is motivated by interpersonal *beliefs*.

Attachment theory (Ainsworth & Bowlby, 1991; Main, 1996) shares common ground with interpersonal theory, and there are some suggestive findings in the literature of a link between attachment patterns, interpersonal style, and psychopathic traits. The theory emphasizes the quality of infant-caregiver attachment during the first year of life as a determinant of later cognitive and social development. This appears to be particularly relevant to psychopathy in view of evidence that psychopaths have commonly experienced abuse as children (Forth & Tobin, 1995; McCord & McCord, 1964). Recent work focuses on adult attachment and recognises a *dismissive* pattern of attachment, a strategy that minimizes distressing thoughts and affects associated with rejection by the attachment figure. Bartholomew and Horowitz (1991) examined the correlates of adult attachment in students, and found that the dismissive pattern was associated with high self-confidence but lack of closeness in personal relationships. On a measure of the interpersonal circle, this pattern was related quite strongly to the cold (hostile) and competitive (coercive) octants. Among hospitalized adolescents, Rosenstein and Horowitz (1996) further found that the dismissive pattern was related to conduct disorder and substance abuse. Dismissive adolescents also scored higher on the antisocial, narcissistic, and paranoid personality disorder scales of the MCMI, and lower on avoidance.

In attachment theory, early attachments affect later relationships outside the family through the internalization of a *working model* of dyadic relationships that dictates expectations of how significant others will respond to the self. A similar cognitive approach underlies accounts of the development of interpersonal styles by interpersonal theorists (Carson, 1970; 1979; Kiesler, 1986; 1988). This model conceptualizes personality disorders as dysfunctional interpersonal styles supported by biased expectations which function as self-fulfilling prophecies through their effects on others.

According to interpersonal theory, a particular behavior *"pulls"* a reaction from the other person, within a limited range, and this is governed by principles of complementarity (Kiesler, 1986). Along the dominance-submission axis, complementarity is reciprocal, *i.e.,* a dominant response pulls a submissive reaction, while along the hostile-friendly axis, the relation is corresponding or congruent, *i.e.,* a hostile response invites a hostile reaction. These will be combined for different behaviors around the circle. For example, hostile-dominant behavior is likely to elicit a hostile-submissive reaction. The effect of a rigid interpersonal style will be for the person to produce many anti-complementary reactions which are aversive to other people.

Carson (1979) argues that the persistence of interpersonal styles across the life-span and across situations can be understood in terms of expectancy confirmation processes. He proposes a causal relation between expectancies, interpersonal style, and the behavior of others. The avoidance of cognitive dissonance is maintained by eliciting behavior from the other in accord with the concept of the self and one's role in the interaction. A particular overture involves verbal and non-verbal behavior which sends a message about the relationship, not necessarily at a conscious level. It invites a complementary response from the other, which if forthcoming, provides feedback confirming the relationship.

Extending this analysis to rigid interpersonal styles, Carson suggests that early interactions create expectations of how others are likely to react to oneself, and these expectations subsequently become self-fulfilling prophecies. Behavior is directed to others to elicit a complementary reaction which then confirms the expectations. Thus, a hostile person expects hostile reactions from others and behaves in a way which gets them. People with strong expectations are thus likely to create interactions which minimize the chance of disconfirming experiences. Extreme interpersonal styles and personality disorders should therefore be associated with particular kinds of expectancies. For example, the coercive style proposed to characterize psychopathy would be expected to be associated with expectations of both hostile-submission and hostile-dominance, according to Carson, and a relative lack of skills for eliciting other reactions. Lack of empathic concern and manipulation of others would readily follow from such beliefs. Friendly-dominance, on the other hand, should be associated with expectations of friendly-submission.

To explore this hypothesis, we constructed a simple measure of social expectations. This asks patients to indicate how often they expect other people to avoid them, criticize them, behave in a hostile way, be sympathetic, and so on, selection of the 32 items being guided by the interpersonal circle. Items were grouped into four scales representing the four quadrants of the circle. A sample of 99 patients was assigned to the four quadrant groups according to CIRCLE interpersonal style and compared on the measures of interpersonal expectations.

There is a significant interaction between interpersonal style and interpersonal expectations, which is most marked for the hostile-dominant and friendly-submissive scales (Table 8). The hostile-dominant group expect others to be hostile-dominant, and tend to have the strongest expectations of hostile-submission ($p < .08$). The friendly-dominant group, in contrast, primarily expect others to be friendly-submissive. These results are broadly in line with Carson's model, although the other two groups do not show distinctive expectations. High scores on the PCL-R would also be predicted to be associated with expectations of hostile-dominance and hostile-submission in others, but this must await future research.

TABLE 8. Means (standardised scores) of CIRCLE groups on Expectations of Others scales

	Group				
Scale	Hostile-Dominant (n = 19)	Hostile-Submissive (n = 24)	Friendly-Dominant (n = 25)	Friendly-Submissive (n = 31)	F(3,89)
HD	.64	-.17	-.11	-.08	3.23*
HS	.54	-.15	-.04	-.12	2.37
FD	.26	-.09	.20	-.13	<1.0
FS	-.32	-.01	.49	-.15	3.01*

Note. HD=Hostile-dominant; HS=Hostile-submissive; FD=Friendly-dominant; FS=Friendly-Submissive.
* = p < .05

Although many clinicians consider psychopaths to be untreatable, firm evidence favoring this view is lacking (Blackburn, 1993c; Dolan & Coid, 1993), and few treatment studies have employed a systematic theory of psychopathy. The cognitive model described has clear implications for treatment interventions with this group. To the extent that dysfunctional styles of relating are supported by biased or distorted expectations, the target for change is the individual's dysfunctional belief system. This is the goal of Beck's cognitive therapy for personality disorders (Beck and Freeman, 1990). However, interpersonal theory offers a more systematic approach to the treatment of personality disorders, and several North American therapists have developed procedures guided explicitly by interpersonal complementarity principles (Carson, 1979; Kiesler, 1988; Safran, 1990). They argue that therapy should focus on disconfirming interpersonal expectations, and that this can be achieved through the medium of the therapist-client relationship. In the case of institutionalized offenders, the model suggests programming the environment to provide not only disconfirming experiences, but also opportunities for developing new interpersonal skills.

CONCLUSIONS

Many of the findings reported in this chapter are no more than suggestive and require replication. However, they support the conceptualization of psychopathy as a dimension of personality disorder linked in turn to the structure of personality as it is currently understood. I have suggested that psychopathy can be understood primarily as the coercive control of interpersonal transactions, and that social cognitive processes may be a possible key to this understanding. In these terms, the behavior of psychopaths is meaningful and, however destructive or *"evil"*, represents their attempts to make sense of the world as they see it. Given our continuing perplexity about this behavior, the interpersonal characteristics of psychopaths seem worth exploring further.

References

Ainsworth, M. D. S., & Bowlby, J. (1991). An ethological approach to personality development. *American Psychologist, 46,* 333-341.

American Psychiatric Association. (1994). *Diagnostic and statistical manual of mental disorders* (4th ed.). Washington, DC: Author.

Andrews, D. A., & Wormith, J. S. (1989). Personality and crime: Knowledge destruction and construction in criminology. *Justice Quarterly, 6,* 289-309.

Bartholomew, K., & Horowitz, L. M. (1991). Attachment styles among young adults: A test of a four category model. *Journal of Personality and Social Psychology, 61,* 226-244.

Beck, A. T., & Freeman, A. (1990). Cognitive therapy of personality disorders. New York: Guilford.

Becker, W. C. (1960). The matching of behavior rating and questionnaire personality factors. *Psychological Bulletin, 57,* 201-212.

Blackburn, R. (1968). Personality in relation to extreme aggression in psychiatric offenders. *British Journal of Psychiatry, 114,* 821-828.

Blackburn, R. (1971). Personality types among abnormal homicides. *British Journal of Criminology, 11,* 14-31.

Blackburn, R. (1975). An empirical classification of psychopathic personality. *British Journal of Psychiatry, 127,* 456-460.

Blackburn, R. (1978). Psychopathy, arousal, and the need for stimulation. In R. D. Hare & D. Schalling (Eds.), *Psychopathic behavior: Approaches to research* (pp. 157-164). Chichester: Wiley.

Blackburn, R. (1979a). Psychopathy and personality: The dimensionality of self-report and behaviour rating data in abnormal offenders. *British Journal of Social and Clinical Psychology, 18,* 111-119.

Blackburn, R. (1979b). Cortical and autonomic arousal in primary and secondary psychopaths. *Psychophysiology, 16,* 143-150.

Blackburn, R. (1986). Patterns of personality deviation among violent offenders: Replication and extension of an empirical taxonomy. *British Journal of Criminology, 26,* 254-269.

Blackburn, R. (1987). Two scales for the assessment of personality disorder in antisocial populations. *Personality and Individual Differences, 8,* 81-93.

Blackburn, R. (1988). On moral judgements and personality disorders: The myth of the psychopathic personality revisited. *British Journal of Psychiatry, 153,* 505-512.

Blackburn, R. (1993a). *The psychology of criminal conduct: Theory, research and practice.* Chichester: Wiley.

Blackburn, R. (1993b). Psychopathic disorder, personality disorders and aggression. In C. Thompson & P. Cowen (Eds.), *Violence: Basic and clinical science* (pp. 101-118). Oxford: Butterworth-Heinemann.

Blackburn, R. (1993c). Clinical programmes with psychopaths. In C. R. Hollin & K. Howells (Eds.), *Clinical approaches to the mentally disordered offender* (pp. 179-208). Chichester: Wiley.

Blackburn, R. (1996). Replicated personality disorder clusters among mentally disordered offenders and their relation to dimensions of personality. *Journal of Personality Disorders, 10,* 68-81.

Blackburn, R. (In press). Relationship of personality disorders to ratings of interpersonal style in forensic psychiatric patients. *Journal of Personality Disorders.*

Blackburn, R., Crellin, M. C., Morgan, E. M., and Tulloch, R. M. B. (1990). Prevalence of personality disorders in a special hospital population. *Journal of Forensic Psychiatry, 1*, 43-52.

Blackburn, R., & Lee-Evans, M. (1985). Reactions of primary and secondary psychopaths to anger evoking situations. *British Journal of Clinical Psychology, 24*, 93-100.

Blackburn, R., & Maybury, C. (1985). Identifying the psychopath; The relation of Cleckley's criteria to the interpersonal domain. *Personality and Individual Differences, 6*, 375-386.

Blackburn, R., & Renwick, S. J. (1996). Rating scales for measuring the interpersonal circle in forensic psychiatric patients. *Psychological Assessment, 8*, 76-84.

Blashfield, R. K. (1980). Propositions regarding the use of cluster analysis in clinical research. *Journal of Consulting and Clinical Psychology, 48*, 456-459.

Carson, R. C. (1970). *Interaction concepts of personality*. Chicago: Aldine.

Carson, R. C. (1979). Personality and exchange in developing relationships. In R. L. Burgess & T. L. Huston (Eds.), *Social Exchange in Developing Relationship* (pp.247-269). New York: Academic Press.

Clark, L. A., Watson, D., & Reynolds, S. (1995). Diagnosis and classification of psychopathology: Challenges to the current system and future directions. *Annual Review of Psychology, 46*, 121-153.

Clarkin, J. F., & Kendall, P. C. (1992). Comorbidity and treatment planning: Summary and future directions. *Journal of Consulting and Clinical Psychology, 60*, 904-908.

Cleckley, H. (1976). *The Mask of Sanity* (6th ed.). St. Louis: Mosby.

Coid, J. W. (1992). DSM-III diagnosis in criminal psychopaths: A way forward. *Criminal Behaviour and Mental Health, 2*, 78-94.

DeJong, C., Brink, W., Jansen, J., & Schippers, G. (1989). Interpersonal aspects of DSM-III Axis II: Theoretical hypotheses and empirical findings. *Journal of Personality Disorders, 3*, 135-146.

Dolan, B., & Coid, J. (1993). *Psychopathic and antisocial personality disorders: Treatment and research issues*. London: Gaskell.

Foa, U. G., & Foa, E. B. (1974). *Societal structures of the mind*. Springfield, IL: Thomas.

Forth, A. E., & Tobin, F. (1995). Psychopathy and young offenders: Rates of childhood maltreatment. *Forum on Corrections Research, 7*, 20-23.

Foulds, G. A. (1971). Personality deviance and personal symptomatology. *Psychological Medicine, 1*, 222-233.

Fowles, D. C. (1988). Psychophysiology and psychopathology: A motivational approach. *Psychophysiology, 25*, 373-391.

Gifford, R. (1994). A lens-mapping framework for understanding the encoding and decoding of interpersonal dispositions in nonverbal behavior. *Journal of Personality and Social Psychology, 66*, 398-412.

Gillham, R. (1978). An investigation of imagery in psychopathic delinquents. Unpublished BSc dissertation, University of Aberdeen, Scotland.

Gough, H. G. (1948). A sociological theory of psychopathy. *American Journal of Sociology, 53*, 359-366.

Gray. J. A. (1987). Perspectives on anxiety and impulsivity. *Journal of Research in Personality, 21*, 493-509.

Hare, R. D. (1980). A research scale for the assessment of psychopathy in criminal populations. *Personality and Individual Differences, 1*, 111-119.

Hare, R. D. (1985). A comparison of procedures for the assessment of psychopathy. *Journal of Consulting and Clinical Psychology, 53*, 7-16.

Hare, R. D. (1991). *The Hare Psychopathy Checklist-Revised*. Toronto: Multi-Health Systems.

Hare, R. D. (In press). Psychopathy: A clinical construct whose time has come. *Criminal Justice and Behavior*.

Hare, R. D., & Cox, D. N. (1978). Clinical and empirical conceptions of psychopathy, and the selection of subjects for research. In R. D. Hare & D. Schalling (Eds.), *Psychopathic behavior: Approaches to research* (pp. 1-21). Chichester: Wiley.

Hare, R. D., Harpur, T. J., Hakstian, A. R., Forth, A. E., Hart, S. D., & Newman, J. P. (1990). The revised Psychopathy Checklist: Reliability and factor structure. *Psychological Assessment: A Journal of Consulting and Clinical Psychology, 2*, 338-341.

Hare, R. D., & Hart, S. D. (1993). Psychopathy, mental disorder, and crime. In S. Hodgins (Ed.), *Mental disorder and crime*. Newbury Park, CA: Sage.

Hare, R. D., Hart, S. J., & Harpur, T. J. (1991). Psychopathy and the DSM-IV criteria for antisocial personality disorder. *Journal of Abnormal Psychology, 100*, 391-398.

Hare, R. D., McPherson, L. M., & Forth, A. E. (1988). Male psychopaths and their criminal careers. *Journal of Consulting and Clinical Psychology, 56*, 710-714.

Harpur, T. J., Hare, R. D., & Hakstian, A. R. (1989). Two-factor conceptualisation of psychopathy: Construct validity and assessment implications. *Psychological Assessment: A Journal of Consulting and Clinical Psychology, 1*, 6-17.

Harpur, T. J., Hart, S. D., & Hare, R. D. (1994). Personality of the psychopath. In P. T. Costa & T. A. Widiger (Eds.) *Personality disorders and the five-factor model of personality*, (pp. 149-173). Washington, DC: American Psychological Association.

Harris, G. T., Rice, M. E., & Cormier, C. A. (1991). Psychopathy and violent recidivism. *Law and Human Behavior, 15*, 625-637.

Harris, G. T., Rice, M. E., & Quinsey, V. L. (1994). Psychopathy as a taxon: Evidence that psychopaths are a discrete class. *Journal of Consulting and Clinical Psychology, 62*, 387-397.

Hart, S. J., Forth, A. E., & Hare, R. D. (1991). The MCMI-II and psychopathy. *Journal of Personality Disorders, 5*, 318-327.

Hart, S. D., & Hare, R. D. (1989). Discriminant validity of the Psychopathy Checklist in a forensic psychiatric population. *Psychological Assessment: A Journal of Consulting and Clinical Psychology, 2*, 338-341.

Hart, S. D., & Hare, R. D. (1994). Psychopathy and the big five: Correlations between observers' ratings of normal and pathological personality. *Journal of Personality Disorders, 8*, 32-40.

Hart, S. D., Hare, R. D., & Forth, A. E. (1994). Psychopathy as a risk marker for violence: Development and validation of a screening version of the revised Psychopathy Checklist. In J. Monahan & H. J. Steadman (Eds.), *Violence and Mental Disorder: Developments in risk assessment* (pp. 81-99). Chicago: University of Chicago Press.

Heilbrun, A. B., & Heilbrun, M. R. (1985). Psychopathy and dangerousness: Comparison, integration, and extension of two psychopathic typologies. *British Journal of Clinical Psychology, 24*, 181-195.

Henderson, M. (1982). An empirical classification of convicted violent offenders. *British Journal of Criminology, 22*, 1-20.

Hogan, R., & Nicholson, R. A. (1988). The meaning of personality test scores. *American Psychologist, 43*, 621-626.

Howard, R. C. (1984). The clinical EEG and personality in mentally abnormal offenders. *Psychological Medicine, 14*, 569-580.

Howard, R. C. (1990). Psychopathy Checklist scores in mentally abnormal offenders: A re-examination. *Personality and Individual Differences, 11*, 1087-1091.

Karpman, B. (1948). The myth of the psychopathic personality. *American Journal of Psychiatry, 104*, 523-534.

Kassebaum, G. C., Couch, A. S., & Slater, P. E. (1959). The factorial dimensions of the MMPI. *Journal of Consulting Psychology, 23*, 226-236.

Kiesler, D. J. (1986). The 1982 interpersonal circle; An analysis of DSM-III personality disorders. In T. Millon & G. Klerman (Eds.), *Contemporary directions in psychopathology: Towards DSM-IV* (pp. 571-598). New York: Guilford Press.

Kiesler, D. J. (1988). *Therapeutic metacommunication: Therapist impact disclosure as feedback in psychotherapy*. Palo Alto, CA: Consulting Psychologists Press.

Kosson, D. S., Smith, S. S., & Newman, J. P. (1990). Evaluating the construct validity of psychopathy on black and white male inmates: Three preliminary studies. *Journal of Abnormal Psychology, 99*, 250-259.

Kuriychuk, M. (1990). *The assessment of psychopathy and risk-taking behavior*. Unpublished doctoral dissertation, Queen's University, Kingston, Ontario.

Leary, T. (1957). *Interpersonal diagnosis of personality*. New York: Ronald Press.

Lorr, M. (1983). *Cluster analysis for social scientists*. San Francisco: Jossey-Bass.

Lykken, D. T. (1957). A study of anxiety in the sociopathic personality. *Journal of Abnormal and Social Psychology, 55*, 6-10.

Main, M. (1996). Introduction to the special section on attachment and psychopathology: 2. Overview of the field of attachment. *Journal of Consulting and Clinical Psychology, 64*, 237-243.

McCord, W. M., & McCord, J. (1964). *The psychopath: An essay on the criminal mind*. New York: Van Nostrand.

McGurk, B. J. (1978). Personality types among normal homicides. *British Journal of Criminology, 18*, 146-161.

McGurk, B. J., & McGurk, R. E. (1979). Personality types among prisoners and prison officers. *British Journal of Criminology, 19*, 31-49.

Megargee, E. I. (1966). Undercontrolled and overcontrolled personality types in extreme antisocial aggression. *Psychological Monographs, 80*, Whole No. 611.

Millon, T. (1981). *Disorders of personality: DSM III: Axis II*. New York: Wiley.

Morey, L. C. (1985). An empirical classification of interpersonal and DSM-III approaches to classification of personality disorders. *Psychiatry, 48*, 358-363.

O'Kane, A., Fawcett, D., & Blackburn, R. (1996). Psychopathy and moral reasoning: Comparison of two methods of assessment. *Personality and Individual Differences, 20*, 504-514.

Peterson, D. R., Quay, H. C., & Cameron, G. R. (1959). Personality and background factors in juvenile delinquency as inferred from questionnaire responses. *Journal of Consulting Psychology, 23*, 295-399.

Pichot, P. (1978). Psychopathic behavior: A historical overview. In R. D. Hare & D. Schalling (Eds.), *Psychopathic behavior: Approaches to research* (pp. 55-70). Chichester: Wiley.

Retzlaff, P. D., & Gibertini, M. (1987). Factor structure of the MCMI basic personality scales and common-item artefact. *Journal of Personality Assessment, 51*, 588-594.

Rosenstein, D. S., & Horowitz, H. A. (1996). Adolescent attachment and psychopathology. *Journal of Consulting and Clinical Psychology, 64*, 244-253.

Safran, J. D. (1990). Toward a refinement of cognitive therapy in light of interpersonal theory: 1. Theory. *Clinical Psychology Review, 10*, 87-105.

Schneider, K. (1950). *Psychopathic personalities* (9th ed.). London: Cassell. (Original work published 1923).

Serin, R. C. (1996). Violent recidivism in criminal psychopaths. Law and Human Behavior, 20, 207-217.

Soldz, S., Budman, S., Demby, A., & Merry, J. (1993). Representation of personality disorders in circumplex and five-factor space: Explorations with a clinical sample. *Psychological Assessment, 5*, 41-52.

Sperry, R. W. (1993). The impact and promise of the cognitive revolution. *American Psychologist, 48*, 878-885.

Sullivan, H. S. (1953). *The interpersonal theory of psychiatry.* New York: Norton.

Tedeschi, J. T. (1983). Social influence theory and aggression. In R. G. Geen & E. I. Donnerstein (Eds.), *Aggression: Theoretical and empirical reviews* (Vol. 1, pp. 1-25). New York: Academic Press.

Trull, T. J. (1992). DSM-III-R personality disorders and the five-factor model of personality: An empirical comparison. *Journal of Abnormal Psychology, 101*, 553-560.

Tyrer, P. (1988a). What's wrong with DSM-III personality disorders? *Journal of Personality Disorders, 2*, 281-291.

Tyrer, P. (1988b). Personality disorders: Diagnosis, management and course. London: Wright.

Widiger, T. A. (1991). Personality disorder dimensional models proposed for DSM-IV. *Journal of Personality Disorders, 5*, 386-398.

Widiger, T. A., & Frances, A. J. (1985). The DSM-III personality disorders: Perspectives from psychology. *Archives of General Psychiatry, 42*, 615-623.

Widiger, T. A., & Frances, A. J. (1994). Toward a dimensional model for the personality disorders. In P. T. Costa & T. A. Widiger (Eds.), *Personality disorders and the five-factor model of personality* (pp. 19-39). Washington, DC: American Psychological Association.

Wiggins, J. S. (1982). Circumplex models of interpersonal behavior in clinical psychology. In P. C. Kendall & J. N. Butcher (Eds.), *Handbook of research methods in clinical psychology* (pp. 183-221). New York: Wiley.

Wiggins, J. S. (1991). Agency and communion as conceptual co-ordinates for the understanding and measurement of interpersonal behavior. In W. M. Grove & D. Cicchetti, (Eds.), *Thinking clearly about psychology: Essays in honor of Paul E. Meehl* (Vol. 2, pp. 89-113). Minneapolis: University of Minnesota Press.

Wiggins, J. S., & Pincus, A. L. (1989). Conceptions of personality disorders and dimensions of personality. *Psychological Assessment: A Journal of Consulting and Clinical Psychology, 1*, 305-316.

Wiggins, J. S., & Pincus, A. L. (1994). Personality structure and the structure of personality disorders. In P. T. Costa & T. A. Widiger (Eds.), *Personality disorders and the five-factor model of personality* (pp. 73-93). Washington, DC: American Psychological Association.

Wiggins, J. S., Phillips, N., & Trapnell, P. (1989). Circular reasoning about interpersonal behavior: Evidence concerning some untested assumptions underlying diagnostic classification. *Journal of Personality and Social Psychology, 56*, 296-305.

Wiggins, J. S., & Trapnell, P. D. (1996). A dyadic-interactional perspective on the five-factor model . In J. S. Wiggins (Ed.), *The five-factor model of personality; Theoretical perspectives* (pp. 88-162). New York: Guilford.

Willner, A. H., & Blackburn, R. (1988). Interpersonal style and personality deviation. *British Journal of Clinical Psychology, 27*, 273-274.

TREATMENT AND MANAGEMENT OF PSYCHOPATHS

FRIEDRICH LÖSEL
Institut Für Psychologie
Der Universität Erlangen - Nürnberg
Germany.

INTRODUCTION

About 20 years ago, Hare and Schalling (1978) edited a book on the results of the first NATO Advanced Study Institute on psychopathy. This volume contained a chapter on *"Approaches to Treatment"* from Suedfeld and Landon (1978) that began as follows: *"Even a quick review of the literature suggests that a chapter on effective treatment should be the shortest in any book concerned with psychopathy. In fact, it has been suggested that one sentence would suffice: 'No demonstrably effective treatment has been found."* (p. 347). In a review from the 1990s, Blackburn (1993, p. 202) drew two main conclusions: *"First, while classical psychopaths have been shown to respond poorly to some traditional therapeutic interventions, it has yet to be established that "nothing works" with this group. Second, some offenders with personality disorders do appear to change with psychological treatment."*

Although the number of conclusions has doubled since 1978, this by no means indicates 100% progress. In contrast, Blackburn (1993), alongside other experts, still emphasizes that no methodologically sound treatment programs have been demonstrated to work with psychopaths (e.g., Hare, 1995; Serin, 1995). Whereas our knowledge on the assessment, classification, etiology, and prediction, as well as the biological, cognitive, emotional, and behavioral correlates of psychopathy is much better than 20 years ago, the topic of treatment is still characterized by many question marks. Despite skepticism, it is necessary to discriminate general doubts from those referring to the current state of research. In the former case, the psychopathic personality is considered to be basically untreatable. Nonetheless, a survey from England revealed that only a very small proportion of more than 500 forensic experts shared this opinion (Tennent et al., 1993). More than two thirds considered that treatment could succeed, even though they did not know an optimal intervention.

The present chapter aims to show that although we do not yet possess sound knowledge about how to treat psychopaths successfully, we have various promising indications regarding which directions practice and research should take. This also includes the issue of which interventions are particularly inadequate or even contra-indicated for psychopaths. Such knowledge is necessary to avoid exposing victims to purportedly rehabilitated offenders. In summary, it has to be remembered that while *"naive optimism doesn't survive long in forensic practice, pessimistic and resigned inertia is a real danger"* (Mullen, 1994, p. 113).

D.J. Cooke et al. (eds.), Psychopathy: Theory, Research and Implications for Society, 303–354.

All previous reviews on the treatment of psychopathy have contained many studies that were not dedicated specifically to this personality disorder but more generally to serious delinquent and criminal behavior. As only a subgroup of psychopaths come into conflict with the law, and the majority of criminals are not psychopaths, this is a problem. Nonetheless, there are various reasons for such an approach: First, very few controlled evaluations specifically address well-defined psychopathy. Second, treatment studies use different concepts of psychopathy that overlap more or less with criminality (e.g., Blackburn, 1992). Third, even precise operationalizations of psychopathy share characteristics with persistent delinquency as indicated in the DSM-IV antisocial personality disorder (Hare, Hart, & Harpur, 1991). Fourth, criminal behavior is the main and legally justified reason for interventions with psychopaths. Although any transfer of findings from general offender treatment has to be weighed carefully, various problems in research and practice are similar. It should also be recalled that skepticism about the treatability of psychopaths has its equivalent in the *"nothing works"* doctrine for the treatment of offenders (Logan et al., 1991; Martinson, 1974). However, recent research integrations on offender treatment reveal a more constructive perspective (Andrews et al., 1990; Lipsey, 1992a; Lösel, 1995a; Palmer, 1992) that may be cautiously applied to the subgroup of psychopaths or persons scaling high on a dimension of psychopathy.

To avoid too much implicit generalization, the present chapter follows such a perspective. Psychopathy is viewed as moderator in the treatment of antisociality that represents a particularly high risk of failure and dangerousness (e.g., Hart, Hare, & Forth, 1994; Rice & Harris, 1995a; Salekin, Rogers, & Sewell, 1996; Serin, 1996). Following such a perspective, I shall give a brief description of basic practical problems involved with therapeutic and other psychosocial interventions for psychopaths. Then, I shall discuss conceptual and methodological problems in evaluation studies. Third, I shall review evaluation research on the treatment of antisocial behavior and psychopathy. After a brief general evaluation, I shall refer particularly to (a) psychotherapy, behavior modification, and educational measures, (b) more complex therapeutic communities, milieu therapy, and social therapy, (c) punishment and deterrence, and (d) pharmacological treatment. The final section will derive practical recommendations for the treatment and management of psychopaths.

I shall rely not just on single studies but on research integrations through meta-analyses. These have several advantages: (a) Systematic procedures reduce implicit selection and weighting biases; (b) The aggregation of single studies with small samples leads to more reliable estimates of efficacy; (c) Computing effect sizes instead of counting significances is a more sensible technique for evaluating the practical relevance of outcomes; (d) The impact of methodological features on results can be tested; (e) The study of outcome moderators provides information for differential indication.

Basic Problems With Psychotherapy for Psychopaths

The particular difficulties involved in carrying out psychotherapy or related psychosocial interventions with psychopaths have been described repeatedly (e.g., Doren, 1987; Yochelson & Samenow, 1977). Already psychoanalysts like Eissler (1949) had considered classical psychotherapy to be inadequate for psychopathic or nonneurotic delinquency. A core problem is the fundamental therapeutic tool of transference and countertransference (Temple, 1996). Transference requires emotional relationships with significant others and with the therapist, and this is precisely where central problems of the psychopathic personality lie (e.g., Cleckley, 1976; Hare, 1995; Yochelson & Samenow, 1976; see for a different view, Vaillant, 1975).

However, other symptoms of psychopathy also confront psychotherapy with particular difficulties. We have to look only at some characteristics of the psychopathic core personality that are mainly represented in Factor 1 of the Psychopathy Checklist-Revised (PCL-R; Hare, 1991): The tendency to engage in pathological lying (PCL-R Item 4) disrupts the preconditions for free association or absolutely honest communication with the therapist. A grandiose sense of self-worth (Item 2) and lack of remorse or guilt (Item 6) hardly permit a real, deep-lying motivation for change to arise. Shallow affect (Item 7) as well as callousness and lack of empathy (Item 8) impede the central work on emotions in therapy. There is a threat that the psychopath will engage in superficial role play and deception, particularly with therapists who have less experience in this domain. Psychopathic glibness and superficial charm (Item 1) and conning or manipulative behavior (Item 5) are further important *"competencies"* in this light. A precondition of successful therapy is to accept responsibility for one's own actions; once more, a trait that is weak in psychopaths (Item 16). Apart from those phases during which psychopaths can engage in self-display, the therapeutic setting with its paucity of action and continuous repetitions is at odds with their need for stimulation and their proneness to boredom (Item 3; Factor 2).

Such and other unfavorable preconditions for therapeutic interventions are not just reflected in the *"talking cure"* of classic psychotherapy. Findings from process research into psychotherapy and behavior modification suggest that the attributes of psychopaths present a particular problem for other "schools" as well. Orlinsky, Grawe, and Parks (1994) have reviewed more than 2,300 findings on psychotherapeutic processes and outcomes. They worked out which process characteristics produced a positive outcome across the various types of interventions, groups of patients, forms of disorder, settings, and so forth. Many variables produced consistent results insofar as the rate of significant positive findings was greater than 50%. Eleven process variables were found to exhibit particularly robust links to outcomes across multiple observation perspectives (patient, therapist, external rater, psychometric measurement). These were: (a) Patient suitability to the specific treatment; (b) patient cooperation versus resistance; (c) global therapeutic bond/group cohesion; (d) patient contribution to bond; (e) patient interactive collaboration versus dependence/ control; (f) patient expressiveness; (g) patient affirmation of therapist; (h) reciprocal affirmation; (i) patient openness versus defensiveness; (j) positive patient impacts in therapeutic realizations; (k) treatment duration (not linearly related to efficacy).

It is apparent that most of these empirically validated characteristics make it hard to carry out effective psychotherapy on psychopathic personalities. This does not just apply to the marker variables in the domain of the therapeutic bond (c to h). Typical psychopathic behaviors like verbal aggression, intimidation, negative comparisons, throwing guilt, demand for trust, purposeful misinterpretation, exaggerations, lying, and playing for sympathy (Doren, 1987) work against most of these process characteristics.

Nonetheless, they should still be taken into account when planning appropriate interventions (see last section).

This also holds for findings in the neurosciences revealing functional processes underlying the psychopathic symptoms (Hare, 1995; Newman & Wallace, 1993a). For example, psychopaths find it difficult to be aware of the emotional significance of experiences or events (e.g., Patrick, 1994; Williamson, Harpur, & Hare, 1991). They show less cardiac, electrodermal, and facial muscle responses to imagined fearful scenes (e.g., Patrick, Cuthbert, & Lang, 1994). Furthermore, their linguistic processes also seem to be superficial: They are less able than others to understand or use the nuances and deeper semantic meanings of language (Williamson et al., 1991). They also have difficulties in shifting attention between different stimuli and are guided more by controlled than automatic cognitive processing (Newman & Wallace, 1993a). It seems as if psychopaths lack a central organizer to plan and monitor what they perceive, think, and say (Gillstrom & Hare, 1988). Although research on neuropsychological foundations and correlates permit only tentative conclusions (Dolan, 1994), the problems in the verbal and executive functions may be related to cerebral dysfunction (Gorenstein & Newman, 1980; Lapierre, Braun, & Hodgins, 1995) that already start to consolidate during childhood (see Farrington, Loeber, & Van Kammen, 1990; Lynam, 1996; Moffitt, 1993).

Such preconditions make it hard to work with the necessary nuances of the therapeutic process. This is joined by motivational problems (e.g., Robertson & Gunn, 1987). Ogloff, Wong, and Greenwood (1990), for example, found that the psychopathic subgroup within a therapeutic community showed less treatment motivation, effort, and improvement than a mixed and nonpsychopathic group (defined in terms of PCL-R). Psychopaths also remained in treatment for a shorter time. The authors considered that the main reason for this is that psychopaths' initial motivation is determined by administrative reasons (in particular, the hope that treatment will make conditional release easier). Such secondary or extrinsic motives also play an important role among nonpsychopathic offenders and drug addicts, and should not be viewed too negatively. Due to a lack of suffering, the classical concept of a primary, intrinsic and *"deep"* motivation to change is less adequate for antisocial clients. Treatment motivation should be differentiated with respect to a goal and means component (Dahle, 1994). Elements of compulsion and expectancies of privileges may be an important first step in the development of treatment motivation (Egg, 1993; Sowers & Daley, 1993). But, as psychopaths typically do not see problems in themselves or their attributional styles, they often fail to engage in the necessary self-examination. Therapy may then become a meaningless and tedious task that they grow to resent (Ogloff et al., 1990). Accordingly, therapies are not only broken off frequently but also burdened with external complications such as more confinements, negative entries, nonfailure misbehaviors, institutional aggression, and other disciplinary problems (e.g., Forth et al., 1990; Rice, Harris, & Cormier, 1992; Salekin et al., 1996). It goes without saying that these factors can have a negative impact on the motivation, expectation, and behavior of therapists as well. Thus, a cycle of disappointment, fear of manipulation, and self-fulfilling prophecy may further reduce treatment efficacy. Nonetheless, all this does not necessarily mean that successful interventions are impossible. The touchstone is controlled outcome evaluations.

METHODOLOGICAL PROBLEMS IN TREATMENT EVALUATIONS

The controlled evaluation of treatments of antisocial behavior and criminality has repeatedly revealed severe conceptual and methodological problems (e.g., Kury, 1986; Lipton, Martinson, & Wilks, 1975; Lösel, Köferl, & Weber, 1987; Sechrest, White, & Brown, 1979; Suedfeld & Landon, 1978). I shall not discuss general design problems and manifold threats to validity in detail. Instead, I shall mainly sketch some problems that are more specific to evaluations of psychopathy treatment.

1. Nonequivalence of control groups

Most older reviews of the literature on correctional treatment concluded that there was a lack of well-controlled experimental designs (e.g., Lipton et al., 1975). Meanwhile, a majority of studies on juvenile delinquency treatment include random assignment (Lipsey, 1992a). However, less progress can be seen regarding control for attrition and many other threats to internal validity. This is particularly the case in the treatment of psychopaths and other serious offenders in prisons or hospitals. Many treatment studies in this field still include quasi-experimental designs with nonequivalent control groups and thus the risk that effects are due to selection, regression, selection x treatment, and so forth (Cook & Campbell, 1979). As the overall relationship between randomization and effect size is small or inconsistent (Lipsey, 1992a; Lösel, 1995a), the consequences of these threats to validity do not seem to be unidirectional. It also has to be considered that the possibilities of randomized and otherwise well-controlled designs are often subject to ethical, legal, or practical constraints. For example, in the case of a heavily disturbed offender, practice can rarely abstain from treatment merely for reasons of experimental control. In comparison with control groups from other institutions, inmates of forensic hospitals or therapeutic prisons may represent either a negative or a positive selection. The latter particularly holds for those clients who terminate a program regularly and often show better effects (e.g., Cullen, 1997; Dolan, 1997). However, would it be fair to count all dropouts to the disadvantage of treatment? In these and other aspects, treatment evaluation should be sensitive to matters of degree. Even an *"untreated"* control group in a regular prison does not receive *"nothing"* but may be exposed to influences that are similar to the evaluated program. Therefore, process information on control conditions is just as necessary as that on the treatment (see below).

2. Heterogeneity of treated groups

While there is a large number of controlled studies on offender treatment (e.g., Gendreau & Goggin, 1996; Lipsey, 1992a; Lösel, 1995a), the situation is much worse in the field of psychopathy. For example, Esteban, Garrido, and Molero (1995) had to apply relatively loose methodological criteria in order to gather the approximately 20 studies needed for a meta-analysis. Although the authors used explicit criteria, the samples in these studies are still rather heterogeneous. In treatment practice, *"psychopathy""* is often defined more vaguely (Blackburn, 1993). Some countries even avoid the concept because it is politically controversial. There is also controversy regarding how far psychopathy represents a clearly distinct taxon (e.g., Harris, Rice, & Quinsey, 1994) or a dimensional concept (e.g., Blackburn, 1975; Lilienfeld, 1994). Estimations of prevalence rates in antisocial groups differ accordingly. In US federal prisons and Canadian penitentiaries, for example, approximately 15 - 25% of adult male inmates have been diagnosed as psychopaths following the PCL cutting point of 30 for high psychopathy (Hare, 1991; Wong, 1996). Cooke (1995, 1996), however, found a much lower rate of 3% in Scottish prisons. In English forensic hospitals, only approximately one quarter of legally defined psychopaths are actually primary psychopaths in the stricter sense (Blackburn, 1996; Copas et al., 1984). Similarly, only a minority of *"antisocial personalities"* in a Canadian forensic hospital met the DSM-III criteria of antisocial personality disorder (Harris, Rice, & Cormier, 1991). Approximately 20 - 30% of inmates with antisocial personality disorder (APD) are estimated to show PCL-R defined psychopathy (Hare, 1995). The prevalence of APD in the USA seems to be particularly high and still rising (Robins & Price, 1991). In many other countries, there is a lack of systematic assessments. Germany, for example, has social-therapeutic prisons designed especially for offenders with personality disorders (Lösel & Egg, 1997), but these do not yet perform specific diagnoses of APD and psychopathy. Even if they did, international comparisons would be complicated because cutting points and various item characteristics of the PCL-R seem to be strongly influenced by cultural differences (Cooke, 1997a; Cooke & Michie, 1997). It is also questionable whether results from mostly Anglo-American samples can be generalized to other ethnic groups or minorities (Salekin et al., 1996).

3. Different concepts and assessments of psychopathy

This point is related directly to the previous one: Some treatment studies use only a legal definition of psychopathy (see Blackburn, 1993; Dolan & Coid, 1993). Others refer to the broader, continental-European concept of *"psychopathy""* introduced by Schneider (1950) that covers the various personality disorders but no specific category of antisocial personality. More frequently, studies use diagnoses of antisocial personality disorder based on DSM or ICD. These focus on the antisocial and impulsive life-style (Factor 2 in the PCL-R) and have to be differentiated from the interpersonal and emotional characteristics of the psychopathic personality assessed in Factor 1 (Hare, 1995; Hare et al., 1991). Although relations between psychopathy and APD are complicated by mixing personality-based and behavior-based approaches (Lilienfeld, 1994), a large subgroup of persons with APD are not psychopaths (Hart & Hare, 1989). However, there are also different concepts of psychopathic personality: The debate on a dimensional versus taxonomic category has already been mentioned. Some authors also discriminate between primary and secondary psychopathy (Blackburn, 1992). Because anxiety and withdrawal are involved in the latter, these conceptual differences are directly relevant to the question of treatability and responsivity (see Serin, 1995). Trait anxiety in psychopaths should also be distinguished from fearfulness (Gray, 1982; Lilienfeld, 1994). In addition to conceptual differences, there are various methods of assessment: (a) Cleckley's criteria and ratings; (b) the PCL or PCL-R; (c) the socialization scale from the California Psychological Inventory; (d) Quay's (1987) behavior classification; (e) the psychopathic deviate scale (Pd) and scale profiles of the MMPI; and (f) the Special Hospitals Assessment of Personality and Socialization (for an overview, see Blackburn, 1992). Because correlations between various measurements are only moderate (Hare, 1985), multiple measures are suggested (e.g., Widiger & Frances, 1987). The problematic use of a pure self-report with psychopaths (Lilienfeld, 1994) also indicates the need for a multiple-setting-multiple-informant approach.

4. Developmental aspects

The majority of studies on offender treatment address juvenile delinquents (Lipsey, 1992a). Controlled studies on the treatment of persistent adult offenders are relatively rare (Lösel, 1995b). This emphasis is understandable from an epidemiological perspective, because crime and antisociality are most frequent in youth (Blumstein, Cohen, & Farrington, 1988). Although a large number of future psychopaths may be among the juvenile delinquents, they are only a small group in comparison with adolescence-limited antisocials (Moffitt, 1993). Mostly, they may be found among the life-course-persistent subtype in which antisocial behavior starts early in childhood (Hodgins et al., this volume; Loeber, 1990; Lynan, 1996; Moffitt, 1993; Robins, 1978). Because different causal mechanisms are considered to be responsible for life-course-persistent versus adolescence-limited antisociality, there is also a strong need for precise diagnostic and developmental data in treatment studies. However, precise assessments of psychopathic traits in childhood or adolescence are rare (Frick et al., 1994; Forth et al., 1990). This makes the question of generalizability of treatment evaluations more difficult to answer than in antisocial adults. If no successful interventions are available, practice may also be reluctant about engaging in early labeling.

5. Comorbidity with other psychiatric disorders

The problem of the Comorbidity of various disorders is rather frequent in forensic therapy. For example, in a study of the inmates of Henderson Hospital (UK), only 3% scored within a single personality disorder cluster (Dolan et al., 1995). Müller-Isberner (1996) reported additional diagnoses for approximately 45% of the inmates in the forensic psychiatric hospital at Haina (Germany). Comorbidity may be partially due to the steady increase in the number of categories in the revisions of DSM and other classification systems. However, it is by no means an artifact that persons who suffer from major mental disorders are also at high risk of committing crimes (Hodgins, 1993; Monahan & Steadman, 1994). When major mental disorders are paired with APD, they are less relevant for criminality and violence (Hodgins & Coté, 1993; Rasmussen & Levander, 1996a). In these cases, the personality disorder seems to be more important. There is fairly strong evidence of an association between APD and several of the Cluster B disorders (American Psychiatric Association, 1994). This particularly holds for histrionic, narcissistic, and borderline personality disorders (e.g., Grove & Tellegen, 1991; Hart & Hare, 1989; Lilienfeld et al., 1986). It is not clear whether this covariation is due to a poor discriminant validity in both the psychopathy construct and the other personality disorders, or whether it reflects an overlap among etiologically different syndromes (Lilienfeld, 1994). Antisociality or psychopathy may not only be paired with other personality disorders, but also with alcoholism and other substance-induced disorders (e.g., Hart & Hare, 1989; Nedopil et al., 1996). Again, the moderate association between psychopathy and drug dependence seems to have more to do with the unstable, antisocial life-style rather than the interpersonal and affective characteristics of psychopathy. Comorbidity with major mental disorders is relatively infrequent for psychopathy (Freese et al., 1996; Nedopil et al., 1996; Rice & Harris, 1995a), but not for APD or in highly selected groups (Rasmussen & Levander, 1996b). Comorbidities may contribute to treatment failure as well as to treatability. For example, Woody et al. (1985) have ascertained better treatment outcomes in patients with APD plus opiate dependence plus major depression than among those with only APD plus opiate dependence (see below).

6. Process data on interventions

Just as with the clients, there are also major conceptual and operational problems with the content of treatment. At times, treatment modalities are sketched only very vaguely, particularly in short journal articles. Reporting a specific label for one single school or direction often reveals little about what actually happened (Lösel et al., 1987; Quay, 1977). Therapy manuals provide some indications on the contents of intervention. But, here as well, implementation may differ. As mentioned above, individual relationship factors make a strong contribution to effectiveness. However, these are rarely documented in forensic treatment studies. Process evaluations become particularly difficult when interventions are more complex. For individual therapies, it is possible to compile course protocols, audiotapes, or video-recordings. However, in a therapeutic community, the effects of psychotherapy, group processes, or educational and vocational measures merge together. Because evaluation addresses a total package and not individual treatment modules, it is often not possible to state specific causes of success or failure. More differentiated as well as comprehensive process data are needed.

7. Treatment integrity

The problem of treatment integrity is closely related to the previous one. Even if a treatment possesses an explicit concept, its implementation may well be insufficient. Efficacy requires not only reliable dependent variables (outcome measures) but also reliable independent variables, that is, program characteristics (Lösel & Wittmann, 1989). Unsuccessful treatment programs have revealed repeatedly that they were not implemented adequately (see Quay, 1977). Meta-analyses show a somewhat smaller effect size for treatments with low integrity (Hill, Andrews, & Hoge, 1991; Lipsey, 1992a). However, this relationship is probably stronger than empirical research has been able to confirm. First, sound information on integrity is rarely reported, and, second, integrity increases efficacy only in programs that are basically adequate. Numerous influences may impair program integrity (Hollin, 1995; Jones, 1997; Lösel, 1996a; Palmer, 1992), for example: lack of a common basic *"philosophy"*, insufficient staff training, organizational barriers, implicit learning processes, deficits in supervision; critical incidents, staff resistance, burnout phenomena, and changes in the political context. To ensure integrity, data are needed regarding the organizational structure, the communication and decision rules, the selection and training of staff, and so forth (e.g., Hollin, 1995; Jones, 1997; Lösel & Bliesener, 1989; Thornton & Hogue, 1993). Although these issues are documented in the forensic treatment literature (e.g., Genders & Player, 1995; Woodward, 1997), they are rarely related to systematic program evaluation (Antonowicz & Ross, 1994).

8. Outcome criteria

Most investigations of the efficacy of treatment for antisociality focus on official measures of reoffending or reconviction. The complications arising from these outcome criteria can only be sketched here (see Lloyd, Mair, & Hough, 1994; Lösel et al., 1987; Sechrest et al., 1979). Official data depend not only on the behavior of the criminals themselves but also on the readiness of the general public to report offenses to the police, the activities of the police, and the practice of the criminal justice system. The high rate of undetected offenses also impairs the validity of official recidivism. Self-report measures, in turn, are primarily appropriate for less severe offenses. They may be particularly inappropriate for psychopaths. Because recidivism data call for a sufficiently long follow-up interval, they reflect the outcomes of treatment after a long delay. Numerous social processes in the natural environment interfere, and may cancel out the changes induced through treatment. Therefore, authors have warned against overrating the value of criminal behavior as an outcome criterion (e.g., Maltz, 1984; Robertson, 1989). This applies particularly to forensic treatment in the clinical sense rather than correctional treatment. Although recidivism data are necessary for practical and theoretical reasons, cognitive, emotional, and behavioral mediating factors that lead to criminal behavior should be included not only for the direct evaluation of treatment efficacy but also for its improvement. It would be desirable to have a coordinated sequence of proximal and distal outcomes and knowledge on the relationship between manipulative key variables (Lipsey, 1995a). However, this is lacking in many evaluation studies. Various measures such as interpersonal adaptation, attitude or personality change, educational or vocational criteria, and criminal behavior only correlate with each other moderately (e.g., Lipsey, 1992b). Therapist's or self-ratings of some of these outcome measures are also relatively *"weak."* Superficial institutional adaptations and treatment-related changes may be present, but they may well fail to impact on subsequent behavior in daily life. Therefore, particular weight should be placed on those evaluation studies that use clinically meaningful as well as behavioral follow-up measures as outcome criteria.

All these factors may impede consistent and substantial effects. Furthermore, most research on the treatment of antisociality is not based on university or analogue settings as is frequently the case in psychotherapy research. Compared with these favorable contexts and clients, the efficacy of daily psychotherapeutic practice is far more moderate than meta-analyses suggest (Matt & Navarro, 1997; Weisz et al., 1995). Broader real-life criteria and longer follow-up periods also reduce treatment efficacy in other fields (e.g. Beelmann, Pfingsten, & Lösel, 1994; Glass & Kliegl, 1983). It must further be taken into account that the statistical optimum of efficacy is not r or phi = 1.0. Due to developmental processes and non-treatment protective factors, failure rates in untreated control groups are often *"only"* about 50%. In this case, the maximum of *phi* is .58. If the base rate is smaller, even effect sizes below Cohen's (1992) criterion of .50 may be *"large."* Deficits in the reliability of treatment and outcome measures further reduce potential effects. Thus, a realistic evaluation of effect sizes in the treatment of antisocial behavior is necessary. About .30 may be an upper limit (Lösel, 1996b). However, even *"small"* effects can be highly relevant for reasons of cost-utility (e.g., Prentky & Burgess, 1992).

GENERAL EVALUATION OF THE TREATMENT OF ANTISOCIALITY

In the last 10 years, more than a dozen meta-analyses have integrated hundreds of studies on the treatment of antisocial behavior (e.g., Andrews et al., 1990; Antonowicz & Ross, 1994; Garrett, 1985; Gendreau & Ross, 1987; Gensheimer et al., 1986; Lipsey, 1992a; Lösel et al., 1987; Redondo, 1994, Whitehead & Lab, 1989; see, for an overview, Lösel, 1995a). Although samples of primary studies overlap in the North American integrations, the material is very heterogeneous. Studies vary in terms of target groups, severity of offending and disorder, modality and length of treatment, institutional context, type of outcome measures, methodological quality, national and juridical background, meta-analytic procedure, and so forth. Definitions of *"treatment"* range from classical psychotherapy and behavior modification over social case work and therapeutic communities to educational and vocational training. Several meta-analyses also include evaluations of formal juridical measures and punishment (e.g., incarceration, probation, scared straight, electronic monitoring).

Despite the wide range of differences, mean effect sizes were remarkably similar. In all meta-analyses on offender treatment in general, the mean effect size (ES) is only small (*r* or *phi* < .30; Cohen, 1992). The overall efficacy suggested in these studies is about .10 +/- .05. According to the Binomial Effect Size Display (Rosenthal & Rubin, 1982), this can be interpreted as a difference in percentage points. If, for example, success in the treated group is 55% compared with 45% in an untreated control group, the resulting effect size is .10. Some analyses show that the mean ES decreases for the following study characteristics: methodologically more appropriate weighting by sample size of the primary studies, control-group instead of pre-post design, institutional setting instead of community, and recidivism as outcome criterion instead of psychological measures with no follow up (Lösel, 1995a; Lösel & Beelmann, 1996). Obviously, not only psychopaths but criminals in general are difficult to change.

However, even within this difficult-to-treat group, psychopaths represent a particular high risk. Psychopathy (as measured by the PCL or PCL-R) predicted violent and nonviolent recidivism not only for individuals released from prison and other nontherapeutic settings (Gendreau et al., 1995) but also for forensic hospitals, therapeutic community programs, or treatment centers for sexual offenders (Salekin et al., 1996). The criminal history and antisocial life-style represented in Factor 2 seems to be more relevant for accurate prediction than the psychopathic core personality assessed in Factor 1 (Salekin et al., 1996). This questions whether psychopathy is more relevant for treatment failure than ASPD. Within a broader definition, Esteban et al. (1995) have analyzed 26 studies on the treatment of *"psychopathy"*. Their diagnostic criteria were based on DSM-APD, PCL, MMPI, or CPI. Many evaluations did not primarily address psychopathy but alcohol and drug problems associated with APD. In a first meta-analysis (A), the authors compared efficacy of the interventions on psychopaths in studies with control groups of nonpsychopathic offenders or participants with other disorders. In another analysis (B), they evaluated pre-posttest treatment efficacy in the psychopathic groups. To improve comparability with other results, I have transformed the ES from d into r. Analysis A showed that psychopaths generally performed worse than the various comparison groups ($r = -.21$). Whereas the difference on the immediate pre-post comparison was low (-.12), it attained -.25 on follow-up measurements, and when recidivism was used as a long-term behavioral outcome, it even reached -.30. The efficacy differences between other treated groups and psychopaths were particularly strong when the PCL was used for the definition of the latter. In the weaker pre-post designs included in Analysis B, however, there was a mean positive effect of .20. In all kinds of posttest measures, this was surprisingly high (.41). On psychological posttest measures, however, it was only .19; and it was no longer present when follow-up criteria were applied (.00). Such moderators should be interpreted with caution because they are based on only a few studies, and some of these have entered the analysis repeatedly. As in other meta-analyses, this raises the threat of artifacts, particularly regarding differential effects.

EVALUATION OF VARIOUS TYPES OF INTERVENTION

Because the general effects are found to be small, it is particularly important to examine differences in the efficacy of treatment modalities. The proportions of variance explained by treatment type vary a great deal in the meta-analyses (e.g., Lipsey, 1992a; Redondo, 1994). However, alongside methodological factors, the type of treatment is most important for the outcome. As mentioned above, mere treatment labels may be rather uninformative and neglect overlaps between different approaches. Therefore, I shall not deal with the various directions of psychotherapy in isolation, but treat them more comparatively. The review focuses on psychotherapy, behavior modification, and educational measures as well as therapeutic communities and milieu therapy. Punishment and formal reactions of the justice system as well as pharmacological treatment will be addressed more briefly.

1. Psychotherapy, Behavior Modification, and Educational Measures

A broad variety of measures are discussed under this heading. They include psychoanalytic treatment, classic methods of behavior modification, cognitive-behavioral therapies, client-centered psychotherapy, nondirective counseling, social skills training, traditional case work, school and other educational measures, employment and vocational training. Treatments are not only individual but also involve group-oriented methods. Compared with the complex therapeutic communities and milieu therapies, these programs are more specific in content. However, it must also be taken into account that, in larger institutions, clients frequently receive various treatments at the same time (e.g., Dell & Robertson, 1988; Lösel et al.,1987).

Meta-analyses referring specifically to social learning treatments and behavioral treatments for delinquent juveniles have shown a larger mean ES compared with the overall mean for all kinds of interventions (Gottschalk et al., 1987; Mayer et al., 1986). This trend is confirmed in Lipsey's (1992a) big analysis of more than 400 studies.

Programs were most effective if they were behavioral, skill-oriented, and multimodal (aiming at multiple risk factors). Although ESs were still small (M = .10 to .16), they were about twice as high as the overall mean. Unstructured case work; individual, group, or family counseling programs; as well as formal justice measures exhibited smaller effect sizes. When the best type of treatment was paired with a higher dosage (more frequent contacts or longer duration) and program monitoring by the researcher (which may have increased integrity), treated groups revealed an average improvement of 25% compared with controls (Lipsey, 1995b). Nonetheless, some treatment programs did not just exhibit small effects but even negative ones (Lipsey, 1992a). In other words, despite of best intentions, controls performed better than the treatment groups (see McCord, 1978).

The highest ES reported in Redondo's (1994) meta-analysis of European studies was also for behavioral and, particularly, cognitive-behavioral programs. At .25, it was well above average, and higher than that for psychodynamic and other therapies or educational measures. Izzo and Ross (1990) reported a higher ES for programs with a cognitive component. In Garrett's (1985) meta-analysis, behavioral and skill-oriented programs did somewhat better than psychodynamic and other treatments, although these differences were confounded with the methodological quality of the primary studies. Whitehead and Lab (1989) found no clear support for better effects of behavioral programs compared with nonbehavioral ones. However, as they counted only studies with an ES greater than .20, their analysis is not very sensitive in this respect.

Andrews et al. (1990) integrated the study sample of Whitehead and Lab (1989) into their analysis, and found better effects in behavioral interventions. These authors also developed a more complex, clinically and theoretically relevant grouping of treatment types. They labeled correctional service as being *"appropriate"* when it met three principles: (a) *The risk principle*: The level of service or intensity of treatment should be matched to the risk of the clients. Higher levels of service are reserved for higher risk cases, whereas lower risk cases do as well with less intensive services. (b) *The need principle*: The targets of services are matched to the specific criminogenic needs of offenders. These include changing antisocial attitudes and feelings, strengthening self-control, improving social skills, curing drug addiction, reducing antisocial peer contacts, enhancing positive social relations, improving cost-utility ratios for noncriminal behavior in various settings, and so forth. (c) *The responsivity principle*: Styles and modes of service are matched to the learning styles and abilities of offenders. This involves less verbal and more concrete measures like anticriminal modeling, role playing, teaching concrete skills, graduate practice, reinforcement, cognitive restructuring, making resources available, use of authority, and so forth.

Appropriate treatment included service delivery to higher risk cases, all behavioral programs (except those for lower risk cases), comparisons reflecting responsivity-treatment relations, and nonbehavioral programs that clearly targeted criminogenic needs and used structured interventions. *Inappropriate* treatment included programs for low risks or mismatching according to need and responsivity, nondirective milieu and group approaches, nondirective or poorly targeted academic or vocational measures, and *"scared straight"* interventions. *Unspecified treatment* included all programs that could not be labeled confidently as appropriate or inappropriate. Independent from other study characteristics, appropriate programs had the best outcomes (.30); unspecified programs showed a weaker positive effect (.13); and inappropriate services even a small negative effect (-.06). These differences have also been confirmed in a more recent analysis of a much larger sample of evaluation studies (see Gendreau & Goggin, 1996). The mean ES was .25 for appropriate programs, .13 for unspecified measures, and -.03 for inappropriate ones.

Lab and Whitehead (1990), Logan et al. (1991), and others have criticized the study of Andrews et al., particularly with regard to circularity problems in the responsivity principle. To some degree, this is justified because we do not know how far knowledge on efficacy had influenced categorization of appropriateness. Nonetheless, the major findings could be confirmed in a meta-analysis based on a different procedure: Antonowicz and Ross (1994) restricted their analysis to studies with particularly good methodological controls. They compared 20 successful programs with 24 unsuccessful ones on the basis of 40 treatment features from the criminological literature. Successful programs more often included a sound conceptual model, the need principle, the responsivity principle, multifaceted treatment, modeling or role-playing techniques, and social-cognitive skills training. The authors were unable to confirm the risk principle. For many other treatment features such as social perspective taking, self-control, interpersonal problem-solving, client motivation, supportive environment, integrity, or staff motivation, there were not enough studies to permit a reliable statement on their moderating effects.

In all, these research syntheses provide a relatively consistent picture that is in line with the results of more qualitative literature reviews (e.g., Basta & Davidson, 1988; Palmer, 1992; Romig, 1978): Structured behavioral, cognitive-behavioral, skill-oriented, and multimodal measures, based on social learning theories have better effects on antisocial behavior than other modes of treatment. Although ESs are not large, they are clearly higher than the small general effects of offender treatment. Naturally, labels such as *"cognitive-behavioral programs," "information-processing approach,"* or *"appropriate treatment"* are not signposts pointing to a royal path to success. However, relatively successful programs should include modules that improve self-control, self-critical thinking, social perspective-taking, victim awareness, anger management, interpersonal problem-solving, social skills, vocational competencies, noncriminal attitudes, experiences of contingent reinforcement, and so forth (see Andrews & Bonta, 1994; Crick & Dodge, 1994; Hollin, 1990; Ross & Ross, 1995). In general, such programs lead to better outcomes than pure psychodynamic or nondirective interventions, unstructured case work, acting out approaches, and other treatments that do not target criminogenic needs so directly. However, these results should not be simplified to a decision between traditional *"schools"* of therapy. Indeed, an emphasis on some basic elements such as a structured approach can be found in otherwise very different psychodynamic approaches (e.g., Berner & Karlick-Bolten, 1986; Vaillant, 1975).

As treatment efficacy also depends on the kind of outcome measure (Lösel, 1995a), another problem is that programs may only lead to improved institutional adjustment but not to long-term successes (Rutter & Giller, 1983). An example of this is reinforcement techniques like the token economies (Ross & Fabiano, 1985). However, several recent meta-analyses specify follow-up measures of recidivism as outcome (e.g., Andrews et al., 1990; Antonowicz & Ross, 1994). In others, the moderator effects of treatment modality can still be confirmed after controlling for methodological differences in the outcome measures (e.g., Lipsey, 1992a; Redondo, 1994).

The lack of confirmation for the risk principle in Antonowicz and Ross (1994) is plausible. When risk is very high, an adequate matching of treatment intensity may well be a necessary but not a sufficient prerequisite of success. It seems more appropriate to assume a curvilinear relationship between risk and efficacy (see Lösel, 1996b). Then, treatment effects on low-risk cases are small, because the comparison group will also not exhibit high failure rates (e.g., due to spontaneous remissions). When risk is very high, antisociality and personality problems are entrenched so strongly that treatability remains questionable even when programs are applied intensively.

This leads to the question on how far these results on criminals can be generalized to the specific subgroup of psychopaths. As mentioned above, classical psychotherapy tends not to be indicated for these groups. Vaillant (1975), however, is less pessimistic about treating psychopaths with psychodynamic approaches. He used case reports to demonstrate that psychopaths are also capable of experiencing anxiety, depression, and motivation for change, although their immature personality and defense structures make them far less accessible. His observations suggest that personality can be changed with treatment approaches integrating a firm behavioral control, confrontation (and less interpretation), support by the therapist and the group, as well as institutional containment. Some more controlled studies on psychotherapy also suggested treatability of offenders with antisocial personalities. For example, Jew, Clanon, and Mattocks (1972) reported a 1-year recidivism rate of only approximately 25% (compared with 33% in the control group) for a residential, structured group therapy. With 28% recidivism in a 9-month follow up, Carney (1977) found a similar rate for group therapy in an outpatient clinic. Nonetheless, this study had no control group. Neither study include precisely defined psychopaths and had only short evaluation periods. With respect to the latter, it is important that positive treatment effects probably improved social adaptation and control of criminal behavior rather than bringing about a fundamental personality change (Carney, 1977). In a combined individual and group therapy for inpatients with a 3-year follow up, Carney (1978) even reported a recidivism rate of only 7% among those who completed treatment. However, this was at an institution (Patuxent) with extremely low general recidivism rates (Wilkins, 1978). Besides other methodological weaknesses (Holder, 1978), selection effects may have posed a severe threat to validity. Bailey and MacCulloch (1992) found much higher failure rates for legally defined psychopaths released from an English special hospital. Within a mean follow-up period of 6 years, 55% of the psychopathic group were reconvicted, about 25% for serious offenses. As in various other studies, psychopaths did worse than patients with major mental illnesses like schizophrenia. Similarly, group therapy for alcoholism was useful for other personality disorders but did not work in antisocial personalities (Poldrugo & Forti, 1988). Failure of about 50-60% of psychopaths has been found in various evaluations of British special hospitals (e.g., Tennent & Way, 1984; Robertson, 1989; see, for an overview, Dolan & Coid,

1993). In Austrian and German forensic hospitals overall recidivism was in the same range and patients with personality disorders or long-term antisociality showed the highest failure rates (Berner & Karlick-Bolten, 1986; Gretenkord, 1994).

That findings differ as a function of the specific disorder and outcome criterion is shown in the relatively well-controlled study of Woody et al., 1985). A total of 110 nonpsychotic opiate addicts were assigned at random to one of three treatment conditions: (a) paraprofessional drug counseling alone (DC), (b) supportive-expressive psychotherapy plus counseling (SE), or (c) cognitive-behavioral psychotherapy plus counseling (CB). Each program lasted 6 months. One month after the end of treatment, pretest-posttest comparisons were performed on 22 outcome criteria. Whereas there were no significant differences between the two psychotherapeutic approaches, both were more successful than counseling alone (Woody et al., 1983). The two psychotherapy groups could be further differentiated in terms of their symptoms into the following subgroups (DSM-III categories): Opiate dependence only (OP Only), opiate dependence plus major depression (OP + DEP), opiate dependence plus major depression plus antisocial personality disorder (OP+DEP+ASP), and opiate dependence plus antisocial personality disorder (OP+ASP). The groups OP+DEP and OP+DEP+ASP performed best across all outcome measures (mean ES: $r = .26$ and .24). For OP Only, there was a mean ES of .20; and for OP+ASP, .09. This indicates that antisocials with no depressive symptoms hardly changed at all. Nonetheless, even the OP+ASP group exhibited better effects in the fields of employment (.29) and legal behavior (.24). However, significant changes were found in only 3 of the 22 single outcome measures, and there were even negative effects in the medical and psychiatric factors (-.16 and -.11 respectively), though these values were similar in other groups because of drug withdrawal. Results on the various outcome factors sometimes varied greatly within the other groups as well. For example, the OP Only group had an ES of only .06 in the area of drug use, but one of .45 in employment. Because groups were small, such differences frequently failed to reach significance. In a pure posttest comparison, the OP+ASP group showed the worst performance on most significant outcomes.

Various other studies have examined behavioral treatments in groups exhibiting personality disorders. Moyes, Tennent, and Bedford (1985) evaluated a combination of token economy, contingency contracting, and social skills training in seriously antisocial juveniles. They found positive outcomes in terms of aggressive behavior and a delay in contacts with the police. Jones et al. (1977) revealed better results compared with controls in a similar program applied to personality-disordered military personnel. However, Cavior and Schmidt (1978) observed neither a total effect in terms of recidivism nor a differential effect for psychopaths in a differentiated token economy program.

More recently, behavioral methods include a stronger cognitive orientation such as cognitive restructuring, problem-solving training, self-control and self-gratification, anger management, or social skills training. Various studies have shown within-treatment or short-term effects on violent offenders (see Serin, 1996). Kadden et al. (1989) found, for example, that in a comparative evaluation of treatments of alcoholics, those who scored higher in psychopathy exhibited better outcomes in a coping skills training. In contrast, interactional therapy was more effective for subjects with lower psychopathy scores. Valliant and Antonowicz (1992) reported on a combination of social skills training and cognitive-behavioral therapy for male sex offenders. There were positive effects in terms of self-esteem and reduced anxiety. However, it is unclear how far these effects relate to later recidivism. As Valliant (1993) showed on a small group of young persons, the positive posttreatment effects of a combined cognitive-behavioral and behavioral therapy could not be maintained over a 2-year follow up (80% recidivism). As far as the direct control of aggressive, disruptive, and other forms of problem behavior is concerned, cognitive-behavioral approaches had some success even in clients with more severe personality disorders or psychopathy (e.g., Beck & Freeman, 1990; Frederiksen & Rainwater, 1981; Levey & Howells, 1990; Templeman & Wollersheim, 1979). However, there are not enough long-term evaluations.

The meta-analysis of Esteban et al. (1995) also provides indications that cognitive-behavioral approaches can be promising for psychopaths. Although psychopaths did generally worse than other groups, cognitive-behavioral measures exhibited the smallest mean ES difference to their disadvantage (-.16). In other forms of psychotherapy, the mean difference in ES was at -.24. The authors also found that individual treatments were superior to group approaches (-.05 vs. -.24). Pretest-posttest designs revealed some differences between treatment modalities; however, these were less than in the group comparisons.

The treatment of sex offenders also points toward cognitive-behavioral approaches. For example, in a review of controlled studies, the effects of cognitive-behavioral measures was higher than the general efficacy of about 10 percentage points difference between treated and untreated groups (Hall, 1996). Thornton (1992) compared evaluation studies of cognitive-behavioral treatment with those of psychodynamic and other types of program. In three of the four cognitive-behavioral programs, the treated group exhibited less sexual reoffending than controls. The relationship inverted in the other types of program. Marques et al. (1994) and Marshall et al. (1991) indicated that comprehensive cognitive-behavioral programs for sex offenders can substantially reduce recidivism. However, Quinsey et al. (1993) have pointed to methodological problems in the primary studies analyzed by Marshall et al. (1991) such as lack of comparison groups, self-selection by the subjects, or doubtful validity of outcome measures. Alongside such criticisms, the composition of the sex offender group may play an important role. For example, results on nonviolent sex offenders (mostly child molesters) seem to be more positive, whereas there is less success with violent rapists (e.g., Marshall & Barbaree, 1988; Marshall et al., 1991; Prentky, 1995). At present, explanations for this are only partial: Barker (1996) suspects, for example, that pro-rape attitudes (rape myths; Hall, 1996) are more widely accepted socially than the idea of sex with children. Therefore, rapists may experience more reinforcement for their distorted ideas about sex and women, and thus be less motivated to accept responsibility and change their behavior. However, another reason could be that there are fewer psychopaths and more neurotic or otherwise personality-disordered personalities among nonviolent sex offenders. In line with this, Prentky et al. (1995) reported that life-style impulsivity, as frequently found among psychopaths, is a particularly negative predictor in sexual offenses. According to Quinsey, Rice, and Harris (1995), rapists with a high score in PCL-R were more at risk for sexual recidivism after release from a forensic treatment center than clients with lower scores. Barbaree et al. (1994) and Serin et al. (1994) reported similar predictions of PCL-R with respect to deviant sexual arousal in prison inmates.

2. Therapeutic Communities, Milieu Therapy, and Social Therapy

This category of treatment modalities can also include some of the specific therapies that were evaluated in the previous section. However, the particular accent is on therapeutically shaping the entire milieu and, in particular, on the group processes in the specific institution. Admittedly, concepts like therapeutic community or milieu should not be taken too literally. The more or less compulsory concentration of persistent antisocials, personality disordered, and dangerous persons in high-security prisons or hospitals is normally not a particularly favorable context for therapy. These concepts have to be conceived in more relative terms: In a setting established for reasons of security, punishment, or retributive justice, an attempt is made to introduce a regime that can achieve a stronger therapeutic impact than simple incarceration. The concept of the therapeutic community (TC) was particularly promoted by Jones (1952) and Main (1946). Since its introduction at Belmont (later Henderson Hospital), it has experienced numerous differentiations and modifications (e.g., Kennard, 1983; Roberts, 1997). What the various approaches seem to have in common is that they (a) establish a more informal atmosphere than in traditional institutions; (b) transfer responsibility for everyday running to the inmates; (c) arrange things so that it is primarily the residential group that provides support, care, and therapeutic processes for individuals; and (d) are open to interchanges with the community. Milieu therapy goes back to the work of Aichhorn (1957), and has been applied particularly to antisocial juveniles (e.g., Redl & Wineman, 1965).

Today, TCs are one of the most prominent approaches to the treatment of serious offenders (Wexler, 1997). Examples are Patuxent (Wilkins, 1978) and the Stay'n Out prison program (Wexler, Falkin, & Lipton, 1990) in the USA, or work at Henderson Hospital (Dolan, 1997; Norton, 1992), Grendon Prison (Cullen, 1997; Genders & Player, 1995; Gunn et al., 1978), and until recently the Barlinnie Special Unit (Cooke, 1989, 1997) in the United Kingdom. In part, the original principles of largely self-imposed control and permissiveness continue to be maintained. For example, at Grendon Prison, emphasis is placed particularly on the combination of voluntary attendance, democratic decision-making, and normative codes of conduct as well as on the tolerance of some deviancy and the encouragement of personal identity (Genders & Player, 1995). In part, however, emphasis is also placed on the necessary structuring, hierarchic organization, and professional standards (e.g., Wexler et al., 1990).

The latter also applies for similar institutions from continental Europe. Typical examples are the Dutch forensic mental hospitals (Koenradt, 1993) and the social-therapeutic prisons in Germany (Lösel & Egg, 1997). The latter were originally conceptualized according to models in the Netherlands like the van der Hoeven Clinic at Utrecht (van der Laan & Janssen, 1996) and the van Mesdag Clinic at Groningen (Hoekstra, 1979) as well as Scandinavian examples like the former therapeutic prison at

Herstedvester (Stürup, 1968). However, placement in the German social-therapeutic prisons is voluntary and the sentence remains determinate (with the possibility of conditional release). Prisoners have to apply for admission and acceptance is based on an assessment of treatment willingness, ability, and necessity. The main target groups are offenders with personality disorders and recidivists with a serious criminal record (including violence and sex offenses). The percentage of psychopaths in the stricter sense is unknown. Although the various institutions do not share a general treatment concept, they all emphasize group processes as well as organizational factors as therapeutic media. Various forms of individual and group therapy are offered. Social training models and educational concepts have become particularly important. After some time and according to progress in the offenders behavior, some major features are work, vocational training and other contacts outside the institution, intensive day-pass and vacation opportunities, as well as specific measures in preparation for release. Although these and other gratifications can also be found in regular prisons, social-therapeutic prisons differ substantially in degree. They generally have not only a more favorable staff-prisoner ratio but also more personnel in social services. Various characteristics indicate that the whole process is indeed more strongly treatment-oriented than in regular prisons (e.g., Egg, 1984; Lösel & Bliesener, 1989; Ortmann, 1994, 1997).

Evaluation studies have shown that TCs impact on psychiatric symptoms, personality, and other psychological variables. For example, they have revealed a strengthening of self-esteem, independence, attitudinal conformity, and morality (McCord, 1982; Norris, 1985); less anxiety, depression, distress, and neuroticism (Dolan, Evans, & Wilson, 1992; Fink, Derby, & Martin, 1969; Gunn et al., 1978; Cullen, 1997); a more internal locus of control and greater sensitivity toward personal responsibility for one's own problems (Genders & Player, 1995, Cullen, 1997); or positive effects on violence and the interaction climate (Cooke, 1989; Cullen, 1994; Peat & Winfree, 1992). These studies are good examples of a positive treatment impact for the institutional management of difficult offenders. However, it has to be asked how far more long-term effects are to be found in the area of antisocial behavior.

Various evaluation studies address antisocial juveniles. For example, McCord and Sanchez (1982) have compared a milieu-therapy setting (Wiltwyck) with a traditional, discipline-oriented reformatory school (Lyman). In the first years, effects on the *"psychopathic"* boys at the former institution were far more favorable. However, long-term comparisons extending into adulthood showed no major differences in terms of criminal recidivism, alcoholism, and the like. McCord (1982) traced this back to negative societal influences subsequent to the original rehabilitation of the Wiltwyck youngsters. Nonetheless, in a similar study, Cornish and Clarke (1975) already found no differences after only a 2-year follow-up interval. Using a randomized design, severely antisocial juveniles were referred either to a TC or to a unit with a traditional disciplined regime. In both cases, recidivism rates were about 70%. Craft, Stephenson, and Granger (1964) made similar observations in a comparison of two different regimes for (legally defined) adolescent psychopaths at Balderton Hospital in England. After a mean follow-up interval of 14 months, they found that *"psychopaths"* (aged between 13 and 25 years) exposed to a self-governing TC approach did not perform better than a comparison group from a unit with a firm, paternalistic, and sympathetic regime.

Reconviction, readmission, and clinical well-being in the latter group was even slightly, but significantly, better.

In a controlled study on TC treatment of adults, Robertson and Gunn (1987) compared 61 men discharged from Grendon with a matched group from other prisons. In a 10-year follow-up, no differences were found regarding frequency or severity of post-discharge convictions. However, more positive results appeared in a subgroup of particularly motivated and relatively intelligent inmates. The authors also reported that the extent of earlier violence, disturbed personal relationships, impulsivity, and alcohol problems correlated positively with the length of subsequent imprisonment, whereas depression and self-esteem showed a negative correlation. The number of pre-Grendon court appearances, lying, and global ratings for personality dysfunctions related to the number of post-discharge court appearances. These differential findings suggest that offenders who were psychopathic in a stricter sense probably benefited least from the approach. In more recent evaluations at Grendon, Cullen (1993) and Newton and Thornton (reported in Cullen, 1997) compared recidivism rates with those from the general prison population serving similar sentences. Results for Grendon were only slightly better. However, it could also be shown that these inmates are a particularly high-risk group. Treatment was more successful for those clients who stayed longer in treatment (> 19 months), had been released directly from Grendon, and were under supervision afterwards (Cullen, 1997).

Indications for differential effects were also found in Copas et al. (1984). This is one of several evaluations of Henderson Hospital (see Dolan, 1997). Their study of 254 patients compared various types of personality disorder: (a) Neurotic (N), showing high anxiety and intropunitiveness; (b) Extrapunitive Neurotic (EN), showing high anxiety and extrapunitiveness; (c) Intropunitive Psychopath (IP), showing intropunitiveness and low anxiety; and (d) Psychopath (P), showing low anxiety and extrapunitiveness. Subjects were followed up over periods of 3 and 5 year after discharge from treatment or nonadmittance to Henderson (one fifth of the group). There was little difference in reconviction or rehospitalization outcome between those not admitted and those who left within the first 4 weeks. But a steady improvement occurred with increasing time spent in treatment. The overall success rate was 41%, and that for subjects staying 9 months or more, 71% (see, also, Whiteley, 1970). The success rates for the N, P, and IP types were similar (about 50% for treatment of more than 6 months). The EN group showed a particularly low success rate (35%), and the disparity between treated and untreated subjects was more pronounced for this type. However, it has to be taken into account that there was no equivalent control group in this study, and it is difficult to compare the subtypes with other categories of psychopathy. In a more recent evaluation at Henderson, Dolan (1997) studied 177 patients. In a 1-year follow-up, of those who stayed longer in treatment, significantly fewer had reoffended or were readmitted as inpatients. The treatment group was also compared with 84 patients not accepted by Henderson, 119 patients who did not attend assessment or whose referral was withdrawn, and 44 patients who were refused treatment funding by their District Health Authority. Whereas 32.8% of the admitted group reoffended or were readmitted, this was the case for 51.8% of the untreated groups. Of the group who stayed more than 12 weeks in treatment, only 19.8% had either reoffended or been readmitted compared with 54.5% of the unfunded group (which was more comparable than the other *"controls"*). Although these results are encouraging, the groups were not specifically psychopaths, and selection, selection x treatment, or other threats to validity have to be taken into account.

In contrast, Ogloff et al. (1990) used the PCL to split their participants into subgroups. They evaluated a TC program in a Canadian forensic hospital. Subjects with a high PCL score (psychopaths) left treatment earlier, showed less motivation, and exhibited less improvement compared with groups with medium to low PCL scores. Whereas follow-up data are not available in this study, Harris et al. (1991) report on a 10-year follow-up study of 169 patients who had spent at least 2 years in a TC program in a maximum security psychiatric hospital. Subjects were classified as violent failures if they incurred any new charge for a criminal offense against persons or were returned to a maximum security institution for violent behavior against persons. Forty percent of the total group and 77% of the psychopaths (defined by a PCL-score of 25) committed a violent offense. The PCL was the best predictor of violent failures.

The results of a controlled evaluation of the TC were even more unfavorable (Rice et al., 1992). For each treated subject, a matched comparison subject was selected who had mostly spent some time in a nontherapeutic correctional institution. In the group of nonpsychopaths, 44% of TC patients were recidivists compared with 58% of the untreated group, and 22% versus 39% exhibited a violent failure (differences significant). Among psychopaths, in contrast, there was no treatment effect. In the treated group, 87% experienced some kind of failure compared with 90% in the untreated group. Of the treated psychopaths, 77% exhibited violent recidivism compared with 55% of the untreated. Obviously, the TC even had negative effects on the psychopaths. This underlines the threat of contra-indicated measures mentioned above. Rice et al. suspected that the TC had tended to promote skills leading to more antisocial behavior among the psychopaths. Nonetheless, this does not explain why the negative effects occurred only in the field of violence. Perhaps, a ceiling effect plays a role in general recidivism. However, it could also be that the treatment activated some cognitive and emotional changes, but because these may not have been processed and controlled sufficiently, they ended up in more violence.

Such findings suggest that although TC programs seem to work with various personality-disordered and other offender groups, they are less suitable for (primary) psychopaths. In line with this, Esteban et al. (1995) found that the highest outcome difference was between psychopaths and nonpsychopaths ($r = -.24$) in the 13 TC programs evaluated in their meta-analysis. This confirms the trend that low structure and permissiveness are inappropriate for psychopaths or high-risk offenders. According to Andrews et al. (1990), inappropriate services include all milieu and group approaches that emphasize within-group communication and lack a clear plan for gaining control over procriminal modeling and reinforcement.

The importance of the specific design of a TC is shown by Wexler et al. (1990) in an outcome evaluation of a prison therapeutic community for substance abuse treatment in New York. They compared a hierarchical TC program with a low-structured milieu treatment, short-term counseling, and a no-treatment control group. The main differences between the TC and milieu therapy were: (a) Time was more structured and activities more regimented, (b) jobs and social roles had a hierarchic order, (c) good conduct was rewarded by giving residents greater responsibilities, and (d) interaction with nonprison TCs was more extensive. In a 3-year follow-up, the percentage of rearrested males was 26.9% for the TC, 34.6% for milieu therapy, 39.8% for counseling, and 40.9% for the untreated group. This indicates 7 to 14 percentage points better outcomes for TC. The positive TC effects could be replicated in a similar program in California with 20 percentage points less recidivism of the treated versus untreated individuals (Wexler, 1997). Even better results were achieved when the prison TC was combined with an aftercare TC in the community (36 percentage points less recidivism). In both cases, however, the present follow-up data only cover 1 year after release.

Such effects of structured TCs correspond to those of social-therapeutic prisons in Germany. Lösel and Köferl (1989) carried out a systematic research integration that was updated by Lösel (1995b). Twelve comparisons used recidivism as outcome criterion with follow-up periods between 2 and 10 years (mostly more than 5 years). The sample size of the treated groups ranged from $N = 30$ to 187. The results varied according to the different definitions of failure. For more severe kinds of recidivism (again a prison sentence), rates were about 40-50%. In comparison with groups from regular prisons, mean effect sizes ranged between one study with a negative outcome of -.04 (Egg, 1990) and positive effects of .16 (Dünkel & Geng, 1994) or .19 (Rehn, 1979). The mean N-weighted ES was *phi* .11. Although the methodologically most sound study of Ortmann (1994) showed an ES of only .01 after 2 years, more recent results of about 7 percentage points difference after 5 years (Ortmann, 1997) were in the typical range. As the differences between the various studies could be attributed to sampling error, German research indicates a relatively consistent but small effect of social therapy. As in the above-mentioned studies from other countries, most evaluations showed that dropouts had the worst outcomes (Lösel et al., 1987). This might be due partially to psychopaths who are less motivated and more difficult to treat. However, two recent studies reported that the outcome differences between those who dropped out from social therapy and those who were discharged regularly from social therapy were less pronounced than in earlier research (Dolde, 1996; Ortmann, 1994, 1997). Perhaps, the practice of transfer as well as that of regular prison regimes has improved since earlier studies. This points to one fundamental problem with any evaluation: Effects depend not only on the evaluated program but also on what happens to the control groups (which is never *"nothing"*).

3. Punishment, Deterrence, and Formal Justice Reactions

Society's traditional reaction to criminality is punishment. It serves various purposes such as the deterrence of other potential offenders and compensation for guilt. However, in most societies, one goal is also deterring the individual from committing further offenses. At times, measures of punishment and deterrence are depicted as the opposite to concepts of treatment. In fact, this is not a dichotomy: On the one hand, most kinds of treatment of antisociality are more or less compulsory and include aspects of punishment, at least by reduced liberty. On the other hand, punishment is an established principle of behavior modification and thus must be regarded as one potential mode of *"treatment"* (e.g., Brennan & Mednick, 1994).

In recent times, particularly in the USA, but also in other countries, the concept of punishment is gaining in significance once more. This is indicated by strong increases in the rates of imprisonment (Kuhn, 1996; Tonry, 1996) as well as less expensive and more specific *"punishment smarter"* strategies. The latter include measures like intensive probation supervision, home confinement, electronic monitoring, shock incarceration, or boot camps.

This is not the right place to discuss how far practice in the justice system violates psychological principles of punishment (e.g., being immediate, intensive, consistent, unavoidable etc.). I also cannot review how far imprisonment and other forms of incarceration have negative effects. High recidivism rates among persons who have been incarcerated are mostly interpreted in this sense. However, recidivism after imprisonment is much less than 100% and declines clearly with age (Lloyd et al., 1994; Lösel, 1994a). Therefore, negative effects of custody must be viewed in a more differential way. Admittedly, it is impossible to say how far a punishment effect is present in those who no longer offend, or whether other psychosocial influences are more important. Negative prisonization effects also do not seem to be as pervasive and strong as often claimed (see Bonta & Gendreau, 1990). Numerous moderators of the person, the context, the regime, and so forth are involved (Lösel, 1993). Although effects of treatment are somewhat better in evaluations of community programs compared with institutional settings (e.g., Andrews et al., 1990; Lipsey, 1992a; Redondo, 1994), the groups of clients are not comparable. Therefore, empirical indications have to be taken from studies that modified either the intensity or the mode of the sanction and compared outcomes with controls:

Several meta-analyses found that pure measures of punishment or deterrence show, at best, weak effects. Lipsey (1992a) reported mean ESs for variations of probation, parole, and release that are clearly below $r = .10$. For programs with an explicitly deterrent component like boot camps or *"scared straight,"* there was even a negative mean ES of -.12. Redondo (1994) reported similar findings. Gendreau and Little (1993) found a slight increase in recidivism of 2% for *"punishment smarter"* programs. Intensive probation supervision programs and other forms of alternative sanctions seem not to be much more effective (Gendreau et al., 1993; Junger-Tas, 1993; Petersilia, Turner, & Dechenes, 1992). There is also no clear evidence that community penalties outperform custody or vice versa (Llloyd et al., 1994; Petersilia, Turner, & Peterson, 1986). Andrews et al. (1990) classified all programs containing only variations in judicial dispositions under the heading of criminal sanctions. These included, for example, restitution, police cautioning versus regular processing, less versus more probation, and probation versus custody. The mean effect size was -.08. In a recent update of this meta-analysis, Gendreau and Goggin (1996) compared separately the results of evaluations of incarceration, intermittent incarceration, restitution, scared straight, electronic monitoring, drug testing, and fines. The percentages of recidivism in the respective punishment and control groups were very similar. The overall mean effect was about zero. Only the restitution programs showed a small mean positive effect of .06.

These and other findings question whether the merely formal variation of criminal justice measures and punishment has a major effect on offenders (Gendreau, 1995). This applies even more strongly to psychopaths because of their lack in anxiety and related problems in learning from negative experiences (Cleckley, 1976; Lykken, 1995). Due to deficits in passive-avoidance learning, less positive effects of traditional reactions by the criminal justice system should be anticipated in psychopaths than in other offenders. Thus, for example, in a study of Hart, Kropp, and Hare (1988), the group with high scores on the PCL-R was least successful on parole or mandatory supervision. The percentage of revoked or reconvicted offenders was smaller in the group with medium PCL-R scores, and low-scoring PCL-R offenders had the most successes. Such unfavorable outcomes for psychopaths were also found in a comprehensive meta-analysis of 133 studies on adult offender recidivism (Gendreau, Little, & Goggin, 1995). The minimum follow-up interval was 6 months, and special treatment studies were excluded. Psychopathy was among the strongest predictors of recidivism. Whereas the mean ES of the best single predictors (like criminogenic needs, family factors) was about .15, *"composite measures"* reached effects of about .30. The latter included measures such as the Level of Survey Inventory-Revised (LSI-R; Andrews & Bonta, 1995) and measures of psychopathy such as the PCL-R. As Loza and Simourd (1994) have shown, there are high correlations between the LSI-R and the PCL-R. However, the PCL-R seems to be particularly sensitive for predicting violent recidivism (Harris, Rice, & Quinsey, 1993; Salekin et al., 1996). Of course, it has to be taken into account that repeated offending and reconvictions enter into the diagnosis of psychopathy, and PCL-Factor 2 seems to be more important for recidivism than Factor 1 (Harpur, Hare, & Hakstian, 1989; Salekin et al., 1996). Thus, the predictive efficacy is in line with criminological research that is not based on the concept of psychopathy. However, it is not only the criminal history but also interpersonal and affective characteristics that contribute to the predictive validity of PCL-R for violence (Hemphill & Hare, 1996).

This body of research suggests that merely formal variations in the traditional measures of the penal justice system or *"punishment smarter"* strategies are less successful for psychopaths than for other offenders. There may be only one exception: When the outcome criterion is not defined as positive behavior change but as protection of the public. In this case, long-term selective incapacitation of psychopaths could be seen as a promising approach. Although the recent toughness in crime policy and rising imprisonment rates is not specifically targeted on psychopaths, it reflects such kinds of reasoning. The Californian *"solution"* of *"Three strikes and you're out"* is its most radical example. Even if ethical aspects are set apart, such practices are not yet well-supported by data (Skolnick, 1994). Parent trainings and graduation incentives, for example, are more cost-effective (Greenwood et al., 1996). That the long-term increase of crime rates and particularly of violent offenses in the USA stopped during the last decade, can not simply be attributed to more or longer imprisonment. Not only economic conditions but also preventive approaches and police control have changed simultaneously. It should also be taken into account that the USA (together with Russia) already had very high rates of imprisonment when their criminality increased (see Kuhn, 1996).

The long-term imprisonment of criminals must be carried out in accordance with basic principles of just punishment, humanity, and liberty in modern societies. Within this framework, the diagnosis of psychopathy can play an important role in deciding on security level and length of placement in custody. We noted earlier that the PCL versions are relatively good predictors of recidivism and dangerousness (Gendreau et al., 1995; Salekin et al., 1996; Serin, 1996; Wong, 1996). However, as Salekin et al. (1996) have shown, the mean predictive validity in 18 studies is not larger than $r = .32$ (.37 for violent behavior and .27 for general recidivism; d coefficients transformed by this author). Combinations with other predictors and the use of receiver operating characteristics can enhance predictive validity for violent recidivism to approximately 40% relative improvement over chance (Rice & Harris, 1995a). Although this may come close to thresholds of predictability in human behavior, substantial problems of misclassification remain. Even if prediction could be further improved, a selective incapacitation of psychopaths would need to be particularly long. On average, their criminal activity fades after age 40 (Hare, McPherson, & Forth, 1988); that is, later than in many other career criminals (Blumstein et al., 1988). Furthermore, violent offences, aggression in the family, alcoholism, vocational problems, or other forms of noncriminal antisociality frequently persist (Robins, 1966). Therefore, a moderate expansion in length of imprisonment would not be a strong benefit for society.

Naturally, in the most serious cases long-term incarceration is unavoidable. As a general strategy, however, it is confronted not only with the demands of human rights, just punishment, and prediction of dangerousness but also with those of economy. For example, a consistent application of the *"three strikes out"* law of 1994 will need 20 more prisons and will consume about 18% of California's budget in only 8 years (Skolnick, 1994). As resources are limited, expanded costs of the prison system may reduce investments in other areas like school or social welfare and thus indirectly contribute to further antisociality in the next generation. All these arguments imply that public opinions like *"lock them up and throw away the key"* are not the best way for societies to cope with problems of psychopathy.

4. Pharmacological treatment

Biological factors and bio-psycho-social interactions can play an important role in the development of persistent violence and criminality (Mednick, Moffitt, & Stack, 1987; Raine, 1993; Raine et al., 1997). Thus, pharmacological treatment of psychopaths may be a promising approach. One main difficulty in evaluating pharmacological treatment is that the respective evaluations refer to a rather broadly defined psychopathy or APD. Another problem is that most studies include patients who have an additional diagnosis of personality disorder (e.g., borderline personality disorder, BPD) or whose primary symptoms are schizotypal features, anxiety, depression, suicidal ideations, and so forth (Dolan & Coid, 1993). Frequently, these psychiatric disorders determine the selection of the respective drugs (Tardiff, 1992). However, Comorbidity with syndromes of the internalizing spectrum raises the issue of specific underlying biological processes (Lilienfeld, 1994).

Pharmacological treatment of psychopathy can be based on Gray's (1982, 1987) concept of brain function. Gray distinguishes three different systems both on the behavioral and neural (anatomic and biochemical) level. Each system is activated by different categories of external stimuli and corresponding to distinguishable behaviors (Birbaumer & Schmidt, 1996). These systems are: (a) the behavioral activation system or approach system (BAS); the mesolimbic dopamine system, activated by conditioned rewards or withdrawal of negative reinforcement stimuli; (b) the behavioral inhibition system (BIS); the septo-hippocampal system with serotonin and norepinephrine (noradrenaline) as transmitters, activated by conditioned punishment and new stimuli; (c) the fight/flight system; amygdala, activated by aversive stimuli like extreme noise or unexpected attacks. Theories of psychopathy that refer to Gray's model suggest a relative dominance of the BAS over the BIS (e.g., Newman & Wallace, 1993b; Quay, 1993). In contrast, individuals with a relative dominance of BIS over BAS are prone to inhibitory psychopathology like anxiety disorders (e.g., Kagan, Reznick, & Snidman, 1988). The dominance of BAS results in impulsive and aggressive behavior, low frustration tolerance, reduced capacity for passive avoidance learning, and the like that are features of the psychopathic personality. Because biochemical evidence suggests a diminished serotonergic and possibly noradrenergic functioning but no increased dopaminergic activity in persons with impulsive aggression (e.g., Markowitz & Coccaro, 1995), the dominance of BAS in psychopaths appears to result more from a weakness of BIS rather than an overactivity of BAS (Quay, 1993).

The differentiation between these systems is important for the efficacy of pharmacological treatment, and, to a certain extent, it is supported by it. In psychopathy, drugs should serve to attenuate dopaminergic functioning in the BAS while enhancing noradrenergic and serotonergic functioning in the BIS (Quay, 1993). In animal experiments, benzodiazepines, barbiturates, and alcohol inhibit the BIS by virtue of their suppressive effect on noradrenergic activation (Birbaumer & Schmidt, 1996; Gray, 1982, 1987). These drugs should further weaken the BIS, reduce anxiety in passive avoidance situations (phobic disorders), and lead to an increase in aggressive and impulsive behavior. Although there are only a few controlled studies on the effect of benzodiazepines (e.g., alprazolam) on behavior and personality disorders (e.g., Dolan & Coid, 1993; Tardiff, 1992), their use in these patients is not supported. There have been reports of observed behavioral dyscontrol such as hostile outbursts, aggressive behavior, suicidal ideations and acts after such treatment (e.g., Browne et al., 1993; Cowdry & Gardner, 1988; Gardner & Cowdry, 1985). Thus, sedative drugs as well as alcohol are contra-indicated in psychopathic personalities. The same holds for sexual offenders (Seto & Barbaree, 1995).

Lithium, however, which serves to increase central serotonin activity, can be thought of as operating to increase BIS inhibition of BAS. This has been partly supported by lithium treatment of patients with explosive, impulsive, and aggressive outbursts and of patients with BPD (e.g., Dolan & Coid, 1993; Goldberg, 1989). Less is known on the therapy of persons with antisocial personality disorders (Wistedt et al., 1994). Some authors have also used lithium successfully for the treatment of undersocialized-aggressive conduct disorder in children (Campbell et al., 1984), whereas others have been unable to confirm a positive effect on this disorder (DeLong & Aldershot, 1987). As lithium shows a relatively narrow therapeutic bandwidth and bears a risk of intoxication, it is not particularly appropriate for acute cases (Hollweg &

Nedopil, 1997). Many patients also discontinue lithium treatment because of the side effects such as diarrhea, weight gain, mental lethargy, tremor, etc. (Markovitz, 1995).

More frequent is the treatment of violent offenders with neuroleptics (Wistedt et al., 1994). As dopamine receptor blockers, neuroleptics can be expected to dampen BAS activity. Support stems from trials that suggest an indication for low-dose neuroleptic therapy (e.g., haloperidol) in psychopaths with overt motor agitation and aggressive behavioral disturbance who also show schizotypal features, such as illusions and paranoid ideations. Improvements were found in schizotypal symptoms as well as in hostility, anger, verbal aggression, and interpersonal sensitivity (e.g., Soloff et al., 1986). Neuroleptics have also been reported to be efficacious in reducing undercontrolled-aggressive conduct disorders in children (Campbell, Cohen, & Small, 1982). Longitudinal studies, however, have shown that the effects of haloperidol are transient and that these patients had a much higher drop-out rate than placebo because of side effects (Cornelius et al., 1993).

Psychostimulants like amphetamines increase turnover of both dopamine and norepinephrine. Thus, their effect is not easily predictable. There are, however, a number of studies reporting a reduction in aggression in children with attention deficit-hyperactivity disorder through the use of psychostimulants (e.g., Barkley et al., 1989). Similarly, they may be useful in subgroups of persons with APD, especially those without schizotypal features (Schulz et al., 1988). At low dosage for behavior disorders, psychostimulants appear to be largely free of unwanted side effects (Dolan & Coid, 1993). However, there is a risk of dependency and further research is needed on their efficacy.

Because depressive symptoms and even major depression are observed in a proportion of patients with APD (Coid, 1992), treatment has also included antidepressants. Here, results are less clear. In some studies, a disturbing clinical deterioration has been observed in a subgroup of patients, such as severe aggressive outbursts, increased hostility, irritability, and behavioral impulsivity (e.g., Soloff et al., 1986). Another double-blind study demonstrated marked improvements in mood, but little change in behavioral dyscontrol (Cowdry & Gardner, 1988). Literature suggests an adverse interaction between DSM-axis I and axis II psychopathology with regard to the outcome of treatment (Reich & Green, 1991). Subjects with pure major depression seem to respond better to tricyclic treatment than subjects with major depression and coexisting personality disorder. This may be due to the biological conditions that suggest disturbances of both the BAS and BIS. On the one hand, these subgroups might respond better to psychological therapy (Ogloff et al., 1990). On the other hand, the "mixed" type has an even worse prognosis for both externalizing problems like aggression, hostility, or substance abuse and internalizing syndromes like anxiety or major depressive disorders (e.g., Windle, 1994). The "shy-aggressive" type identified in childhood literature (see Windle & Windle, 1993) also appears to develop more pervasive internalizing and externalizing problems in adolescence and adulthood. Thus, pharmacological treatment of this type needs further clarification in carefully controlled trials.

In antisocial subjects with atypical depression or with features of hysteroid dysphoria, monoamine oxidase inhibitors (MAOIs) may be a treatment of choice

(Dolan & Coid, 1993). However, there are divergent views as to whether the beneficial effects on personality disorder are due to their antidepressant or psychostimulant effects (Stein, 1992). Because there is a serious risk of side effects (e.g., hypotension, weight gain, agitation, poor sleep) and an observed unreliability in treated patients with severe personality disorder, a trial of MAOIs may only be appropriate after other treatments have failed. These patients, however, should not abuse alcohol or other substances (like cocaine, amphetamine, etc.) because the use of these drugs with MAOIs can prove lethal (Markovitz, 1995). Among anticonvulsants, only carbamazepine has been shown to reduce behavior symptoms such as overactivity, aggression, and poor impulse control in patients with borderline personality disorder (BPD; Cowdry & Gardner, 1988).

A more recent and promising approach is suggested by treatment with serotonin re-uptake inhibitors (SRIs; e.g., fluoxetine, sertraline). In a prospective study with sertraline, Kavoussi, Liu, and Coccaro (1994) found relatively positive effects on the impulsive-aggressive behavior of personality disordered patients. In another study of fluoxetine in patients with BPD, Markovitz et al. (1991) also noted improvement in hostility, obsessiveness, anxiety, depression psychosis and interpersonal skills. Perhaps, this may become a more specific path to the pharmacological treatment of impulsive aggressive and eventually also auto-aggressive behavior (Hollweg & Nedopil, 1997). However, more controlled studies on different personality disorders are necessary for an adequate evaluation.

In the field of sexual offending, hormone treatment with antiandrogens is suggested. Testosterone antagonists like cyproterone acetate and medroxyprogesterone acetate are applied with some success (Berner, 1997; Gottesman & Schubert, 1993). As testosterone is not only related to sexuality in the narrow sense but also to dominant, aggressive, and impulsive behavior, antiandrogens would fit to the versatile antisociality of many sex offenders. However, it is not clear whether a high testosterone level is a cause or consequence of aggressive dominance (Archer, 1991). In addition, studies showed that plasma testosterone was within normal limits in all but a subgroup of the most violent paraphilias (Hucker & Bain, 1990). Thus, testosterone antagonists may be indicated in the long-term treatment of specific cases of sexual violence, their broader use in acute therapy, however, is not recommended (Hollweg & Nedopil, 1997). More controlled replications and reductions of unwanted side effects are necessary.

Furthermore, studies suggest that the effect of hormones (the cellular mechanisms) may be at the level of monoamine receptors, namely the modulation of serotonin (5-HT), dopamine and norepinephrine, because "sex" hormones can induce alterations in the binding of monoamine neurotransmitters in the limbic systems (Everitt, 1983). It has been shown that decreased 5-HT may disinhibit or promote sexual behavior, whereas decreased central dopaminergic functioning reduces motivation as well as drive behavior, including male sexual behavior (Kafka, 1995). It is most likely that hormones and monoamine neurotransmitter interact in a dynamic fashion that determines the form and intensity of drive (including sexual) behaviors (Everitt, 1983). Thus, the use of selective SRIs represents a promising addition to the pharmacotherapy of sexual impulse disorders with antiandrogens (e.g., Kafka & Prentky, 1992).

As various reviews have shown, there is not yet one specific drug for the treatment of aggression, impulsivity, and related disorders (e.g., Browne et al., 1993; Marcovitz, 1995; Wistedt et al., 1994). However, despite a paucity of studies on which to assess the potential pharmacological effect on *"core"* features of psychopathic disorder, pharmacotherapy is one area of treatment that does show some promise for the future (Dolan & Coid, 1993). For legal and ethical reasons, pharmacological treatment will rarely be the first and only choice. Normally, combinations with psychotherapy and social measures are indicated. In contrast to ideological and professional conflicts, the successful combination of cognitive psychotherapy and pharmacotherapy in the treatment of depression may function as a model for further attempts in the field of antisociality.

CONCLUSIONS AND PERSPECTIVES FOR PRACTICE

Whereas this review reveals a substantial body of research on the treatment of antisociality and criminality in general, there is a lack of well-controlled studies on interventions into psychopathy. Nonequivalence of control groups, heterogeneity of treated groups, different concepts and assessments of the disorder, developmental aspects, Comorbidity, lack of data on treatment processes, integrity deficits, and problems of effect criteria further impair methodologically sound conclusions. However, some relatively consistent patterns of results appear: Small to medium efficacy can be demonstrated for cognitive-behavioral programs, multimodal treatment, structured TC programs and social therapy for serious and personality-disordered offenders. In contrast, psychopathy proves to be a moderator that generally reduces positive outcomes. Although no measure is clearly successful with psychopaths, further developments of various approaches seem to be promising. Due to their negative effects, other measures are even contra-indicated. Although such results indicate not yet a big knowledge change since earlier reviews, the pattern now looks more differentiated: General typologies of treatment (like psychotherapy or therapeutic community) are less indicated than specific characteristics of programs. Research on the treatment of antisociality suggests differentiated pathways that may lead to more successful interventions with at least some groups of psychopaths under particular conditions. What we need now is a new generation of theoretically and methodologically sound evaluations of well-planned interventions in this field (Lösel, 1995c). Naturalistic studies of the development of cohorts of clients could play an important role for their development (Dolan & Coid, 1993).

Due to the lack of well-controlled evaluations, differences in dangerousness, variations in Comorbidity, and other problems, it is not yet appropriate to emphasize only one single concept or program. Instead, a broader set of principles should guide the development of concepts that must be tested empirically (see also Andrews, 1995; Gendreau, 1995; Howells, et al., 1997). Although psychopaths do not necessarily become criminals and are only a small high-risk group among offenders, principles of effective correctional intervention should be used for this development. Well-established programs like the Reasoning and Rehabilitation approach (Ross & Fabiano, 1985; Ross et al., 1989; Ross & Ross, 1995) and more specific concepts for psychopaths (Hare, 1992) can serve as a basis for local interventions. In the following, a number of relevant principles will be briefly described. They focus not only on the individual client but also include the staff and institutional level as well as relations to the community and society level. The principles are based on the empirical research reviewed above as well as on generalizations from practice.

1. Theoretically sound conceptualization

Although basic knowledge on psychopathy has increased, we still do not have a coherent theory. Research on the treatment of antisociality, however, shows that the most successful programs are based on empirically supported hypotheses on the etiology and maintenance of problem behavior (Andrews & Bonta, 1994; Antonowicz & Ross, 1994). Interventions should not focus exclusively on specific schools or traditions of psychotherapy but on what is known about the causes of antisociality and recidivism. This is in line with modern concepts of integrative or eclectic psychotherapy (Garfield & Bergin, 1994). A majority of programs that have proven to be most appropriate for various groups of offenders are based on cognitive social learning theory (Andrews & Bonta, 1994). Such a cognitive-behavioral approach seems to be transferable to the psychopathic clientele. Probably, concepts must focus more intensively on deficits in information processing and emotional understanding than they need to be with other offenders. A sound theoretical approach also needs to consider kinds of Comorbidity (e.g., alcohol dependence) as well as eventual subtype characteristics (e.g., anxiety in secondary psychopaths). For example, when more emotionality is present, elements of classical psychotherapy may be less inadequate than in other cases. Similarly, it is suggested that it is worthwhile to include physiological hypotheses and respective pharmacological treatment for some groups of psychopaths. This particularly holds for specific comorbidities or kinds of offending (like violent and sexual crimes). Within a broader evaluation theory (Chen, 1990), the concept must also include realistic indicators of goal attainment. For example, working on specific thinking patterns, teaching concrete skills for prosocial behavior, or reducing substance abuse are more adequate than too broad aims of changing the psychopathic core personality. Last but not least, such a theoretical concept should contain assumptions about positive rewards for the psychopaths as well as the risks of abusing program elements.

2. Thorough dynamic assessment of the client

A theoretically sound concept for intervention must be based on an accurate and detailed assessment of the individual case. This is initially necessary for a diagnosis of risk, dangerousness, and treatability that leads to an adequate placement in more or less secure institutions. Standardized instruments like the PCL-R, PCL-SV, LSI-R, and the Risk Appraisal Guide are indicated here. Although these methods prove to be relatively accurate, there seem to be upper limits of predictability of about $r = .40$ (Monahan & Steadman, 1994; Menzies & Webster, 1995). Furthermore, actuarial predictions tell us not enough about individuals, particularly when base rates are relatively low (Grubin & Wingate, 1996). Cutting points are also not fully clear, neither within nor across cultures (Cooke, 1996; Salekin et al., 1996). For individual decisions, a comprehensive and dynamic clinical assessment of psychopathic disorder is necessary. Dolan and Coid

(1993) suggest three elements: *1. Personality disorder*: At least one of the following informations: (a) DSM-IV axis II categorization; (b) ICD-10 categorization; (c) PCL-R score, (d) MMPI or SHAPS profiles, (e) structured clinical interview for a psychodynamic formulation of character disorder. *2. Clinical syndromes (DSM axis I)*: Analysis of all major mental disorders, including paraphilias and substance abuse, within a lifetime perspective (not only present state analysis). *3. Behavioral disorder*: At least information on (a) criminal history, (b) noncriminalized antisocial and aggressive behavior, (c) ability to form and maintain relationships with others, (d) occupational functioning. In addition, for reasons of comparability and validity, the PCL-R should generally be assessed as a central marker. With respect to the planning of interventions, the schedule must be completed by detailed assessments of treatment motivation and of problems associated with specific kinds of offenses. In the case of sexual offenses, for example, assessment of sexual arousal, sexual fantasies, rationalizing cognitions, and victim empathy are relevant (e.g., Briggs, 1994). An analysis of violent offenses should include information on the offense such as the type, victim, motivation, and trigger events; information on risk factors like alcohol consumption, preoccupation with weapons, hostility biases, coping behavior; and manifestations of risk behavior in the institution (McDougall, Clark, & Fisher, 1994). Such offense-specific information may give insight into the links between antisocial behavior and the psychopathic core personality and thinking patterns. As far as possible, dynamic assessment must rely on multiple sources and never the psychopath alone.

3. Intensive service

Whether in prison, forensic and other psychiatric hospitals, or even in ambulatory treatment, psychopaths regularly will need an intensive level of service. This is due not only to the characteristics of their personality disorder but also to their low motivation for change. Normally, psychopaths will not appear in ambulatory practice or only if an immediate reward is expected (e.g. parole or an otherwise milder sentence). As they are frequently persistent offenders, most interventions must take place in institutional settings. Taking the above-mentioned results on treatment motivation and dropout into account, a closed prison or high-security hospital will be the most frequent choice. Subjects with a high PCL-R score even show criminal career profiles that may require a super-maximum security environment (Wong, 1996). Developing at least some primary motivation for change often takes rather a long time. Collaboration may be forced by a cautious delivering of gratifications. Thus, a successful program will need more time than *"normal"* offender treatment. While 3 to 9 months may be sufficient for other offenders (Gendreau, 1995), at least one year will be necessary with psychopaths. The principle of matching the high risk for recidivism with an intensive level of service (Andrews et al., 1990) is also supported by better effects of high dosage in offender treatment (Lipsey, 1995b) as well as in psychotherapy in general (Orlinsky et al., 1994). As shown above, a longer duration of treatment was associated repeatedly with less failures for personality-disordered offenders (see Cullen, 1997; Dolan, 1997). However, even for this group, dosage does not have a linear relation to outcome (e.g., Jones, 1997). For some clients, a short intervention can already be sufficient; for others, a very long treatment may indicate stagnation and failure. Overall, regularly terminated longer treatments reveal less recidivism (e.g., Jones, 1997; Lösel et al., 1987). As treatment is often terminated due to misbehavior or motivational problems of the client (Jones, 1997; Rice et al., 1992), dosage cannot be varied flexibly. However, if dynamic assessment shows that a critical event is associated with a sensitive period and some progress in treatment, termination should be avoided as far as possible. In contrast, early termination due to superficial adaptation of psychopaths must also be avoided. Similarly, in the case of juvenile offenders, the usual short-term interventions or diversion measures would be inappropriate for clients whose developmental assessment suggests that they are on the track to adult psychopathy.

4. Clearly structured and distinct setting

Decisions like those just mentioned must avoid the typical external attributions, blamings, negotiations, and manipulations of psychopaths. For these and other reasons, a clearly structured institutional setting is indicated. To ensure the specific therapeutic conditions that are necessary for psychopaths, the institution or department should be separated from regular prisons (Hare, 1992; Lösel & Egg, 1997). As the review of evaluations has shown, low structured forms of therapeutic community or milieu therapy are less successful or even counterproductive. Structured, hierarchical therapeutic communities or social-therapeutic prisons are more adequate. Clear rules, regulations, rights, duties, and responsibilities have two main aims: First, they help the client directly; Psychopaths with deficits in shifting attention between different stimuli and in flexible cognitive processing (Newman & Wallace, 1993a) may be less overstretched if they can follow a clear institutional structure. Second, this helps the staff and other inmates to reduce the psychopaths' attempts to obtain environmental control. Their typical behaviors may become more ineffective when institutional life is based on clear structures and rules and their cognitive distortions are continuously confronted with the reality by others. Although this is a basic principle for programs with psychopaths, nuances should be included to avoid too much thinking in black-and-white categories. This can be achieved, for example, by differentiated gratifications (specific leisure programs, visits, disposal for money, work outside, day-pass, or holidays). In cases of misbehavior, possibilities for retribution by objective endeavors (not only verbally) may also be included. In any case, these differentiations should be fixed in advance to avoid the above-mentioned traps in the interpersonal style of psychopaths. If a client shows substantial progress, regulations may be reduced to improve learning of the emotional significances and behavioral nuances that are often deficient (Hare, 1995).

5. Development of a prosocial institutional climate and regime

Although a clear-structured setting as well as firm and consistent staff behavior are particularly necessary for the treatment of psychopathy, the institutional regime must be interpersonally sensitive, constructive and supportive (Hare, 1992; Porporino & Baylis, 1993; Woowdard, 1997). Organizational structure and climate can have rather different influences in otherwise comparable prisons or hospitals (e.g., Akers, Hayner, & Gruninger, 1977; Moos, 1975; Wing, 1993). Results in the family, schools, and residential welfare institutions have also shown that an accepting/supportive as well as demanding/controlling ("*authoritative*") educational climate is most healthy for social development (Baumrind, 1989; Lösel, 1994b; Rutter et al., 1979). The behavior of psychopaths easily leads to conflicts and interpersonal problems that worsen institutional climate. For example, the positive aspects of a clearly structured regime may become cold and hostile. Thus, the psychopaths' interpersonal style will be indirectly reinforced. To counteract their antisocial expectations, the institutional climate must continuously be a focus of attention and self-regulation. Systematic instruments like the scales from Moos (1975) should be used for assessment. Paying attention to social climate and culture is also necessary with respect to interdepartmental consistency and mutual support between different agencies (Roberts, 1995).

6. Following the need principle

The evaluations have shown that appropriate targeting of specific criminogenic factors is one of the most important features in the treatment of antisociality. There are no reasons why this principle could not be transferred to psychopaths. Although individual needs have to be derived from the dynamic assessment, a variety of them are particularly relevant. Andrews and Bonta (1994), Gendreau (1995), and others suggest promising intermediate targets like changing antisocial attitudes; modifying antisocial attributions, neutralizations, and other thinking patterns; reducing antisocial feelings; increasing anger management, impulse-control, and problem solving-skills; replacing the skills of lying, stealing, aggression, and manipulation with more prosocial alternatives; improving victim awareness; reducing alcohol and other chemical dependencies; reducing comorbidities that are relevant for antisocial behavior; promoting familial affection, monitoring, and supervision; promoting association with anticriminal role models; shifting the density of the personal, interpersonal, and other rewards and costs for antisocial and prosocial activities toward the noncriminal spectrum; ensuring that the client is able to recognize risky situations and has a concrete and well rehearsed plan for dealing with those situations. As many of these kinds of intermediate targets are the same as the deep-rooted problems of psychopathy, one might object that changes are too difficult. However, need-oriented programs have the advantage of concentrating interventions on a limited number of specific objectives like improvement of social skills, control of anger or reduction of alcohol consumption.

Contingent reinforcement of positive attempts towards these targets is more promising than punishment of misbehavior, although the latter must be included in behavior contracts. Even psychopaths do not generally show negative behavior and are sensitive to reinforcers of positive behaviors (material goods, activities, attention, praise, etc.). There may also be less defense against interventions if "*only*" the control of specific problems and not the whole "*self*" is under question. Need-oriented targets should be arranged in a hierarchical manner. As psychopaths are occupied with immediate goals and have difficulties in understanding complex and subtle issues (Hare 1995; Kosson, 1996), improvement of information processing and cognitive functioning is a central target (e.g., Serin & Browne, 1996). Born (1997) compares this with developing from Piaget's level of concrete operations to the level of formal operations. Thinking processes should be improved toward more distance from the here and now, delay of gratification, generalization of experiences, critical self-reflection, and less egocentricism. Although better cognitive functioning is among the central needs of psychopaths, many nonpsychopathic people exhibit similar cognitive and moral problems. Results on the relation between level of moral reasoning and antisocial behavior are also not consistent (e.g., Goldsmith, Throfast, & Nilsson, 1989). If improved cognitive functioning is not accompanied by prosocial changes in attitudes, negative treatment outcomes like those reported in Rice et al. (1992) may occur. Chandler and Moran (1990), for example, found that scores on moral reasoning, social convention understanding, interpersonal awareness, socialization, empathy, and autonomy were combined differently in young psychopaths than in other groups. Psychopaths felt themselves to be autonomous without having developed serious commitments to society. Thus, the client must move from a strategy of unqualified self-interest to one of qualified self-interest (Beck & Freeman, 1990).

7. Following the responsivity principle, particularly with cognitive-behavioral methods

The consolidated problems of psychopaths suggest that it is primarily comprehensive multimodal approaches that might be able to alter criminogenic thinking patterns and behavior styles. As in the treatment of nonpsychopathic violent offenders, it is necessary to implement combinations of behavioral and cognitive-behavioral programs. They seem to be most appropriate to change the cognitive distortions, denials, minimizations, and so forth (Serin & Kuriychuk, 1994). As the responsivity principle includes matching treatment mode x offender type x staff style, no general package is suggested. However, existing programs or concepts (e.g., Beck & Freeman, 1990; Hare, 1992; Ross & Ross, 1995) are applicable and can be supplemented or accentuated for specific problems (like sexual offending or alcohol problems). The broad array of classical behavioral and modern cognitive behavioral techniques cannot be discussed here. Contingency contracting, cognitive restructuring, problem-solving training, social skills training, self-instruction and self-reinforcement, prosocial modeling, guided discussions, and various other techniques may be useful (e.g., McGuire & Priestley, 1995). If individuals are not totally cold-blooded, anger management (Novaco, 1997) and stress inoculation techniques (Meichembaum, 1985) should also be included. As mentioned above, each element of intervention has to be checked to see whether it is susceptible to misuse. Although empirical evaluations do not suggest classical psychotherapy, psychodynamic, nondirective, or otherwise low-structured approaches for working with psychopaths, one of their most important elements must be included in any kind of successful treatment: the therapeutic bond (see Orlinsky et al., 1994). Probably, in psychopathy treatment this grows much more slowly and more as a consequence and less as a condition of other changes. However, it can not be basically denied (Vaillant, 1975). An adequate matching with an accepting but firm and consistent staff member may be particularly important.

8. Realizing treatment integrity

As I noted above, lack of integrity is an important cause of failure in potentially successful programs. Having no well-developed concept or treatment manual is one source of this problem. Another derives from deficits or inconsistencies in skills, attitudes, motivation, and subjective theories among staff members. Furthermore, in the treatment of psychopaths, the clients also share responsibility for reduced integrity. Their various manipulations frequently question the behavior of individual staff members and contribute to group processes that weaken consistency in program implementation. Thus, monitoring the quality and quantity of the program must be a principle in any kind of treatment (Hollin, 1995; Thornton & Hogue, 1993). Information on program integrity should be based on direct observer recording as well as practitioner and (eventually) client report. Records include both quantitative aspects (e.g., length or frequency of sessions) and qualitative aspects (e.g., therapeutic process variables). The Correctional Program Evaluation Inventory (Gendreau & Andrews, 1994) is a broad instrument tested for various institutions and aspects of service delivery in Canada. A more specific attempt to record integrity has been made in Wales (Knott, 1995). Regularly assessments of integrity can not only be used for improving the general quality of treatment but also for case conferences. On the one hand, they make manipulative actions of psychopaths more transparent. On the other hand, monitoring can help to detect negative attitudes and counter-transferences in specific staff-client relations. Emphasizing integrity does not mean that programs should not be changed. Learning by experience and program adaptation are even particularly important for innovative treatments of psychopaths. However, reasons and contents of any major changes must follow empirically sound principles, be well documented and monitored.

9. Thorough selection, training, and supervision of staff

All principles discussed so far require well selected, sensitive, competent, and multidisciplinary staff members. Selection should not just be oriented toward general and special professional qualifications but try to match personal characteristics to the specific clientele. For example, relatively anxious, apprehensive, or verbal-nonpragmatic persons could be misplaced in work with psychopaths. Age and sex relations should also be taken into account. Intensive training must impart detailed knowledge on psychopathy and treatment skills. Continuos supervision is relevant for improving professional skills and attitudes on the job (Woodward, 1997). It is also necessary to avoid typical inconsistencies or destructive interpersonal processes in the work with psychopaths, for example: (a) battling to win, (b) becoming the advocate, (c) believing what you hear, (d) fearing manipulations, and (e) becoming fascinated (Doren, 1987). To find the right way between naive trust and disappointed cynicism is an important task in staff training and supervision. This must be encouraged by ongoing social support from the agency and community (Andrews, 1995; Roberts, 1995), particularly when critical events have occurred.

10. Neutralization of unfavorable social networks

Relations to deviant peers and affiliation with criminal subgroups are major risks in the development and maintenance of antisocial behavior (e.g., Caspi & Moffitt, 1995; Elliott, Huizinga, & Menard, 1989). Therefore, appropriate programs should neutralize these reinforcing and modeling influences. Unfortunately, correctional institutions, forensic hospitals, and even ambulatory settings promote unfavorable peer influences through the concentration of individuals with similar problems. However, even under such circumstances a reliable group atmosphere is not impossible. For psychopaths, the peer network has to be focused for an additional reason: Although they are not closely related to the group, they are influential because of their glibness, manipulation, institutional experience, antisocial career, and so forth. Frequently, such individuals may take over central roles in housekeeping, merchandising, smuggling, or gambling (Hürlimann, 1993). Staff must be aware of such social processes and counteract exploitative relationships through an adequate replacement of inmates. Groups should also develop explicit behavior norms. Here, principles from structured therapeutic communities are relevant (Wexler, 1997). Elements from bully-victim programs (Olweus, 1993) can also used to reduce antisocial and manipulative interactions within the group. Relatively firm and prosocial inmates can also take an important role in confronting the psychopath with reality. They may also function as a kind of co-trainer (Hare, 1992).

11. Strengthening natural protective mechanisms

Most research and practice on the treatment of antisociality is primarily oriented toward risks. However, studies on the natural history of antisocial behavior reveal processes of resilience and desistance that are linked to the protective functions of individual or social resources (e.g., Lösel & Bliesener, 1994; Stattin, Romelsjö, & Stenbacka, 1996; Stouthamer-Loeber et al., 1993). Such protective processes are often similar to those in successful treatment. Like professional interventions, they can help to create turning points in a criminal career. Although research on resilience has expanded in various fields, we know very little about protective processes in the natural history of psychopathy. As psychopaths manipulate their environment, the development of protective resources will be more difficult than in other cases. A warm-hearted but firm and consistent spouse, a clear-structured *"authoritative"* educational climate at work, relatively low impulsivity, or specific competencies and talents may have such a function (e.g., Lösel, 1994b; Rutter, 1990; Werner & Smith, 1992). Treatment staff should try to figure out potential protective resources that support professional interventions and neutralize criminogenic social relations (e.g., Ditchfield, 1994; Motiuk, 1995). For this, it is necessary to assess thoroughly whether an otherwise protective factor like social support will not represent a risk under specific circumstances (Bender & Lösel, 1997).

12. Relapse prevention and aftercare

Treatment of antisocial behavior often has only surface or short term-effects. The present review suggests that this is particularly the case for psychopaths. As research on sex offenders, substance abusers, and other groups has shown, a thorough planning and implementation of relapse prevention and aftercare are essential for more long-term positive outcomes (Annis, 1986; Laws, 1989; Prentky, 1995). This is also suggested for personality-disordered offenders (e.g., Cullen, 1997), although community supervision has not been generally successful (e.g., Bailey & MacCulloch, 1992). As in the intra-institutional interventions, the content and structure of the program should be individualized. Generally there is a need to control whether positive changes in interpersonal style, social relations and cognitions are maintained under the challenges of life in the community (Serin, 1995). This also includes a thorough assessment of potential abuse of the skills and competencies acquired during the treatment program. Again, assessment should not just rely on information from the subject, but include actuarial data, work records, and information from the family. In specific cases, like sexual or drug addicted offenders, plethysmographic, polygraphic, or drug testing examinations may be indicated to monitor the avoidance of high-risk situations or behaviors. Electronic monitoring may also be appropriate in some cases. The diagnostic component in aftercare must be combined with interventions or booster sessions to improve or maintain self-regulation in the community. There are various prerequisites for a successful implementation of such aftercare. First, probation officers, social workers, psychologists, or other staff who are in contact with the individual must be familiar with the specific disorders of psychopaths. Second, the network between services and family members should be closely interrelated to reduce manipulation and influences of criminal peers. Third, relapse prevention and aftercare must be enforced legally.

13. Early intervention

Although psychopathy and antisocial personality disorder are categories of adult psychopathology, conduct disorders in childhood and antisocial behavior in adolescence are frequent precursors (Hodgins et al., this volume; Lynam, 1996; Moffitt, 1993; Robins, 1978). The Psychopathy Checklist Youth Version can be used to measure psychopathic characteristics in adolescence (Forth et al., 1990). Frick et al. (1994) assessed a callous-unemotional subgroup of children with conduct disorders that even misbehaved under conditions of good parenting (see also Frick, 1996). The differentiation between a psychopathic-motivational pathway and a poor parental socialization pathway to conduct problems is promising. More long-term prospective studies on early starting, persistent antisociality reveal a cumulative risk or snowball effect of factors like genetic dispositions; pre-, peri-, or postnatal complications; neurospsychological deficits; a difficult temperament; stress factors in a multiproblem-milieu; poor parental behavior; problems in bonding; early disruptive behavior; achievement and social deficits at school; problematic peer relations; and, in consequence, early delinquency (Moffitt, 1993). Regardless of the further differentiation of pathways, it seems most adequate to intervene into fledgling psychopathy before too many risks have cumulated. Recent research reviews suggest that this can be rather successful (Farrington, 1994; Tremblay & Craig, 1995; Yoshikawa, 1994). Even early prevention programs for preschool children have demonstrated long-term effects on antisocial behavior in adulthood (e.g., Schweinhart, Barnes, & Weikart, 1993). Successful measures for children at-risk must include elements for improving cognitive and social competencies and reducing impulsivity and attention deficits. However, programs that only target the child often do not have a long-term impact (e.g., Beelmann et al., 1994). They must be accompanied by intensive measures that improve parental behavior, reduce their coercion and aggression, and promote consistency and supervision (e.g., Patterson, Reid, & Dishion, 1992).

Multimodal, long-lasting, and early starting programs seem to be particularly promising (Tremblay & Craig, 1995). As in the treatment of adult psychopaths, there is still a lack of well-controlled early prevention studies. Furthermore, programs must cope thoroughly with the stigmatization of children and families. However, when all the psychosocial and financial costs that arise from long-lasting psychopathic behavior are considered, more investment in early intervention would be particularly beneficial.

14. Reducing societal reinforcement

Attempts to counteract psychopathic behavior also have to take the wider societal and cultural context into account (Hare, 1993). As Cooke (1996, 1997a) has concluded from his comparison between North America and Scotland, it is likely that cultural factors will serve either to suppress or to reinforce the expression of psychopathic behavior. Individualistic cultures may transmit or amplify psychopathic characteristics because, for example, their high competitiveness supports deceptive and manipulative behavior. One-sided emphasis on self- and social independence can reinforce psychopathic tendencies of exhibiting grandiosity, glibness, callousness and a parasitic lifestyle. In business life, the pace of technological change has accelerated so much that old rules and relations break down rapidly, management controls loosen up, organizations become less rigid and bureaucratic, and managers must take greater risks (Babiak, 1996). At least for some time, and particularly in rapid growth or downsize situations, such transitional organizations provide a platform for psychopathic lifestyles. Probably, economic globalization and emphasis on shareholder value also reduce social bonds and social responsibilities. The modern possibilities of high mobility and electronic communication may have a similar side effect. In private life, short-term marital relationships are becoming more and more frequent. Some sectors of society see promiscuity not as a problem of value and bonding but only as a medical risk for HIV infection. Triggered or reinforced by mass media and the leisure-time industry, there are subcultures that emphasize an impulsive, trivial and short-term oriented lifestyle. Yellow journalism and dozens of television channels promote the superficial *"good story,"* while shouldering little responsibility for its truth and relevance in the longer run. In many Hollywood movies, nuances of social relationships, emotionality and speech are overwhelmed by role stereotypes, pure action, dynamite, and blood. To avoid misunderstanding, the pathways to antisocial behavior are naturally much more complicated, and I do not want to emphasize a cultural pessimism like Postman (1985). However, when dealing with the treatment of psychopathy, we also must learn to understand and cautiously to modify macro-level processes that sustain and reward its behavioral expression.

References

Aichhorn, A. (1957). *Verwahrloste Jugend*, 4. Aufl. Stuttgart: Huber.

Akers, R.L., Hayner, N.S., & Gruninger, W. (1977). Prisonization in five countries: Types of prison and inmate characteristics. *Criminology, 14*, 527-554.

American Psychiatric Association (1994). *Diagnostic and Statistical Manual of Mental Disorders, 4th ed.* Washington, DC: American Psychiatric Association.

Andrews, D. (1995). The psychology of criminal conduct and effective treatment. In J. McGuire (Ed.), *What works: Reducing reoffending* (pp. 35-62). Chichester: Wiley.

Andrews, D.A., & Bonta, J. (1994). *The psychology of criminal conduct.* Cincinatti, OH: Anderson.

Andrews, D., & Bonta, J. (1995). *LSI-R: The Level of Service Inventory-Revised.* Toronto: Multi-Health Systems.

Andrews, D.A., Zinger, I., Hoge, R.D., Bonta, J., Gendreau, P., & Cullen, F.T. (1990). Does correctional treatment work? A clinically-relevant and psychologically informed meta-analysis. *Criminology, 28,* 369-404.

Annis, H. (1986). A relapse prevention model for treatment of alcoholics. In W.E. Miller & N. Heather (Eds.), *Treating Addictive Behaviors* (pp. 407-435). New York: Plenum.

Antonowicz, D., & Ross, R.R. (1994). Essential components of successful rehabilitation programs for offenders. *International Journal of Offender Therapy and Comparative Criminology, 38,* 97-104.

Archer, J. (1991). The influence of testosterone on human aggression. *British Journal of Psychology, 82,* 1-28.

Babiak, P. (1996). Psychopathic manipulation in organizations: pawns, patrons, and patsies. *Issues in Criminological and Legal Psychology, 24,* 12-17.

Bailey, J., & MacCulloch, M. (1992). Patterns of reconviction in patients discharged directly to the community from a special hospital: Implications for after-care. *Journal of Forensic Psychiatry, 3,* 445-461.

Barbaree, H.E., Seto, M.C., Serin, R.C., Amos, N.L., & Preston, D.L. (1994). Comparison between sexual and nonsexual rapist subtypes: Sexual arousal to rape, offense precursors and offense characteristics. *Criminal Justice and Behavior, 21,* 95-114.

Barker, M. (1996). What works with sex offenders? In G. McIvor (Ed.), *Working with offenders* (pp. 107-119). London: Jessica Kingsley.

Barkley, R.A., McMurray, M.B., Edelbrock, C.S., & Robbins, K. (1989). The response of aggressive and nonaggressive ADHD children to two doses of methylphenidate. *Journal of the American Academy of Child and Adolescent Psychiatry, 28,* 873-881.

Basta, J.M., & Davidson II, W.S. (1988). Treatment of juvenile offenders: Study outcomes since 1980. *Behavioral Sciences and the Law, 6,* 353-384.

Baumrind, D. (1989). Rearing competent children. In W. Damon (Ed.), *Child development today and tomorrow* (pp. 349-378). San Francisco: Jossey-Bass.

Beck, A.T., & Freeman, A. (1990). *Cognitive therapy of personality disorders.* New York: Guilford Press.

Beelmann, A., Pfingsten, U., & Lösel, F. (1994). Effects of training social competence in children: A meta-analysis of recent evaluation studies. *Journal of Clinical Child Psychology, 23,* 260-271.

Bender, D., & Lösel, F. (1997). Protective and risk effects of peer relations and social support on antisocial behaviour in adolescents from multi-problem milieus. *Journal of Adolescence, 20,* in press.

Berner, W. (1997). *Diagnostik und stationäre Therapie bei Sexualstraftätern.* Beitrag zur Fachtagung "Stand und Aufgaben der forensischen Forschung", 12.-14. Juni 1997, Berlin.

Berner, W., & Karlick-Bolten, E. (1986). Verlaufsformen der Sexualkriminalität. Stuttgart: Enke.

Birbaumer, N., & Schmidt, R.F. (1996). *Biologische Psychologie.* Heidelberg: Springer.

Blackburn, R. (1975). An empirical classification of psychopathic personality. *British Journal of Psychiatry, 127,* 456-460.

Blackburn, R. (1992). *The psychology of criminal conduct.* Chichester: Wiley.

Blackburn, R. (1993). Clinical programs with psychopaths. In K. Howells & C.R. Hollin (Eds.), *Clinical approaches to metally disordered offenders* (pp. 179-208). Chichester: Wiley.

Blackburn, R. (1996). Psychopathy and personality disorder: implications of interpersonal theory. *Issues in Criminological and Legal Psychology, 24,* 18-23.

Blumstein, A., Cohen, J., & Farrington, D,P. (1988). Criminal career research: Its value for criminology. *Criminology, 26*, 57-74.

Bonta, J., & Gendreau, P. (1990). Reexamining the cruel and unusual punishment of prison life. *Law and Human Behavior, 14*, 347-372.

Born, P. (1997). *Ein Behandlungskonzept für schwerst Dissoziale*. Beitrag zur Fachtagung Forensische Psychiatrie aktuell, 15.-16. Mai 1997, Giessen.

Brennan, P.A., & Mednick, S.A. (1994). Evidence for the adaptation of a learning theory approach to criminal deterrence: A preliminary study. In E. Weitekamp & H.-J. Kerner (Eds.), *Cross-national longitudinal research on human development and criminal behavior* (pp. 371-379). Dordrecht, NL: Kluwer.

Briggs, D.J. (1994). Assessment of sexual offenders. In M. McMurran & J. Hodge (Eds.), *The assessment of criminal behaviours of clients in secure settings* (pp. 53-67). London: Jessica Kingsley.

Browne, F., Gudjonsson, G., Gunn, J., Rix, G., Sohn, L., & Taylor, P.J. (1993). Principles of treatment of the mentally ill offender. In J. Gunn & P. Taylor (Eds.), *Forensic psychiatry: Clinical, legal and ethical issues* (pp. 646-690). Oxford: Butterworth-Heinemann.

Campbell, M., Cohen, I.L., & Small, A.M. (1982). Drugs in aggressive behavior. *Journal of the American Academy of Child Psychiatry, 21*, 107-117.

Campbell, M., Small, A.M., Green, W.H., Jennings, S.J., Perry, R., Bennett, W.G., & Anderson, L. (1984). Behavioral efficacy of haloperidol and lithium carbonate. *Archives of General Psychiatry, 41*, 650-656.

Carney, F.L. (1977). Out-patient treatment of the aggressive offender. *American Journal of Psychotherapy, 31*, 265-274.

Carney, F.L. (1978). In-patient treatment programs. In W.H. Reid (Eds.), *The psychopath: A comprehensive study of antisocial disorders and behaviors*. New York: Brunner & Mazel.

Caspi, A., & Moffitt, T.E. (1995). The continuity of maladaptive behavior: From description to understanding in the study of antisocial behavior. In D. Cicchetti & D.J. Cohen (Eds.), *Developmental psychopathology, vol. 1: Theory and methods* (pp. 472-511). New York: Wiley.

Cavior, H.E., & Schmidt, A. (1978). Test of the effectiveness of a differential treatment strategy at the Robert F. Kennedy Centre. *Criminal Justice and Behavior, 5*, 131-139.

Chandler, M., & Moran, T. (1990). Psychopathy and moral development: A comparative study of delinquent and nondelinquent youth. *Development and Psychopathology, 2*, 227-246.

Chen, H.T. (1989). *Theory-driven evaluations*. Newbury Park, CA: Sage.

Cleckley, H. (1976). *The mask of sanity*, 5th. ed. St. Louis, MO: Mosby.

Cohen, J. (1992). A power primer. *Psychological Bulletin, 112*, 155-159.

Coid, J.W. (1992). DSM-III diagnosis in criminal psychopaths: a way forward. *Criminal Behaviour and Mental Health, 2*, 78-79.

Cook, T., & Campbell, D.T. (1979). *Quasi-experimentation*. Boston: Houghton Mifflin Company.

Cooke, D.J. (1989). Containing violent prisoners: An analysis of the Barlinnie Special Unit. *British Journal of Criminology, 29*, 129-143.

Cooke, D.J. (1995). Psychopathic disturbance in Scottish prison population: The cross-cultural generalizability of the Hare Psychopathy Checklist. *Psychology, Crime, and Law, 2*, 101-108.

Cooke, D.J. (1996). Psychopathic personality in different cultures. What do we know? What do we need to find out? *Journal of Personality Disorders, 10*, 23-40.

Cooke, D. J. (1997a). Psychopaths: oversexed, overplayed but not over here? *Criminal Behaviour and Mental Health, 7*, 3-11.

Cooke, D.J. (1997b). The Barlinnie Special Unit: The rise and fall of a therapeutic experiment. In E. Cullen, L. Jones, & R. Woodward (Eds.), Therapeutic communities for offenders (pp. 101-120). Chichester: Wiley.

Cooke, D.J., & Michie, C. (1997). Psychopathy across cultures: an item response theory evaluation of Hare's Psychopathy Checklist. *Psychological Assessment, 9*, 3-14.

Copas, J.B., O'Brien, M., Roberts, J., & Whiteley, S. (1984). Treatment outcome in personality disorder: The effect of social, psychological and behavioral variables. *Personality and Individual Differences, 5*, 565-573.

Cornelius, J.R., Soloff, P.H., Perel, J.M., & Ulrich, R.F. (1993). Continuation pharmacotherapy of borderline personality disorder with haloperidol and phenelzine. *American Journal of Psychiatry, 150*, 1843-1848.

Cornish, D.B., & Clarke, R.V.G. (1975). Residential treatment and its effects on delinquency. London: Home Office Research Studies, No. 32.

Cowdry, R., & Gardner, D.C. (1988). Pharmacotherapy of borderline personality disorder. *Archives of General Psychiatry, 45*, 111-119.

Craft, M., Stephenson, G., & Granger, C. (1964). A controlled trial of authoritarian and self-governing regimes with adolescent psychopaths. *American Journal of Orthopsychiatry, 34*, 543-554.

Crick, N.R., & Dodge, K.A. (1994). A review and reformulation of social information--processing mechanisms in children's social adjustment. *Psychological Bulletin, 115*, 74-101.

Cullen, E. (1993). The Grendon reconviction study, part 1. *Prison Service Journal, 90*, 35-37.

Cullen, E. (1994). Grendon: the therapeutic prison that works. *Journal of Therapeutic Communities, 15*, 4, 301-311.

Cullen, E. (1997). Can a prison be a therapeutic community? The Grendon template. In E. Cullen, L. Jones, & R. Woodward (Eds.), *Therapeutic communities for offenders* (pp. 75-99). Chichester: Wiley.

Dahle, K.-P. (1994) Therapiemotivation inhaftierter Straftäter. In M. Steller, K.-P. Dahle, & M. Basqué (Eds), *Straftäterbehandlung* (S. 227-246). Pfaffenweiler: Centaurus.

Dell, S., & Robertson, G. (1988). *Sentenced to hospital. Offenders in Broadmoor.* Oxford: University Press.

DeLong, G.R., & Aldershot, A.L. (1987). Long-term experience with lithium treatment in childhood: Correlation with clinical diagnosis. *Journal of the American Academy of Child and Adolescent Psychiatry, 26*, 389-394.

Ditchfield, J. (1994). Family ties and recidivism: Main findings of the literature. *Research Bulletin of the Home Office Research and Statistics Department, 36*, 1-9.

Dolan, B. (1997). A community based TC: The Henderson hospital. In E. Cullen, L. Jones, & R. Woodward (Eds.), *Therapeutic communities for offenders* (pp. 47-74). Chichester: Wiley.

Dolan, B., & Coid, J. (1993). *Psychopathic and antisocial personality disorders.* London: Gaskell.

Dolan, B., Evans, C., & Norton, K. (1995). The multiple axis-II diagnosis of personality disorders. *British Journal of Psychiatry, 166*, 107-112.

Dolan, B.M., Evans, C.D., & Wilson, J. (1992). Therapeutic community treatment for personality disordered adults: Changes in neurotic symptomatology on follow-up. *International Journal of Social Psychiatry, 38*, 243-250.

Dolan, M. (1994). Psychopathy: A neurobiological perspective. *British Journal of Psychiatry, 165*, 151-159.

Dolde, G. (1996). Zur "Bewährung" der Sozialtherapie im Justizvollzug von Baden-Württemberg: Tendenzen aus einer neueren Rückfalluntersuchung. *Zeitschrift für Strafvollzug und Straffälligenhilfe, 45*, 290-297.

Doren, D.M. (1987). *Understanding and treating the psychopath.* Toronto: Wiley.

Dünkel, F., & Geng, B. (1994). Rückfall und Bewährung von Karrieretätern nach Entlassung aus dem sozialtherapeutischen Behandlungsvollzug und aus dem Regelvollzug. In M. Steller, K.-P. Dahle, & M. Basqué (Hrsg.), *Straftäterbehandlung* (S. 35-59). Pfaffenweiler: Centaurus.

Eissler, K.R. (1949). Some problems of delinquency. In K.R. Eissler (Ed.), *Searchlights on delinquency* (pp. 3-25). New York: International Universities Press.

Egg, R. (1984). *Straffälligkeit und Sozialtherapie.* Köln: Heymanns.

Egg, R. (1990). Sozialtherapeutische Behandlung und Rückfälligkeit im längerfristigen Vergleich. *Monatsschrift für Kriminologie und Strafrechtsreform, 73,* 358-368.

Egg, R. (1993). Drogenabhängige Straftäter. Therapiemotivation durch justitiellen Zwang? *Bewährungshilfe, 40,* 26-37.

Elliott, D.S., Huizinga, D., & Menard, S. (1989). *Multiple problem youth.* New York: Springer.

Esteban, C., Garrido, V., & Molero, C. (1995). *The effectiveness of treatment of psychopathy: A meta-analysis.* Paper presented at the NATO Advanced Study Institute on Psychpathy, November 1996, Alvor, Portugal.

Everitt, B.J. (1983). Monoamines and the control of sexual behavior. *Psychology and Medicine, 13,* 715-720.

Farrington, D.P. (1992). Explaining the beginning, progress and ending of antisocial behavior from birth to adulthood. In J. McCord (Ed.), *Facts, frameworks and forecasts: Advances in criminological theory, vol. 3* (pp. 253-286). New Brunswick, NJ: Transaction Press.

Farrington, D.P. (1994) Early developmental prevention of juvenile delinquency. *Criminal Behaviour and Mental Health, 4,* 209-227.

Farrington, D.P., Loeber, R., & Van Kammen, W.B. (1990). Long-term criminal outcomes of hyperactivity-impulsivity-attention deficit and conduct problems in childhood. In L.N. Robins & M. Rutter (Eds.), *Straight and deviant pathways from childhood to adulthood* (pp. 62-81). Cambridge: Cambridge University Press.

Fink, L., Derby, W.N., & Martin, J.P. (1969). Psychiatry's new role in corrections. *American Journal of Psychiatry, 126,* 124-128.

Forth, A.E., Hart, S.D., & Hare, R.D. (1990). Assessment of psychopathy in male young offenders. *Psychological Assessment: A Journal of Consulting and Clinical Psychology, 2,* 342-344.

Frederiksen, L.W., & Rainwater, N. (1981). Explosive behavior: A skill development approach to treatment. In R.B. Stuart (Eds.), *Violent behavior: Social learning approaches to prediction, management and treatment* (pp. 265-288). New York: Brunner/Mazel.

Freese, R., Müller-Isberner, R., & Jöckel, D. (1996). Psychopathy and co-morbidity in a German hospital order population. *Issues in Criminological and Legal Psychology, 24,* 45-46.

Frick, P.J. (1996). Callous-unemotional traits and conduct problems: a two-factor model of psychopathy in children. *Issues in Criminological and Legal Psychology, 24,* 47-51.

Frick, P.J., O'Brien, B.S., Wootton, J.M., & McBurnett, K. (1994). Psychopathy and conduct problems in children. Journal of Abnormal Psychology, 103, 700-707.

Gardner, D.C., & Cowdry, R.W. (1985). Alprazolam-induced dyscontrol in borderline personality disorder. *American Journal of Psychiatry, 142,* 98-100.

Garfield, S.L., Bergin, A.E. (1994). Introduction and historical overview. In A.E. Bergin & S.L. Garfiled (Eds.), *Handbook of psychotherapy and behavior change, 4th ed.* (pp. 3-18). New York: Wiley.

Garrett, P. (1985). Effects of residential treatment of adjudicated delinquents: A meta-analysis. *Journal of Research in Crime and Delinquency, 22,* 287-308.

Genders, E., & Player, E. (1995). *Grendon: A study of a therapeutic prison.* Oxford: Clarendon Press.

Gendreau, P. (1995). The principles of effective intervention with offenders. In A.J. Harland (Ed.), *Choosing correctional options that work: Defining the demand and evaluating the supply* (pp.117-136). Thousand Oaks, CA: Sage.

Gendreau, P., & Andrews, D.A. (1994). *The Correctional Program Assessment Inventory, 6th ed.* Saint John: University of New Brunswick.

Gendreau, P., & Goggin, C. (1996). Principles of effective programming. *Forum on Corrections Research, 8(3)*, 38-41.

Gendreau, P., & Little, T. (1993). *A meta-analysis of the effectiveness of sanctions on offender recidivism.* Unpublished manuscript. Saint John: University of New Brunswick.

Gendreau, P., Little, T., & Goggin, C. (1995). *A meta-analysis of the predictors of adult offender recidivism: Assessment guidelines for classification and treatment.* Ottawa: Corrections Branch, Ministry Secretariat, Solicitor General of Canada.

Gendreau, P., Paparozzi, M., Little, T., & Goddard, M. (1993). Does "punishment smarter" work? An assessment of the new generation of alternative sanctions in probation. *Forum on Corrections Research, 5*, 31-34.

Gendreau, P., & Ross, R.R. (1987). Revivication of rehabilitation: Evidence from the 1980s. *Justice Quarterly, 4*, 349-407.

Gensheimer, L.K., Mayer, J.P., Gottschalk, R., & Davidson II, W.S. (1986). Diverting youths from the juvenile justice system: A meta-analysis of intervention efficacy. In S.J. Apter & A. Goldstein (Eds.), *Youth violence: Programs and prospects* (pp. 39-57). Elmsford: Pergamon Press.

Gillstrom, B., & Hare, R.D. (1988). Language-related hand gestures in psychopaths. *Journal of Personality Disorders, 2*, 21-27.

Glass, G.V., & Kliegl, R.M. (1983). An apology for research integration in the study of psychotherapy. *Journal of Consulting and Clinical Psychology, 51*, 28-41.

Goldberg, S.C. (1989). Lithium in the treatment of borderline personality disorder. *Pharmacological Bulletin, 25*, 550-555.

Goldsmith, R.W., Throfast, G., & Nilsson, P.-E. (1989). Situational effects on the decision of adolescent offenders to carry out delinquent acts. Relations to moral reasoning, moral goals, and personal constructs. In H. Wegener, F. Lösel, & J. Haisch (Eds.), *Criminal behavior and the justice system: Psychological perspectives* (pp. 81-102). New York: Springer.

Gorenstein, E.E., & Newman, J.P. (1980). Disinhibitory psychopathology: A new perspective and a model for research. *Psychological Review, 87*, 301-315.

Gottesman, H.G., & Schubert, D.S.P. (1993). Low-dose oral medroxyprogesterone acetate in the management of paraphilias. *Journal of Clinical Psychiatry, 54*, 182-187.

Gottschalk, R., Davidson II, W.S., Gensheimer, L.K., & Mayer, J.P. (1987). Community-based interventions. In H.C. Quay (Ed.), *Handbook of juvenile delinquency* (pp. 266-289). New York: Wiley.

Gray, J.A. (1982). *The neuropsychology of anxiety: An enquiry into the function of the septo-hippocampal system.* New York: Oxford University Press.

Gray, J.A. (1987). *The psychology of fear and stress.* New York: Cambridge University Press.

Greenwood, P.W., Model, K.E., Rydell, C.P., & Chiesa, J. (1996). *Diverting children from a life to crime: Measuring costs and benefits.* Santa Monica, CA: Rand Corporation.

Gretenkord, L. (1994). Gewalttaten nach Massregelvollzug (§ 63 StGB). In M. Steller, K.-P. Dahle, & M. Basqué (Eds.), *Straftäterbehandlung* (pp. 75-89). Pfaffenweiler: Centaurus.

Grove, W.M., & Tellegen, A. (1991). Problems in the classification of personality disorders. *Journal of Personality Disorders, 5*, 31-42.

Grubin, D., & Wingate, S. (1996). Sexual offence recidivism: prediction versus understanding. *Criminal Behaviour and Mental Health, 6*, 349-359.

Gunn, J., Robertson, G., & Dell, S. (1978). *Psychiatric aspects of imprisonment.* London: Academic Press.

Hall, G.C.N. (1996). *Theory-based assessment, treatment, and prevention of sexual aggression*. New York: Oxford University Press.

Hare, R.D. (1985). A comparison of procedures for the assessment of psychopathy. *Journal of Consulting and Clinical Psychology, 53*, 7-16.

Hare, R.D. (1991). *The Hare Psychopathy Checklist-Revised*. Toronto, Ontario: Multi-Health Systems.

Hare, R.D. (1992). *A model program for offenders at high risk for violence*. Ottawa: Correctional Service of Canada.

Hare, R.D. (1993). *Without conscience: The disturbing world of the psychopaths among us*. New York: Simon & Schuster.

Hare, R.D. (1995). Psychopathy: A clinical construct whose time has come. *Criminal Justice and Behavior, 23*, 25-54.

Hare, R.D., Hart, S.D., & Harpur, T.J. (1991). Psychopathy and the DSM-IV criteria for antisocial personality disorder. *Journal of Abnormal Psychology, 100*, 391-398.

Hare, R.D., McPherson, L.E., & Forth, A.E. (1988). Male psychopaths and their criminal careers. *Journal of Consulting and Clinical Psychology, 56*, 710-714.

Hare, R.D., & Schalling, D. (Eds.)(1978). *Psychopathic behavior: Approaches to research*. Chichester: Wiley.

Harpur,T.J., Hare, R.D., & Hakstian, A.R. (1989). Two-factor conceptualization of psychopathy: Construct validity and assessment implications. *Psychological Assessment: A Journal of Consulting and Clinical Psychology, 1*, 6-17.

Harris, G.T., Rice, M.E., & Cormier, C.A. (1991). Psychopathy and violent recidivism. *Law and Human Behavior, 15*, 625-637.

Harris, G.T., Rice, M.E., & Quinsey, V.L. (1993). Violent recidivism of mentally disordered offenders: The development of a statistical prediction instrument. *Criminal Justice and Behavior, 20*, 315-335.

Harris, G.T., Rice, M.E., & Quinsey, V.L. (1994). Psychopathy as a taxon: Evidence that psychopaths are a discrete class. *Journal of Consulting and Clinical Psychology, 62*, 387-397.

Hart, S.D., & Hare, R.D. (1989). Discriminant validity of the Psychopathy Checklist in a forensic psychiatric population. *Psychological Assessment: A Journal of Consulting and Clinical Psychology, 1*, 211-218.

Hart, S.D., Hare, R.D., & Forth, A.E. (1994). Psychopathy as a risk marker for violence: Development and validation of a screening version of the Revised Psychopythy Checklist. In J. Monahan & H. Steadman (Eds.), *Violence and mental disorder: Developments in risk assessment* (pp. 81-98). Chicago: University of Chicago Press.

Hart, S.D., Kropp, P.R., & Hare, R.D. (1988). Performance of male psychopaths following conditional release from prison. *Journal of Consulting and Clinical Psychology, 56*, 227-232.

Hemphill, J.F., & Hare, R.D. (1996). Psychopathy Checklist factor scores and recidivism. *Issues in Criminological and Legal Psychology, 24*, 68-73.

Hill, J.K., Andrews, D.A., & Hoge, R.D. (1991). Meta-analysis of treatment programs for young offenders: The effect of clinically relevant treatment on recidivism. *Canadian Journal of Program Evaluation, 6*, 97-109.

Hodgins, S. (1993). The criminality of mentality disordered persons. In S. Hodgins (Ed.), *Mental disorder and crime* (pp. 1-21). Newbury Park, CA: Sage.

Hodgins, S., & Coté, G. (1993). Major mental disorder and APD: A criminal combination. *Bulletin of the American Academy of Psychiatry and the Law, 21*, 155-160.

Hoekstra, R.C. (1979). Entwicklung und Behandlungsergebnisse der Mesdag-Klinik. *Monatsschrift für Kriminologie und Strafrechtsreform, 62*, 91-98.

Holder, T. (1978). A review and perspective of human resource development programs in corrections. *Criminal Justice Review, 2*, 7-16.

Hollin, C.R. (1990). *Cognitive-behavioral interventions with young offenders.* Elmsford: Pergamon Press.

Hollin, C.R. (1995). The meaning and implications of 'programme integrity'. In J. McGuire (Ed.), *What works: Reducing reoffending* (pp. 195-208). Chichester: Wiley.

Hollweg, M., & Nedopil, N. (1997). Die pharmokologische Behandlung aggressiv-impulsiven Verhaltens. *Psycho, 23*, 308-318.

Howells, K., Watt, B., Hall, G., & Baldwin, S. (1997). Developing programmes for violent offenders. *Legal and Criminological Psychology, 2*, 117-128.

Hucker, S.J., & Bain, J. (1990). Androgenic hormones and sexual assault. In W.L. Marshall, D.R. Laws, & H.E. Barbaree (Eds.), *Handbook of sexual assault* (pp. 93-102). New York: Plenum Press.

Hürlimann, M. (1993). *Führer und Einflussfaktoren in der Subkultur des Strafvollzugs.* Pfaffenweiler: Centaurus.

Izzo, R.L., & Ross, R.R. (1990). Meta-analysis of rehabilitation programs for juvenile delinquents. A brief report. *Criminal Justice and Behavior, 17*, 134-142.

Jew, C.C., Clanon, T.L., & Mattocks, A.L. (1972). The effectiveness of group psychotherapy in a correctional institution. *American Journal of Psychiatry, 129*, 602-605.

Jones, F.D., Stayer, S.J., Wichlaz, C.R., Thomes, L., & Livingstone, B.L. (1977). Contingency management of hospital diagnosed character and behavior disorder in soldiers. *Journal of Behavior Therapy and Experimental Psychiatry, 8*, 33.

Jones, L. (1997). Developing models for managing treatment integrity and efficacy in a prison-based TC: The Max Glatt Centre. In E. Cullen, L. Jones, & R. Woodward (Eds.), *Therapeutic communities for offenders* (pp. 121-157). Chichester: Wiley.

Jones, M. (1952). *Social psychiatry in practice: The idea of a therapeutic community.* Harmondsworth: Penguin.

Junger-Tas, J. (1993). Alternatives to prison: myth and reality. In NISCALE (Ed.), *Report on the workshop on criminality and law enforcement* (pp. 104-131). Leiden: Netherlands Institute for the Study of Criminality and Law Enforcement.

Kadden, R.M., Cooney, N.L., Getter, H., & Litt, M.D. (1989). Matching alcoholics to coping skills or interactional therapies: Posttreatment results. *Journal of Consulting and Clinical Psychology, 57*, 698-704.

Kafka, M.P. (1995). Sexual impulsivity. In E. Hollander & D.J. Stein (Eds.), *Impulsivity and aggression* (pp. 201-228). Chichester: Wiley.

Kafka, M.P., & Prentky, R. (1992). Fluoxetine treatment of nonparaphilic sexual addictions and paraphilias in men. *Journal of Clinical Psychiatry, 53*, 351-358.

Kagan, J., Reznick, S., & Snidman, N. (1988). Biological bases of childhood shyness. *Science, 240*, 167-171.

Kavoussi, R.J., Liu, L., & Coccaro, E.F. (1994). An open trial of sertraline in personality disordered patients with impulsive aggression. *Journal of Clinical Psychiatry, 55*, 137-141.

Kennard, D. (1983). *An introduction to therapeutic communities.* London: Routledge.

Knott, C. (1995). The STOP programme: Reasoning and rehabilitation in a British setting. In J. McGuire (Ed.), *What works: Reducing reoffending* (pp. 115-126). Chichester: Wiley.

Koenradt, F. (1993). Forensic mental hospitals according to Dutch standards. *Criminal Behaviour and Mental Health, 3*, 322-334.

Kosson, D.S. (1996). Psychopathic offenders display performance deficits but not over-focusing under dual-task conditions of unequal priority. *Issues in Criminological and Legal Psychology, 24*, 82-89.

Kuhn, A. (1996). Incarceration rates: Europe versus USA. *European Journal on Criminal Policy and Research, 4(3)*, 46-73.

Kury, H. (1986). *Die Behandlung Straffälliger*. Berlin: Duncker & Humblot.

Lab, S.P., & Whitehead, J.T. (1990). From 'nothing works' to 'the appropiate works': The latest stop on the search for the secular grail. *Criminology, 28*, 405-417.

Laws, D.R. (1989). *Relapse prevention with sex offenders*. New York: Guilford Press.

Lapierre, D., Braun, C.M., & Hodgins, S. (1995). Ventral frontal deficits in psychopathy: Neuropsychological test findings. *Neuropsychologia, 33*, 139-151.

Levey, S., & Howells, K. (1990). Anger and its management. *Journal of Forensic Psychiatry, 1*, 305-327.

Lilienfeld, S.O. (1994). Conceptual problems in the assessment of psychopathy. *Clinical Psychology Review, 14*, 17-38.

Lilienfeld, S.O., Van Valkenburg, C., Larntz, K., & Akiskal, H.S. (1986). The relationship of histrionic personality disorder to antisocial personality disorder and somatization disorders. *American Journal of Psychiatry, 143*, 718-721.

Lipsey, M.W. (1992a). Juvenile delinquency treatment: A meta-analytic inquiry into variability of effects. In T.D. Cook, H. Cooper, D.S. Cordray, H. Hartmann, L.V. Hedges, R.L. Light, T.A. Louis, & F. Mosteller (Eds.), *Meta-analysis for explanation* (pp. 83-127). New York: Russell Sage Foundation.

Lipsey, M.W. (1992b). The effect of treatment on juvenile delinquents: Results from meta-analysis. In F. Lösel, D. Bender, & T. Bliesener (Eds.), *Psychology and law: International perspectives* (pp. 131-143). Berlin: De Gruyter.

Lipsey, M.M. (1995a). *Using linked meta-analysis to build policy models for juvenile delinquency*. Paper presented at the Annual Meeting of the American Society of Criminology, November 1995, Boston.

Lipsey, M.W.(1995b). What do we learn from 400 research studies on the effectiveness of treatment with juvenile delinquents. In J. McGuire (Ed.), *What works: Reducing reoffending* (pp. 63-78). Chichester: Wiley.

Lipton, D.S., Martinson, R., & Wilks, J. (1975). *The effectiveness of correctional treatment. A survey of treatment evaluation studies*. New York: Praeger.

Lloyd, C., Mair, G., & Hough, M. (1994). *Explaining reconviction rates: A critical analysis*. London: Home Office.

Loeber, R. (1990). Development and risk factors of juvenile antisocial behavior and delinquency. *Clinical Psychology Review, 10*, 1-41.

Logan, C.H., Gaes, G.G., Harer, M., Innes, C.A., Karacki, L., & Saylor, W.G. (1991). *Can meta-analysis save correctional rehabilitation?* Washington, DC: Federal Bureau of Prison.

Lösel, F. (1993). The effectiveness of treatment in institutional and community settings. *Criminal Behaviour and Mental Health, 3*, 416-437.

Lösel, F. (1994a) Educating - punishing - helping: What do young offenders need? In G. Brianti, A. Dunant, E. Mouravieff-Apostol, C. Noll, G. Rubeiz, & F. Rüegg (Eds.), *Children and youth in conflict with the law* (pp. 53-66). Geneva, CH: International Catholic Child Bureau.

Lösel, F. (1994b). Protective effects of social resources in adolescents at high risk for antisocial behavior. In H.-J. Kerner & E.G.M. Weitekamp (Eds.), *Cross-national longitudinal research on human development and criminal behavior* (pp. 283-301). Dordrecht: Kluwer.

Lösel, F. (1995a). The efficacy of correctional treatment: A review and synthesis of meta-evaluations. In J. McGuire (Ed.), *What works: Reducing reoffending* (pp. 79-111). Chichester: Wiley.

Lösel, F. (1995b). Increasing consensus in the evaluation of offender rehabilitation? Lessons from research syntheses. *Psychology, Crime and Law, 2*, 19-39.

Lösel, F. (1995c). Evaluating psychosocial interventions in prison and other penal contexts. In European Committee on Crime Problems (Ed.), *Psychosocial interventions in the criminal justice system* (pp. 79-114). Strasbourg: Council of Europe.

Lösel, F. (1996a). Working with young offenders: The impact of meta-analyses. In C.R. Hollin & K. Howells (Eds.), *Clinical approaches to working with young offenders* (pp. 57-82). Chichester: Wiley.

Lösel, F. (1996b). Changing patterns in the use of prisons: An evidence-based perspective. *European Journal on Criminal Policy and Research, 4 (3)*, 108-127.

Lösel, F. (1997). Management of psychopaths. *Issues in Criminological and Legal Psychology, 24*, 100-106.

Lösel, F., & Beelmann, A. (1996). *Early intervention and protective factors in the development of delinquency.* Paper presented at the Conference on Prevention of Antisocial Behavior, December 1996, Stockholm.

Lösel, F., & Bliesener, T. (1989). Psychology in prison: Role assessment and testing of an organizational model. In H. Wegener, F. Lösel, & J. Haisch (Eds.), *Criminal behavior and the justice system: Psychological perspectives* (pp. 419-439). New York: Springer.

Lösel, F., & Bliesener, T. (1994). Some high-risk adolescents do not develop conduct problems: A study of protective factors. *International Journal of Behavioral Development, 17*, 753-777.

Lösel, F., & Egg, R. (1997). Social-therapeutic institutions in Germany: Description and evaluation. In E. Cullen, L. Jones, & R. Woodward (Eds.), *Therapeutic communities for offenders* (pp. 181-203). Chichester: Wiley.

Lösel, F. (1989). Evaluation research on correctional treatment in West Germany: A meta-analysis. In H. Wegener, F. Lösel, & J. Haisch (Eds.), *Criminal behavior and the justice system: Psychological perspectives* (pp. 334-355). New York: Springer.

Lösel, F., Köferl, P., & Weber, F. (1987). *Meta-Evaluation der Sozialtherapie.* Stuttgart: Enke.

Lösel, F., & Wittmann, W.W. (1989). The relationship of treatment integrity to outcome criteria. In R.F. Conner & M. Hendricks (Eds.), *International innovations in evaluation methodology* (pp. 97-108). San Francisco: Jossey-Bass.

Loza, W., & Simourd, D.J. (1994). Psychometric evaluation of the Level of Supervision Inventory (LSI-R) among male Canadian federal offenders. *Criminal Justice and Behavior, 21*, 468-480.

Lykken, D.T. (1995). *The antisocial personalities.* Hillsdale, NJ: Lawrence Erlbaum.

Lynan, D.R. (1996). Early identification of chronic offenders: Who is the fledgling psychopath? *Psychological Bulletin, 120*, 209-234.

Main, T.F. (1946). The hospital as a therapeutic institution. *Bulletin of the Menninger Clinic, 10*, 66-70.

Maltz, M. (1984). *Recidivism.* London: Academic Press.

Markovitz, P. (1995). Pharmacotherapy of impulsivity, aggression, and related disorders. In E. Hollander & D.J. Stein (Eds.), *Impulsivity and aggression* (pp. 263-287). Chichester: Wiley.

Markovitz, P.J., Calabrese, J.R., Schulz, S.C., & Meltzer, H.Y. (1991). Fluoxetine in border-line and schizotypal personality disorder. *American Journal of Psychiatry, 148*, 1064-1067.

Markowitz, P.I., & Coccaro, E.F. (1995). Biological studies of impulsivity, aggression, and suicidal behavior. In E. Hollander & D.J. Stein (Eds.), *Impulsivity and aggression* (pp. 71-90). Chichester: Wiley.

Marques, J.K., Day, D.M., Nelson, C., & West, M.A. (1994). Effects of cognitive-behavioral treatment on sex offender recidivism. Preliminary results of a longitudinal study. *Criminal Justice and Behavior, 21*, 28-54.

Marshall, W.L., & Barbaree, H.E. (1988). The long-term evaluation of a behavioral treatment program for child molesters. *Behavior Research and Therapy, 26*, 499-511.

Marshall, W.L., Jones, R., Ward, T., Johnston, P., & Barbaree, H.E. (1991). Treatment outcome with sex offenders. *Clinical Psychology Review, 11*, 465-485.

Martinson, R. (1974). What works? Questions and answers about prison reform. *The Public Interest, 10*, 22-54.

Matt, G.E., & Navarro, A.M. (1997). What meta-analyses have and have not taught us about psychotherapy effects: A review and future directions. *Clinical Psychology Review, 17*, 1-32.

Mayer, J.P., Gensheimer, L.K., Davidson II, W.S., & Gottschalk, R. (1986). Social learning treatment within juvenile justice: A meta-analysis of impact in the natural environment. In S.J. Apter & A. Goldstein (Eds.), *Youth violence: Programs and prospects* (pp. 24-38). Elmsford, NY: Pergamon Press.

McCord, J. (1978). A thirty-year follow-up of treatment effects. *American Psychologist, 33*, 284-289.

McCord, W. (1982). *The psychopath and milieu-therapy: A longitudinal study*. New York: Academic Press.

McCord, W., & Sanchez, J. (1982). The Wiltwyck-Lynan Project: A twenty-five-year follow-up study of milieu therapy. In W. McCord (Ed.), *The psychopath and milieu therapy: A longitudinal study* (pp. 229-296). New York: Academic Press.

McDougall, C., Clark, D.A., & Fisher, M.J. (1994). Assessment of violent offenders. In M. McMurran & J. Hodge (Eds.), *The assessment of criminal behaviors of clients in secure settings* (pp. 68-93). London: Jessica Kingsley.

McGuire, J., & Priestley, P. (1995). Reviewing 'what works': Past, present and future. In J. McGuire (Ed.), *What works: Reducing reoffending* (pp. 3-34). Chichester: Wiley.

Mednick, S.A., Moffitt, T.E., & Stack, S.A. (Eds.)(1987). *The causes of crime. New biological approaches*. Cambridge: Cambridge University Press.

Megargee, E.I., & Bohn, M.J. (1979). *Classifying criminal offenders*. Beverly Hills, CA: Sage.

Mellerup, E.T., & Plenge, P. (1990). The side-effect of lithium. *Biological Psychiatry, 28*, 464-466.

Menzies, R., & Webster, C.D. (1995). Construction and validation of risk assessments in a six-year follow-up of forensic patients: A tridimensional analysis. *Journal of Consulting and Clinical Psychology, 63*, 766-778.

Moffitt, T.E. (1993). Adolescence-limited and life-course-persistent antisocial behavior: A developmental taxonomy. *Psychological Review, 4*, 674-701.

Monahan, J., & Steadman, H. (Eds.)(1994). *Violence and mental disorder: Developments in risk assessment*. Chicago: University of Chicago Press.

Moos, R. (1975). *Evaluationg correctional and community settings*. New York: Wiley.

Motiuk, L.L. (1995). Using familial factors to assess offender risk and need. *Forum on Corrections Research, 7 (2)*, 19-22.

Moyes, T., Tennent, T.G., & Bedford, A.P. (1985). Long-term follow-up of a ward based behaviour modification programme for adolescents with acting out and conduct problems. *British Journal of Psychiatry, 147*, 300-305.

Mullen, P.E. (1994). Treatment. *Criminal Behaviour and Mental Health, 4*, 111-130.

Müller-Isberner, J.R. (1996). Forensic psychiatric aftercare following hospital order treatment. *International Journal of Law and Psychiatry, 19*, 81-86.

Nedopil, N., Hollweg, M., Hartmann, J., & Jaser, R. (1996). Comorbidity of psychopathy with major mental disorders. *Issues in Criminological and Legal Psychology, 24*, 115-118.

Newman, J.P., & Wallace, J.F. (1993a). Psychopathy and cognition. In K.S. Dobson & P.C. Kendall (Eds.), *Psychopathology and cognition* (pp. 293-349). Orlando: Academic Press.

Newman, J.P., & Wallace, J.F. (1993b). Diverse pathways to deficient self-regulation: Implications for disinhibitory psychopathology in children. *Clinical Psychology Review, 13*, 699-720.

Norris, M. (1985). Changes in patients during treatment at Hendersen Hospital therapeutic community during 1977-1981. *British Journal of Medical Psychology, 56*, 135-143.

Norton, K. (1992). Treating personality disordered individuals: the Henderson hospital model. *Criminal Behaviour and Mental Health, 2*, 180-191.

Novaco, R.W. (1997). Remediating anger and aggression with violent offenders. *Legal and Criminological Psychology, 2*, 77-88.

Ogloff, J.R.P., Wong, S., & Greenwood, A. (1990). Treating criminal psychopaths in a therapeutic community program. *Behavioral Sciences and the Law, 8*, 181-190.

Olweus, D. (1993). *Bullying at school*. Oxford: Blackwell.

Orlinsky, D.E., Grawe, K., & Parks, B.K. (1994). Process and outcome in psychotherapy In A.E. Bergin & S.L. Garfield (Eds.), *Handbook of psychotherapy and behavior change, 4th ed.* (pp. 270-376). New York: Wiley.

Ortmann, R. (1994). Zur Evaluation der Sozialtherapie. Ergebnisse einer experimentellen Längsschnittstudie zu Justizvollzugsanstalten in Nordrhein-Westfalen. *Zeitschrift für die gesamte Strafrechtswissenschaft, 106*, 782-821.

Ortmann, R. (1997). Resozialisierung im Strafvollzug. Eine vergleichende Längsschnittstudie zu Regelvollzugs- und sozialtherapeutischen Modellanstalten in Nordrhein-Westfalen. In *Kriminologische Projektberichte 1996* (S. 6-32). Freiburg i.Br.: Max-Planck-Institut für ausländisches und internationales Strafrecht.

Palmer, T. (1992). *The re-emergence of correctional intervention*. Newbury Park: Sage.

Patrick, C.J. (1994). Emotion and psychopathy: Some startling new insights. *Psychophysiology, 31*, 319-330.

Patrick, C.J., Cuthbert, B.N., & Lang., P.J. (1994). Emotion in the criminal psychopath: Fear image processing. *Journal of Abnormal Psychology, 103*, 523-534.

Patterson, G.R., Reid, J.B., & Dishion, T.J. (1992). *Antisocial boys*. Eugene, OR: Castalia.

Peat, B.J., & Winfree, L.T. (1992). Reducing intra-institutional effects of "prisonization". A study of a therapeutic community for drug-using inmates. *Criminal Justice and Behavior, 19*, 206-225.

Petersilia, J., Turner, & Dechenes, E.P. (1992). The costs and effects of intensive supervision for drug offenders. *Federal Probation, 61*, 12-17.

Petersilia, J., Turner, S., & Peterson, J. (1986). *Prison versus probation in California*. Santa Monica, CA: Rand Corporation.

Poldrugo, F., & Forti, B. (1988). Personality disorders and alcoholism treatment outcome. *Drug and Alcohol Dependence, 21*, 171-176.

Porporino, F., & Baylis, E. (1993). Designing a progressive penology: the evolution of Canadian federal correction. *Criminal Behaviour and Mental Health, 3*, 268-289.

Postman, N. (1985). *Amusing ourselves to death. Public discourse in the age of show business*. New York: Viking-Penguin, Inc.

Prentky, R.A. (1995). A rationale for the treatment of sex offenders: Pro bono publico. In J. McGuire (Ed.), *What works: Reducing reoffending* (pp. 155-172). Chichester: Wiley.

Prentky, R., & Burgess, A.W. (1992). Rehabilitation of child molesters: A cost-benefit analysis. In A.W. Burgess (Ed.), *Child trauma I: Issues and research* (pp. 417-442). New York: Garland.

Prentky, R.A., Knight, R.A., Lee, A.F.S., & Cerce, D. (1995). Predictive validity of lifestyle impulsivity for rapists. *Criminal Justice and Behavior, 22*, 106-128.

Quay, H.C. (1977). The three faces of evaluation: What can be expected to work. *Criminal Justice and Behavior, 4*, 341-354.

Quay, H. (1987). Patterns of delinquent behavior. In H.C. Quay (Ed.), *Handbook of juvenile delinquency* (pp. 118-138). New York: Wiley.

Quay, H.C. (1993). The psychobiology of undersocialized aggressive conduct disorder: A theoretical perspective. *Development and Psychopathology, 5*, 165-180.

Quinsey, V.L., Harris, G.T, Rice, M.E., & Lalumière, M.L. (1993). Assessing treatment efficacy in outcome studies of sex offenders. *Journal of Interpersonal Violence, 8*, 512-523.

Quinsey, V.L., Rice, M.E., & Harris, G.T. (1995). Actuarial prediction of sexual recidivism. *Journal of Interpersonal Violence, 10*, 85-105.

Raine, A. (1993). *The psychopathology of crime*. San Diego: Academic Press.

Raine, A., Farrington, D.P., Brennan, P., & Mednick, S.A. (Eds.)(1997). *Biosocial bases of violence*. New York: Plenum Press (in press).

Redl, F., & Wineman, D. (1965). *Children who hate, 2nd ed*. New York: Free Press.

Redondo, S. (1994). *El tratamiento de la delinqencia en Europa: Un estudio meta-analatico [Delinquency treatment in Europe: A meta-analysis]*. Tesis Doctoral. Universidad de Barcelona.

Rehn, G. (1979). *Behandlung im Strafvollzug*. Weinheim: Beltz.

Reich, J.H., & Green, A.I. (1991). Effect of personality disorders on outcome of treatment. *Journal of Nervous and Mental Disease, 179*, 74-82.

Rasmussen, K., & Levander, S. (1996a). Crime and violence among psychiatric patients in a maximum security psychiatric hospital. *Criminal Justice and Behavior, 23*, 455-471.

Rasmussen, K., & Levander, S. (1996b). Symptoms and personality characteristics of patients in a maximum security psychiatric unit. *International Journal of Law and Psychiatry, 19*, 27-37.

Rice, M.E., & Harris, G.T. (1995a). Violent recidivism: Assessing predictive validity. *Journal of Consulting and Clinical Psychology, 63*, 737-748.

Rice, M.E., & Harris, G.T. (1995b). Psychopathy, schizophrenia, alcohol abuse, and violent recidivism. *International Journal of Law and Psychiatry, 18*, 333-342.

Rice, M.E., Harris, G.T., & Cormier, C.A. (1992). An evaluation of a maximum security therapeutic community for psychopaths and other mentally disordered offenders. *Law and Human Behavior, 16*, 399-412.

Roberts, C. (1995). Effective practice and service delivery. In J. McGuire (Ed.), *What works: Reducing reoffending* (pp. 221-236). Chichester: Wiley.

Roberts, J. (1997). History of the therapeutic community. In E. Cullen, L. Jones, & R. Woodward (Eds.), *Therapeutic communities for offenders* (pp. 3-22). Chichester: Wiley.

Robertson, G. (1989). Treatment of offender patients: How should success be measured. *Medicine, Science and the Law, 29*, 303-307.

Robertson, G., & Gunn, J. (1987). A ten-year follow-up of men discharged from Grendon Prison. *British Journal of Psychiatry, 151*, 674-678.

Robins, L.N. (1966). *Deviant children grown up: A sociological and psychiatric study of sociopathic personality*. Baltimore: Williams & Wilkins.

Robins, L.N. (1978). Sturdy predictors of adult antisocial behavior: Replications from longitudinal studies. *Psychological Medicine, 8*, 611-622.

Robins, L.N., & Price, R.K. (1991). Adult disorders predicted by childhood conduct problems: Results from the NIMH epidemiologic catchment area project. *Psychiatry, 54*, 116-132.

Romig, A.D. (1978). *Justice for our children. An examination of juvenile delinquent rehabilitation programs*. Lexington, MA: Lexington Books.

Rosenthal, R., & Rubin, D.B. (1982). A simple general purpose display of magnitude of experimental effect. *Journal of Educational Psychology, 74*, 166-169.

Ross, R.R., & Fabiano, A.A. (1985). *Time to think: A cognitive model of delinquency prevention and offender rehabilitation*. Johnson City: Institute of Social Sciences and Arts.

Ross, R.R., Fabiano, E.A., & Ross, B. (1989). *Reasoning and rehabilitation: A handbook for teaching cognitive skills*. Ottawa: The Cognitive Centre.

Ross, R.R., & Ross, B. (Eds.)(1995). *Thinking straight*. Ottawa: Cognitive Centre.

Rutter, M. (1990) Psychosocial resilience and protective mechanisms. In J. Rolf, A. Masten, D. Cicchetti, K. Nuechterlein, & S. Weintraub (Eds.), *Risk and protective factors in the development of psychopathology* (pp. 181-214). Cambridge: Cambridge University Press.

Rutter, M., & Giller, H. (1983). *Juvenile delinquency: Trends and perspectives*. New York: Guilford.

Rutter, M., Maughan, B., Mortimore, P., & Ouston, J. (1979). *Fifteen thousand hours: Secondary schools and their effects on children*. Cambridge, MA: Harvard University Press.

Salekin, R.T., Rogers, R., & Sewell, K.W. (1996). A review and meta-analysis of the Psychopathy Checklist and Psychopathy Checklist-Revised: Predictive validity of dangerousness. *Clinical Psychology: Science and Practice, 3*, 203-215.

Schneider, K. (1950). *Die psychopathischen Persönlichkeiten*, 9. Aufl. Wien: Franz Deuticke.

Schulz, S.C., Cornelius, J., Schulz, P.M., & Soloff, P.M. (1988). The amphetamine challenge test in patients with borderline personality disorder. *American Journal of Psychiatry, 145*, 809-814.

Schweinhart, L.J., Barnes, H.V., & Weikart, D.P. (1993). *Significant benefits: The High/Scope Perry Preschool Study through age*. Ypsilanti, MI: High/Scope Press.

Sechrest, L.B., White, S.O., & Brown, E.D. (1979). *The rehabilitation of criminal offenders: Problems and prospects*. Washington, DC: National Academy of Sciences.

Serin, R. (1995). Treatment responsivity in criminal psychopaths. *Forum on Corrections Research, 7(3)*, 23-26.

Serin, R. (1996). Violent recidivism in criminal psychopaths. *Law and Human Behavior, 20*, 207-217.

Serin, R., & Brown, S. (1996). Strategies for enhancing the treatment of violent offenders. *Forum on Corrections Research, 8(3)*, 45-48.

Serin, R.C., & Kuriychuk, M. (1994). Social and cognitive processing deficits in violent offenders: Implications for treatment. *International Journal of Law and Psychiatry, 17*, 431-441.

Serin, R.C., Malcolm, P.B., Khanna, A., & Barbaree, H.E. (1994). Psychopathy and deviant sexual arousal in incarcerated sexual offenders. *Journal of Interpersonal Violence, 9*, 3-11.

Seto, M.C., & Barbaree, H.E. (1995). The role of alcohol in sexual aggression. *Clinical Psychology Review, 15*, 545-566.

Skolnick, J.H. (1994). What not to do about crime. *Criminology, 33*, 1-15.

Soloff, P.H., George, A., Nathan, R.S., Schulz, P.M., Ulrich, R.F., & Perel, J.M. (1986). Progress in pharmacotherapy of borderline disorders: A double-blind study of amitriptyline, haloperidol and placebo. *Archives of General Psychiatry, 43*, 691-697.

Sowers, W.E., & Daley, D.C. (1993). Compulsory treatment of substance use disorders. *Criminal Behaviour and Mental Health, 3*, 403-415.

Stattin, H., Romelsjö, A., & Stenbacka, M. (1997). Personal resources as modifiers of the risk for future criminality: an analysis of protective factors in the relation to 18-year-old boys. *British Journal of Criminology, 37*, 198-222.

Stein, G. (1992). Drug treatment of the personality disorders. *British Journal of Psychiatry, 161*, 167-184.

Stouthamer-Loeber, M., Loeber, R., Farrington, D.P., Zhang, Q., van Kammen, W., & Maguin, E. (1993). The double edge of protective and risk factors for delinquency: Interrelations and developmental patterns. *Development and Psychopathology, 5*, 683-701.

Stürup, G.K. (1968). *Treating the "untreatable". Chronic criminals at Herstdedvester*. Baltimore: John Hopkins Press.

Suedfeld, P., & Landon, P.B. (1978). Approaches to treatment. In R.D. Hare & D. Schalling (Eds.), *Psychopathic behavior: Approaches to research* (pp. 347-376). Chichester: Wiley.

Swanson, J.W., Borum, R., Swartz, M.S., & Monahan, J. (1996). Psychotic symptoms and disorders and the risk of violent behaviour in the community. *Criminal Behaviour and Mental Health, 6,* 309-329.

Tardiff, K. (1992). The current state of psychiatry in the treatment of violent patients. *Archives of General Psychiatry, 49,* 493-499.

Temple, N. (1996). Transference and countertransference. General and forensic aspects. In C. Cordess & M. Cox (Eds.), *Forensic psychotherapy, vol. I* (pp. 23-39). London: Jessica Kingsley.

Templeman, T.L., & Wollersheim, J.P. (1979). A cognitive-behavioral approach to the treatment of psychopathy. *Psychotherapy: Theory, Research and Practice, 16,* 132-139.

Tennent, G., Tennent, D., Prins, H., & Bedford, A. (1993). Is psychopathic disorder a treatable condition? *Medicine, Science, and the Law, 33,* 63-66.

Tennent, G., & Way, C. (1984). The English Special Hospital: A 12-17 year follow-up study. *Medicine, Science and the Law, 24,* 81-91.

Thornton, D. (1992). *Long-term outcome of sex offender treatment.* Paper given at the 3rd European Conference on Psychology and Law, Oxford, England.

Thornton, D., & Hogue, T. (1993). The large-scale provision of programmes for imprisoned sex offenders: Issues, dilemmas and progress. *Criminal Behaviour and Mental Health, 3,* 371-380.

Tonry, M. (1996). Controlling prison population size. *European Journal on Criminal Policy and Research, 4(3),* 26-45.

Tremblay, R.E. & Craig, W.M. (1995). Developmental prevention of crime. In N. Morris & M. Tonry (Eds.), *Building a safer society: Strategic approaches to crime prevention* (pp. 151-236). Chicago: University of Chicago Press.

Vaillant, G.E. (1975). Sociopathy as a human process. A viewpoint. *Archives of General Psychiatry, 32,* 178-183.

Valliant, P.M. (1993). Cognitive and behavioral therapy with adolescent males in a residential treatment centre. *Journal of Child and Youth Care, 8,* 41-49.

Valliant, P.M., & Antonowicz, D.H. (1992). Rapists, incest offenders, and child molestors in treatment: Cognitive and social skills training. *International Journal of Offender Therapy and Comparative Criminology, 36,* 221-230.

Van der Laan, M.C., & Janssen, M.G.P. (1996). Addressing drug abuse in a Dutch forensic hospital. *Criminal Behaviour and Mental Health, 6,* 157-166.

Weisz, J.R., Donenberg, G.R., Han, S., & Weiss, B. (1995). Bridging the gap between laboratory and clinic in child and adolescent psychotherapy. *Journal of Consulting and Clinical Psychology, 63,* 688-701.

Werner, E.E., & Smith, R.S. (1992). *Overcoming the odds.* Ithaca: Cornell University Press.

Wexler, H. (1997). Therapeutic communities in American prisons. In E. Cullen, L. Jones, & R. Woodward (Eds.), *Therapeutic communities for offenders* (pp. 161-179). Chichester: Wiley.

Wexler, H.K., Falkin, G.P., & Lipton, D.S. (1990). Outcome evaluation of a prison therapeutic community for substance abuse treatment. *Criminal Justice and Behavior, 17,* 71-92.

Whitehead, J.T., & Lab, S.P. (1989). A meta-analysis of juvenile correctional treatment. *Journal of Research in Crime and Delinquency, 26,* 276-295.

Whiteley, J.S. (1970). The response of psychopaths to a therapeutic community. *British Journal of Psychiatry, 116,* 517-529.

Widiger, T.A., & Frances, A. (1987). Interviews and inventories for the measurement of personality disorders. *Clinical Psychology Review, 7,* 47-75.

Wilkins, L. (1978). "Treatment" on trial: the case of Patuxent. In N. Johnston & L. Savitz (Eds.)., *Justice and corrections* (pp. 670-687). New York: Wiley.

Williamson, S., Harpur, T.J., & Hare, R.D. (1991). Abnormal processing of affective words by psychopaths. *Psychophysiology, 28*, 260-273.

Wing, J.K. (1993). Institutionalism revisited. *Criminal Behaviour and Mental Health, 3*, 441-451.

Windle, M. (1994). Temperamental inhibition and activation: Hormonal and psychosocial correlates and associated psychiatric disorders. *Personality and Individual Differences, 17*, 61-70.

Windle, M., & Windle, R.C. (1993). The continuity of behavioral expression among disinhibited and inhibited childhood subtypes. *Clinical Psychology Review, 13*, 741-761.

Wistedt, B., Helldin, L., Omerov, M., & Palmstierna, T. (1994). Pharmacotherapy for aggressive and violent behaviour: A view of practical management from clinicians. *Criminal Behaviour and Mental Health, 4*, 328-340.

Wong, S. (1996). Recidivism and criminal career profiles of psychopaths: a longitudinal study. *Issues in Criminological and Legal Psychology, 24*, 147-152.

Woodward, R. (1997). Selection and training of staff for the therapeutic role in the prison setting. In E. Cullen, L. Jones, & R. Woodward (Eds.), *Therapeutic communities for offenders* (pp. 223-252). Chichester: Wiley.

Woody, G.E., McLellan, A.T., Luborsky, L., & O'Brien, C.P. (1985). Sociopathy and psychotherapy outcome. *Archives of General Psychiatry, 42*, 1081-1086.

Yochelson, S., & Samenow, S.E. (1976). *The criminal personality, vol. 1: A profile for change.* New York: Jason Aronson.

Yochelson, S., Samenow, S.E. (1977). *The criminal personality, vol. 2: The change process.* New York: Jason Aronson.

Yoshikawa, H. (1994). Prevention as cumulative protection: Effects of early family support and education on chronic delinquency and its risks. *Psychological Bulletin, 115*, 28-54.

PSYCHOPATHY AND RISK FOR VIOLENCE

STEPHEN D. HART
Department of Psychology and
Mental Health, Law, and Policy Institute
Simon Fraser University
Vancouver, Canada.

INTRODUCTION

The clinical concept of psychopathy is linked inextricably to criminal behavior, and in particular to criminal violence. For those of us who work with psychopaths, this link is both a blessing and a curse. On the one hand, it is a stark reminder of the tremendous social, psychological, and economic costs associated with psychopathy and it reinforces the motivation of researchers and clinicians to understand the disorder. But, on the other hand, it proves distracting at times. It is common for people to assume, naively and incorrectly, that all psychopaths commit crime and that anyone who routinely engages in antisocial behavior must be a psychopath. This has lead some to reject psychopathy as simply a moral judgment or a tautology, one that can be misused dangerously in forensic contexts (Hart & Hare, 1996).

In this chapter, I will discuss the association between psychopathy and violence. The first major section begins with a review of the historical, conceptual, and empirical facets of the association, and ends with an attempt to summarize, in relatively simple quantitative terms, the ability of psychopathy assessments to predict future violence. In the second section, I evaluate the practical importance of psychopathy in clinical assessments of risk for violence. This task necessitates a rather broad discussion of methodological issues in research on violence predictions and the evaluation of interventions. I finish the chapter by drawing some general conclusions regarding the importance of psychopathy in the explanation and prediction of violence.

THE NATURE OF THE LINK BETWEEN PSYCHOPATHY AND VIOLENCE

Historical Facet

A simple historical review of the concept of psychopathy is made difficult by inconsistencies in the use of the term (Lewis, 1974; Millon, 1981; Pichot, 1978). Literally *"disease of the mind,"* psychopathy originally referred to mental disorder in general; as Berrios (1996) notes, *"[d]uring the late nineteenth century, the adjective 'psychopathic' meant 'psychopathological' and applied to any and all forms of mental disorder"* (p. 429; emphasis in original). Around this time, and continuing into the twentieth century, descriptive psychopathologists increasingly recognized types of mental disorder. One trend was the identification of varieties of "total insanity," illnesses that appeared to result in a general disintegration or deterioration of mental

D.J. Cooke et al. (eds.), Psychopathy: Theory, Research and Implications for Society, 355–373.

functions. Another, supported by faculty psychology — a theory that argued the human mind comprised discrete functional units — was the identification of relatively specific impairments of intellect, emotion, or volition (Berrios, 1996). Influential alienists, including Pinel and Pritchard, described cases characterized by a disturbance of emotion or volition in the absence of intellectual deficits. The terms used to refer to such conditions included *manie sans délire, monomanie*, moral insanity, and *folie lucide* (Millon, 1981; Pichot, 1978). Although unrelated to modern conception of psychopathy (Whitlock, 1967, 1982), these case descriptions reinforced the notion that mental disorder could exist even when reasoning was intact.

One condition identified around this time is of particular relevance to the present discussion. *Impulsion* (or *impulsive insanity*) was conceptualized as a volitional disturbance characterized by unreflective or involuntary aggression and the absence of other symptoms. According to Berrios (1996), it *"provided the kernel around which the notion of psychopathic personality was eventually to become organised"* (p. 428). It is interesting to note that part of the motivation for developing the concept of emotional or volitional disturbances in general, and more specifically the notion of impulsion, was forensic: For the testimony of alienists to be legally relevant, their expertise had to extend beyond the realm of *"total insanity"* (Berrios, 1996).

In the first half of the twentieth century, the concept of psychopathy was narrowed to refer to personality disorder in general. Personality disorder itself was defined as a chronic disturbance of emotion or volition, or a disturbance of their integration with intellectual functions, that resulted in socially disruptive behavior. As Blackburn (1993) notes, this represents a fascinating shift from viewing psychopaths as *"damaged"* to *"damaging"* (p. 80). Although there was little agreement among alienists concerning the specific variants of personality disorder they identified, or in the names given to these disorders, there was consensus that one important cluster was characterized by impulsive, aggressive, and antisocial behavior. For example, Schneider described *"labile," "explosive,"* and *"wicked"* psychopaths; Kahn described a cluster of *"impulsive," "weak,"* and *"sexual"* psychopaths; and Henderson described a cluster of psychopaths with "predominantly aggressive" features (Berrios, 1996; pp. 431-433).

In the last half of the twentieth century, with the development of fixed and explicit diagnostic criteria, the importance of violence in psychopathic symptomatology has become even more clear. Hart and Dempster (1997) reviewed three major criteria sets: those for antisocial personality disorder in the fourth edition of the American Psychiatric Association's *Diagnostic and Statistical Manual of Mental Disorders* (*DSM-IV*; American Psychiatric Association, 1994); those for dissocial personality disorder in the tenth edition of the *International Classification of Diseases* (*ICD-10*; World Health Organization, 1992); and those for psychopathy in the Hare Psychopathy Checklist-Revised (PCL-R; Hare, 1991) and the Screening Version of the PCL-R (PCL:SV; Hart, Cox, & Hare, 1995). Each set contained one criterion that was directly related to a history of irritability, hostility, and aggression, including overt physical violence. In addition, each set contained several criteria that were indirectly related to violence (e.g., callousness, lack of remorse).

It is worth noting here that the historical link between psychopathy and violence is not one peculiar to Western psychiatry. Indeed, psychopathy is a disorder that apparently occurs in every culture, and violence always is considered symptomatic of the disorder (Cooke, 1996, this volume; Tyrer & Ferguson, 1988).

Conceptual Facet

Even if one omitted symptoms directly related to violence from criteria sets for diagnosing psychopathy, it seems that the remaining symptoms — such as grandiosity, shallow affect, lack of empathy, projection of blame, impulsivity — virtually doom psychopaths to become involved in violent crime (Hare, 1993, 1996; Hart & Hare, 1996, in press). The conceptual link is strong enough that psychopathy has been described as a *"mini-theory"* of violence (Steadman et al., 1994).

TABLE 1. Some important factors that (may) influence decisions to act violently

Domain	Specific Examples
Biological	• Hormonal abnormality (e.g., ↑ testosterone)
	• Neurotransmitter dysfunction (e.g., ↓ serotonin, ↑ MAO)
	• Neurological insult (e.g., intoxication, perinatal trauma)
Psychological	• Psychosis (e.g., mania, delusions, hallucinations)
	• Personality disorder (e.g., psychopathy, impulsivity)
	• Cognitive impairment (e.g., low intelligence, learning deficits)
Social	• Attitudes supporting violence (e.g., male prerogative, misogyny)
	• Exposure to violent models (e.g., childrearing, mass media)
	• Resource conflicts (e.g., lack of employment or education)

Does psychopathy *cause* violence? And if so, are psychopaths morally culpable for the violence they perpetrate? A full answer to these questions would require philosophical and legal discourse beyond the scope of this chapter (see Ogloff and Lyon, this volume). It is possible to avoid such discourse, at least temporarily, if we entertain the notion that violence is the end result of a conscious and (quasi-) rational decision. A decision-making model of violence is consistent with general models of human behavior and, perhaps more to the point, with major theories of criminality (e.g., Andrews & Bonta, 1993; Gottfredson & Hirschi, 1990; Wilson & Herrnstein, 1985).

The decision-making process is itself influenced by a host of biological, psychological, and social factors, a few of which I have attempted to summarize in Table 1. According to this model, then, the proximal cause of violence is not psychopathy, but rather a decision to act violently; psychopathy is one of many distal or indirect causal factors that exert a strong influence on the decision-making process. The strength of this model is, I believe, that it discourages us from viewing the link between psychopathy and violence in simplistic terms. The relevant question now becomes, How do psychopathic symptoms influence decisions to act violently?

The new, improved question is one that facilitates scientific analysis. Unfortunately, we cannot answer it at the present time. As my colleagues and I have discussed previously, though, there are at least three potential mechanisms that could account for the link between psychopathy and violence (Hart & Dempster, 1997; Hart & Hare, 1996, in press). The first is cognitive. It is possible that psychopaths are more likely than others to have antisocial cognitions (e.g., thoughts, fantasies, urges). More specifically, with respect to violence, psychopaths may have cognitive schemata that predispose them to perceive hostile intent in the actions of others; they may also have cognitive schemata (e.g., Meloy, 1988; Serin, 1991) and attentional deficits (e.g., Newman & Wallace, 1993) that lead them to evaluate the commission of violent acts as potentially rewarding. The second mechanism is affective. Psychopaths appear to suffer from a generalized affective deficit (Hare, 1993, 1996); and because affects such as empathy, guilt, and fear, may naturally inhibit the expression of violent impulses (e.g., Blair, 1995; Blair et al., 1995; Patrick & Zempolich, in press), psychopaths may be less likely than others to consider the commission of violent acts as threatening to their own physical, psychological, and social well-being. This mechanism sounds similar in many ways to the cognitive one described above, but there is an important difference: The cognitive mechanism results from positive symptoms (i.e., characteristics that are pathological when present), whereas the affective mechanism results from negative symptoms (which are deficits, or characteristics pathological by their absence). Put simply, the antisocial cognitions shouldn't occur, but do; and the affects should occur, but do not. The third mechanism is behavioral. Psychopaths appear to suffer from pronounced impulsivity, that is, a tendency to commit harmful acts without forethought or planning that results in impaired social functioning (Hart & Dempster, 1997). It may be that psychopaths are predisposed to committing all kinds of acts, including violence, before they engage in much consideration or processing of internal cognitive and affective cues. It may also be that psychopaths impulsively engage in irresponsible behaviors, such as substance use, that indirectly increase the chances they will become involved in violence.

Before proceeding further, I should emphasize that the discussion above is highly speculative. It is possible that all of the mechanisms described exist and influence the behavior of psychopaths, or that none of them exist and some other mechanism is responsible. However, I find it fascinating that it is so easy to develop reasonable conceptual models to explain the link between psychopathy and violence.

Empirical Facet

If there did not exist an empirical association between psychopathy and violence, any discussion of historical and conceptual issues would be moot. Fortunately, both narrative reviews of the research literature (e.g., Hart & Hare, 1996, in press; Hart, Hare, & Forth, 1994; Patrick & Zempolich, in press) and meta-analytic reviews (e.g., Hemphill, Templeman, Wong & Hare, this volume; Salekin, Rogers, & Sewell, 1996; Simourd, Bonta, Andrews, & Hoge, 1990) have concluded that this association does exist. Here, I will attempt to review research that used the PCL-R or related assessment procedures.

General criminality. As noted by Hart and Hare (1996), psychopaths are high-density, versatile offenders. The research they reviewed demonstrated that psychopaths commit more offenses and more types of offenses than do nonpsychopaths, regardless of whether they are living in the community or in an institution (e.g., Cooke, 1994; Hare, 1981; Wong, 1985). Also, the criminal careers of psychopaths begin at an earlier age and persists longer than do those of nonpsychopaths (e.g., Hare, Forth, & Strachan, 1992). Thus, any discussion of the violence committed by psychopaths should recognize that these offenders are not at all criminal specialists (or, perhaps more correctly, that psychopaths specialize even less than do most offenders).

Violent criminality. Psychopaths are more likely than nonpsychopaths to have a documented history of violence in the community or in institutions (e.g., Hare, 1981; Hare & McPherson, 1984; Serin, 1991), including family and sexual violence (e.g., Dempster, Lyon, Sullivan, Hart, & Boer, 1997; Quinsey, Rice, & Harris, 1995). In addition to committing more violence, psychopaths also appear to have different motivations for violence, with the result that the behavioral topography of their criminal conduct (i.e., their victimology or *modus operandi*) also is different. For example, when nonpsychopaths commit violence, they are likely to target people known to them, especially vulnerable victims (e.g., women and children), and the violence is likely to occur in the context of intoxication or strong emotional arousal. In contrast, psychopaths are especially likely to target strangers, and the violence they commit often is impulsive and motivated by material gain, revenge, or sadism (e.g., Cornell et al., 1996; Dempster et al., 1996; Williamson, Hare, & Wong, 1987). As Dempster et al. (1996) put it, the violence of psychopaths appears to be *"impulsively instrumental."* Theoretical musings about psychopathy and violence must take into account not only the frequency with which psychopaths commit violence, but the type of violence they commit.

Predictions of violence

Studying the predictive validity of psychopathy is complicated by the fact that some psychopathic symptoms are directly related to crime. Unless steps are taken to control for these symptoms, it is impossible to determine whether the disorder *per se* is predictive, or whether it is simply that past criminal behavior predicts future criminal behavior. Using the PCL-R, there are at least three methods that researchers can (and do) use to control for past crime. One is to exclude from statistical analyses those PCL-R items related to the outcome of interest (e.g., Hart, Kropp, & Hare, 1988). A second is to use all items from the PCL-R, but to control statistically for past crime (e.g., Hart et al., 1988; Harris, Rice, & Cormier, 1993). A third is to use all items from the PCL-R, but to control statistically for risk of future crime as assessed by actuarial scales scored on the basis of past crime (e.g., Serin, Peters, & Barbaree, 1990). These studies demonstrate that psychopathy does indeed predict future crime, and that its predictive validity cannot be explained away solely in terms of the extent to which it reflects past crime.

It is interesting that psychopathy may predict violence more robustly than it does general criminality (e.g., Salekin et al., 1996). Research suggests that psychopathy predicts a wide range of violence, including institutional and sexual violence (e.g., Heilbrun et al., in press; Quinsey et al., 1995); and that it predicts in diverse groups, including offenders, forensic psychiatric patients, and civil psychiatric patients (e.g., Douglas, 1996; Hill, Rogers, & Bickford, 1996; Serin & Amos, 1995). Despite wide variation in methodology across studies, meta-analyses conducted by Hemphill, Templeman, Wong and Hare (this volume) and Salekin et al. (1996) show that it is possible to summarize the predictive validity of psychopathy (more accurately, PCL-R total scores) with respect to violence in terms of a single number, known technically as an *"effect size."* The results of these meta-analyses are not identical, as they used different procedures to select studies and estimate effect sizes; readers interested in details should consult the original sources. Hemphill, Templeman, Wong and Hare, using very conservative procedures, obtained an effect size of $r = .27$, which corresponds to a Cohen's d of about .56. Salekin et al., using less conservative procedures and with access to a larger database of studies, obtained a Cohen's d of .79, which corresponds to a Pearson r of about .37. For the purpose of discussion, on the basis of these meta-analyses, I estimate that the predictive validity of the PCL-R with respect to violence is about $r = .35$ or $d = .75$ (Hart & Hare, 1996).

THE PRACTICAL IMPORTANCE OF PSYCHOPATHY IN ASSESSING RISK FOR VIOLENCE

To this point, my discussion has been primarily theoretical: I have tried to make the point that there are good reasons to believe that, although psychopathy and violence are distinct and separable constructs, psychopathy plays an important role in decisions to act violently. Indeed, in my view (and that of many others, notably Hare, 1993, 1996; Newman & Wallace, 1993; Patrick & Zempolich, in press), the association between them is so important that its scientific analysis may help us to understand something fundamental about each construct.

But there are other, more practical reasons for studying psychopathy. Those of us who work in corrections and forensic mental health agencies are confronted daily with large numbers of individuals who have committed serious criminal and violent acts. Our task is to identify those who are at risk for future violence, either in an institution or in the community, and to develop strategies for managing this risk. It is a sobering task, because we know that human suffering, even loss of life, may result from failing to detect risk where it exists or from assuming risk where none exists. Others have written more generally about the problems associated with the clinical assessment of risk for violence (e.g., Borum, 1996; Hart, Webster, & Menzies, 1993; Litwack & Schlesinger, 1987, in press; Monahan, 1981; Monahan & Steadman, 1994; Mossman, 1994; Rice & Harris, 1995; Webster et al., 1994). My goal here is to review some of the points raised in these reviews and to attempt to answer the following question: Is the association between psychopathy and violence sufficiently large and important that clinicians can, and should, incorporate the PCL-R into the process of clinical risk assessment?

Methodological Issues

As most readers are no doubt aware, there is a rather substantial empirical literature that examines the accuracy of clinical predictions of violence, as well as the demographic, clinical, and criminal history variables on which the predictions are based (e.g., Monahan & Steadman, 1994). The most common research design is to assess a cohort of offenders or psychiatric patients, make predictions of violence, follow up the cohort over some period of time, determine which cohort members were or were not violent at the end of the follow-up, and then calculate a statistical index of the accuracy of predictions made during the assessment phase. If this design appears simple, then appearances are deceiving; the interpretation of findings is made difficult by the complex nature of the predictions, the outcome variable (i.e., violence), the follow-up, and even statistical indices of accuracy.

Predictions

There is tremendous variability across studies with respect to how predictions of violence are made, how they are expressed, and who makes them. The assessment that is conducted to gather information may comprise a fixed battery of standardized tests, or it may be tailored to the individual being assessed. It may occur at various points in time (e.g., at sentencing, at admission to or discharge from an institution, or at regular intervals during the follow-up). The assessment may focus on a few specific factors, or it may be extremely broad in scope. The decision-makers may be asked to consider and weight the assessment results in a highly structured manner, and asked to make predictions in a specific context (e.g., focusing on a single form of violence, a certain location or time period), or the decisions may be completely unstructured. The predictions themselves may be expressed in a metric that is categorical or continuous; they may specify the likelihood for various forms of violence, over various periods of time; and they may specify certain conditions that might increase or decrease the likelihood of violence. Finally, the decision-makers may be clinicians, criminal justice professionals, or researchers, with varying degrees of training and experience, working alone or in teams.

Violence

There is no simple way to define and measure violence. Violence may be assessed via official records (e.g., police reports, hospital records), by self-report, or by reports from collateral sources. The definition may or may not include property damage, verbal threats, and self-directed aggression. It is quite common to differentiate among violent acts on the basis of acquaintanceship with the victims (e.g., family members versus friends versus strangers) or the severity of harm suffered by the victims (e.g., psychological harm versus physical injury versus death). Some researchers make a distinction between sexual and nonsexual violence; others do not. The context of the violence may be examined to identify the motivation of the perpetrator or situational precipitants of the violence, such as intoxication, psychosis, or victim provocation. Finally, it is worth noting that violence can be coded in a metric that is categorical (e.g., yes versus no, time to first violence) or continuous (e.g., number of incidents during the follow-up, or number per time at risk).

Follow-up

The most obvious way in which the follow-up differs across studies is length. Some studies look at predictions over the short-term, with time periods as short as one or two weeks; others have follow-ups of moderate length, ranging from several months to a year; and still others have long-term follow-ups, ranging from 3 or 4 years to 20 years or longer. Given this variability, it is not surprising that studies also differ in the degree to which they record and control for events that occur during the follow-up, including changes in mental health status, (re-) institutionalization, level of supervision by criminal justice agencies, treatments received from mental health agencies, changes in socio-demographic status (divorce, unemployment) — even injury and death. Although some factors are static in nature, and are expected to change little or even not at all over long periods of time, many are inherently dynamic and are in a near-constant state of flux; yet, few (if any) studies routinely monitor these latter variables during the follow-up period.

   Statistical indices. Most commonly-used statistical indices of predictive accuracy compare the likelihood of violence among subjects sharing some common characteristic (e.g., a prediction that they will be violent) to that among subjects without that characteristic. The statistical index can be multivariate, incorporating multiple aspects of the prediction, controlling for nuisance factors, or examining predictive accuracy as a function of time. It may also accord differential weights to various prediction errors (e.g., false positives versus false negatives). The magnitude or effect size of the statistic may be interpreted relative to chance (p level; that is, the probability of obtaining an effect size of magnitude x in a sample of size y if, in fact, there existed no association between prediction and outcome). Alternatively, the effect size may be interpreted relative to some other criterion, such as perfection or the *status quo.*

Research Examples

How have scientists responded to the bewildering complexity of research on violence predictions? I have attempted to characterize our response in Figure 1, the basic structure of which is familiar to anyone who has read a paper on violence prediction. As the figure indicates, most studies cleave the prediction into a dichotomous metric in a Procrustean — even psychopathic — manner, with callous disregard for its richness and complexity; the poor outcome variable suffers a similar fate. Notice that time, a crucial aspect of the basic research design, is not reflected in the figure at all. The simplistic manner in which the data are summarized allows one to define easily prediction *"successes,"* which are identified with a happy face, and *"failures,"* identified with a sad face (although I doubt victims of violence would agree with the definition of success and failure used by scientists here). It is now a relatively trivial matter to assign arbitrary numeric values to the predictions (say, *"low risk"* = 0 and *"high risk"* = 1) and to the outcomes (say, *"not violent"* = 0 and *"violent"* = 1), and calculate one's preferred statistical index of association.

Outcome:

Not Violent   Violent

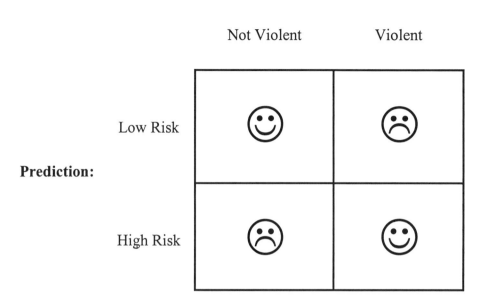

Prediction:

Low Risk

High Risk

Figure 1. Science responds to complexity.

Not to belabour the point further, it is clear that a tremendous amount of potentially valuable information is lost — not aggregated or simplified, but gone forever — when the data are summarized as in Figure 1. The crucial point is this: *Lost information results in the under-estimation of predictive accuracy.* I cannot imagine any circumstance in which artificially dichotomizing predictor and outcome, ignoring time as a factor, ignoring nuisance variables, and so forth will systematically increase the apparent accuracy of violence predictions.

Despite the underestimation of accuracy, it is very common to observe better-than-chance predictions of violence when data are summarized as in Figure 1. Take, for example, a study conducted by Harris, Rice, and Cormier (1991), which examined the association between psychopathy and violence in a cohort of forensic psychiatric patients who completed an institutional treatment program. Psychopathy was assessed using the PCL-R; violence was coded from police and hospital records; and the follow-up period averaged about 10 years, with no regular monitoring. PCL-R scores and follow-up data were available for 166 patients. Patients with scores of 25 and greater were considered psychopathic (high risk); those with scores of 24 and lower were considered nonpsychopathic (low risk). Everyone who had an arrest for offences against persons, or whose hospital files indicated that they committed an act that could have resulted in such an arrest, was deemed violent. The association between the PCL-R and violence during follow-up is presented in Figure 2.

Outcome:

Not Violent   Violent

	Not Violent	Violent
Low Risk	90	24
High Risk	12	40

Prediction:

Figure 2. Association between psychopathy and violence in Harris et al (1991).

That there is an association between psychopathy and violence in Figure 2 is apparent even to the naked eye. Here are some statistical indices of the magnitude of the association: overall accuracy, 78%; accuracy of positive predictions, 77%; accuracy of negative predictions, 79%; relative improvement over chance, .62; chance corrected agreement (Cohen's κ), .53; correlation (phi), .53; and odds ratio, 12.5.

Optimists will note these findings indicate that, relative to chance, predictions of violence based on a single variable, the PCL-R, were reliably accurate — that is, reliably better than nothing. To pessimists, this is hardly a strong endorsement. They are likely to point out that, relative to perfection, the predictions leave much to be desired. Technically, of course, both groups are correct. But I would like to make three observations.

First, the statistical indices in the paragraph above are based on a gross simplification of the original data. More sophisticated and appropriate analyses are likely to reveal a stronger association between psychopathy and violence. For example, receiver operating characteristic analysis (e.g., Rice & Harris, 1995; Mossman, 1994) is most appropriate for examining the association between a continuous predictor and a dichotomous outcome over a fixed time period. If there is a dichotomous outcome and several predictors, or a single predictor and several nuisance variables, then logistic regression may be indicated (e.g., Hart et al., 1988). If violent incidents are analyzed as a count or rate variable, then nonlinear regression analysis is appropriate (Gardner, Mulvey, & Shaw, 1995). If time to violence is an important consideration, survival analysis (e.g., Hart et al., 1988; Rice & Harris, 1995) can identify variables that predict the rapidity of violence, defined dichotomously, during follow-up. Survival analysis is well-suited for situations where the length of the follow-up is variable across subjects or when there is a need to control for nuisance variables; it can also be used to analyze or control for variables that change status during the follow-up (i.e., time-dependent covariates).

Second, the original data themselves do not capture fully the complexity of the predictions, the violence, and the follow-up. For example, if self-reports or collateral reports of violence were used in addition to official records, it is likely that the rate of violence during follow-up would have increased substantially; indeed, the rate of violence among psychopaths may have approached 100%. Also, the association between psychopathy and violence was observed despite any supervision or treatment delivered during the follow-up. Interventions may have reduced the overall rate of violence, particularly among those at high risk (as those at low risk are subject to a floor effect), thereby reducing the magnitude of the association.[1]

Third, the magnitude of the association is large in terms of effect size. Perhaps the simplest effect size indicator is the familiar Pearson correlation, r. The r between psychopathy and violence in the Harris et al. (1991) study is .53, which is considered large in absolute terms (e.g., Cohen, 1988). It is somewhat unusual to find a large effect size in research on psychopathology, even in highly-controlled laboratory research. To find a large correlation between psychopathy and violence — despite measurement problems, despite a 10-year follow-up, despite intervening life events — is, to me, quite amazing. Even if one takes the more typical correlation between psychopathy and violence discussed earlier, $r = .35$ and $d = .75$, then the magnitude of the association is at least moderate in absolute terms; and this is a lower-bound estimate.[2]

Characterizing the Status Quo

So, according to the discussion above, violence predictions based on the PCL-R are significantly better than chance, considerably worse than perfection, and, in absolute

---

[1] This is a rather misunderstood point, discussed at some length by Litwack and Schlesinger (in press). In much of the research literature, predictions of violence are not passive assessments but rather decisions that influenced the services delivered to individuals. Clinicians are bound — morally, ethically, and legally — to try to prove themselves wrong when they *"predict"* violence; they must take every reasonable action to ensure that those at high risk for violence do not act violently. If clinicians predicted violence with perfect accuracy on the basis of an assessment at discharge from hospital, then it would mean that community-based interventions were completely useless at reducing risk for violence in psychiatric patients.

[2] It is also worth noting here that the maximum value of the correlation between two dichotomous variables is often substantially less than unity (1.0). Unity is the maximum only when the base rates of the predictor and the outcome are identical. To illustrate, I will use an example provided by Professor Lösel at the NATO conference in Portugal (Lösel, 1996). Suppose we assign 200 offenders at random either to a correctional treatment or to a no-treatment control group. The treated group is deemed *"low risk,"* and the untreated group *"high risk."* All offenders subsequently are released from prison. During the follow-up, half of the untreated offenders (50 of 100, or 50%) recidivate. In contrast, virtually none of the treated offenders (1 of 100, or 1%). Treatment almost eliminated violence, reducing the recidivism rate by nearly 50 percentage points. Yet, the correlation between treatment and reduction in recidivism is only .56!

terms, at least moderate in magnitude. But earlier I raised the possibility of comparing the predictive accuracy of the PCL-R to the *status quo*. The problem is that the *status quo* is difficult to identify. It may be of some limited interest to point out that the PCL-R appears to be the most robust and best predictor of violence identified to date in the empirical literature, or to note that the predictive accuracy of other known risk factors for violence is considerably lower (e.g., the correlation between psychosis and violence averages about $r = .20$; Douglas & Hart, 1996). Skeptics might argue, though, that perhaps the PCL-R is just the best predictor of a bad lot. A more relevant criterion might be the ability to predict other outcomes of interest to human beings, such as response to treatment for physical disease or mental disorder, or the degree of benefit resulting from various social programs.

Luckily, Lipsey and Wilson (1993) conducted a review of 302 meta-analyses that evaluated the impact of various psychological, correctional, and educational interventions; they also compared these with meta-analyses of medical interventions. For those unfamiliar with the term, meta-analysis is a set of statistical procedures that attempts to find the typical or average effect size observed in a body of research studies.

TABLE 2. Average effect sizes for various interventions

Intervention	Effect Size	
	d	r
Psychological		
Cognitive behavioral therapy, effects on depression (Dobson, 1989)	.99	.44
Psychotherapy, effects on all outcomes (Smith, Glass, & Miller, 1980)	.85	.39
Correctional treatment-adults, effects on all outcomes (Lösel & Koferl, 1989)	.25	.12
Educational		
Student tutoring, effects on academic achievement(Cohen, Kulik, & Kulik, 1982)	.40	.20
Small class size, effects on achievement (Hedges & Stock, 1983)	.20	.10
Mass media campaigns, effects on seatbelt use (Moore, 1990)	.14	.07
Medical		
Cardiac bypass surgery, effects on angina pain (Lynn & Donovan, 1980)	.80	.37
Cyclosporine, effects on organ rejection (Rosenthal, 1991)	.39	.15
Cardiac bypass surgery, effects on mortality (Lynn & Donovan, 1980)	.15	.07

Note. From Lipsey & Wilson (1993).

To ease interpretation of the findings, Lipsey and Wilson translated all the meta-analytic results into a common effect size, Cohen's d. The net result is that one can consult Lipsey and Wilson (1993) and determine, for example, that the interventions reviewed typically were moderately effective; the median d was .47, which corresponds to about $r = .23$. Table 2 presents selected effect sizes from meta-analyses reviewed by Lipsey and Wilson. From the lengthy list, I tried to choose examples of good (i.e., relatively effective), bad (i.e., relatively ineffective), and typical interventions within the fields of psychotherapy, education, and medicine. To facilitate comparisons with research on the PCL-R, the table also presents the r corresponding to each d. As the table indicates, the accuracy of violence predictions using the PCL-R is only slightly lower than the accuracy of predictions that cognitive behavioral therapy will reduce symptoms of depression, psychotherapy will improve general well-being, or cardiac bypass surgery will reduce angina pain. Violence predictions using the PCL-R are more accurate, often substantially more accurate, than predictions that smaller class sizes will lead to improved academic achievement, correctional treatment will improve the well-being of offenders, cardiac bypass surgery will reduce mortality, or public education will increase seatbelt use.

Based on a strict statistical criterion, then, it would be hypocritical to support cardiac bypass surgery, small class sizes, or correctional treatment programs as promoting social good without also supporting violence predictions.[3] When I have brought up this example in the past, some people have objected to sole reliance on a statistical criterion to judge importance, saying that it is impossible to compare studies with such diverse outcomes and that even small effects can be practically important when the outcome is serious (e.g., as in medical research). My response is that I am trying to compare the accuracy of predictions, not the nature of the outcomes. Also, I think it is quite reasonable to compare the outcome of violence predictions with that of many medical interventions; in both cases, prediction errors may result in suffering or death. I think the general public would view the occurrence of criminal violence to be as important a social outcome as improved classroom climate or increased use of seatbelts.

DISCUSSION

Conclusions

As promised in the Introduction, I draw two general conclusions on the basis of the literature reviewed in this chapter. My first conclusion is that, by any standard, psychopathy is of great theoretical importance in the explanation of criminal violence. Please note that I am not blaming all violence on psychopaths, nor am I stating that risk for violence is the essence of psychopathy. Rather, my point is that the two are so intimately connected that a full understanding of violence is impossible without consideration of the role played by psychopathy.

---

[3] Interestingly, I don't know anyone who has turned down cardiac bypass surgery when it was recommended by a physician, but I know many people who still claim it is impossible to predict violence reliably.

My second conclusion is that, by any standard (save perhaps perfection), psychopathy is of great practical importance in the assessment of risk for violence. Even on its own, the PCL-R predicts future violence reliably better than chance; better than do other demographic, clinical, and criminal history risk factors that have been studied; and as well as or better than we are able to predict outcomes of interest in other fields of human endeavor, such as education and medicine. Violence predictions based on the systematic integration of PCL-R results with other assessment data may be better still (e.g., Webster et al., 1994).

Implications for Practice

Science can tell us what is possible, not what is preferable; so even though it appears we *can* use the PCL-R to assess violence risk, it is not clear that we *should* use it for this purpose. Decisions about what we *"should"* do in risk assessments must be influenced as much by legal and pragmatic principles as they are by empirical research (e.g., Hart, 1996). Together with my colleagues at Simon Fraser University, I have been involved in several attempts to develop general clinical guidelines for violence risk assessments in various contexts (e.g., Boer, Wilson, Gauthier, & Hart, 1997; Kropp, Hart, Webster, & Eaves, 1995; Webster, Douglas, Eaves, & Hart, 1997). We have reached five general conclusions about the role of psychopathy in risk assessment:

1. **Psychopathy is a factor that should be considered in any assessment of violence risk.** With respect to the three principles identified earlier, psychopathy should be considered because it is empirically related to future violence, it is theoretically important in the explanation of violence, and it is pragmatically relevant is making decisions about risk management. Indeed, failure to consider psychopathy when conducting a risk assessment may be unreasonable (from a legal perspective) or unethical (from a professional perspective).

2. **Psychopathy should be assessed using the PCL-R.** Almost all research that supports the predictive validity of psychopathy assessments has used the PCL-R (or PCL:SV). Also, it is clear from research that other procedures for the assessment of psychopathy are, at best, moderately correlated with the PCL-R; at worst, they may be completely uncorrelated with the PCL-R (Hare, 1991).

3. **Psychopathy should be assessed by appropriately qualified and trained personnel.** The PCL-R is a psychological test, and the use of such tests is governed by a variety of ethical and legal considerations (see Ogloff & Lyon, this volume). Guidelines for evaluating the qualification and training of test users are provided in the PCL-R manual (Hare, 1991), although it must be remembered that these are basic or minimum standards. Agencies that include the PCL-R in standardized risk assessments must take steps to ensure that the test is used properly; this might include routine monitoring or evaluation of the quality of assessments.

4. **The presence of extreme psychopathic traits compels a conclusion of high risk.** The rate of violent recidivism in psychopaths is so high that extreme psychopathic traits (assessed using the PCL-R or PCL:SV) may be considered a sufficient basis for concluding that an individual is at high risk for future

violence, at least over time periods of three to five years or longer. In this respect, a diagnosis of psychopathy is similar to other rare clinical factors, such as expressed homicidal ideation/intent or a history of sexual sadism. I should emphasize here that the level of psychopathic traits should be high in absolute terms, not in relative terms (e.g., Litwack & Schlesinger, in press; Salekin et al., 1996). Some researchers may define *"psychopathy"* as scores above the sample mean on the PCL-R, which may be as low as 15 or 20. In contrast, the diagnostic cutoff for psychopathy specified in the PCL-R manual is 30 (Hare, 1991). Taking into account the standard error of measurement on the PCL-R, it seems that extremely high levels of psychopathic traits should be defined as PCL-R scores of 34 and greater, a score that would place the individual in the top 5% of all offenders and forensic patients in the PCL-R normative samples (Hare, 1991).

5.   **The absence of psychopathy does not compel a conclusion of low risk.** Although extreme psychopathic traits may be sufficient, they are not necessary to conclude that an individual is high risk. Even people with very low scores on the PCL-R may be at high risk for violence (e.g., if they express serious homicidal ideation/intent or have a history of sexual sadism, as noted above). This is particularly true when assessing the risk for specific forms of violence, such as sexual or spousal assault, in which psychopathy may play a rather circumscribed role.

Implications for Research

There is still much we need to know about the association between psychopathy and violence. No doubt, researchers will continue to conduct follow-up studies to determine the risk for violence associated with psychopathy in various contexts, as well as the co-factors that may increase or attenuate this risk. We are particularly in need of studies that closely monitor individuals over time, so that we can identify important dynamic risk factors. (Some of the statistical procedures discussed earlier, such as survival analysis with time-dependent covariates, offer great potential in this regard.) We also need to determine why a small subgroup of psychopaths (comprising about 10% to 20% of those diagnosed) appears to spontaneously desist from further criminal and violent behavior after release from prison. It may be that these individuals have found a prosocial (or less overtly anti-social) alternative to violence. Alternatively, it may be that they continue to act violently, but that this violence is not noted in formal records (e.g., because they have moved to another jurisdiction or learned how to avoid arrest). Finally, it may be that they are dead, but that this event has escaped the notice of researchers (e.g., researchers failed to search death records, or death records were filed under an alias).

It would be a mistake to over-focus on follow-up studies, however. They are inherently descriptive, and are of limited value in identifying or testing causal mechanisms. We need research that attempts to explore further the proximal affective, cognitive, and behavioral factors that lead psychopaths to the decision to act violently. We also need to conduct intervention studies that target these (putative) factors in psychopaths; evidence from well-controlled studies that intervention systematically decreases risk for future violence is strong evidence that an important causal mechanism has been identified.

References

American Psychiatric Association. (1994). *Diagnostic and statistical manual of mental disorders*, 4th edition. Washington, DC: Author.

Andrews, D. A., & Bonta, J. (1993). *The psychology of criminal conduct*. Cincinnati: Anderson.

Berrios, G. E. (1996). *The history of mental symptoms: Descriptive psychopathology since the nineteenth century*. Cambridge, UK: Cambridge University Press.

Blair, R. J. R. (1995). A cognitive developmental approach to morality: Investigating the psychopath. *Cognition, 57*, 1-29.

Blair, R. J. R., Sellars, C., Strickland, I., Clark, F., Smith, M., & Jones, L. (1995). Emotional attributions in the psychopath. *Personality and Individual Differences, 19*, 431-437.

Blackburn, R. (1993). *The psychology of criminal conduct: Theory, research, and practice*. Chichester, England: Wiley.

Boer, D. P., Wilson, R. J., Gauthier, C. M., & Hart, S. D. (1997). Assessing risk for sexual violence: Guidelines for clinical practice. In C. D. Webster & M. A. Jackson (Eds.), *Impulsivity and violence: Principles and practice*. New York: Guilford.

Borum, R. (1996). Improving the clinical practice of violence risk assessment: Technology, guidelines, and training. *American Psychologist, 51*, 945-956.

Cohen, J. (1988). *Statistical power analysis for the behavioral sciences*. New York: Academic Press.

Cohen, P. A., Kulik, J. A., & Kulik, C. C. (1982). Educational outcomes of tutoring: A meta-analysis of findings. *American Educational Research Journal, 19*, 237-248.

Cooke, D. J. (1994). *Psychological disturbance in the Scottish Prison System: Prevalence, precipitants, and policy*. Edinburgh: Scottish Home and Health Department.

Cooke, D. J. (1996). Psychopathic personality in different cultures: What do we know? What do we need to find out? *Journal of Personality Disorders, 10*, 23-40.

Cornell, D., Warren, J., Hawk, G., Stafford, E., Oram, G., & Pine, D. (1996). Psychopathy in instrumental and reactive violent offenders. *Journal of Consulting and Clinical Psychology, 64*, 783-790.

Dempster, R. J., Lyon, D. R., Sullivan, L. E., Hart, S. D., Smiley, W. C., & Mulloy, R. (1996, August). *Psychopathy and instrumental aggression in violent offenders*. Paper presented at the Annual Meeting of the American Psychological Association, Toronto, Ontario.

Dobson, K. S. (1989). A meta-analysis of the efficacy of cognitive therapy for depression. *Journal of Consulting and Clinical Psychology, 57*, 414-419.

Douglas, K. (1996). *Assessing the risk of violence in psychiatric outpatients: The predictive validity of the HCR-20 risk assessment scheme*. Unpublished Master's thesis, Simon Fraser University, Burnaby, British Columbia.

Douglas, K., & Hart, S. D. (1996, March). *Major mental disorder and violent behavior: A meta-analysis of study characteristics and substantive factors influencing effect size*. Paper presented at the Biennial Meeting of the American Psychology-Law Society (APA Div. 41), Hilton Head, South Carolina.

Gardner, W., Mulvey, E. P., & Shaw, E. C. (1995). Regression analyses of counts and rates: Poisson, overdispersed Poisson, and negative binomial models. *Psychological Bulletin, 118*, 392-404.

Gottfredson, M. R., & Hirschi, T. (1990). *A general theory of crime*. Stanford, CA: Stanford University Press.

Hare, R. D. (1981). Psychopathy and violence. In J. R. Hays, T. K. Roberts, & K. S. Soloway (Eds.), *Violence and the violent individual* (pp. 53-74). Jamaica, NY: Spectrum.

Hare, R. D. (1991). *The Hare Psychopathy Checklist-Revised.* Toronto, Ontario: Multi-Health Systems.

Hare, R. D. (1993). *Without conscience: The disturbing world of the psychopaths among us.* New York: Simon & Schuster.

Hare, R. D. (1996). Psychopathy: A clinical construct whose time has come. *Criminal Justice and Behavior, 23*, 25-54.

Hare, R. D., Forth, A. E., & Strachan, K. (1992). Psychopathy and crime across the lifespan. In R. DeV. Peters, R. J. McMahon, & V. L. Quinsey (Eds.), *Aggression and violence throughout the life span* (pp. 285-300). Newbury Park, CA: Sage.

Hare, R. D., & McPherson, L. M. (1984). Violent and aggressive behavior by criminal psychopaths. *International Journal of Law and Psychiatry, 7*, 35-50.

Harris, G. T., Rice, M. E., & Cormier, C. A. (1991). Psychopathy and violent recidivism. *Law and Human Behavior, 15*, 625-637.

Hart, S. D. (1996, March). *Conceptual issues in predicting violence: Some unasked and unanswered questions about risk assessment.* Paper presented at the Biennial Meeting of the American Psychology-Law Society (APA Div. 41), Hilton Head, South Carolina.

Hart, S. D., Cox, D. N., & Hare, R. D. (1995). *Manual for the Hare Psychopathy Checklist-Revised: Screening Version (PCL:SV).* Toronto: Multi-Health Systems, Inc.

Hart, S. D., & Dempster, R. J. (1997). Impulsivity and psychopathy. In C. D. Webster & M. A. Jackson (Eds.), *Impulsivity and violence: Principles and practice.* New York: Guilford.

Hart, S. D., & Hare, R. D. (in press). Psychopathy: Assessment and association with criminal conduct. In D. M. Stoff, J. Brieling, & J. Maser (Eds.), *Handbook of antisocial behavior.* New York: Wiley.

Hart, S. D., & Hare, R. D. (1996). Psychopathy and risk assessment. *Current Opinion in Psychiatry.*

Hart, S. D., Hare, R. D., & Forth, A. E. (1994). Psychopathy as a risk marker for violence: Development and validation of a screening version of the Revised Psychopathy Checklist. In J. Monahan & H. Steadman (Eds.), *Violence and mental disorder: Developments in risk assessment* (pp. 81-98). Chicago: University of Chicago Press.

Hart, S. D., Kropp, P. R., & Hare, R. D. (1988). Performance of psychopaths following conditional release from prison. *Journal of Consulting and Clinical Psychology, 56*, 227-232.

Hart, S. D., Webster, C. D., & Menzies, R. J. (1993). A note on portraying the accuracy of violence predictions. *Law and Human Behavior, 17*, 695-700.

Hedges, L. V., & Stock, W. (1983). The effects of class size: An examination of rival hypotheses. *American Educational Research Journal, 20*, 63-85.

Heilbrun, K., Hart, S. D., Hare, R. D., Gustafson, D., Nunez, C., & White, A. (in press). Inpatient and post-discharge aggression in mentally disordered offenders: The role of psychopathy. *Journal of Interpersonal Violence.*

Hill, C. D., Rogers, R., & Bickford, M. E. (1996). Predicting aggressive and socially disruptive behavior in a maximum security forensic psychiatric hospital. *Journal of Forensic Sciences, 41*, 56-59.

Kropp, P. R., Hart, S. D., Webster, C.W., & Eaves, D. (1995). Manual for the Spousal Assault Risk Assessment Guide, 2nd ed. Vancouver, BC: British Columbia Institute on Family Violence.

Lewis, A. (1974). Psychopathic personality: A most elusive category. *Psychological Medicine, 4*, 133-140.

Lipsey, M. W., & Wilson, D. B. (1993). The efficacy of psychological, educational, and behavioral treatment: Confirmation from meta-analysis. *American Psychologist, 48*, 1181-1209.

Litwack, T., & Schlesinger, L. B. (in press). Dangerousness risk assessments: Research, legal, and clinical considerations. In I. B. Weiner & A. K. Hess (Eds.), *Handbook of forensic psychology*. New York: Wiley.

Litwack, T., & Schlesinger, L. B. (1987). Assessing and predicting violence: Research, law, and applications. In I. B. Weiner & A. K. Hess (Eds.), *Handbook of forensic psychology* (pp. 205-207). New York: Wiley.

Lösel, F. (1996). Management of psychopaths [Abstract]. In D. J. Cooke, A. E. Forth, J. P. Newman, & R. D. Hare (Eds.), *Issues in Criminological and Legal Psychology: No. 24, International perspectives on psychopathy* (pp. 100-106). Leicester, UK: British Psychological Society.

Lösel, F., & Koferl, P. (1989). Evaluation research on correctional treatment in West Germany: A meta-analysis. In H. Wegener, F. Lösel, & J. Haisch (Eds.), *Criminal behavior and the justice system: Psychological perspectives* (pp. 334-355). New York: Springer.

Lynn, D. D., & Donovan, J. M. (1980). Medical versus surgical treatment of coronary artery disease. *Evaluation in Education, 4*, 98-99.

Meloy, J. R. (1988). *The psychopathic mind: Origins, dynamics, and treatments*. Northvale, NJ: Jason Aronson Inc.

Millon, T. (1981). *Disorders of personality: DSM-III Axis II*. New York: Wiley.

Monahan, J. (1981). *The clinical prediction of violent behavior*. Beverly Hills, CA: Sage.

Monahan, J., & Steadman, H. (1994). (Eds.), *Violence and mental disorder: Developments in risk assessment*. Chicago: University of Chicago Press.

Moore, S. D. (1990). A meta-analytic review of mass media campaigns designed to change automobile occupant restraint behavior (Doctoral dissertation, University of Illinois at Urbana-Champaign, 1989). *Dissertation Abstracts International, 50*, 1840A.

Mossman, D. (1994). Assessing predictions of violence: Being accurate about accuracy. *Journal of Consulting and Clinical Psychology, 62*, 783-792.

Newman, J. P., & Wallace, J. F. (1993). Divergent pathways to deficient self-regulation: Implications for disinhibitory psychopathology in children. *Clinical Psychology Review, 13*, 699-720.

Patrick, C. J., & Zempolich, K. A. (in press). Emotion and aggression in the psychopathic personality. *Aggression and Violent Behavior*.

Pichot, P. (1978). Psychopathic behavior: A historical overview. In R. D. Hare & D. Schalling (Eds.), *Psychopathic behavior: Approaches to research* (pp. 55-70). Chichester, UK: Wiley.

Quinsey, V. L., Rice, M. E., & Harris, G. T. (1995). Actuarial prediction of sexual recidivism. *Journal of Interpersonal Violence, 10*, 85-105.

Rice, M. E., & Harris, G. T. (1995). Violent recidivism: Assessing predictive validity. *Journal of Consulting and Clinical Psychology, 63*, 737-748.

Rosenthal, R. (1991). Meta-analysis: A review. *Psychosomatic Medicine, 53*, 247-271.

Salekin, R., Rogers, R., & Sewell, K. (1996). A review and meta-analysis of the Psychopathy Checklist and Psychopathy Checklist-Revised: Predictive validity of dangerousness. *Clinical Psychology: Science and Practice, 3*, 203-215.

Serin, R. C. (1991). Psychopathy and violence in criminals. *Journal of Interpersonal Violence, 6*, 423-431.

Serin, R. C., & Amos, N. L. (1995). The role of psychopathy in the assessment of dangerousness. *International Journal of Law and Psychiatry, 18*, 231-238.

Serin, R. C., Peters, R. D., & Barbaree, H. E. (1990). Predictors of psychopathy and release outcome in a criminal population. *Psychological Assessment: A Journal of Consulting and Clinical Psychology, 2*, 419-422.

Simourd, D., Bonta, J., Andrews, D., & Hoge, R. D. (1990). Criminal behavior and psychopaths: A meta-analysis [Abstract]. *Canadian Psychology, 31*, 347.

Smith, M. L., Glass, G. V., & Miller, T. I. (1980). *The benefits of psychotherapy*. Baltimore: Johns Hopkins University Press.

Steadman, H., Monahan, J. A., Applebaum, P. S., Grisso, T., Mulvey, E. P., Roth, L. H., Robbins, P. C., & Klassen, D. (1994). Designing a new generation of risk assessment research. In In J. Monahan & H. Steadman (Eds.), *Violence and mental disorder: Developments in risk assessment* (pp. 297-318). Chicago: University of Chicago Press.

Tyrer, P., & Ferguson, B. (1988). Development of the concept of abnormal personality. In P. Tyrer (Ed.)., *Personality disorders: Diagnosis, management, and course* (pp. 1-11). London: Wright.

Webster, C. D., Douglas, K. S., Eaves, D., & Hart, S. D. (1997). *HCR-20: Assessing risk for violence*, version 2. Burnaby, British Columbia: Simon Fraser University.

Webster, C. D., Harris, G. T., Rice, M. E., Cormier, C. A., & Quinsey, V. L. (1994). *The Violence Prediction Scheme: Assessing dangerousness in high risk men*. Toronto: Centre of Criminology, University of Toronto.

Whitlock, F. A. (1967). Prichard and the concept of moral insanity. *Australian and New Zealand Journal of Psychiatry, 1*, 72-79.

Whitlock, F. A. (1982). A note on moral insanity and psychopathic disorders. *Bulletin of the Royal College of Psychiatry, 6*, 57-59.

Williamson, S. E., Hare, R. D., & Wong, S. (1987). Violence: Criminal psychopaths and their victims. *Canadian Journal of Behavioral Science, 19*, 454-462.

Wilson, J. Q., & Herrnstein, R. J. (1985). *Crime and human nature*. New York: Simon and Schuster.

Wong, S. (1985). *Criminal and institutional behaviors of psychopaths*. Ottawa, Ontario: Programs Branch Users Report, Ministry of the Solicitor General of Canada.

World Health Organization (1992). *The ICD-10 classification of mental and behavioral disorder: Clinical descriptions and diagnostic guidelines*. Geneva: Author.

Author's notes

The material in this chapter is an integration of ideas with which I have struggled in various articles, chapters, and conference presentations over the past few years. My thoughts — at least, any useful ones I may have had — are the result of conversations and single malt scotch shared with many friends and colleagues, notably David Cooke, Robert Hare, Christopher Webster, Randy Kropp, and Douglas Boer; and a group of outstanding graduate students at SFU, including Rebecca Dempster, Kevin Douglas, David Lyon, and Lynne Sullivan.

Preparation of this chapter was supported in part by grants from the British Columbia Health Research Foundation and from the Social Sciences and Humanities Research Council of Canada. The views expressed herein are mine and do not necessarily reflect those of the funding agencies. Address correspondence to the Department of Psychology, Simon Fraser University, Burnaby, British Columbia, Canada, V5A 1S6. E-mail should be addressed to SHART@arts.sfu.ca.

PSYCHOPATHY AND CRIME: RECIDIVISM AND CRIMINAL CAREERS

JAMES F. HEMPHILL
Department of Psychology
University of British Columbia
Vancouver, British Columbia, Canada
RON TEMPLEMAN
Colonsay, Saskatchewan, Canada
STEPHEN WONG
Regional Psychiatric Centre (Prairies)
Saskatoon, Saskatchewan, Canada
ROBERT D. HARE
Department of Psychology
University of British Columbia
Vancouver, British Columbia, Canada

1. INTRODUCTION

In this chapter we address two of the most significant methodological problems hampering predictions of criminal and violent behaviors: the lack of theoretically relevant predictor variables and weak criterion variables (Monahan & Steadman, 1994). To address the limitation of atheoretical predictor variables, we summarize the association between the construct of psychopathy and recidivism. Consistent with current clinical and research practice, our operational definition of psychopathy is the Hare Psychopathy Checklist (PCL; Hare 1980); its revision, the Hare Psychopathy Checklist-Revised (PCL-R; Hare, 1991); a version of the PCL-R modified for use with adolescents (Forth, Hart, & Hare, 1990; Forth, Kosson, & Hare, in press); and a French translation of the PCL-R (Hare, 1996a). We also compare the predictive utility of the PCL/PCL-R with key demographic and criminal history variables, personality disorder diagnoses, and actuarial risk scales. To address the limitation of weak criterion variables, we describe two methods of measuring and analyzing criminal behaviors: survival analyses and Criminal Career Profiles (CCPs; Templeman, 1995; Wong, Templeman, Gu, Andre, & Leis, 1997). We emphasize the strengths of the newly developed CCP methodology for providing an overall measure of criminal behaviors. To illustrate the benefits of the CCP methodology for conceptualizing, coding, analyzing, and presenting criminal behaviors, we present 10-year outcome data from a random sample of federal offenders.

2. PSYCHOPATHY AND RECIDIVISM: META-ANALYSES

Psychopathy is an important predictor of recidivism, and is consistently associated with a variety of socially deviant behaviors, presumably because of the persisting and enduring constellation of interpersonal, affective, and behavioral characteristics that define the disorder (Harpur & Hare, 1994; Litwack & Schlesinger, 1987; Widiger &

D.J. Cooke et al. (eds.), Psychopathy: Theory, Research and Implications for Society, 375–399.
© 1998 *Kluwer Academic Publishers. Printed in the Netherlands.*

Trull, 1994). Psychopaths are interpersonally manipulative and exploitive; they are callous, with shallow, poorly integrated affective experiences; and they are impulsive, often violating societal rules and conventions (Cleckley, 1976; Hare, 1991; McCord & McCord, 1964). These distinctive interpersonal, affective, and behavioral characteristics are first observed in childhood (Frick, this volume; Frick, O'Brien, Wootton, & McBurnett, 1994; McBurnett & Pfiffner, this volume) and are well-defined by early adolescence (Forth & Burke, this volume). Many of the characteristics that define psychopathy--lack of empathy, impulsivity, little capacity for close emotional bonds, and so forth--are associated with antisocial and aggressive behaviors (Miller & Eisenberg, 1988). Logically, therefore, the PCL/PCL-R should be an important predictor of recidivism.

Two recent, independent meta-analyses have examined the association between the PCL/PCL-R and recidivism (Hemphill, Hare, & Wong, in press; Salekin, Rogers, & Sewell, 1996). Here we focus on the results of the Hemphill et al. (in press) meta-analyses because they addressed four methodological limitations of the Salekin et al. study. First, despite their caution that researchers should "avoid using postdictive-type studies when discussing predictions of dangerousness" (Salekin et al., 1996, p. 212), Salekin et al. included both predictive and postdictive studies in their meta-analyses whereas Hemphill et al. (in press) included only predictive studies.

Second, Hemphill et al. (in press) included only recidivism studies in which effect sizes were estimated from independent samples of subjects, consistent with the recommendation that researchers select only one estimate of effect size per sample (Rosenthal, 1991; Wolf, 1986). Salekin et al. (1996) included several studies based on the same sample of offenders. For example, some of the studies by the Oak Ridge research group (Harris, Rice, & Cormier, 1991; Harris, Rice, & Quinsey, 1993, 1994; Quinsey, Rice, & Harris, 1995; Rice & Harris, 1992, 1995a, 1995b, 1997; Rice, Harris, & Cormier, 1992; Rice, Harris, & Quinsey, 1990), and several conducted by Serin and colleagues (Barbaree, Seto, Serin, Amos, & Preston, 1994; Serin, 1991, 1992, 1996; Serin & Amos, 1995; Serin, Malcolm, Khanna, & Barbaree, 1994; Serin, Peters, & Barbaree, 1990), were not based on independent, mutually exclusive samples of offenders.

Third, Hemphill et al. (in press) limited their selection of recidivism studies to those with behavioral outcomes; recidivism typically was coded from criminal records or from institutional behaviors. However, Salekin et al. (1996) included in their meta-analyses several studies that examined the association between the PCL/PCL-R and various measures of deviant sexual behavior or arousal that were not based on recidivism indices. For example, Barbaree et al. (1994) compared PCL-R scores of subtypes of rapists, whereas Serin et al. (1994) computed correlations between PCL-R scores and phallometric measures of deviant sexual arousal. Fourth, the meta-analyses conducted by Hemphill et al. (in press) included data from several unpublished studies not available to Salekin et al. (1996).

Below we briefly describe the method and results from the Hemphill et al. (in press) meta-analyses. Results are presented separately for general recidivism and for violent recidivism.

2.1. Method

2.1.1. PROCEDURE
2.1.1.1. Selecting studies and statistical values

Studies that met the following criteria were included: (1) analyses were predictive in nature (that is, PCL/PCL-R ratings were completed before a prospective follow-up period and calculation of outcome); (2) Within each meta-analysis, samples of offenders were independent from each other. For single databases reanalyzed several times, one statistical value per database was selected based on the largest sample size for each respective type of recidivism (general, violent); and (3) Outcome was measured behaviorally. Reconviction measures were selected for studies that reported several behavioral outcome variables.

2.1.1.2. Assessment of psychopathy

Most of the studies discussed below used the PCL-R for the assessment of psychopathy. However, some researchers assessed psychopathy with the 22-item PCL (Hart, Kropp, & Hare, 1988a, 1988b; Heilbrun et al., in press), an 18-item version of the PCL-R modified for use with adolescent offenders (Forth et al., in press, 1990), or with a French translation of the 20-item PCL-R (Hare, 1996a; Ross, Hodgins, & Côté, 1992). Each PCL/PCL-R item is scored on a 3-point scale: 2 indicates the item definitely applies, 1 indicates it may or may not apply, and 0 indicates it definitely does not apply, to the individual. Items are summed, and total scores represent the degree to which the subject matches the prototypical psychopath. The recommended cutoff score for a diagnosis of psychopathy on the PCL-R is 30 (Hare, 1991).

2.1.2. SUBJECTS
Much of the research on psychopathy and recidivism has been conducted with offenders in Canadian institutions, either in a provincial facility (offenders with a sentence of less than two years) or a federal institution (offenders with a sentence of two years or more). In Canada, research on recidivism is greatly facilitated by a central computer system that enables researchers to keep track of an offender's contacts with the criminal justice system.

The findings presented below are based on samples from diverse populations, including adult and adolescent offenders, sex offenders, and mentally disordered offenders. Most of the samples consisted of persistent offenders whose convictions included serious, often violent offenses.

2.2. Results

2.2.1. PSYCHOPATHY AND RECIDIVISM
Two sets of meta-analyses were performed that examined the association between psychopathy and both general and violent recidivism. In one set of analyses, continuous scores on the PCL/PCL-R were correlated with outcome. In the other set, the

distribution of PCL/PCL-R scores were subdivided to form two or three groups of offenders.

2.2.1.1. Continuous PCL/PCL-R scores and recidivism

Each correlation between scores on the PCL/PCL-R and recidivism (yes, no) was subjected to a Fisher z to r transformation, weighted by its N - 3 degrees of freedom, averaged across studies, and converted back to r. Across seven studies (Forth et al., 1990; Hart et al., 1988a; Heilbrun et al., in press; Hemphill, 1992; Rice et al., 1992; Ross et al., 1992; Serin & Amos, 1995) involving 1,275 male offenders, the average correlation between the PCL/PCL-R and general recidivism was .27. The average correlation between the PCL/PCL-R and violent recidivism also was .27, for 1,374 offenders across six studies (Forth et al., 1990; Harris et al., 1993; Heilbrun et al., in press; Hemphill, 1992; Ross et al., 1992; Serin & Amos, 1995). The association between the PCL-R and sexual recidivism was examined in only one independent sample of 178 offenders (Quinsey et al., 1995), and the correlation between the PCL-R and sexual recidivism was .23.

Magnitudes of the correlations between PCL/PCL-R scores and both general and violent recidivism were heterogeneous across studies. This heterogeneity might reflect individual differences in study methodology (e.g., length of follow-up, method of coding recidivism) or offender characteristics within each sample (e.g., age, race, socioeconomic background) that moderate the magnitudes of psychopathy/recidivism associations (see Hemphill et al., in press, for a discussion).

2.2.1.2. PCL/PCL-R groups and recidivism

Several studies have compared the recidivism rates of offenders subdivided into two or three groups on the basis of their scores on the PCL/PCL-R. With the PCL-R, the high and low psychopathy groups are typically defined, respectively, by a score of 30 or above and by a score of 20 or below. Several studies (Harris et al., 1991; Quinsey et al., 1995; Rice et al., 1992; Rice & Harris, 1995a, 1997) classified subjects into only two PCL-R groups; for convenience, subjects scoring at or above the respective PCL-R cutpoint were treated as high PCL-R group members and those scoring below the respective PCL-R cutpoint were treated as low PCL-R group members.

Statistical associations between psychopathy and outcome were determined by computing (a) the average phi coefficient (weighted by degrees of freedom) between psychopathy group (low, high) and recidivism (no, yes); and (b) the average odds ratio, considered to be the preferred summary statistic for determining the degree of association in 2 x 2 contingency tables (Fleiss, 1994). Here, the odds ratio is defined as the odds that a member of the high psychopathy group will recidivate divided by the odds that a member of the low psychopathy group will recidivate.

Across five studies (Hart et al., 1988a; Hemphill, 1992; Rice et al., 1992; Ross et al., 1992; Serin & Amos, 1995) involving a total 1,021 male offenders, the general recidivism rates (%) during the entire outcome period for the low, medium, and high PCL/PCL-R groups, respectively, were 39.7, 54.9, and 74.1. The mean phi coefficient was .36 and the mean odds ratio was 5.31 (both statistics based on Ns = 651). Because the average length of follow-up varied considerably from study to study, Hemphill et al.

(in press) estimated failure rates at one year by aggregating across studies failure rates from survival analyses. (The study by Rice et al., 1992, was excluded from this analysis because they did not present results from survival analyses.) Survival analyses, described in more detail below, are powerful statistical procedures that circumvent problems associated with unequal follow-up times by estimating risk across a range of follow-up periods (Morita, Lee, & Mowday, 1989). At one year, the estimated mean general recidivism rates for 733 offenders in four studies were 20.4, 42.1, and 59.3 for the low, medium, and high PCL/PCL-R groups. The mean phi coefficient was .41 and the mean odds ratio was 6.23 ($\underline{N}$s = 363).

Similar analyses were completed for violent recidivism reported in four studies (Hemphill, 1992; Rice & Harris, 1995a; Ross et al., 1992; Serin & Amos, 1995). During the entire follow-up period, mean violent recidivism rates for 1,089 offenders in the low, medium, and high PCL-R groups, respectively, were 20.2, 21.4, and 45.7. The mean phi coefficient was .27 and the mean odds ratio was 3.82 ($\underline{N}$s = 813). At one year, violent recidivism rates estimated from survival functions for the Hemphill (1992; $\underline{N}$ = 106) study were approximately 14, 32, and 37, respectively, for the low, medium, and high PCL-R groups. Corresponding values for the Quinsey et al. (1995; $\underline{N}$ = 178) study were 3 for the low PCL-R group and 16 for the high PCL-R group. The mean phi coefficient was .23 and the mean odds ratio was 4.57 ($\underline{N}$s = 237).

2.2.1.3. Additional PCL-R recidivism studies

Several additional prospective PCL-R recidivism studies, available since Hemphill et al. (in press) conducted their meta-analyses, obtained similar results with adolescent offenders (Gretton, 1997; Gretton, McBride, O'Shaughnessy, & Hare, 1995; Toupin, Mercier, Déry, Côté, & Hodgins, 1996), female offenders (Loucks, 1995; Zaparniuk & Paris, 1995), male federal offenders (Zamble & Palmer, 1996), forensic psychiatric offenders (Hill, Rogers, & Bickford, 1996; Wintrup, Coles, Hart, & Webster, 1994), civil psychiatric patients (Douglas, Ogloff, & Nicholls, 1997), African American offenders (Hemphill, Newman, & Hare, 1997), and sex offenders (Rice & Harris, 1997).

Three additional recidivism studies have been conducted with adolescent offenders using a modified version of the PCL-R (see Forth et al., 1990, in press) to rate psychopathy. Gretton et al. (1995) studied 220 adolescent male sex offenders who attended a treatment program. Psychopathy assessments were conducted from extensive file information and recidivism was coded from official criminal records. Participants were followed-up for an average 4.7 years. Psychopaths committed sexual, violent, and nonviolent offenses at a higher rate than did nonpsychopaths (odds ratios ranged from 3.4 to 7.8), and survival analyses indicated psychopaths failed at a higher and faster rate than did nonpsychopaths. Failure rates (%) estimated at two years from survival analyses were 36 for the nonpsychopaths and 72 for the psychopaths. Moreover, the combination of deviant phallometric arousal and high PCL-R score was a powerful predictor of general recidivism: at 56 months, the failure rate estimated from survival analyses was 83 for the deviant psychopaths and was 45 for the remaining subjects. Using similar coding procedures in a general sample of 157 adolescent offenders,

Gretton (1997) found that during a 10-year follow-up period PCL-R scores correlated .30 with violent failure (yes, no) and .49 with number of conduct disorder symptoms. Toupin et al. (1996) administered a French translation of the PCL-R (Hare, 1996a) to 52 male adolescents. Subjects were receiving treatment in rehabilitation centers, day centers, or special educational programs, and 42 participants were later reinterviewed. During the 1-year follow-up period, Toupin et al. found that PCL-R scores correlated .43 with delinquency, .30 with aggressive behavior, .32 with alcohol use, and .28 with number of aggressive conduct disorder symptoms.

Zaparniuk and Paris (1995) used survival analyses to estimate general failure rates among a sample of 75 female offenders. PCL-R scores were rated from both interview and collateral file information and recidivism was coded from official criminal records. At one year, failure rates were approximately 20, 35, and 60, respectively, for the low, medium, and high PCL-R groups. Loucks (1995) studied 100 federally incarcerated adult female offenders. PCL-R scores were rated from interview and file information, and institutional behaviors were rated for the period six months prior to and six months subsequent to the PCL-R assessments. PCL-R scores correlated .63 with institutional convictions, .59 with institutional behavior problems, and .38 with institutional violence.

In a sample of 106 adult male federal offenders, Zamble and Palmer (1996) separately classified subjects into low- and high-risk groups for each of three predictor variables: the PCL-R; the Statistical Information on Recidivism (SIR; Nuffield, 1982, 1989) scale, an actuarial instrument used by the National Parole Board of Canada to estimate release risk; and Parole Board decisions to grant or deny early release. Failure was defined as a new revocation or conviction and was coded after a 2.5 year follow-up. The researchers examined the predictive utility of each measure. Both the PCL-R groups and the SIR groups were substantially more accurate at predicting outcome than were Parole Board decisions: Relative Improvement Over Chance (Loeber & Dishion, 1983) statistics were, respectively, 45.1, 41.2, and 25.6.

Wintrup et al. (1994) followed-up 80 males remanded for assessments of fitness to stand trial at a forensic psychiatric facility (see Hart and Hare, 1989, for sample details). Mean time at risk was 5.0 years, and outcome was coded from official criminal records and from health care records. The PCL-R correlated .38 (N = 72) with total number of charges and convictions and .25 (N = 79) with number of violent charges and convictions. From survival analyses (N = 72), Wintrup et al. estimated that failure rates at one year for the low, medium, and high PCL-R groups were, respectively, 7, 32, and 43. Hill et al. (1996) studied 55 male adult offenders, most of whom were found incompetent to stand trial or Not Guilty By Reason of Insanity. They assessed psychopathy with the screening version of the PCL-R (PCL:SV; Hart, Cox, & Hare, 1995) and conducted a six month follow-up review of institutional files. Hill et al. reported results from two stepwise regression analyses in which four predictor variables (PCL:SV scores, age, type of charge, substance abuse/dependence) were used to predict two types of outcome (aggression; treatment noncompliance). Neither age nor type of charge (property, person) significantly predicted outcome. PCL:SV score was the only significant predictor of treatment noncompliance, and PCL:SV score improved upon history of substance abuse/dependence for predicting aggression (multiple $\underline{R}$ = .43). PCL:SV diagnoses (yes, no) correlated .69 with aggression and .30 with treatment noncompliance. During the follow-up period, the number of institutional incidents recorded were 29.7 for psychopaths and 10.7 for nonpsychopaths.

Douglas et al. (1997) used a median split on the PCL:SV (Hart et al., 1995) to classify 279 involuntary civil psychiatric patients into two psychopathy groups. Participants were followed-up for an average of two years post-release. The odds ratio between PCL:SV group (psychopath, nonpsychopath) and arrest for a violent offense (yes, no) was 9.9.

In a recent study of 189 sex offenders, Rice and Harris (1997) classified each subject into a PCL-R (low, high) group and into a deviant sexual arousal (low, high) group based on phallometric arousal scores. PCL-R group classification alone was a strong predictor of violent recidivism, and deviant sexual arousal group classification failed to contribute to the prediction of violent recidivism beyond that offered by the PCL-R. From survival analyses, violent failure rates estimated at one year were 5 for the nonpsychopaths and 30 for the psychopaths; respective values at five years were 35 and 85. Of particular interest was the pattern of results for sexual recidivism. The combination of high PCL-R score and high deviant sexual arousal score resulted in substantially faster and higher rates of sexually reoffending than did a high score on a single measure: psychopaths with low deviant phallometric arousal scores, and nonpsychopaths (regardless of deviant phallometric arousal scores), were at much lower risk to sexually reoffend. Survival analyses indicated that the sexual failure rates at five years were approximately 60 for the deviant psychopaths and 30 for the three other groups.

2.2.2. PCL/PCL-R FACTORS
The PCL/PCL-R contains two correlated factors that have distinct patterns of intercorrelations with other variables. PCL/PCL-R Factor 1 describes a constellation of interpersonal and affective traits commonly considered fundamental to most clinical descriptions of the psychopath, whereas PCL/PCL-R Factor 2 describes a chronically unstable, antisocial, and socially deviant lifestyle (Hare et al., 1990; Harpur, Hakstian, & Hare, 1988; Harpur, Hare, & Hakstian, 1989; Templeman & Wong, 1994). After examining the patterns of correlations between the PCL/PCL-R Factors and recidivism, Hemphill et al. (in press; see also Hemphill & Hare, 1996) concluded that PCL/PCL-R Factor 2 was more strongly associated with general recidivism than was PCL/PCL-R Factor 1. However, results indicated that both PCL/PCL-R Factors were important predictors of violent recidivism (see also Harpur & Hare, 1991).

3. COMPARISONS OF THE PCL/PCL-R WITH OTHER PREDICTOR VARIABLES
The preceding analyses indicate that the PCL and the PCL-R by themselves are significant predictors of reoffending. However, an important issue is their ability to add to the predictive validity of other, more traditional, variables. Some investigators (e.g., Sechrest, 1963) consider the demonstration of incremental predictive validity crucial

for evaluating the utility of any psychometric instrument intended to assist decision-makers. Do PCL/PCL-R scores contribute unique information to the prediction of reoffending beyond that offered by demographic and criminal history variables, personality disorder diagnoses, and standard actuarial risk scales developed specifically to predict reoffending?

3.1. Demographic and Criminal History Variables

The ability of the PCL/PCL-R to predict recidivism, independent of the contribution of key demographic and criminal history variables, has been evaluated several ways. Perhaps the simplest procedure has been to delete items from the PCL/PCL-R that reflect criminal history. Both Harris et al. (1991) and Serin (1996) found that the association between the PCL-R and recidivism was essentially the same whether or not items that measured criminal activities were deleted.

Several researchers have compared the magnitude of the association between PCL-R scores and recidivism with the magnitude of the association between demographic/criminal history variables and recidivism. In each case, the PCL-R was among the strongest single predictors of both sexual and violent recidivism (Harris et al., 1991, 1993; Quinsey et al., 1995; Rice et al., 1990; Serin, 1996). PCL-R scores alone correctly classified violent recidivists as accurately as did a multivariate combination of 16 variables (Harris et al., 1991). Similarly, a combination of high PCL-R score and high deviant phallometric arousal score correctly classified rapists into sexual recidivism (yes, no) and violent recidivism (yes, no) groups as accurately as did a combination of variables statistically selected from over 30 study variables (Rice et al., 1990). These findings are particularly important because a small number of variables, carefully chosen and theoretically relevant (such as the PCL/PCL-R), are more likely to cross-validate on new samples than is a multivariate combination of a large number of predictor variables (Wiggins, 1973).

A stringent test of the incremental predictive validity of the PCL/PCL-R is to force demographic and criminal history variables into a hierarchical multiple regression analysis and to permit the PCL/PCL-R to enter the regression equation only if it adds unique information to the prediction of outcome. All five prediction studies that performed such analyses (Harris et al., 1991; Hart et al., 1988a; Heilbrun et al., in press; Rice et al., 1990; Ross et al., 1992) found that PCL/PCL-R scores provided significant incremental validity to the prediction of outcome.

3.2. Personality Disorder Diagnoses

Several researchers (Harris et al., 1991; Hart et al., 1988b) reported that the PCL/PCL-R was more strongly related to recidivism than was a diagnosis of antisocial personality disorder, or a diagnosis of any personality disorder (Harris et al., 1991, 1993; Quinsey et al., 1995), as defined by criteria listed in the third edition of the American Psychiatric Association's Diagnostic and Statistical Manual of Mental Disorders (DSM-III; American Psychiatric Association, 1980). (See Hemphill et al., in press, for reanalyses of these studies.)

3.3. Actuarial risk scales

Perhaps the most relevant comparison for establishing the incremental predictive validity of the PCL/PCL-R is to compare it with actuarial scales designed specifically to predict reoffending. Actuarial risk scales include the Base Expectancy Score (BES; Gottfredson & Bonds, 1961), the Level of Supervision Inventory (LSI; Andrews, 1982), the Salient Factor Score (SFS; Hoffman, 1983; Hoffman & Beck, 1974), the SIR scale (Nuffield, 1982, 1989), and the Violence Risk Appraisal Guide (VRAG; Harris et al., 1993; Rice & Harris, 1995b).

Four independent research groups have reported predictions of general recidivism and violent recidivism from both PCL/PCL-R ratings and from one or more of these actuarial risk scales (Harris et al., 1993; Hart et al., 1988b; Hemphill, 1992; Rice & Harris, 1992; Serin, 1996). Hemphill et al. (in press) compared the predictive validity of the PCL/PCL-R and the actuarial scale used in each of these studies. They concluded that, overall, the PCL/PCL-R and the actuarial scales performed equally well in the prediction of general recidivism, but that the PCL-R predicted violent recidivism significantly better than did actuarial scales.

4. MEASURING AND ANALYZING CRIMINAL BEHAVIORS

Although the PCL and PCL-R were constructed simply to measure the clinical construct of psychopathy, they have turned out to be strong predictors of recidivism and violence. This should not be surprising, given that the 20 items in the PCL-R capture most of the traits and behaviors important to understanding and predicting criminal behavior. The PCL/PCL-R thus provides a theoretically and clinically meaningful basis for assessing dangerousness and risk for reoffending.

We now turn to the issue of weak criterion or outcome variables designed to measure criminal behavior (Monahan & Steadman, 1994). Despite evidence that histories of violence and social deviance are good predictors of future criminal behaviors (Blomhoff, Seim & Friis, 1990; Klassen & O'Connor, 1994; Monahan, 1981), researchers have lacked systematic or generally agreed upon ways of operationalizing, measuring, and combining criminal behaviors (see Blumstein, Cohen, Roth & Visher, 1986; Hare, McPherson, & Forth, 1988; Monahan & Steadman, 1994). For example, some of the many indices of criminal behaviors include age at first conviction, number of previous convictions, number of convictions committed per year free, and time to first reconviction.

The lack of a generally accepted criterion variable, or set of criterion variables, has made it difficult to directly compare results from different studies. There is need for a single summary index that accurately reflects an offender's criminal career. Such an index should be capable of facilitating the cross-validation of prediction instruments and might strengthen the observed associations between predictor and criterion variables.

Researchers typically conceptualize and analyze criminal behaviors with retrospective and prospective research designs; the former analyzes behaviors that occurred prior to the index offense or clinical assessment, whereas the latter looks at behaviors that occur subsequent to the index offense or clinical assessment. For each of these designs, researchers often classify offenses into broader subgroups such as nonviolent, violent, and sexual. A common set of statistical procedures for prospective research is survival analyses, which we briefly describe here. Then we describe Criminal Career Profiles (CCPs), a new method for summarizing individual and group criminal careers from combined prospective and retrospective data.

4.1. Survival Analyses

Survival analyses are a set of statistical procedures well-suited for analyzing data from prospective research designs, particularly when different groups of offenders are followed-up for unequal lengths of time. Indeed, Schmidt and Witte (1988) have described survival analysis as "one of the major methodological innovations in justice research" (p. 2). Because researchers often use survival analyses to estimate time to first reoffense following release from incarceration, survival analyses have an important statistical advantage (Morita et al., 1989) over traditional dichotomous (yes, no) estimates of recidivism. However, survival analyses tell us little about an offender's criminal activities before the time period involved in the analyses and subsequent to the first reoffense. This limitation is particularly important when dealing with individuals, such as psychopaths, whose criminal histories are more serious and extensive, and their recidivism rates higher, than those of other offenders (for reviews, see Hare, 1996b; Hart & Hare, 1997).

4.2. Criminal Career Profiles

4.2.1. STRENGTHS OF THE CCP METHODOLOGY

In addition to estimating time to first failure, clearly the number of offenses committed and length of incarcerations are key variables for assessing seriousness of a criminal history and for assessing each offender's risk to reoffend. Unfortunately, survival analyses only estimate time to first failure while neglecting these other important variables. To address the limitations of survival analyses, Wong and colleagues (Templeman, 1995; Wong et al., 1997) developed the CCP methodology of conceptualizing, estimating, and presenting criminal behaviors.

The CCP methodology maintains three primary strengths of survival analyses: (1) to incorporate into the statistical analyses the time interval between criminal behaviors; (2) to reduce the impact on statistical results of varying follow-up lengths between groups; and (3) to provide statistical comparisons of criminal behaviors simultaneously across a range of time periods and between groups. Moreover, CCP slope provides a continuous measure of criminal behaviors--rather than a dichotomous estimate provided by survival analyses--suggesting that statistical analyses using the CCP methodology with adequate follow-up periods will be more powerful than results obtained using survival analyses.

4.2.2. TWO CCP EXAMPLES

For illustrative purposes, CCPs and CCP slopes are graphically represented in Figure 1 separately for fictional inmates A and B. Time Out lines are plotted parallel to the horizontal axis and Time In lines are plotted parallel to the vertical axis. Each Time Out line represents time the offender is at risk to reoffend or is not serving time for a conviction or set of convictions, and each Time In line represents time the offender is incarcerated for respective conviction periods or for conditional release violations. Data coordinates for each inmate are sequentially joined by horizontal lines to represent Time Out periods and by vertical lines to represent Time In periods.

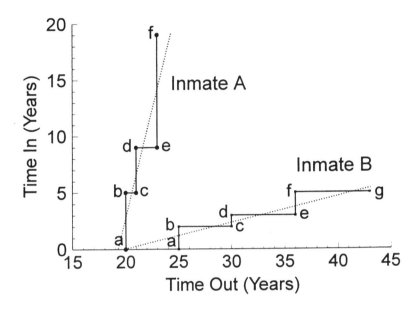

Figure 1. Example Criminal Career Profiles of Fictional Inmates A and B.

Data point "a" represents the age at first conviction or set of convictions (AFC) appearing on the criminal record. Inmate A was first convicted at age 20, indicated by the coordinate (20, 0); inmate B was first convicted at age 25, indicated by the coordinate (25, 0). Data point "b" represents the actual or estimated time of release from the first incarceration period. Coordinate (20, 5) indicates inmate A served five years for the first conviction or set of convictions, and coordinate (25, 2) indicates inmate B served two years for the first conviction or set of convictions. Data point "c" represents the time from first release to second admission. Coordinate (21, 5) indicates inmate A was readmitted one year after the first release, and coordinate (30, 2) indicates inmate B was readmitted five years after the first release. For each inmate, subsequent times between each release and readmission are represented in this manner for all offenses appearing on the criminal record. At the end of the study period, inmate A was 42 years-old and spent 19 years incarcerated; inmate B was 48 years-old and spent 5 years incarcerated. Although conceptually easy to understand, the CCP methodology is statistically involved and for most practical purposes requires specialized computer software to convert and extract conviction information.

4.2.3. CCP SLOPE

A linear regression line that minimizes squared differences between observed and estimated CCP coordinates is calculated for each subject. The slope of this regression line measured in degrees--termed CCP slope--is used as a single overall index of criminal behavior for each individual. CCP slope is a function of the time each offender is, and is not, incarcerated. The steeper CCP slope (graphically depicted in Figure 1 by a dotted line) of inmate A than of inmate B reflects the more extensive criminal career of inmate A. With adequate follow-up periods, the CCP slope is a robust estimate of criminal career and presumably reflects overall severity of a single criminal career or of averaged criminal careers. The finding that CCP slope and time incarcerated are strongly correlated (see Wong et al., 1997) provides validity for CCP slope as a good single measure of criminal career. We now present results from a recent study in which survival analyses and CCP analyses were conducted. A manuscript with more detailed descriptions, analyses, and results from this data set may be obtained from James F. Hemphill.

5. TEN-YEAR FOLLOW-UP OF WONG'S (1984) SAMPLE

Wong (1984) examined the association between psychopathy and criminal and institutional behaviors among a random sample of 15% of inmates serving sentences of two or more years in Canada's Prairie Region. In the current paper, we report results from a further 10-year prospective follow-up period for Wong's (1984) sample. Specifically, the association between the PCL and recidivism was estimated using survival analyses, and the association between the PCL and criminal career was calculated using CCPs and CCP slope. CCP measures incorporate criminal convictions both before and after PCL ratings were conducted.

5.1. Method

5.1.1. SUBJECTS

Details of subject selection and sample demographics are available elsewhere (Wong, 1984, 1997). Briefly, all subjects had been convicted of one or more criminal offenses and were serving sentences of two or more years. Unless otherwise indicated, all the following analyses are based on 274 subjects for whom we obtained official criminal records (see below). Inmates were an average 32.9 ($\underline{SD}$ = 9.71) years-old when first released from prison after the PCL assessment. The racial composition of the sample was 68.6% Caucasian, 27.7% Native, and 3.6% other. Length of follow-up, or time at risk, was calculated for each offender by subtracting the age when the inmate was first released from the data collection date. Subjects were prospectively followed-up for 10.1 ($\underline{SD}$ = 2.87) years.

5.1.2. PROCEDURE
5.1.2.1. Assessment of psychopathy

After raters reviewed comprehensive case files, each subject was rated on psychopathy using Hare's (1980) 22-item PCL; no interview was conducted. Interrater reliability for PCL ratings conducted by two independent raters was r = .86 (n = 244). We averaged independent PCL ratings when two ratings were available; coefficient alpha was .85. Mean PCL score was 25.3 (SD = 5.87) and values ranged from 6.0 to 40.0. Subjects with PCL scores between 0 and 19.99, between 20 and 29.99, and between 30 and 44, were respectively placed into low, medium, and high PCL groups. Factor analyses of the 22 PCL items for the current data set yielded two factors (Templeman & Wong, 1994) that were strongly associated with the stable and replicable 2-factor solution described by Harpur et al. (1988). We computed PCL Factor scores by summing together items that respectively loaded on the two factors identified by Harpur et al. (1988). The mean score on PCL Factor 1, the interpersonal/affective facet of psychopathy, was 10.2 (SD = 2.96). The mean score on PCL Factor 2, the social deviance facet of psychopathy, was 13.1 (SD = 3.65). The two PCL Factors correlated .42 with each other. The low PCL group was significantly older when released from prison than was the medium PCL group. The high PCL group was composed of significantly more Caucasian offenders than would be expected by chance, and the low PCL group was followed-up for significantly less time than was the medium PCL group.

5.1.2.2. Obtaining criminal records

The Royal Canadian Mounted Police (RCMP) maintains a central registry on each offender convicted of violating the Canadian Criminal Code. To ensure every entry in the criminal record is associated with the correct offender, each offender's identity is first confirmed by fingerprints and then his or her criminal data are entered into the conviction registry. We obtained official criminal records from the RCMP for 87.0% (N = 274) of the 315 subjects previously assessed in 1983 (Wong, 1984). In terms of age, racial composition, and mean PCL scores, the 274 subjects with valid criminal records were similar to the entire sample of 315 subjects and to the population from which the samples were drawn (see Wong, 1984).

5.1.2.3. Coding criminal records

CrimeWare (Templeman, 1995) is a computer software program designed to convert criminal records into spreadsheet form so researchers can compute measures of criminal behaviors. Each Canadian Criminal Code conviction was coded into nonviolent convictions (break and enter, theft, possession of stolen property, fraud, nonviolent sexual offenses [e.g., indecent exposure], driving while intoxicated, narcotics convictions, breach of conditional release, failure to comply, miscellaneous convictions) and violent convictions (murder, attempted murder, manslaughter, sexual assault, kidnapping, robbery, weapons-related convictions, assault, threatening behavior, escape, dangerous use of an automobile, criminal negligence). After we used

CrimeWare to code criminal records, we computed AFCs, CCPs, and CCP slopes for each subject and for the low, medium, and high PCL groups.

5.2. Results

We first present results from retrospective AFC analyses, then from prospective recidivism analyses, and finally from combined retrospective and prospective CCP analyses.

5.2.1. AGE AT FIRST CONVICTION

AFC was computed for each offender by subtracting his date of birth from the first conviction appearing on his adult criminal record. As shown in Table 1, Total PCL scores and PCL Factor 2 scores correlated negatively with AFC, but PCL Factor 1 scores were uncorrelated with AFC. These findings indicate that inmates with higher PCL scores and that those who exhibit more socially deviant behaviors are first convicted at an earlier age. The three PCL groups had significantly different mean AFC scores (see Table 1); the medium and high PCL groups received their first convictions at a younger age than did the low PCL group.

5.2.2. PROSPECTIVE FAILURE

After release from incarceration, three-quarters (77.4%) of offenders received a new conviction. Most (70.1%) subjects were convicted of a nonviolent offense and more than half (53.6%) were convicted of a violent offense. Point-biserial correlations were computed between continuous PCL (Total, Factor 1, Factor 2) scores and recidivism (yes, no; see Table 1). PCL Total scores and PCL Factor 2 scores--but not PCL Factor 1 scores--correlated significantly with both measures of recidivism (any, violent). Failure rates among the three PCL groups were significantly different for both measures of recidivism (see Table 1). Because of the high reconviction rates across the 10-year follow-up period, we calculated recidivism rates during the first year of the prospective follow-up period. Conviction rates (%) for new offenses during the first year after release were 13.0, 35.3, and 41.0, respectively, for the low, medium, and high PCL groups. Taken together, these results indicate psychopaths were convicted earlier and at a higher rate than were nonpsychopaths.

5.2.3. SURVIVAL ANALYSES

Survival functions were computed (Norusis and SPSS Inc., 1994) for each of the low, medium, and high PCL groups. We calculated time to first failure during the prospective follow-up period for each offender by subtracting the first date of release after the PCL rating was conducted from the date of the first respective conviction.
5.2.3.1. Any recidivism

Survival functions, plotted in Figure 2 for the low, medium, and high PCL groups, were significantly different overall from each other indicating that these groups were reconvicted at different rates. Proportionately fewer inmates in the low PCL group than in the medium PCL group or than in the high PCL group were reconvicted. Median survival times (the respective time points at which half the cases are expected to

Table 1 Associations Between the Psychopathy Checklist (PCL) and Criminal Behaviors

| | PCL groups | | | | Correlations | | |
| | Low | Medium | High | | PCL scores, $\underline{N}$ = 274 | | |
	$\underline{n}$ = 46	$\underline{n}$ = 167	$\underline{n}$ = 61		Total	Factor 1	Factor 2
Age at first conviction	24.33 (9.68)	19.50 (5.89)	18.62 (4.74)	$\underline{F}$(2, 271) = 12.18**	-.31**	.00	-.48**
Recidivism during follow-up[a]							
Any new conviction	50.00%	84.43%	78.69%	χ^2(2) = 24.50**	.19**	.07	.26**
Violent conviction	30.43%	58.08%	59.02%	χ^2(2) = 12.00*	.20**	.09	.27**
Median survival time (years)							
Any new conviction	7.32	1.82	1.32				
Violent conviction	12.00+	6.60	5.99				

Note: PCL = Hare's (1980) 22-item Psychopathy Checklist. Values enclosed in parentheses under the heading "PCL groups" represent standard deviations. [a]Recidivism defined by convictions (yes, no) observed during the prospective 10-year follow-up period.
*p < .01. **p < .001

recidivate) were about 7 years for the low PCL group and about 1.5 years for the medium and high PCL groups (see Table 1). At one year, 13.5% of the low PCL group, 35.8% of the medium PCL group, and 41.7% of the high PCL group were estimated from survival functions to have reoffended. (Values were obtained by subtracting estimates in survival tables of individuals not reoffending from 1.00.) These values estimated from survival tables at the maximum time of 13 years were, respectively, 60.6%, 87.9%, and 82.5%.

Table 2 Mean Ages at First Conviction and Mean Criminal Career Profile (CCP) Slopes for Various Inmate Groups.

Inmate Groups[a]	n	Age at First Conviction		CCP Slope	
		Mean	SD	Mean	SD
Low PCL group	46	24.33	9.68	13.34	11.61
Females	70	25.86	9.52	19.24	25.06
Random sample	555	20.73	7.72	22.51	16.68
Medium PCL group	167	19.50	5.89	24.84	15.04
Violent	172	17.93	2.40	32.00	19.24
High PCL group	61	18.62	4.74	33.25	16.13

Note: CCP = Criminal Career Profile (Templeman, 1995; Wong et al., 1997); PCL = Hare's (1980) 22-item Psychopathy Checklist.
[a]Groups sorted in ascending order by magnitude of CCP slope.

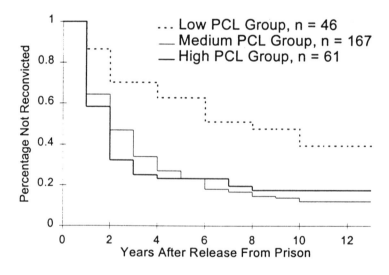

Figure 2. Estimated Percentages of Subjects in the Low, Medium, and High Psychopathy Checklist (PCL) Groups Not Reconvicted Following Release.

5.2.3.2. Violent recidivism

Survival functions plotted in Figure 3 for the low, medium, and high PCL groups were significantly different overall from each other, indicating that these groups were convicted of violent offenses at different rates. Fewer inmates in the low PCL group than in the medium PCL group or than in the high PCL group were convicted of violent offenses. As shown in Table 1, median survival times for violent convictions were about 12+ years for the low PCL group and about 6 years for the medium and high PCL groups. At one year, 4.5% of the low PCL group, 13.9% of the medium PCL group, and 13.3% of the high PCL group were estimated from survival functions to have offended violently. These values estimated from survival tables at the maximum time of 13 years were, respectively, 35.9%, 61.4%, and 64.9%.

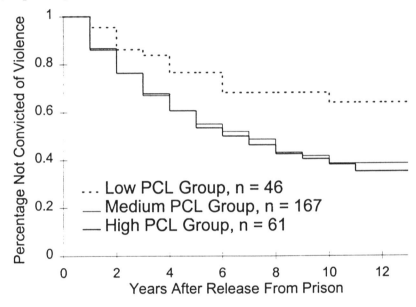

Figure 3. Estimated Percentage of Subjects in the Low, Medium, and High Psychopathy Checklist (PCL) Groups Not Convicted of a Violent Offense Following Release.

5.2.4. CRIMINAL CAREER PROFILE ANALYSES
5.2.4.1. PCL Analyses

CCP slopes correlated .37 with PCL Total scores, .17 with PCL Factor 1 scores, and .45 with PCL Factor 2 scores (all $ps < .01$), indicating that offenders with higher PCL scores had more extensive criminal careers. CCP data points for the low, medium, and high PCL groups are plotted in Figure 4 with solid markers. Mean CCP slopes for the three PCL groups (see Table 2) were significantly different overall, and pairwise, from each other.

5.2.4.3. Comparisons of Criminal Behaviors Among Offender Samples

In addition to analyses computed by PCL groups, we computed AFCs and CCP slopes
for three diverse Canadian inmate samples (see Wong et al., 1997, for detailed sample
descriptions): a randomly selected sample of 555 male offenders who received

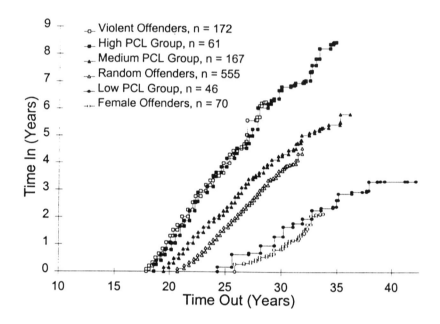

Figure 4. Criminal Career Profiles for Three Psychopathy Checklist (PCL) Groups
(Low, Medium, High) and Three Inmate Samples (Female Offenders, Random Sample
of Offenders, Violent Offenders).

sentences of at least two years, a sample of 172 male offenders incarcerated in a super-
maximum security institution for committing serious violent behaviors while
incarcerated (Wong, Leis, Andre, & Gordon, 1995), and a sample of 70 female
offenders with fewer violent and nonviolent convictions than the randomly selected
male inmate sample.

We reasoned that the most serious and persistent offenders would have earlier
AFCs and steeper CCP slopes and that the least serious and persistent offenders would
have later AFCs and less steep CCP slopes. Specifically, we hypothesized that
respective mean criminal behavior indices (AFCs, CCP slopes) would be similar for the
following pairs of groups: (1) the low PCL group and the female sample; (2) the
medium PCL group and the random offender sample; and (3) the high PCL group and
the violent offender sample. We also hypothesized that the criminal behavior indices

(AFCs, CCP slopes) for these pairs of groups would differ significantly from the other four offender samples. Mean AFCs and CCP slopes--sorted in ascending order by magnitude of CCP slope--are presented in Table 2 for the three PCL groups and for the three comparison samples. Results were consistent with our predictions for both AFCs and CCP slopes. Similarities of CCPs between respective pairs of samples (i.e., low PCL group, female sample; medium PCL group, random offender sample; high PCL group, violent offender sample) are graphically depicted in Figure 4. Data points for the three PCL groups are represented by solid markers and for the three comparison samples are represented by hollow markers.

6. SUMMARY AND DISCUSSION

In this chapter we addressed two of the most significant methodological problems hampering predictions of criminal and violent behaviors: the lack of theoretically relevant predictor variables and weak criterion variables (Monahan & Steadman, 1994). We summarized results using the theoretically meaningful construct of psychopathy, measured by Hare's (1980, 1991) PCL/PCL-R, to predict recidivism. Then, we described CCPs (Templeman, 1995; Wong et al., 1997) and the strengths of this new methodology for conceptualizing, coding, analyzing, and presenting criminal behaviors. Finally, for a random sample of 274 Canadian male offenders, we presented results from AFCs, survival analyses, and CCP analyses.

Results indicate that Hare's (1980, 1991) PCL/PCL-R is a potent predictor of recidivism. The magnitude of the association between the PCL/PCL-R and criminal behaviors compares favorably with other well-established behavioral and biomedical research findings (Rosenthal, 1990, 1991) and the association is highly robust. It is found in diverse inmate samples, for general and violent criminal behaviors, using a variety of statistical procedures and methodologies. Of great practical and theoretical importance, the PCL/PCL-R contributes unique information to the prediction of recidivism beyond that offered by other key predictor variables. For example, the PCL/PCL-R improves upon the contribution of demographic and criminal history variables for predicting recidivism, and correlations between PCL/PCL-R scores and recidivism are larger than correlations between personality disorder diagnoses and recidivism. PCL/PCL-R scores predict general recidivism as accurately as actuarial instruments designed specifically to predict recidivism, and across studies PCL/PCL-R scores are stronger predictors of violent recidivism than are actuarial risk scales. Mental health practitioners and researchers--particularly those working within the criminal justice system--should consider the PCL-R a primary instrument for guiding predictions of dangerousness and criminal recidivism.

In our sample, survival functions for the medium and high PCL groups were not clearly differentiated from each other. This lack of discrimination between the medium and high PCL/PCL-R groups is atypical of recidivism results typically found (e.g., Hart et al., 1988a; Hemphill, 1992; Quinsey et al., 1995; Ross et al., 1992; Serin & Amos, 1995), and is particularly surprising for recidivism rates estimated at shorter (e.g., < 1.5 years) follow-up periods. (We might expect survival functions for the three PCL/PCL-R groups to converge over longer follow-up periods because survival analyses only estimate time to <u>first</u> failure. Subjects in the low and medium PCL/PCL-R groups are often first reconvicted years after release, a time when many subjects in the high PCL/PCL-R group have already received multiple reconvictions.) The exclusive use of files to conduct PCL ratings may at least partly explain this lack of a medium-high PCL group difference. Perhaps the interpersonal and affective characteristics of psychopathy are less adequately assessed without an interview than are the social deviance characteristics. A poorer measure of the interpersonal/affective facet, which presumably contributes to the persistence and stability of criminal behaviors and violence, may result in less discrimination between serious antisocial individuals. (Quinsey et al., 1995, and Rice & Harris, 1997, also used file-only ratings to assess psychopathy. However, because they categorized subjects into only low and high PCL-R groups when calculating recidivism rates and survival analyses, it is difficult to evaluate the influence of file-only ratings on their results.)

Despite the similarities among the medium and low PCL groups of general and violent recidivism estimated from survival analyses, our CCP analyses clearly differentiated failures among the low, medium, and high PCL groups. These results suggest survival analyses may be statistically less sensitive than CCP analyses for detecting behaviors that reliably occur at different rates among groups but that also occur with similar binary (yes, no) frequency among the groups across time. The CCP methodology may detect different rates and patterns of criminal reoffending among offender groups because, in part, the CCP methodology incorporates many sentencing periods into its summary measure. Also, the finding of isomorphic CCPs among each of three similar pairs of groups (the low PCL group and the female sample; the medium PCL group and the random offender sample; the high PCL group and the violent offender sample) provides further validity and indicates the CCP methodology shows considerable promise as an overall measure of criminal behaviors.

References

American Psychiatric Association. (1980). <u>Diagnostic and statistical manual of mental disorders</u> (3rd ed.). Washington, DC: Author.

Andrews, D. A. (1982). <u>The Level of Supervision Inventory (LSI).</u> Toronto, Canada: Ontario Ministry of Correctional Services.

Barbaree, H. E., Seto, M. C., Serin, R. C., Amos, N. L., & Preston, D. L. (1994). Comparisons between sexual and nonsexual rapist subtypes: Sexual arousal to rape, offense precursors, and offense characteristics. <u>Criminal Justice and Behavior, 21,</u> 95-114.

Blomhoff, S., Seim, S., & Friis, S. (1990). Can prediction of violence among psychiatric inpatients be improved? <u>Hospital and Community Psychiatry, 41,</u> 771-775.

Blumstein, A., Cohen, J., Roth, J. A., & Visher, C. A. (Eds.). (1986). <u>Criminal careers and "career criminals"</u> (Vols. I and II). Washington, DC: National Academy Press.

Cleckley, H. (1976). <u>The mask of sanity</u> (5th ed.). St. Louis, MO: Mosby.

Douglas, K. S., Ogloff, J. R. P., & Nicholls, T. L. (1997, June). Personality disorders and violence in civil psychiatric patients. In C. D. Webster (Chair), Personality disorders and violence. Symposium conducted at the meeting of the Fifth International Congress on the Disorders of Personality, Vancouver, British Columbia, Canada.

Fleiss, J. L. (1994). Measures of effect size for categorical data. In H. Cooper & L. V. Hedges (Eds.), The handbook of research synthesis (pp. 245-260). New York: Russell Sage Foundation.

Forth, A. E., Hart, S. D., & Hare, R. D. (1990). Assessment of psychopathy in male young offenders. Psychological Assessment: A Journal of Consulting and Clinical Psychology, 2, 342-344.

Forth, A. E., Kosson, D., & Hare, R. D. (in press). The Hare Psychopathy Checklist: Youth Version. Toronto, Canada: Multi-Health Systems.

Frick, P. J., O'Brien, B. S., Wootton, J. M., & McBurnett, K. (1994). Psychopathy and conduct problems in children. Journal of Abnormal Psychology, 103, 700-707.

Gottfredson, D. M., & Bonds, J. A. (1961). A manual for intake base expectancy scoring. San Francisco, CA: California Department of Corrections, Research Division.

Gretton, H. M. (1997). Psychopathy and recidivism from adolescence to adulthood: A ten year retrospective follow-up. Dissertation in preparation, University of British Columbia, Vancouver, British Columbia, Canada.

Gretton, H. M., McBride, M., O'Shaughnessy, R., & Hare, R. D. (1995, October). Psychopathy in adolescent sex offenders: A follow up study. Paper presented at The Fourteenth Annual Research and Treatment Conference for the Association for the Treatment of Sexual Abusers, New Orleans, LA.

Hare, R. D. (1980). A research scale for the assessment of psychopathy in criminal populations. Personality and Individual Differences, 1, 111-119.

Hare, R. D. (1991). The Hare Psychopathy Checklist-Revised. Toronto, Canada: Multi-Health Systems.

Hare, R. D. (1996a). L'Échelle de Psychopathie de Hare-Révisée (PCL-R): Guide de cotation. Toronto, Canada: Multi-Health Systems.

Hare, R. D. (1996b). Psychopathy: A clinical construct whose time has come. Criminal Justice and Behavior, 23, 25-54.

Hare, R. D., Harpur, T. J., Hakstian, A. R., Forth, A. E., Hart, S. D., & Newman, J. P. (1990). The Revised Psychopathy Checklist: Reliability and factor structure. Psychological Assessment: A Journal of Consulting and Clinical Psychology, 2, 338-341.

Hare, R. D., McPherson, L. M., & Forth, A. E. (1988). Male psychopaths and their criminal careers. Journal of Consulting and Clinical Psychology, 56, 710-714.

Harpur, T. J., Hakstian, A. R., & Hare, R. D. (1988). Factor structure of the Psychopathy Checklist. Journal of Consulting and Clinical Psychology, 56, 741-747.

Harpur, T. J., & Hare, R. D. (1991, August). Psychopathy and violent behavior: Two factors are better than one. Paper presented at the 99th Annual Meeting of the American Psychological Association, San Francisco, CA.

Harpur, T. J., & Hare, R. D. (1994). Assessment of psychopathy as a function of age. Journal of Abnormal Psychology, 103, 604-609.

Harpur, T. J., Hare, R. D., & Hakstian, A. R. (1989). Two-factor conceptualization of psychopathy: Construct validity and assessment implications. Psychological Assessment: A Journal of Consulting and Clinical Psychology, 1, 6-17.

Harris, G. T., Rice, M. E., & Cormier, C. A. (1991). Psychopathy and violent recidivism. Law and Human Behavior, 15, 625-637.

Harris, G. T., Rice, M. E., & Quinsey, V. L. (1993). Violent recidivism of mentally disordered offenders: The development of a statistical prediction instrument. Criminal Justice and Behavior, 20, 315-335.

Harris, G. T., Rice, M. E., & Quinsey, V. L. (1994). Psychopathy as a taxon: Evidence that psychopaths are a discrete class. Journal of Consulting and Clinical Psychology, 62, 387-397.

Hart, S. D., Cox, D. N., & Hare, R. D. (1995). The Hare Psychopathy Checklist: Screening Version (PCL:SV). Toronto, Canada: Multi-Health Systems.

Hart, S. D., & Hare, R. D. (1989). Discriminant validity of the Psychopathy Checklist in a forensic psychiatric population. Psychological Assessment: A Journal of Consulting and Clinical Psychology, 1, 211-218.

Hart, S. D., & Hare, R. D. (1997). Psychopathy: Assessment and association with criminal conduct. In D. M. Stoff, J. Breiling, & J. D. Maser (Eds.), Handbook of antisocial behavior (pp. 22-35). New York: Wiley.

Hart, S. D., Kropp, P. R., & Hare, R. D. (1988a). Performance of male psychopaths following conditional release from prison. Journal of Consulting and Clinical Psychology, 56, 227-232.

Hart, S. D., Kropp, P. R., & Hare, R. D. (1988b). [Prediction of outcome on conditional release: Relative efficiency of the Psychopathy Checklist, antisocial personality disorder diagnoses, and the Salient Factor Score]. Unpublished raw data.

Heilbrun, K., Hart, S. D., Hare, R. D., Gustafson, D., Nunez, C., & White, A. J. (in press). Inpatient and post-discharge aggression in mentally disordered offenders. Journal of Interpersonal Violence.

Hemphill, J. F. (1992). Recidivism of criminal psychopaths after therapeutic community treatment. Unpublished master's thesis, University of Saskatchewan, Saskatoon, Saskatchewan, Canada.

Hemphill, J. F., & Hare, R. D. (1996). Psychopathy Checklist factor scores and recidivism. In D. J. Cooke, A. E. Forth, J. Newman, & R. D. Hare (Eds.), International perspectives on psychopathy (pp. 68-73). Leicester, England: The British Psychological Society.

Hemphill, J. F., Hare, R. D., & Wong, S. (in press). Psychopathy and Recidivism: A Review. Legal and Criminological Psychology.

Hemphill, J. F., Newman, J., & Hare, R. D. (1997). [Psychopathy and recidivism among Black offenders]. Unpublished raw data.

Hill, C. D., Rogers, R., & Bickford, M. E. (1996). Predicting aggressive and socially disruptive behavior in a maximum security forensic psychiatric hospital. Journal of Forensic Sciences, 41, 56-59.

Hoffman, P. B. (1983). Screening for risk: A revised Salient Factor Score (SFS 81). Journal of Criminal Justice, 11, 539-547.

Hoffman, P. B., & Beck, J. L. (1974). Parole decision-making: A Salient Factor Score. Journal of Criminal Justice, 2, 195-206.

Klassen, D., & O'Connor, W. A. (1994). Demographic and case history variables in risk assessment. In J. Monahan & H. J. Steadman (Eds.), Violence and mental disorder: Developments in risk assessment (pp. 229-257). Chicago: University of Chicago Press.

Litwack, T. R., & Schlesinger, L. B. (1987). Assessing and predicting violence: Research, law, and applications. In I. B. Weiner & A. K. Hess (Eds.), Handbook of forensic psychology (pp. 205-257). New York: Wiley.

Loeber, R., & Dishion, T. (1983). Early predictors of male delinquency: A review. Psychological Bulletin, 94, 68-99.

Loucks, A. D. (1995). Criminal behavior, violent behavior, and prison maladjustment in federal female offenders. Unpublished doctoral dissertation, Queen's University, Kingston, Ontario, Canada.

McCord, W., & McCord, J. (1964). The psychopath: An essay on the criminal mind. Princeton, NJ: Van Nostrand.

Miller, P. A., & Eisenberg, N. (1988). The relation of empathy to aggressive and externalizing/antisocial behavior. Psychological Bulletin, 103, 324-344.

Monahan, J. (1981). Predicting violent behavior: An assessment of clinical techniques. Beverly Hills, CA: Sage.

Monahan, J., & Steadman, H. J. (Eds.). (1994). Violence and mental disorder: Developments in risk assessment. Chicago: University of Chicago Press.

Morita, J. G., Lee, T. W., & Mowday, R. T. (1989). Introducing survival analysis to organizational researchers: A selected application to turnover research. Journal of Applied Psychology, 74, 280-292.

Norusis, M. J., and SPSS Inc. (1994). SPSS Advanced Statistics 6.1. Chicago: SPSS.

Nuffield, J. (1982). Parole decision-making in Canada: Research towards decision guidelines. Ottawa, Canada: Communication Division, Solicitor General of Canada.

Nuffield, J. (1989). The 'SIR Scale': Some reflections on its applications. Forum On Corrections Research, 1(2), 19-22.

Quinsey, V. L., Rice, M. E., & Harris, G. T. (1995). Actuarial prediction of sexual recidivism. Journal of Interpersonal Violence, 10, 85-105.

Rice, M. E., & Harris, G. T. (1992). A comparison of criminal recidivism among schizophrenic and nonschizophrenic offenders. International Journal of Law and Psychiatry, 15, 397-408.

Rice, M. E., & Harris, G. T. (1995a). Psychopathy, schizophrenia, alcohol abuse, and violent recidivism. International Journal of Law and Psychiatry, 18, 333-342.

Rice, M. E., & Harris, G. T. (1995b). Violent recidivism: Assessing predictive validity. Journal of Consulting and Clinical Psychology, 63, 737-748.

Rice, M. E., & Harris, G. T. (1997). Cross-validation and extension of the Violence Risk Appraisal Guide for child molesters and rapists. Law and Human Behavior, 21, 231-241.

Rice, M. E., Harris, G. T., & Cormier, C. A. (1992). An evaluation of a maximum security therapeutic community for psychopaths and other mentally disordered offenders. Law and Human Behavior, 16, 399-412.

Rice, M. E., Harris, G. T., & Quinsey, V. L. (1990). A follow-up of rapists assessed in a maximum-security psychiatric facility. Journal of Interpersonal Violence, 5, 435-448.

Rosenthal, R. (1990). How are we doing in soft psychology? American Psychologist, 45, 775-777.

Rosenthal, R. (1991). Meta-analytic procedures for social research (Rev. ed.). Newbury Park, CA: Sage.

Ross, D., Hodgins, S., & Côté, G. (1992). The predictive validity of the French Psychopathy Checklist: Male inmates on parole. Unpublished manuscript.

Salekin, R. T., Rogers, R., & Sewell, K. W. (1996). A review and meta-analysis of the Psychopathy Checklist and Psychopathy Checklist-Revised: Predictive validity of dangerousness. Clinical Psychology: Science and Practice, 3, 203-215.

Schmidt, P., & Witte, A. D. (1988). Predicting recidivism using survival models. New York: Springer-Verlag.

Sechrest, L. (1963). Incremental validity: A recommendation. Educational and Psychological Measurement, 23, 153-158.

Serin, R. C. (1991). Psychopathy and violence in criminals. Journal of Interpersonal Violence, 6, 423-431.

Serin, R. C. (1992). The clinical application of the Psychopathy Checklist-Revised (PCL-R) in a prison population. Journal of Clinical Psychology, 48, 637-642.

Serin, R. C. (1996). Violent recidivism in criminal psychopaths. Law and Human Behavior, 20, 207-217.

Serin, R. C., & Amos, N. L. (1995). The role of psychopathy in the assessment of dangerousness. International Journal of Law and Psychiatry, 18, 231-238.

Serin, R. C., Malcolm, P. B., Khanna, A., & Barbaree, H. E. (1994). Psychopathy and deviant sexual arousal in incarcerated sexual offenders. Journal of Interpersonal Violence, 9, 3-11.

Serin, R. C., Peters, R. DeV., & Barbaree, H. E. (1990). Predictors of psychopathy and release outcome in a criminal population. Psychological Assessment: A Journal of Consulting and Clinical Psychology, 2, 419-422.

Templeman, R. (1995). CrimeWare (Patent pending) [Computer software]. Available from Ron Templeman, Optima Research Inc., Box 147, Colonsay, Saskatchewan, Canada, S0K 0Z0.

Templeman, R., & Wong, S. (1994). Determining the factor structure of the Psychopathy Checklist: A converging approach. Multivariate Experimental Clinical Research, 10, 157-166.

Toupin, J., Mercier, H., Déry, M., Côté, G., & Hodgins, S. (1996). Validity of the PCL-R for adolescents. In D. J. Cooke, A. E. Forth, J. Newman, & R. D. Hare (Eds.), International perspectives on psychopathy (pp. 143-145). Leicester, England: The British Psychological Society.

Widiger, T. A., & Trull, T. J. (1994). Personality disorders and violence. In J. Monahan & H. J. Steadman (Eds.), Violence and mental disorder: Developments in risk assessment (pp. 203-226). Chicago: University of Chicago Press.

Wiggins, J. S. (1973). Personality and prediction: Principles of personality assessment. Reading, MA: Addison-Wesley.

Wintrup, A., Coles, M., Hart, S., & Webster, C. D. (1994). The predictive validity of the PCL-R in high-risk mentally disordered offenders [Abstract]. Canadian Psychology, 35, 47.

Wolf, F. M. (1986). Meta-analysis: Quantitative methods for research synthesis. Newbury Park, CA: Sage.

Wong, S. (1984). The criminal and institutional behaviors of psychopaths (Programs Branch User Report). Ottawa, Canada: Ministry of the Solicitor General of Canada.

Wong, S. (1997) Ten year follow-up of a random sample of offenders assessed using the Psychopathy Checklist. Manuscript in preparation.

Wong, S., Leis, T., Andre, G., & Gordon, A. (1995). A preliminary study of offenders incarcerated at the Special Handling Unit [Abstract]. Canadian Psychologist, 36(2a), 23.

Wong, S., Templeman, R., Gu, D., Andre, G., & Leis, T. (1997). Criminal Career Profile: A methodology to derive a quantitative index of criminal violence. Manuscript in preparation.

Zamble, E., & Palmer, W. (1996). Prediction of recidivism using psychopathy and other psychologically meaningful variables. In D. J. Cooke, A. E. Forth, J. Newman, & R. D. Hare (Eds.), International perspectives on psychopathy (pp. 153-156). Leicester, England: The British Psychological Society.

Zaparniuk, J., & Paris, F. (1995, April). Female psychopaths: Violence and recidivism. Paper presented at conference on "Mental Disorder and Criminal Justice: Changes, Challenges, and Solutions," Vancouver, British Columbia, Canada.

Author Note

James F. Hemphill, Department of Psychology; Ron Templeman, Optima Research Inc.; Stephen Wong, Research Unit; Robert D. Hare, Department of Psychology.

Preparation of this manuscript was supported by a Medical Research Council of Canada Studentship to James F. Hemphill. We gratefully aknowledge the support and cooperation of the Correctional Service of Canada. We thank Drs. S. D. Hart and P. D. Trapnell for comments on earlier versions of this paper, and Dr. D. Gu for his assistance with some of the statistical analyses.

Correspondence concerning this article should be addressed to James Hemphill or Robert Hare, Department of Psychology, University of British Columbia, 2136 West Mall, Vancouver, British Columbia, Canada, V6T 1Z4.

LEGAL ISSUES ASSOCIATED WITH THE CONCEPT OF PSYCHOPATHY

JAMES R. P. OGLOFF and DAVID R. LYON
Department of Psychology and
Mental Health, Law, and Policy Institute
Simon Fraser University
Vancouver, Canada.

It is noteworthy that the title of the NATO ASI from which this book emerged was *"Psychopathy: Theory, Research, and Implications for Society."* As the other chapters make clear, over the course of 10 days there was much discussion of theory and research concerning psychopathy. While some of the presentations and discussions addressed the behavior of psychopathy and its effect on society, there was relatively little mention of the implications of the concept for society. In other words — how can or should our knowledge of psychopathy affect society?

To the extent that the law controls, regulates or, at the very least, sets the parameters for the behavior of people in society (Ogloff, 1990; Ogloff, Tomkins, & Bersoff, 1996), a consideration of how the concept of psychopathy can be used by the law is crucial to any discussion of the implications of psychopathy for society. Based on what was presented during the ASI, and for those of us who actually work or have worked with psychopaths, there is little doubt that, as a group, psychopaths *"are responsible for a markedly disproportionate amount of the serious crime, violence, and social distress in every society"* (Hare, 1996, p. 26).

It is clear from the literature that psychopaths are more likely than others, including other offenders, to be violent (Hare & McPherson, 1984), to recidivate violently (Harris, Rice & Cormier, 1991; Rice, Harris & Cormier, 1992; Serin, 1996), and to cause problems not only in society (Hare, Forth, & Strachan, 1992; Hare & McPherson, 1984; Hare, McPherson, & Forth, 1988), but in the institutions in which they are incarcerated (Wong, 1984). Indeed, they may appropriately be called — as Hare has termed them — *"intraspecies predators who use charm, manipulation, intimidation, and violence to control others and to satisfy their own selfish needs"* (Hare, 1996, p. 26).

Given their antisocial and oftentimes devastating behavior, it may seem almost *"obvious"* that psychopaths should be treated differently than non-psychopathic offenders within the legal system. For example, it might seem fitting for psychopaths, when compared to non-psychopaths, to be: denied bail, found guilty more often, deserving of more serious sentences, justifiably denied parole, and, in some jurisdictions, to be detained even after their sentences expire. To the extent that the cause of psychopathy may be, at least in part, genetic (Livesley, this volume) and those with the disorder may be beyond rehabilitation (Harris et al., 1992; Ogloff, Wong, &

D.J. Cooke et al. (eds.), Psychopathy: Theory, Research and Implications for Society, 401–422.

Greenwood, 1990), an argument even could be made that psychopaths should be detained on a preventative basis. In fact, we may have heard the solution of how to rid society of the ills of the psychopath early on in the conference when we heard about the Inuit solution of pushing the *"psychopaths"* in their society — those suffering from *"Kunlangeta"* — off ice flows. Certainly, even a cursory review of the death penalty case law in the United States would suggest that this tradition is not limited to the Inuit since the term *"psychopath,"* and those related, are very often linked with those men who are sentenced to death (*Barefoot v. Estelle*, 1983; *Earhart v. State*, 1991; *Satterwhite v. Texas*, 1988; *Smith v. Estelle*, 1977).

Regardless of what we believe or even know to be true regarding psychopathy, there are many problems, from a legal perspective, associated with the reasoning of Inuit approach to dealing with psychopaths. Over the past few years we have been collecting and reading the reported cases in Canada and the United States that refer to psychopathy, sociopathy, dissocial and antisocial personality disorder. This project has provided much insight about the uses and misuses of psychopathy, and related terms, in the legal system. It is worth saying that it is surprising that so little attention has been paid to psychopathy and related disorders by legal scholars. This is unfortunate because it appears psychopathy can exert a strong influence on case decisions and dispositions although often evidence of the disorder is misconstrued or inappropriately applied.

Just as lawyers and judges may be naive about psychopathy, so too are mental health professionals naive about law — and about the potential for misuse of their work in the legal system. In an attempt to discuss information relating to psychopathy and the implications for the law, we will cover three main topics in the remainder of this chapter. First, we will highlight six legal dilemmas or areas of concern that we believe arise from the concept of psychopathy and the way it has been or might be employed in the legal system: (1) group norms vs. individual rights; (2) psychopathy vs. Mental disorders; (3) legal vs. psychological nomenclature; (4) protection of society vs. individual rights; (5) preventive incapacitation or detention; and, (6) misuse of the label *"psychopathy."* Second, we will describe the rules governing the legal admissibility of expert evidence relating to psychopathy to provide some background about appropriate limitations for the use of the concept. Finally, we will close with a brief discussion of the propriety of using the concept of psychopathy in the legal arena.

LEGAL DILEMMAS OR AREAS OF CONCERN ARISING FROM PSYCHOPATHY

Group norms vs. individual cases

A fundamental difference between psychology — indeed with science — and with law is that science deals with normative data while the law must deal with individual cases. This is why researchers are so obsessed with sample size and replication, and why statutes are written in an intentionally vague manner. What this means for the law is that while psychopathy is a good predictor of many things, including violent recidivism, it likely never will be entirely satisfactory for the law. This is because, in any individual case, the law does not concern itself with how *"most people with similar psychopathy scores behave,"* but, rather, with how the *particular* individual in question will behave.

Unfortunately, though, the cases are replete with examples of how individual psychiatrists and psychologists have used the term psychopathy as though it were synonymous with whatever legal issue was in question. Perhaps the best example of this is the infamous Dr. Grigson from Texas who has very often testified that he was absolutely certain that a particular offender would reoffend violently if he was not sentenced to death (*Gholson v. Estelle*, 1982; *Satterwhite v. Texas*, 1988; *Smith v. Estelle*, 1977). Although in *Satterwhite v. Texas* (1988) the United States Supreme Court held that Dr. Grigson's testimony was improperly admitted, the Supreme Court's summary of the case facts illustrates the extreme nature of his testimony. Dr. Grigson was the State's final witness. His testimony stands out both because of his qualifications as a medical doctor specializing in psychiatry and because of the powerful content of his message. . . . He stated unequivocally that, in his expert opinion, Satterwhite *"will present a continuing threat to society by continuing acts of violence."* He explained that Satterwhite has a *"lack of conscience"* and is *"as severe a sociopath as you can be."* Dr. Grigson concluded his testimony on direct examination with perhaps his most devastating opinion of all: he told the jury that Satterwhite was beyond the reach of psychiatric rehabilitation (p. 1799).

The point here, of course, is that very often Grigson, and many like him, justify their opinion with the *"fact"* that the person has antisocial personality disorder, sociopathy, or is a psychopath. Psychopathy undoubtedly is an important consideration in the criminal justice system, and in some cases it may even be the most salient consideration, but it must never become the *only* consideration. Psychopathy is only one of many factors which should be evaluated within the forensic context and mental health professionals — and the courts — must ensure they do not focus on psychopathy to the exclusion of other important considerations.

Psychopathy vs. Mental disorders

For several thousand years now, the law has considered mental illness and, of course, the product of this has been the development of concepts such as fitness or competency to stand trial, the insanity defense, involuntary civil commitment, hospital or treatment orders (see Perlin, 1989; Walker, 1968, 1985). As psychopaths formally were just considered to be *"bad"* rather than *"mad,"* the law has not developed any special considerations for them (Campbell, 1992). Indeed, it is not a conventional mental disorder. Instead, psychopathy has been synonymous with *"bad"* and, as many, many cases show, evidence of psychopathy — via the testimony of an expert — leads to harsher treatment by the legal system.

However, the closer we get to a model of psychopathy that is biologically or genetically based, the closer we come to believe that the behavior of psychopaths is at least to some extent deterministic. As Figure 1 shows, under traditional jurisprudential constructs, the closer human behavior comes to being deterministic, the less people are held criminally responsible. Indeed, during the NATO ASI from which this book grew, we heard the words *"compelled,"* *"determined,"* and *"involuntary organismic impairment"* used to describe psychopaths or psychopathy. Of course, the difference between psychopaths and mentally ill persons who typically are found to be legally *"insane"* or otherwise not criminally responsible, is that psychopaths are not cognitively impaired; however, there now is evidence that even this may not be true

(Hare, Williamson, & Harpur, 1988; Raine, O'Brien, Smiley, Scerbo, & Chan, 1990; Williamson, Harpur, & Hare, 1991).

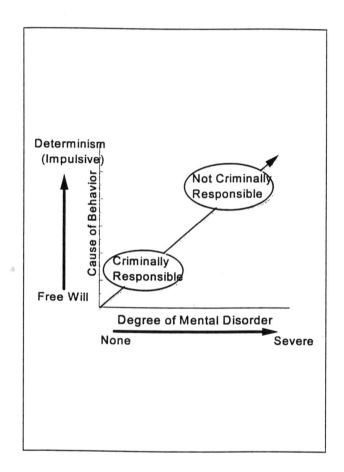

Figure 1. The General Relationship in the Law Between Mental Illness and Determinism

Nonetheless, it would be highly problematic if psychopaths were not held criminally responsible and, therefore, careful attention must be paid to how the law should construe psychopathy. The answer to this dilemma may stem from how we consider children or youth with characteristics of psychopathy.

Special concerns for children and youth

As the literature shows, there has been considerable interest in antisocial behavior in children and youth (Myers, Burket, & Harris, 1995; Robbins, 1966). More recently, a modified version of the PCL-R has been developed for use with young people (PCL:YV; Forth, Kosson, & Hare, in press). Finally, a number of studies have investigated the presence of psychopathy in young children (Frick, O'Brien, Wootton, & McBurnett, 1994) and efforts are now underway to develop a measure of psychopathy suitable for this population (Lynam, 1996).

This movement poses some great concerns. Of course, the researchers involved are well-intentioned and during the NATO ASI and at other times, we heard explicitly that the underlying goal of identifying psychopathy in early childhood is to maximize the possibility that we can intervene or treat them to prevent future behavioral problems. However, how many times has the law overlooked the intentions and good nature of the social science and mental health professions?

Without getting into too much detail here, we will provide two examples from American case law that demonstrate the ease with which the law overlooks the good intentions, and even warnings, of mental health professionals. First, in the infamous case of *Barefoot v. Estelle* (1983), the United States Supreme Court ignored the advice of the APA that psychiatric testimony pertaining to future dangerousness was wholly unreliable. In delivering the opinion of the majority, Justice White stated: *"we are no more convinced now that the view of the APA should be converted into a constitutional rule barring an entire category of expert testimony. We are not persuaded that such testimony is almost entirely unreliable and that the fact finder and the adversary system will not be competent to uncover, recognize, and take due account of its shortcomings"* (p. 1108). Although our ability to predict violence has improved during the intervening period (e.g., Borum, 1996), it still is far from perfect. But, the point is that the Supreme Court disregarded the empirical findings and advice of social scientists.

Similarly, in *McCleskey v. Kemp* (1987) the United States Supreme Court dismissed the appeal of a black defendant who claimed his death sentence violated his constitutional rights despite empirical research presented in court which showed a black man convicted of killing a white victim was 4.3 times more likely to receive the death penalty than a white man convicted of killing a black victim (Baldus, Pulaski & Woodworth, 1983). In the ruling of the majority, Justice Powell stated that at most, the Baldus study indicates a discrepancy that appears to correlate with race. Apparent disparities in sentencing are an inevitable part of our criminal justice system. As this Court has recognized, any mode for determining guilt or punishment *"has its weaknesses and the potential for misuse."* Specifically, *"there can be no perfect procedure for deciding in which cases governmental authority should be used to impose death."* Despite these imperfections, our consistent rule has been that constitutional guarantees are met when *"the mode for determining guilt or punishment itself has been surrounded with safeguards to make it as fair as possible."* (p. 1778)

The message here is that, like so many other areas of the law, we can only expect the worst from its use of our knowledge. Therefore, we can imagine scales like the PCL:YV and Psychopathy Screening Device being used inappropriately by school systems, social service systems, and youth criminal justice services.

When we think back to the problem between group norms and individual cases, it is apparent that in many cases decisions about children and youth will be made not based on an extensive individual assessment — but on the basis of a score from a test (like IQ and special education placement, etc.). This is very disconcerting, especially since there is no absolute agreement in the field regarding what an appropriate cut-off score for psychopathy should be — particularly in a population of youth. Given the track record of countries like the United States and Canada, what would happen if we could reliably predict that a child — or group of children — would become or already are psychopaths who will harm others? Would we try to treat them, or would we try to *"get rid of them"* — at least figuratively?

If we construe child or youth antisocial behavior as a *"learning disability"*, or some such thing, then attempts could be made to use a mental disability model of psychopathy rather than a mental illness model — which does not fit — or the punishment model that most assuredly will be developed. Such an approach could be beneficial for young people who demonstrate characteristics of psychopathy since there would be an onus on society to provide some intervention — rather than to wait for some crisis to occur and then punish the person.

This may not be as radical a departure from existing legal models as might first appear to be the case. The Education for All Handicapped Children Act (EAHCA) was enacted in the United States in 1975 and together with its successor, the Individuals with Disabilities Education Act (IDEA, 1993), it could serve as a possible prototype — with appropriate revision — for the mental disability model of psychopathy we propose. Among the provisions of the EAHCA, every child with a qualifying disability is guaranteed a free and appropriate education. And, although judicial decisions following the enactment of the EAHCA have ruled that qualified children are not necessarily entitled to the best or most ideal education (e.g., see *Board of Education v. Rowley*, 1982), they are entitled to an education which is capable of providing demonstrable educational gains. One of the notable effects of the legislation, from our perspective here, was that it imposed on the state the responsibility of creating, implementing and operating, individualized educational programs for children with disabilities (Parry, 1996). From this starting point, it is not an inconceivable leap to suggest that the state also could be mandated to provide individualized and on-going intervention programs for young people who are *"psychopaths"*. Interestingly enough, *"medically oriented"* services typically fall outside the boundaries of the EAHCA, but in some circumstances the courts have ruled that psychotherapy is consistent with the meaning and intention of the act, and presumably the IDEA, and, therefore, these services must be provided (e.g., see *Papacoda v. State*, 1981; *T.G. v. Board of Education,* 1983).

In short, by considering psychopathy as analogous to a learning disability, rather than being akin to a mental illness for which one is found not criminally responsible, the law may begin to construe psychopathy in a more constructive manner. Under this model, psychopaths would not be exculpated for their criminal actions nor would the state be allowed to wait idly by while young people, who show characteristics of psychopathy, become serious societal problems and be formally pushed into the criminal justice system. Instead, there would be an onus on the state to provide individualized intervention programs for these people proactively.

Legal vs. Psychological Nomenclature

In law, the term *"psychopathy," per se* is irrelevant. Psychopathy is a psychological term, not a legal one. When it is used in statutes, as it is or has been in several countries, it is given its own unique legal definition. To use psychopathy — or any other term — as though it was equated with a legal construct is simply wrong. It never really matters to the law whether an individual is a psychopath. What does matter, of course, is an assessment of the individual's behavior and cognitive processes and, if one is a psychopath, how that affects the individual person's behavior in matters that are relevant to the legal issues in question.

As an example, let us reflect on the relationship between schizophrenia and the insanity defense. Although most insanity acquittees — at least in North America — are schizophrenic, schizophrenia is not a necessary nor sufficient condition to find one legally insane (Ogloff, Roberts, & Roesch, 1993; Ogloff, Schweighofer, Turnbull, & Whittemore, 1992). Indeed, no case or statute requires one to be a schizophrenic to be found insane, nor limits legal insanity to persons with schizophrenia.

Likewise, a diagnosis of psychopathy, in and of itself, really is quite irrelevant to the law. Unfortunately, though, what has already happened in many cases is that the condition of psychopathy is used as direct evidence that a person is guilty, dangerous, or even deserving of execution. Thus, we must be mindful of the differences between legal and psychological use of terms — sometimes, as the term *"psychopathic disorder"* in the English Mental Health Act (see Baker & Crichton, 1995) or the term *"sexual psychopath"* in some of the old US (Minnesota Statute 253B.02 (18a)) and Canadian statutes (s. 43 Criminal Code Amendment Act, 1948) illustrate, the legal and psychological terminology may be identical but the concepts behind such terms can be very different.

The *"sexual psychopathic personality"* referred to in Minnesota's statutes serves as a useful example of this dichotomy. According to Minnesota's statute a sexual psychopathic personality refers to the existence in any person of such conditions of emotional instability, or impulsiveness of behavior, or lack of customary standards of good judgment, or failure to appreciate the consequences of personal acts, or a combination of any of these conditions, which render the person irresponsible for personal conduct with respect to sexual matters, if the person has evidenced, by a habitual course of misconduct in sexual matters, an utter lack of power to control the person's sexual impulses and, as a result, is dangerous to other persons (Minnesota statute 253B.02 (18a)). It is evident from the statute that the legal conception of a sexual psychopathic personality has no correspondence to clinical conceptions of psychopathy. Admittedly, many of the individuals considered psychopaths from a clinical perspective will fit the legal definition of a sexual psychopathic personality; however, like the example of schizophrenia and insanity given earlier, the presence of a psychopathic disorder is neither a necessary nor sufficient condition for determining whether a person legally constitutes a sexual psychopathic personality. That is, not every clinical psychopath will satisfy the legal criteria and, conversely, not every person satisfying the legal criteria will be considered a psychopath in clinical terms. It is imperative for two reasons that we, as mental health professionals, are aware of, and understand these distinctions. First, we must be cognizant of the applicable legal standards to ensure our testimony addresses the legal issues in question. Second, we need to educate lawyers and judges about the differences which exist between the legal and psychological constructs.

Protection of Society vs. Individual Rights

In so-called free societies, there is no greater value than liberty. Indeed, as the well-known jurist William Blackstone wrote, *"it is better that ten guilty people escape than that one innocent suffer"* (1765, p. 27). With this value statement as a foundation, it is easy to see why concepts such as due process and natural justice are so important. The true measure of a justice system is not how it deals with the *"easy"* cases — but how it deals with the most *"difficult"* ones. Indeed, as the noted American jurist Oliver Wendell Holmes wrote, *"great cases like hard cases make bad law"* (Northern Securities Co. v. U.S., 1904, p. 400).

In terms of psychopathy, the importance of protecting individual rights relates back to the differences between group norms and individual cases. It may be worthwhile to illustrate this point using our right to bail as an example. On the surface it appears *"logical"* to deny psychopaths bail because we know that as a group they re-offend violently at an alarmingly disproportionate rate compared to non-psychopaths; yet, we do not know for certain *which* psychopaths will re-offend and which will not. It is this problem which strikes at the very heart of the dilemma which exists between individual rights and the protection of society. As a society and as individuals, we place a high value on our rights and freedoms and it is from this desire to protect our own rights that we must, by necessity, protect the rights of the collective group — even if this means protecting the rights of society's most reprehensible members. Thus, even though the evidence indicates psychopaths are the *"worst of the worst,"* they have the right to the same procedural justice that we all do.

Preventive Incapacitation or Detention

There are very few situations in a free society where people are detained not because of what they did — i.e., committing a crime, being found guilty, and being sentenced — but for what they *might* do. This is called preventive incapacitation or preventive detention. Some examples of its use are involuntary civil commitment, and the denial of bail or bond in the criminal justice system.

Given society's increasing fear of, and intolerance toward, dangerous offenders, attempts have been made to confine people because they may be dangerous in the future. As might be expected, of course, the concept of psychopathy has been used in such situations as *"proof"* or *"support"* for an individual's dangerousness. In 1992 the United States Supreme Court dealt with such a case in *Foucha v. Louisiana*. Typically, to be held involuntarily under civil commitment laws, a person must be both mentally ill and dangerous either to themselves or others. The issue in this case was whether an insanity acquittee, who is no longer mentally ill, can be detained solely on the basis of dangerousness. In *Foucha*, a man who was found NGRI was detained in hospital for four years. According to Louisiana law, a hospital review panel can make a recommendation for releasing a patient being held NGRI. Following such a recommendation, a hearing is held to determine whether the person should be released. In this case, the hospital review panel recommended Foucha's release, noting that he did not suffer from a mental illness and was, in fact, *"mentally healthy."* The opinion of two physicians was sought for the hearing. Both physicians testified that he was not mentally ill. However, one physician noted that Foucha had an anti-social personality, a condition he stated that is not a mental disorder and is untreatable. And, as a result of the anti-social personality, he would not feel comfortable certifying that Foucha was no longer dangerous to either himself or others. For that reason, Foucha was not released from custody. On eventual appeal to the United States Supreme Court, the State of Louisiana argued that it was permissible to detain a person found NGRI based on a finding that the person was dangerous, even though the person was no longer mentally ill. In a five/four decision, the Supreme Court did not agree with this reasoning, holding that such a scheme violated Foucha's due process rights. Notably, though, four of the nine justices on the Supreme Court would have allowed Foucha's detention to be continued — based at least in part on the physician's testimony in the case that he *"would not feel comfortable in certifying that [Foucha] would not be a danger to himself or other people"* (p. 1782).

How comfortable can we be knowing that people could be detained on a preventive basis, based on what we know about psychopathy and, in the case of *Foucha*, on the basis of a diagnosis of APD? Think of the false positives and the high rate of APD in a prison sample. Ironically, in a dissenting opinion, Justice Thomas wrote that *"I believe that it is unwise, given our present understanding of the human mind, to suggest that a determination that a person has 'regained sanity' is precise. Psychiatry is not an exact science, and psychiatrists disagree widely and frequently on what constitutes mental illness."* (p. 1801)

Nonetheless, based on the testimony of the physicians, Justice Thomas would have allowed Foucha's detention to continue — even where the physician would say no more than that he would hesitate to certify that Foucha would not be dangerous to himself or others. Indeed, such opinion is reliable enough for civil commitments, the insanity defense, fitness or competency to stand trial determinations, etc.

Misuse of the Label *"Psychopathy"*

One of the difficulties currently plaguing this field is the lack of consensus over the most appropriate diagnostic scheme or assessment instruments for evaluating psychopathy (e.g., Hare & Hart, 1995; Widiger & Corbitt, 1995). As a result of the PCL-R's reliability and predictive power it is becoming increasingly popular in the field, but there are several other measures with widespread acceptance. In 1995 we conducted a survey of the methods employed by mental health professionals to assess psychopathy and related constructs in forensic settings. We surveyed all the members of the Criminal Justice Section of Canadian Psychological Association, all the self-identified forensic psychologists in the Canadian Health Registry of Service Providers in Psychology; and all the Forensic Psychiatrists in the Canadian Association.[1] Respondents identified no fewer than 34 different assessment instruments which had been used for this purpose. The 15 most frequently employed assessment instruments are listed in Figure 2.

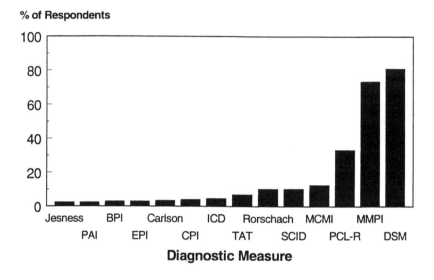

% of Respondents

Diagnostic Measure

* Jesness=Jesness Inventory, PAI=Personality Assessment Inventory, BPI=Basic Personality Inventory, EPI=Eysenck Personality Inventory, Carlson=Carlson Psychological Survey, CPI=California Personality Inventory, ICD=International Classification of Diseases and Causes of Death, TAT=Thematic Aperception Test, SCID=Structured Clinical Interview for DSM, MCMI=Millon Clinical Multiaxial Inventory, PCL-R=Hare's Psychopathy Checklist-Revised, MMPI=Minnesota Multiphasic Personality Inventory, DSM=DSM-IIIR and/or DSM-IV.
** Because many respondents reported using more than one assessment measure the percentages do not sum to 100%.

Figure 2. Assessment Measures used to Diagnose Psychopathy/APD by Survey Respondents

---

[1] A total of 921 surveys were mailed out between September and December 1994. Of the surveys sent out, 383 were completed and returned for a response rate of just over 42%. Sixty-four percent of the respondents (n=245) indicated they had testified about psychopathy, sociopathy or anti-social personality during the course of their careers. A smaller percentage, 46%, (n=174) reported providing such information to the courts within the 24 month period prior to the survey. The figures presented here, are based on this narrow group of respondents who had provided information to the courts within the past 24 months.

The presence of so many, and such varied, assessment instruments is troublesome because different methods identify different populations. Research shows the diagnostic agreement among some of these measures is only poor to moderate, with greater discordance reported among self-report measures than among clinical-behavioral measures (Hare, 1985). Even among clinical-behavioral measures which exhibit relatively good agreement, such as the DSM-III-R and the PCL-R, there can be marked diagnostic differences. For example, while approximately 70-75 percent of all federal inmates in Canada meet the DSM-III-R criteria for anti-social personality disorder (Correctional Service of Canada, 1990) only 15 to 30% would be considered psychopaths using the PCL-R (Hare, 1996). The high prevalence of APD among federal offenders raises doubts over the utility of the DSM criteria within this population because it does not provide a meaningful basis on which to discriminate members of this group.

Despite differences in criteria, the diagnostic labels *"anti-social personality disorder," "psychopathy," "dissocial personality disorder,"* and *"sociopathy"*, often are used interchangeably — even synonymously. Unfortunately, the DSM-IV makes no attempt to clarify these diagnostic distinctions and goes so far as to state that the pattern of behavior characterized by APD *"has also been referred to as psychopathy, sociopathy, or dissocial personality disorder"* (p. 645). It should come as no surprise, then, to find that the confusion and misuse of these terms within psychology has spilled over into the law and the terms seem to be used indiscriminantly in legal cases. This confusion is aptly demonstrated in a recent Canadian case in which the defendant had *"received a DSM-III-R psychiatric diagnosis of personality disorder apparently based on a scoring on the Hare Revised Psychopathy Checklist"* (*R. v. Young*, 1994). Just as curious, are recent examples of expert witnesses referring to defendants as *"sociopaths"* (e.g., *R. v. Charest*, 1990) even though this has not existed as a formal diagnosis since the APA revised the DSM-II in 1968 (APA, 1968).

In many cases the precise *"label"* given to a defendant is irrelevant because it is the person's behavior and cognitive processes and their implications for the specific legal issues in question that is critical for the law. But, in other cases the distinction between diagnostic labels may be important. For example, such a distinction was essential in *Regina v. Small* (1993) because the court was directed to a specific study which examined recidivism and *"burn out"* in PCL-R defined psychopaths. In this case, *if* the defendant had been diagnosed with APD in conjunction with the references made to the relationship between the PCL-R and recidivism, the court could have been led perilously astray. Fortunately, this did not occur in the case cited, but it does serve to inform us of the potential consequences of using incorrect or imprecise diagnostic labels.

Perhaps what is even more discomforting about our survey's results than the sheer number of instruments utilized, is the inappropriate reliance of many survey respondents on self-report or projective measures (e.g., Rorschach, MMPI-2 etc.) for assessing psychopathy (see Figure 2). A review of the case law supports the survey's finding. There are examples of defendants who were diagnosed as psychopathic or anti-social personality disordered based only on self-report or projective tests (e.g., in the

U.S. see *Edwards v. State*, 1983; *In re Kunshier*, 1994; *People v. Davis*, 1995; in Canada see *R. v. L. (B.R.)*, 1987; *In re G.M.*, 1992). Moreover, the evidence of psychopathy or APD offered in these cases was frequently relied upon to support juvenile transfers to adult court, dangerous offender designations, and capital sentences. In other cases, ordinarily appropriate instruments have been employed with populations or for purposes for which they have not been validated. Our survey indicated that just over 11 percent of the respondents had testified in court about assessments they had conducted in adolescent populations using the PCL-R, despite an explicit warning contained in the test manual that *"[t]he PCL-R (and the PCL before it) has been extensively validated only with samples of males drawn from prison and forensic psychiatric populations . . . and until sufficient reliability and validity data are available, the PCL-R should be used with other populations only for research purposes"* (Hare, 1991, p. 63).

As the preceding discussion suggests, it is essential that mental health professionals are forthright about what, if any, diagnosis applies, the basis for their diagnosis, and what implications this diagnosis does and does not have for the legal issues at hand. Furthermore, mental health professionals must ensure the assessment method employed is appropriate for the population in which it is used and the purpose for which it is conducted.

In summary, whenever the concept of psychopathy is brought into the courtroom, it raises a host of legal dilemmas. Mental health professionals who choose to act as expert witnesses in such cases need to be cognizant of these dilemmas to assure that their testimony is informed, relevant and ethical. It is incumbent upon the courts to determine whether the testimony of a mental health professional is indeed warranted and, in those cases where it is warranted, to ensure that the testimony provided addresses the legal issues in dispute. To gain a better understanding of the legal considerations governing expert evidence and the appropriate limitations which necessarily flow from them, we will turn to this next.

ADMISSIBILITY OF EXPERT TESTIMONY CONCERNING PSYCHOPATHY

In Canada, the criteria for determining the admissibility of evidence, and hence expert testimony, were reviewed and clarified recently in the Supreme Court of Canada's decision in *R. v. Mohan* (1994).[2] Interestingly enough, *Mohan* involved the issue — and again we would argue the misuse — of psychopathy. In this case, a doctor was charged with four counts of sexual assault against four female patients aged 13 to 16 years. At trial, his counsel wanted to introduce testimony of a psychiatrist who would say that the perpetrator of the offenses would be either a person who suffers from a major mental disorder (which the accused did not) or a sexual psychopath (which he declared the accused was not). The trial judge refused to admit the psychiatrist's testimony into evidence. On appeal, the Ontario Court of Appeal ruled that the evidence should have been included, and ordered a new trial. Finally, in the case to which we will be

---

[2] The ensuing discussion of *Mohan* and the Canadian rules of admissibility draws on an earlier work of the principle author (Ogloff & Polvi, in press).

referring, the Supreme Court of Canada overturned the decision of the Court of Appeal, and held that the expert testimony should indeed have been excluded, as the original trial judge had ruled. From the decision in *R. v. Mohan*, the Supreme Court of Canada has formulated the following four criteria governing the admissibility of expert evidence: 1) relevance; 2) necessity in assisting the trier of fact; 3) the absence of an exclusionary rule; and, 4) a qualified expert. These criteria are presented in Table 1.

TABLE 1. Decision model for assessing the admissibility of expert testimony about psychopathy in Canada

---

I.   Is Admission of Expert Testimony about Psychopathy Relevant to the Case?

   Will Admission of Testimony Establish or Dispose of a Fact at Issue in the Case?
   If NO — STOP, Testimony is INADMISSIBLE
   If YES — CONTINUE

II.   Do the Benefits of the Expert Testimony about Psychopathy Outweigh its Cost?

   A.   Is the Probative Value of the Expert Testimony Greater than the Prejudicial Effect of the Testimony?
      If NO — STOP, Testimony is INADMISSIBLE
      If YES — CONTINUE

   B.   Will the Expert Testimony involve an Inordinate Amount of Time Which is not Commensurate with its Value?
      If NO — STOP, Testimony is INADMISSIBLE
      If YES — CONTINUE

   C.   Is the Expert Testimony Misleading (i.e., Will its Effect be Out of Proportion to its Reliability)?
      If NO — STOP, Testimony is INADMISSIBLE
      If YES — CONTINUE

III.   Is the Proposed Expert Testimony about Psychopathy Necessary for Assisting the Trier of Fact in its Determination?

   A.   Does the Expert Evidence Provide Information Which is Likely to be Outside the Experience and   Knowledge of the Judge and/or Jury?
      If NO — STOP, Testimony is INADMISSIBLE
      If YES — CONTINUE

   B.   Will the Expert Testimony Address an Ultimate Issue in the Case?
      If NO — STOP, Testimony is INADMISSIBLE
      If YES — CONTINUE

IV.   Does the Expert Testimony Violate an Exclusionary Rule Which is Separate and Apart from the Opinion Evidence Rule?

      If NO — STOP, Testimony is INADMISSIBLE
      If YES — CONTINUE

V.   Is the Witness a Properly Qualified Expert?

      If NO — STOP, Testimony is INADMISSIBLE
      If YES — Testimony is ADMISSIBLE

For any evidence to be admitted at trial, including expert witness opinion, the first threshold which must be crossed is that the evidence must have some *"logical relevance"* to the case at hand. Stated quite simply, a judge will only admit evidence which tends to establish or dispose of a fact at issue in the case. In practice the threshold for relevance is not difficult to meet and, therefore, the breadth of evidence considered in a case may be quite extensive.

The mere relevance of an expert witness' testimony to a matter at issue in the case does not assure the testimony will be allowed into court. As Sopinka, J. stated for the majority in *Mohan*, decisions of admissibility must also necessarily involve *"a cost benefit analysis, that is 'whether its value is worth what it costs'"* (p. 21). Three specific factors which must be considered in this cost-benefit analysis were laid down by the court in *Mohan*. The first factor to be considered is whether the probative value of the expert testimony is greater than the prejudicial effect of the testimony. Thus, the value of the expert testimony in resolving an issue in the case must outweigh any prejudicial impact resulting from it. The second factor specified in the Court's cost-benefit analysis is whether the expert testimony will require *"an inordinate amount of time which is not commensurate with its value"* (p. 21). In other words, if the merit of the expert testimony in question does not warrant the additional court time that will be required to hear it, then the testimony should not be admitted. The final cost-benefit factor a judge must consider before admitting expert testimony is whether *"its effect on the trier of fact, particularly a jury, is out of proportion to its reliability"* (p. 21). If the testimony is likely to be confusing or if jurors are likely to place undue weight upon it in reaching their verdict, the testimony should not be allowed.

Moving beyond the cost-benefit analysis, the testimony of an expert witness will be permitted only if it is necessary to assist the trier of fact; that is, the information provided by the expert must be beyond the experience and knowledge of a judge or jury. Moreover, any information furnished by the expert must not usurp the functions of the judge or jury. It is the responsibility and duty of the judge or jury to decide the *"ultimate issue"* (i.e., the central issue on which the verdict rests) of a case and consequently judges are very careful to examine the admissibility of expert testimony which could encroach upon the ultimate issue.

Even expert testimony that satisfies the aforementioned rules may still be held inadmissible if there is an exclusionary rule that precludes it. While it is beyond the scope of this chapter to examine any of these rules in depth, it will suffice to say that exclusionary rules govern specific types of evidence that are not permitted at trial. As an example, expert testimony relating to the character or disposition of a defendant is typically not admitted into court.

Finally, before the court will receive expert testimony it must be shown that the proposed expert has *"acquired special or peculiar knowledge through study or experience in respect to the matters on which he or she undertakes to testify"* (*Mohan*, 1994, p. 25). Although it is not necessary that the expertise be gained through formal study or experience, this will almost certainly be the case for mental health professionals.

The situation is somewhat more complicated in the United States because the rules governing admissibility vary according to the jurisdiction. To simplify matters somewhat, the discussion here will focus on the Federal Rules of Evidence (FRE, 1976) with an emphasis on the U.S. Supreme Court's interpretation of these rules handed down in *Daubert v. Merrel Dow Pharmaceutical, Inc.* (1993). Based on the FRE and the ruling in *Daubert*, for expert testimony to be admissible at the federal court level in the United States the following four criteria must be satisfied: 1) relevance; 2) the probative value must outweigh the prejudicial impact; 3) it must assist the trier of fact in its determination; and, 4) the expert must be qualified.

Because the rules governing the admissibility of expert testimony in Canada and the United States are quite similar and we have already reviewed the Canadian rules in some detail, our discussion of the American rules will be fairly brief.[3] The evidentiary rules for the United States have been outlined in Table 2 and it may be useful for the reader to refer to this as the rules are discussed below.

TABLE 2. Decision model for assessing the admissibility of expert testimony about psychopathy in the United States

---

I. Is Admission of Expert Testimony about Psychopathy Relevant to the Case?

    A. Will Admission of Evidence about Psychopathy Make Some Fact More Probable or Less Probable Than it Would Be Without the Evidence?

        If NO — STOP, Testimony is INADMISSIBLE
        If YES — CONTINUE

II. Is the Probative Value of the Expert Testimony about Psychopathy Outweighed by its Prejudicial Impact?

        If NO — STOP, Testimony is INADMISSIBLE
        If YES — CONTINUE

III. Will the Proposed Expert Testimony about Psychopathy Assist the Trier of Fact in its Determination?

    A. Is the Method of Assessing/Diagnosing Psychopathy Valid?*

        If NO — STOP, Testimony is INADMISSIBLE
        If YES — CONTINUE

    B. Is the Evidence of Psychopathy Relevant to the Matters at Issue in the Case?

        If NO — STOP, Testimony is INADMISSIBLE
        If YES — CONTINUE

IV. Does the Witness Qualify as an Expert on Psychopathy?

        If NO — STOP, Testimony is INADMISSIBLE
        If YES — Testimony is ADMISSIBLE

---

[3] The discussion of *Daubert* and the American rules of admissibility relies upon an earlier work of the principle author (Ogloff, 1995).

*In some states, the *Frye* Test may still be employed to determine whether the method of assessing/diagnosing psychopathy has gained general acceptance in psychology or psychiatry for the purposes of addressing the question at issue in the case.

The American versions of the broad rule surrounding the *"relevance"* of evidence (see FRE 402) and the requirement that *"the probative value of the expert testimony outweigh its prejudicial impact"* (see FRE 403) are remarkably similar to the corresponding rules in Canada and need no further elaboration here. In addition, both countries require that the expert testimony assist the trier of fact (FRE 702) in some matter that is beyond the common knowledge or understanding of the ordinary person (*Dyas v. United States*, 1977). However, at this point, the American and Canadian rules depart — in Canada, no further inquiry is made along these lines. The *Daubert* case in the United States examined the specific question of the admissibility of expert testimony about novel scientific evidence.[4] The court ruled that the question of whether the expert testimony will assist the trier of fact can only be answered by determining if the expert testimony has 1) a reliable foundation, and, 2) is relevant to the matters at issue in the case (*Daubert*, 1993).

It is apparent from the Supreme Court decision in *Daubert* (1993) that the evidentiary reliability referred to in this ruling comports closely to what social scientists would term *"validity."* In determining if the expert testimony has a reliable foundation the judge must ascertain whether the expert's assessment of psychopathy is scientifically valid. In other words, does the assessment method or scheme utilized by the expert allow one to properly draw conclusions about the presence or absence of psychopathy? If the judge is not confident that the assessment method(s) employed by the expert yields valid information regarding psychopathy, then the testimony of that expert will not be admitted into evidence.

The second question which emerges in relation to whether the expert testimony will assist the trier of fact is whether psychopathy is relevant to the matters at issue in the case. For the expert testimony to be admissible, there must be some scientifically justifiable basis for linking the results of the expert's psychopathy assessment to one (or more) of the issues in the case. In terms of mental health professionals, this rule appears to present much more of a hurdle for testimony relating to specific psychological tests

---

[4] The ruling in *Daubert* replaces an earlier decision in *Frye v. United States* (1923) and the *"Frye Test"* which emanated from that case. The standard for admitting scientific evidence laid out in the *Frye Test* stated *"[j]ust when a scientific principle or discovery crosses the line between the experimental and demonstrable stages is difficult to define. Somewhere in this twilight zone the evidential force of the principle must be recognized, and while courts will go a long way in admitting expert testimony deduced from a well-recognized scientific principle or discovery, the thing from which the deduction is made must be sufficiently established to have gained general acceptance in the particular field in which it belongs"* (p. 1014). Because *Daubert* is a federal case, its jurisdiction does not extend to state evidentiary laws and, therefore, the *Frye Test* may still be applicable in some states.

(i.e., MMPI) than it does for mental illnesses or disorders like psychopathy (see Ogloff, 1995).

The final rule governing the admissibility of expert testimony in the United States specifies that the proposed expert has the appropriate education, training, or experience to qualify him or her as an expert in the eyes of the court. This rule is virtually identical to the Canadian version stated in *Mohan* (1994).

It is apparent from the case law of both Canada and the United States that the courts consider evidence of psychopathy to be relevant to a large number of legal issues including insanity, juvenile transfer proceedings, sentencing dispositions, child custody disputes, etc. Unfortunately, though, in determining the admissibility of psychopathy related testimony, the courts in both countries appear to place far too much emphasis on the qualifications of the expert testifying and insufficient emphasis on the other rules governing admissibility. In particular, the probative value of this evidence must be carefully measured against its prejudicial impact — as *Satterwhite v. Texas* so clearly illustrates, the prejudicial impact can be very great indeed.

Also, the basis for the expert's testimony on psychopathy could be subjected to much closer scrutiny. This is especially true of the jurisdictions in the United States where existing admissibility rules specifically assign judges the task of ensuring that 1) the assessment procedures undertaken by the expert are scientifically valid and, 2) there is some scientific basis for raising evidence of psychopathy in relation to an issue in the case. In view of these rules, lawyers should be mindful of whether the proposed expert followed empirically validated assessment procedures, and whether the results yielded by these assessment procedures have any empirically validated relationship to the issue in question. The existing case law suggests that these rules could be applied with a great deal more rigor.

CONCLUSION: THE PROPRIETY OF USING THE CONCEPT OF PSYCHOPATHY IN THE LEGAL ARENA

Based on the six legal issues relating to psychopathy which were elucidated earlier, together with the rules surrounding the admissibility of expert testimony, a number of general concluding comments can be made regarding the propriety of using the concept of psychopathy in the legal arena.

Psychopathy is a psychological term, not a legal one and the issues must not become confused

As mentioned above, psychopathy, as we use it, is not a legal term and should never be equated with any legal term. In cases where confusion is likely to arise because the legal terminology is very similar, or even identical to the psychological terminology, mental health professionals need to educate their legal counterparts regarding the differences between the psychological and legal nomenclature. Moreover, mental health professionals who frame their testimony around the legal questions under examination are likely to be of greater service to the courts than those who merely present their testimony more generally. However, to perform both of these tasks, mental health professionals need to be familiar with the legal issues and standards applicable in the case. Those individuals who insist on testifying but do not familiarize themselves with the relevant aspects of the law not only risk performing a disservice to their client but may also fail to meet their professional ethical standards.[5]

Psychopathy is but one aspect of an assessment of an offender

Related to the above point, it is not the fact that one is diagnosed or identified as a psychopath that is relevant to the law but, rather, the global description of the person and how his or her behavior relates to the matters at issue. Mental health professionals have an obligation to conduct thorough and comprehensive assessments and to report all of the relevant findings.[6] Thus, while psychopathy may be an important piece of evidence because it is such a powerful predictor of future violence, it is still only one aspect of an overall assessment and therefore expert witnesses should try to give testimony that is comprehensive, balanced and not unduly focused on psychopathy to the exclusion of other pertinent evidence.[7] Evaluations of psychopathy should utilize well defined, established assessment schemes with empirically demonstrated validity and reliability. Finally, self-report and projective tests generally should be avoided or used only as ancillary measures in favor of clinical-behavioral assessment schemes which possess greater reliability and validity.

It is important not to go beyond the current bounds of knowledge

To ensure they do not venture beyond the current bounds of knowledge, mental health professionals must be cognizant of the current state of the scientific literature in the field[8] and any conclusions made during the course of testimony must be supported by

---

[5] The APA Ethical Principles and Code of Conduct states *"[p]sychologists provide services, teach, and conduct research only within the boundaries of their competence"* (APA, 1992, Ethical Standard 1.04, p. 1600).

[6] The APA Ethical Principles and Code of Conduct stipulates that *"[p]sychologists' forensic assessments, recommendations, and reports are based on information and techniques sufficient to provide appropriate substantiation for their findings"* (APA, 1992, Ethical Standard 7.02, p. 1600).

[7] According to the APA Ethical Principles and Code of Conduct *"[i]n forensic testimony and reports, psychologists testify truthfully, honestly, and candidly and, consistent with applicable legal procedures, describe fairly the bases for their testimony and conclusions"* and *"[w]henever necessary to avoid misleading, psychologists acknowledge the limits of their data or conclusions"* (APA, 1992, Ethical Standard 7.04, p. 1610).

[8] *"Psychologists who engage in assessment, therapy, teaching, research, organizational consulting, or other professional activities maintain a reasonable level of awareness of current scientific and professional information in their fields of activity"* (APA, 1992, Ethical Standard 1.05, p. 1600).

literature.[9] Relatedly, mental health professionals should readily testify about the limitations of their assessments and the opinions they offer. Stated succinctly, mental health professionals need to be humble, conservative and ethical. In a related matter, researchers need to be aware of the implications of their work and the potential for its misuse and abuse. Researchers can take steps to dissuade others from using their work inappropriately, such as candidly stating its limitations and the purposes for which it may, and may not, reasonably be used.

Ultimate opinion testimony/reports must be avoided

Finally, mental health professionals must — wherever possible — avoid providing the court or legal system with a definitive statement of the ultimate legal issue. Ultimate opinion testimony is inappropriate for two reasons.[10] First, it is the trier of fact (the judge or jury) who is to draw conclusions from the facts presented. Thus, ultimate opinion testimony undermines this function by presenting conclusionary statements which already answer the central question in the case. The end result is the trial becomes nothing more than a battle of experts with the trier of fact relegated to the role of referee — they merely decide which expert to accept. Second, mental health professionals are not legal decision makers, and as such we are not qualified to make such decisions.

References

American Psychiatric Association (1968). *Diagnostic and statistical manual of mental disorders* (2nd ed.). Washington, DC: author.

American Psychiatric Association (1987). *Diagnostic and statistical manual of mental disorders* (3rd ed., rev.). Washington, DC: author.

American Psychiatric Association (1994). *Diagnostic and statistical manual of mental disorders* (4th ed.). Washington, DC: author.

American Psychological Association (1991). Specialty guidelines for forensic psychologists. *Law and Human Behavior*, 15(6), 655-664.

American Psychological Association (1990). Ethical principles of psychologists and code of conduct. *American Psychologist*, 47, 1597-1611.

Baker, E., & Crichton, J. (1995). Ex parte A: psychopathy, treatability and the law. *Journal of Forensic Psychiatry*, 6(1), 101-119.

---

[9] The Ethical Principles and Code of Conduct of the APA requires that *"[p]sychologists rely on scientifically and professionally derived knowledge when making scientific or professional judgements"* (APA, 1992, Ethical Standard 1.06, 1600).

[10] In fact, the Specialty Guidelines for Forensic Psychologists state that *"[f]orensic psychologists are aware that their essential role as expert to the court is to assist the trier of fact to understand the evidence or to determine a fact in issue. In offering expert evidence, they are aware that their own professional observations, inferences, and conclusions must be distinguished from legal facts, opinions, and conclusions"* (APA, 1991, Guideline VII(E), p. 665).

Baldus, D. C., Pulaski, C. A., & Woodworth, G. (1983). Comparative review of death sentences: An empirical study of the Georgia experience. *Journal of Criminal Law and Criminology, 74*, 661- 753.

Barefoot v. Estelle, 463 U.S. 880 (1983).

Blackstone, W. (1765). *Commentaries on the law of England.* volume IV (9th ed.). London: Printed for W. Strahan, 1783.

Board of Education v. Rowley, 458 U.S. 176 (1982).

Borum, R. (1996). Improving the clinical practice of violence risk assessment. *American Psychologist, 51*, 945-956.

Campbell, E. (1992). The psychopath and the definition of "mental disease or defect" under the Model Penal Code test of insanity: A question of psychology or a question of law? In J. R. P. Ogloff (Ed.), *Law and psychology: The broadening of the discipline* (pp. 139-170). Durham, NC: Carolina Academic Press.

Correctional Service of Canada (1990). A mental health profile of federally sentenced offenders. *Forum on Corrections Research, 2*, 7-8.

Criminal Sexual Psychopath., S.C. 1948, c.39, s. 43

Daubert v. Merrel Dow Pharmaceuticals, 727 F. Supp. 570 (S.D. Cal. 1989), *aff'd*, 951 F.2d 1128 (9th Cir. 1990), *vacated*, 113 S. Ct. 2786 (1993).

Dyas v. United States, 376 A.2d 827 (D.C. 1977).

Earhart v. State, 823 S.W.2d 607 (Tex.Cr.App. 1991).

Education for All Handicapped Children Act, 20 U.S.C. s1400 (1975).

Edwards v. State, 441 So.2d 84 (S.Ct. Miss., 1983).

Federal Rules of Evidence, 28 U.S.C. s101-1103 (1976).

Forth, A. E., Kosson, D., & Hare, R. D. (in press). *Manual for the youth version of the Hare Psychopathy Checklist-Revised (PCL:YV).* Toronto: Multi-Health Systems.

Foucha v. Louisiana, 112 S.Ct. 1780 (1992).

Frick, P. J., O'Brien, B., Wootton, J., & McBurnett, K. (1994). Psychopathy and conduct problems in children. *Journal of Abnormal Psychology, 103*, 700-707.

Frye v. United States, 293 F. 1013 (D.C. Cir. 1923).

Gholson v. Estelle, 675 F.2d 734 (5th Cir. 1982).

Hare, R.D., (1985) A comparison of procedures for the assessment of psychopathy. *Journal of Consulting and Clinical Psychology, 53*, 7-16.

Hare, R. D. (1991). *Manual for the Hare Psychopathy Checklist-Revised.* Toronto: Multi-Health Systems.

Hare, R. D. (1996). Psychopathy: A clinical construct whose time has come. *Criminal Justice and Behavior, 23(1)*, 25-54.

Hare, R. D., Forth, A. E., & Strachan, K. (1992). Psychopathy and crime across the lifespan. In R. DeV. Peters, R. J. McMahon, & V. L. Quinsey (Eds.), *Aggression and violence throughout the lifespan* (pp. 285-300). Newbury Park, CA: Sage.

Hare, R. D., & Hart, S. D. (1995). Commentary on antisocial personality disorder: The DSM-IV field trial. In W. J. Livesley (Ed.), *The DSM-IV personality disorders* (pp. 127-134). New York: Guilford.

Hare, R. D., & McPherson, L. M. (1984). Violent and aggressive behavior in criminal psychopaths. *International Journal of Law and Psychiatry, 7*, 35-50.

Hare, R. D., McPherson, L. M., & Forth, A. E. (1988). Male psychopaths and their criminal careers. *Journal of Consulting and Clinical Psychology, 56*, 710-714.

Hare, R. D., Williamson, S. E., & Harpur, T. J. (1988). Psychopathy and language. In T. E. Moffitt & S. A. Mednick (Eds.), *Biological contributions to crime causation* (pp. 68-92). Dordrecht, The Netherlands: Martinus Nijhoff.

Harris, G. T., Rice, M.E., & Cormier, C. A. (1991). Psychopaths and violent recidivism. *Law and Human Behavior, 15*, 625-637.

Individuals with Disabilities Education Act, 20 U.S.C. s1400 (1990).

In re G.M., Alta. Prov. Ct. (DRS 93-11665, Feb. 12, 1992).

Lynam, D. R. (1996). Early identification of chronic offenders: Who is the fledging psychopath? *Psychological Bulletin, 120*, 209-234.

In re Kunshier, 521 N.W.2d 880 (Minn. App., 1994).

McCleskey v. Kemp, 107 S.Ct. 1756 (1987).

Minnesota Statutes Annotated s253B.02 (18a) (1994).

Myers, W. C., Burket, R. C., & Harris, E. H. (1995). Adolescent psychopathy in relation to delinquent behaviors, conduct disorder, and personality disorders. *Journal of Forensic Sciences, 40*, 436-440.

Northern Securities Co. v. U.S., 193 U.S. 197 (1904).

Ogloff, J. R. P. (1990). Law and psychology in Canada: The need for training and research. *Canadian Psychology, 31,* 61-73.

Ogloff, J. R. P. (1995). The legal basis of forensic applications of the MMPI-2. In Y. S. Ben-Porath, J. R. Graham, C. N. Hall, R. D. Hirschman, M. S. Zargoza (Eds.), *Forensic applications of the MMPI-2.* (p. 18-47). CA, Thousand Oaks: Sage Publications.

Ogloff, J. R. P., & Polvi, N. H. (in press). Legal evidence and expert testimony. In D. Turner & M. Uhlemann (Eds.), *A legal handbook for the helping profession (2nd ed.).* Victoria BC: The Sedgewick Society for Consumer and Public Education.

Ogloff, J. R. P., Roberts, C.F., & Roesch, R. (1993). The insanity defense: Legal standards and clinical assessment. *Applied and Preventive Psychology, 2*, 163-178.

Ogloff, J. R. P., Schweighofer, A., & Turnbull, S., & Whittemore, K. (1992). Empirical research and the insanity defense: How much do we really know? In J. R. P. Ogloff (Ed.). *Psychology and law: The broadening of the discipline* (pp. 171-210). Durham, NC: Carolina Academic Press.

Ogloff, J. R. P., Tomkins, A. J., & Bersoff, D. N. (1996). Education and training in law/criminal justice: Historical foundations, present structures, and future developments. *Criminal Justice and Behavior, 23*, 200-235.

Ogloff, J. R. P., Wong, S., & Greenwood, A. (1990). Treating criminal psychopaths in a therapeutic community program. *Behavioral Sciences and Law, 8*, 181-190.

Papacoda v. State, 528 F. Supp. 68 (DC, 1981).

Parry, J. W. (1996). Mental and physical disability rights: The formative years and future prospects. *Mental and Disability Law Reporter, 20*, 627-630.

People v. Davis, 896 P.2d 119 (S.Ct. Cal., 1995).

Perlin, M. L. (1989). *Mental disability law: Civil and criminal.* Charlottesville, VA: The Mitchie Company.

R. v. Charest, 57 C.C.C. 312 (Que. C.A., 1990).

R. v. L. (B. R.), Man. Q.B. (Suit no. 85-01-01160, May 20, 1987).

R. v. Mohan, [1994] 2 S.C.R. 9

R. v. Young, NFLD. S.Ct. (DRS 94-14193, June 16, 1994).

Raine, A., O' Brien, M., Smiley, N., Scerbo, A., & Chan, C. J. (1990). Reduced lateralization in verbal dichotic listening in adolescent psychopaths. *Journal of Abnormal Psychology, 99*, 272-277.

Rice, M. E., Harris, G. T., & Cormier, C. A. (1992). An evaluation of a maximum security therapeutic community for psychopaths and other mentally disordered offenders. *Law and Human Behavior, 16(4)*, 399-412.

Robbins, L. N. (1966). *Deviant children grow up.* Baltimore: William & Wilkins.

Satterwhite v. Texas, 108 S.Ct. 1792 (1988).

Serin, R. C. (1996). Violent recidivism in criminal psychopaths. *Law and Human Behavior, 20(2)*, 207-217.

Smith v. Estelle, 445 F.Supp. 647 (1977).

T. G. v. Board of Education, (DC NJ, 1983).

Walker, N. (1968). *Crime and insanity in England, Vol. I: The historical perspective.* Edinburgh: Edinburgh University Press.

Walker, N. (1985). The insanity defense before 1800. *The annals of the American Academy of political and social science, 477*, 25-30.

Widiger, T. A., & Corbitt, E. (1995). Antisocial personality disorder: Proposals for DSM-IV. In W. J. Livesley (Ed.), *The DSM-IV personality disorders* (pp. 127-134). New York: Guilford.

Williamson, S. E., Harpur, T. J., & Hare, R. D. (1991). Abnormal processing of affective words by psychopaths. *Psychophysiology, 28*, 260-273.

Wong, S. (1984). *Criminal and institutional behaviors of psychopaths* (Programs branch users report). Ottawa: Ministry of the Solicitor-General of Canada.

INDEX

LIST OF CONTRIBUTORS

BRITT AF KLINTEBERG
Department of Psychology
Stockholm University
S-106 91 Stockholm
Sweden

RONALD BLACKBURN
Department of Clinical Psychology
University of Liverpool
Liverpool
United Kingdom L69 3BX

HEATHER C. BURKE
Department of Psychology
Carleton University
Ottawa
Ontario
Canada K1S 5B6

DAVID J COOKE
Douglas Inch Centre
2 Woodside Terrace
Glasgow
United Kingdom G3 7UY

GILLES CÔTÉ
Department of Psychology
Université du Québec à Trois-Rivières
Trois-Rivières
Quebec
Canada

ADELLE E. FORTH
Department of Psychology
Carleton University
Ottawa
Ontario
Canada K1S 5B6

PAUL J. FRICK
Department of Psychology
University of Alabama
Tuscaloosa,
United States of America AL 35487

ROBERT D. HARE
Department of Psychology
University of British Columbia
Vancouver
Canada V6T 1Z4

STEPHEN D. HART
Department of Psychology
Simon Fraser University
Burnaby
British Columbia
Canada V5A 1S6

JULIA HARTMANN
Abteilung fur Firensische Psychiatric/
Nervenclinik der Universitat Munchen
8000 Muchen 2
Germany

JAMES F. HEMPHILL
Department of Psychology
University of British Columbia
Vancouver
British Columbia
Canada V6T 1Z4

SHEILAGH HODGINS
Department of Psychology
Université de Montréal
Montréal (Québec)
Canada H3C 3J7

428

MATTHIAS HOLLWEG
Abteilung fur Firensische Psychiatric/
Nervenclinik der Universitat Munchen
8000 Muchen 2
Germany

ROBERT JASER
Abteilung fur Firensische Psychiatric/
Nervenclinik der Universitat Munchen
8000 Muchen 2
Germany

W. JOHN LIVESLEY
Department of Psychiatry
University of British Columbia
2136 West Mall
Vancouver
British Columbia
Canada V6T 1Z4

FRIEDRICH LÖSEL
Institut Für Psychologie
Der Universität Erlangen
Nürnberg
Germany

DAVID R. LYON
Department of Psychology
Simon Fraser University
Burnaby
British Columbia
Canada

KEITH MCBURNETT
University of California, Irvine
UCI Child Development Center
Newport Beach,
United States of America CA 92715

NORBERT NEDOPIL,
Abteilung für Forensische Psychiatrie,
Psychiatrische Klinik der Universität
München
Germany

JOSEPH P. NEWMAN
Department of Psychology
University of Wisconsin, Madison
United States of America

JAMES R. P. OGLOFF
Department of Psychology and
Mental Health, Law, and Policy Institute
Simon Fraser University
Burnaby, British Columbia
Vancouver
Canada

LINDA PFIFFNER
University of California
Irvine
United States of America

RON TEMPLEMAN
Optima Research Inc
Colonsay
Saskatchewan
Canada

JEAN TOUPIN
Department of Special Education
Université de Sherbrooke
Sherbrooke
Canada J1K 2RI

THOMAS A. WIDIGER
Department of Psychology
University of Kentucky
115 Kastle Hall
Lexington, KY, 40506-0044
United States of America

STEPHEN WONG
Research Unit
Regional Psychiatric Centre (Prairies)
Saskatoon
Saskatchewan
Canada S7K 3X5